Minimally Invasive Surgery of the Foot and Ankle

Nicola Maffulli • Mark Easley
(Editors)

Minimally Invasive Surgery of the Foot and Ankle

Springer

Editors
Nicola Maffulli
Centre for Sports and Exercise Medicine
Queen Mary University of London
Barts and The London School of Medicine and Dentistry
Mile End Hospital, London
England, UK

Mark Easley
Duke Health Center
Crutchfield Street 407
27704-2726 Durham North Carolina
USA

ISBN 978-1-4471-6857-7 ISBN 978-1-84996-417-3 (eBook)
DOI 10.1007/978-1-84996-417-3
Springer London Dordrecht Heidelberg New York

British Library Cataloguing in Publication Data
A catalogue record for this book is available from the British Library

Softcover re-print of the Hardcover 1st edition 2011

Cover design: eStudioCalamar, Figueres/Berlin

Springer is part of Springer Science+Business Media (www.springer.com)

Preface

Orthopedic surgeons have already embraced minimally invasive procedures such as total and partial knee replacements, total hip replacements, and rotator cuff repairs. Inevitably, the technical challenge, the requests of patients and the imagination of surgeons has prompted more and more of us to perform surgery through small incisions in the foot and ankle. We already routinely perform arthroscopy of the ankle, subtalar, and first metatarsophalangeal joints, and many surgeons have become conversant with soft tissue endoscopy of the hindfoot and tendoscopy of the peroneal, the tibialis posterior, and the flexor hallucis longus tendons. These have the clear advantages of less morbidity and faster recovery than the equivalent open procedures, and there is enough scientific background to justify their use. Traditionally, the Achilles tendon lends itself to less invasive surgical approaches, and many surgeons have developed less invasive techniques to repair acute ruptures, reconstruct chronic ruptures, and deal with Achilles tendinopathy.

In the field of forefoot surgery, the concept of not having to perform extensive soft tissue dissection and perform extra-articular surgery is appealing. For example, in hallux valgus surgery there are several procedures which, using a subcapital osteotomy with marked lateral displacement of the capital fragment, avoid excision of the bunion, and therefore remain totally extraarticular. Theoretically, they should minimize post-operative stiffness. Sparing of soft tissue, less post-operative pain, less problems with wounds, better cosmesis, shorter operating times, shorter hospital stay are all benefits of minimally invasive procedures.

Minimally invasive techniques are not free of complications. The main problems are connected to poor knowledge of anatomy, and, in osteotomies, to less than optimal placement of the osteotomy. Less invasive techniques are not 'better' than traditional, open techniques: at best, they are equivalent in terms of patients' satisfaction and objective outcome measures, with hopefully less soft tissue complications and better cosmesis.

With this in mind, we present in this book procedures by many of the pioneers in less invasive surgery of the foot and ankle. These techniques can be powerful, and should not be embraced without full knowledge of the open procedures, and without appropriate anatomical knowledge and supervised training. The list of techniques presented is by no means exhaustive, and in this vibrant field we expect that may more will be described soon. Above all, we report a new philosophy of less and minimally invasive surgery, prompting the reader to understand that which procedure to use in a particular patient is very much a question of horses for courses, and of surgical skills and training.

Nicola Maffulli
Mark Easley

Contents

Contributors

FrancescoA llegra,M D Department of Orthopaedics, Università La Sapienza, Roma, Italy

Joseph M. Anain Jr., DPM, FACFAS PodiatricM edicinea ndS urgery Sisters of Charity Hospital, Buffalo, NY, USA

Ozgür Ahmet Atay, MD Department of Orthopedics and Sports Medicine, Hacettepe University, Sihhiye, Ankara, Turkey

Thomas Bauer, MD Ambroise Paré Hospital, West Paris University, Department of Orthopedic Surgery, Boulogne, France

Murat Bozkurt, MD Department of Orthopedics and Sports Medicine, Hacettepe University, Sihhiye, Ankara, Turkey

Stefan Buchmann, MD Department of Orthopedic Sports Medicine, Klinikum Rechts der Isar, University of Munich, Munich, Germany

Christophe Cermolacce, MD L'Institut de Chirurgie Orthopédique et Sportive, Marseille, France

Jen Yves Colliard, MD Clinique du Parc Lyon, Stalingrad, Lyon, France

Paul Hamilton Cooke, MB, ChB, ChM, FRCS Nuffield Orthopaedic Centre, Headington, Oxford, UK

Christophe de Lavigne, MD Sport Medical Center, Department of Orthopedic Surgery, Merignac, France

Peter Albert Johannes de Leeuw, MSc AcademicM edicalC enter, University of Amsterdam, Amsterdam, The Netherlands

Mariano de Prado, MD Department of Orthopedics, Hospital USP San Carlos, Murcia, Spain

Vincenzo Denaro, MD Department of Orthopedic and Trauma Surgery, Campus Biomedico University, Rome, Italy

Patrice Determe, MD Clinique du Parc, Toulouse, France

Lawrence A. Di Domenico, DPM, FACFAS ReconstructiveR earfoota ndA nkle Surgical Fellowship, Ankle and Footcare Centre, Ohio College of Podiatric Medicine, Cleveland, OH, USA

Christopher Di Giovanni Department of Orthopedic Surgery, The Warren Alpert School of Medicine at Brown University, Rhode Island Hospital, Providence, Providence, RI, USA

Mahmut Nedim Doral, MD Department of Orthopedics and Sports Medicine, Hacettepe University, Faculty of Medicine, Sihhiye, Ankara, Turkey

Austin T. Fragomen, MD Weill Medical College of Cornell University, New York, USA

Pau Golanó, MD Department Pathology and Experimental Therapeutics, University of Barcelona, Spain

Stéphane Guillo, MD Research and Study Group for Mini-invasive Surgery of the Foot, Mérignac, France

Shuji Horibe, MD, PhD Department of Orthopedic Sports Medicine, Osaka Rosai Hospital, Sakai, Osaka, Japan

Andreas B. Imhoff, MD, PhD Department of Orthopedic Sports Medicine, Klinikum Rechts der Isar, University of Munich, Munich, Germany

Stephen A. Isham, MD, DPM, DrHC San Francisco Hospital, Sanatorio San Francisco, Mexico DF, Mexico

Keisuke Kita, MD, PhD Department of Orthopedic Surgery, Yao Municipal Hospital, Yao, Osaka, Japan

Michael D. LaCivita, DPM Buffalo,N Y,U SA

Olivier Laffenetre, MD Department of Orthopedic Surgery, Bordeaux University Hospital Pellegrin, Bordeaux, France

Bradley M. Lamm, DPM, FACFAS International Center for Limb Lengthening, Rubin Institute for Advanced Orthopedics, Sinai Hospital of Baltimore, Baltimore, MD, USA

Umile Giuseppe Longo, MD Department of Trauma and Orthopaedic Surgery, University of Rome, Rome, Italy

Tun Hing Lui, MBBS (HK), FRCS (Edin), FHKAM, FHKCOS Departmentof Orthopaedics and Traumatology, North District Hospital, Hong Kong SAR, China

Nicola Maffulli, MD, MS, PhD, FRCS(Orth) Centre for Sports and Exercise Medicine, Queen Mary University of London, Barts and The London School of Medicine and Dentistry, Mile End Hospital, London, England, UK

Sheldon Nadal, BSc, DPM 586, Eglinton Avenue East, Suite 501, Toronto, Canada

Orlando E. Nunez, MD, DPM del Cesar Clinic, Valledupar - Cesar, Colombia Coeur d'Alene Foot & Ankle Surgery Center, Coeur d'Alene, Idaho, USA

James A. Nunley II, MD Duke University Medical Center, Durham, NC, USA

Francesco Oliva, MD, PhD Department of Trauma and Orthopaedic Surgery, University' of Rome, Rome, Italy

Chandrusekar Ramamurthy, MD Department of Trauma and Orthopaedic Surgery, University Hospital of North Staffordshire, Keele University School of Medicine, Stoke on Trent, UK

Martinus Richter, MD, PhD Department for Trauma, Orthopaedic and Foot Surgery, Coburg Clinical Center and Hospital Hildburghausen, Coburg and Hildburghausen, Germany

Pedro-Luis Ripoll, MD Hospital San Carlos, Murcia, Spain

Michael M. Romash, MD United Services University of Health Sciences, Bethesda, MD, USA

Mario Ronga, MD Department of Orthopedics and Trauma Sciences, Ospedale di Circolo, Varese, Italy

S. Robert Rozbruch, MD Limb Lengthening and Reconstruction, Hospital for Special Surgery, Weill Medical College of Cornell University, New York, USA

Amol Saxena, DPM, FACFAS Department of Sports Medicine, PAFMG, Palo Alto, CA, USA

Murali Krishna Sayana, MRCS Department of Trauma and Orthopaedic Surgery, University Hospital of North Staffordshire, Keele University School of Medicine, Stoke on Trent, UK

Aaron T. Scott, MD Department of Orthopaedic Surgery, Wake Forest University Baptist Medical Center, NC, USA

Chezhiyan Shanmugam, MRCS Department of Trauma and Orthopedic Surgery, Dumfries and Galloway Royalty, Dumfries, Scotland, UK

Filippo Spiezia, MD Department of Orthopedic and Trauma Surgery, Campus Biomedico University, Rome, Italy

Vittorino Testa, MD Olympic Center, Angri, Salerno, Italy

Egemen Turhan, MD Department of Orthopedics and Sports Medicine, Hacettepe University, Sihhiye, Ankara, Turkey

Cornelis Nicolaas van Dijk, MD, PhD AcademicM edicalC enter, University of Amsterdam, Amsterdam, The Netherlands

Maayke Nadine van Sterkenburg, MD Department of Orthopedic Surgery, Academic Medical Center, University of Amsterdam, Amsterdam, The Netherlands

Javier Vaquero, MD Department of Orthopedic Surgery, Hospital General Universitatrio Greorio Maranon, Madrid, Spain

Jonathan S. Young, MRCS Department of Trauma and Orthopaedic Surgery, University Hospital of North Staffordshire, Keele University School of Medicine, Stoke on Trent, UK

Part I

Generalities

Minimally Invasive Foot Surgery: AP aradigmS hift

1

Mariano de Prado

Over the last few years, Foot Surgery has come to be recognised as a major Orthopaedic subspecialty.

The understanding of biomechanics, the growing social demands and the technological developments in surgery have produced techniques to manage many foot conditions which were swept under the carpet by traditional orthopaedic surgeons.

The current goal of surgical treatment of deformities of the feet is correct all elements that produce the deformity, and promote the maintenance and functional biomechanics of the foot. To be effective using traditional techniques, one has to be prepared to use extensive surgical approaches and aggressive techniques (Fig. 1.1).[6]

Modern orthopaedic surgery tends to use minimally invasive techniques to minimize some of the problems posed by open surgery, reducing complications and improving and shortening postsurgical recovery.

Arthroscopy has been a pioneer in the techniques of minimally invasive surgery. Born in the first half of the twentieth century to provide a clearer understanding of the state of the synovium, cartilage and other intra-articular structures, since the 1970s it has been possible to tackle a vast array of conditions in the knee (Fig. 1.2), shoulder and ankle (Fig. 1.3).

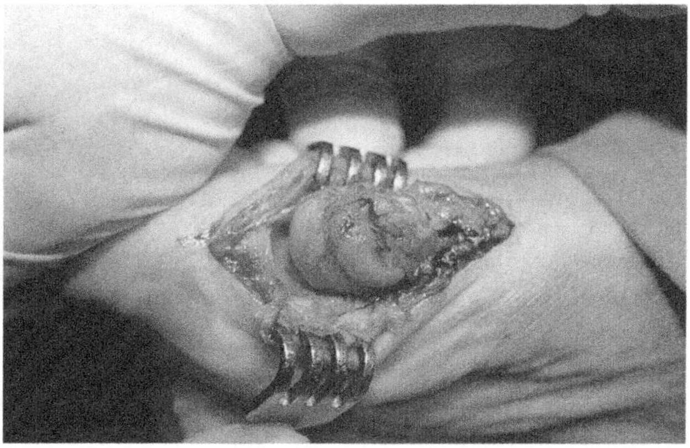

Fig.1. 1 To be effective using traditional techniques, one has to be prepared to use extensive surgical approaches and aggressive techniques(Fig. 1.1)

M. de Prado
DepartmentofO rthopaedics, HospitalU SPS anC arlos, Murcia, España
e-mail:de prado@hospitalsancarlos.net

N. Maffulli and M. Easley (eds.), *Minimally Invasive Surgery of the Foot and Ankle*,
DOI: 10.1007/978-1-84996-417-3_1, © Springer-Verlag London Limited 2011

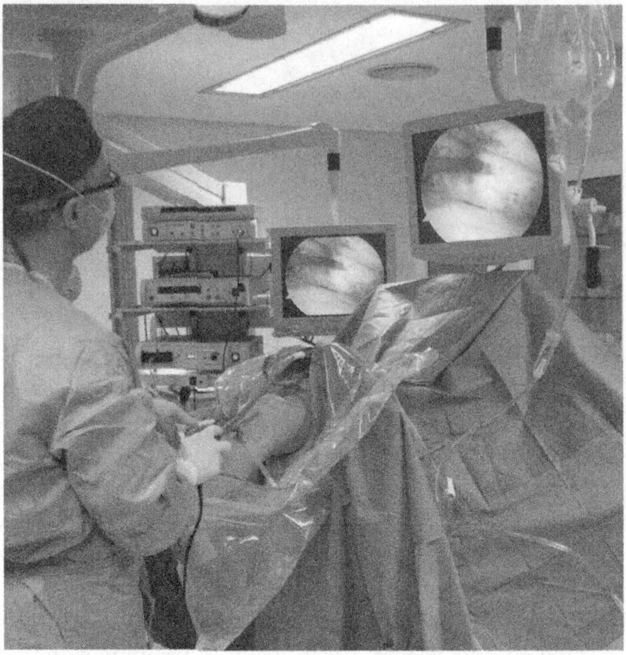

Fig. 1.2 Arthroscopyc an tackle a vast array of conditionsi nt hekne e

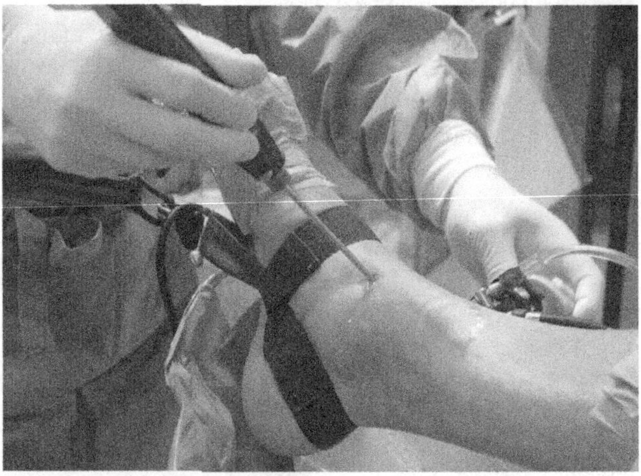

Fig. 1.3 Arthroscopyc an tackle a vast array of conditions in the shoulder anda nkle

Surgery of the spine and entrapment syndromes of peripheral nerves have seen the evolution of equally popular minimally invasive techniques.

In foot surgery, the minimally invasive surgical approach allows surgery through small incisions, without direct exposure of surgical planes, causing minimal trauma to the tissues, using radiographic control.[1,4,7]

These techniques were born when, in 1945, Morton Polokoff introduced subdermal surgery using tiny as chisels and scalpels. These were connected to a galvanic current generator, and, through a small incision, they accessed the nail matrix and, through the action of the current, destroyed it. Subsequently, the authors stopped using galvanic current, and began using small cobs, similar to those used in plastic surgery to perform rhinoplasty, expanding the indications for these minimally invasive surgical techniques for removal of exostoses in different locations.

Polokoffs ideas were later incorporated by other foot surgeons, and, in the 1960s, Edwin Probber introduced new tools and techniques, describing more aggressive procedures.

Simultaneously, Bernard S. Weinstock began to use an electric motor with small sterilizable burrs which allowed more effective interventions and minimal tissue damage in neighboring structures. This use of an electric motor led Brown, in 1968, to their use to excision a calcaneal spur.

In the 1970s, Pritt, Addante and Hymes boosted this minimally invasive surgery techniques, and in 1974, the first course of surgical techniques in minimally invasive surgery of the foot was held in the Pensylvannia College of Podiatric Medicine.

In the 1980s, Partel, Robert Strauss and White dramatically expanded the indications for minimally invasive surgery. At the end of the 1980s and especially in the 1990s, Stephen Isham desceibed techniques for the treatment of hallux valgus, tailors bunions, and deformities of the lesser toes.

In Europe Bosch, in 1990, proposes a modification of the Hohmann osteotomy by minimally invasive techniques for hallux valgus correction. In Spain, also in the 1990s, M. Prado and P. L. Ripoll began to perform the techniques proposed by Isham, expanding their indications and adapting some techniques. Their experience culminated in a book published in 2003, in Spanish, and in 2009 in English.[2,3]

Magnan and Montanari, in Italy, following Boschs ideas, reported their results in 1997, and began to conduct workshops for the dissemination of percutaneous surgery of the foot. In 2003, Sandro Giannini and 2005 Nicola Maffulli present their work with modifications to this technique. Since the mid 1990, Nicola Maffulli has reported a vast array of techniques aimed at dealing with a variety of soft tissue and bony conditions of the foot and ankle using minimally invasive techniques.

1.1 General Principles Percutaneous Surgery of the Foot

In the foot surgery, a minimally invasive surgical approach allows interventions through minimal incisions. As direct exposure of the structures to operate on, the surgeon has to have profound knowledge of the local anatomy, and will need three essential conditions:

- The anatomy of the foot should be deeply known to adopt the most appropriate approach to minimise the risk of injury to other structures, avoiding causing iatrogenic injuries.
- Appropriate equipment allows efficient and effective surgery. Dedicated instruments have now been produced, and instructional courses have been designed to teach how to use them correctly.
- Image intensification should be used intraoperatively to check the exact position of the surgical instruments to prevent complications arising from the lack of direct vision of thes urgicalf ield.

The complications that occurred in many patients operated using minimally invasive surgery in the 1980s in the United States led to discourage or ban these techniques. A small group of podiatrists gathered around the Academy of Ambulatory Foot Surgery (AAFAS), who continued the practice and refinement of these techniques reaching accuracy and results comparable to traditional open surgery.[5,8,9]

The poor performance of minimally invasive surgery of the foot in those early years resulted from incorrect indications, the use of non-dedicated instruments, and a lack of technical preparation for this type of surgery, compounded by a lack of appropriate scientific literature.

Not all foot operations can be performed using minimally invasive techniques: minimally invasive surgery is a method in the hands of the surgeon and not an end in itself, and surgeons should be experienced in both traditional and minimally invasive surgery to fully understand the patho-anatomy of the conditions they seek to treat.

Surgeons beginning to use minimally invasive foot surgery techniques should adaptat to the loss of three-dimensionality. Surgery is performed through small incisions (portals) through which we introduce the surgical instruments which will reach parts remote from the entry portals. Hence, the need to appreciate and respect the anatomical structures not just at the point of surgery but also along the route followed by the instruments used.

1.2 Planning

Surgeons must plan how to perform surgery in a precise and effective fashion, choosing the most appropriate incision, calculating the distance from the incision to the point of surgery, and the angle at which the bony and soft tisue structures are to be approached.

1.2.1 Incision

First, the incision is made at a point which does not injury vessels, nerves, ligaments or tendons. When possible, the skin incision is produced along the lines of Langier, regardless of the subsequent direction to the point of surgical performance. We suggest not to plave the incision in the areas of pressure footwear, as this would favour the development of hypertrophic scars or keloids, and postoperative pain. The size of the incision should be large enough to introduce easily the surgical instruments, without damage the skin surface, and to allow the extrusion of bone debris following exostosectomy or osteotomy. This will prevent local inflammatory reactions and calcifications.

1.2.2 Angleo fA pproach

The distance between point of entry and the area where the surgery is actually performed should be such that the cutting portion of instrument is fully covered by skin and soft tissues, thus preventing iatrogenic skin injury. Unless specifically required, the angle of approach should not be perpendicular to articular surfaces. For example, to remove an exostosis the burr should be parallel to the surface of the bone that is being removed (Fig. 1.4).

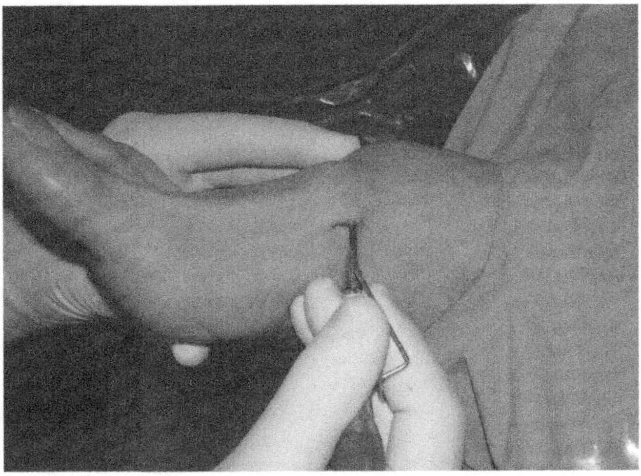

Fig. 1.4 Removinga n exostosis showing the burr parallel to the surface of the bonetha tis be ingre moved

1.2.3 ApproachP ath

The path from the skin incision to the area of surgery should be unique. Multiple passages will injury the soft tissues, and risk neurovascular and musculoskeletal compromise. The maximum angular pivoting of the instrument around the entry portal should be 60°.

After surgery has been completed, bone fragments and blood should be gently expressed from the area of surgery, the skin incision closed, and a compression bandage applied.

Both soft tissues and bony surgery can be performed using minimally invasive techniques:

1. Softt issues urgery:
   - Tenotomy
   - Tendonl engthening
   - Tendona ndj ointde bridement
   - Capsulotomy
2. Bones urgery:
   - Exostosectomy
   - Osteotomy

1.3 Percutaneous Surgery for Soft Tissue

1.3.1 Subcutaneous Tenotomy

Tenotomy of the extensor digitorum is an example of this type of intervention. It is performed on subcutaneous tendons (Fig. 1.5), asking the patient to contract the relevant muscle against digital resistance of the surgeon. The incision is centered on the tedon

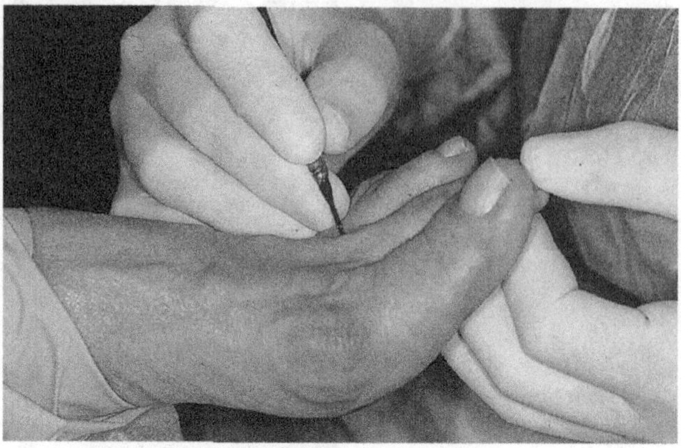

Fig. 1.5 Tenotomyofthe extensor digitorum performed on subcutaneous tendons

itself, sparing the neurovascular structures which may lie close to the tendons, using the small minimally invasive blades. This will be introduced parallel to the long acis of the tendon tendon, rotated 90°, and with progressive gentle pressure on the tendon this will be tenotomised, with impossibility to resist the digital force applied by the surgeon.

1.3.2 Deep Tenotomy

It is practiced, for example, in the abductor hallucis. In this instance, the tendon can not be palpated, and we suggest to use image intensification to visualise relevant landmarks.In the case of adductor tenotomy in hallux valgus, the incision is made on the metatarsophalangeal joint of the hallux.

1.3.3 TendonL engthening

Selective lengthening of a tendon can be performed by minimally invasive techniques, provided tendon has a sufficiently long subcutaneous path.

The incisions should be at lest 2 cm apart. A lateral is perfomed through of is perfomed through one, and a medial is perfomed through through the other, progresively and forcibly stretching the tendon, observing how it slides on itself within its sheath (Fig. 1.6).

At other times, three or more incisions 1.5 cm apart are performed, alternating a lateral to a medial hemisection.

1.3.4 TendonDe bridement

When previous operations or other tendon injuries (partial tears, or traumatic wounds adhesions may hinder the function of the affected tendon. In these patients, an

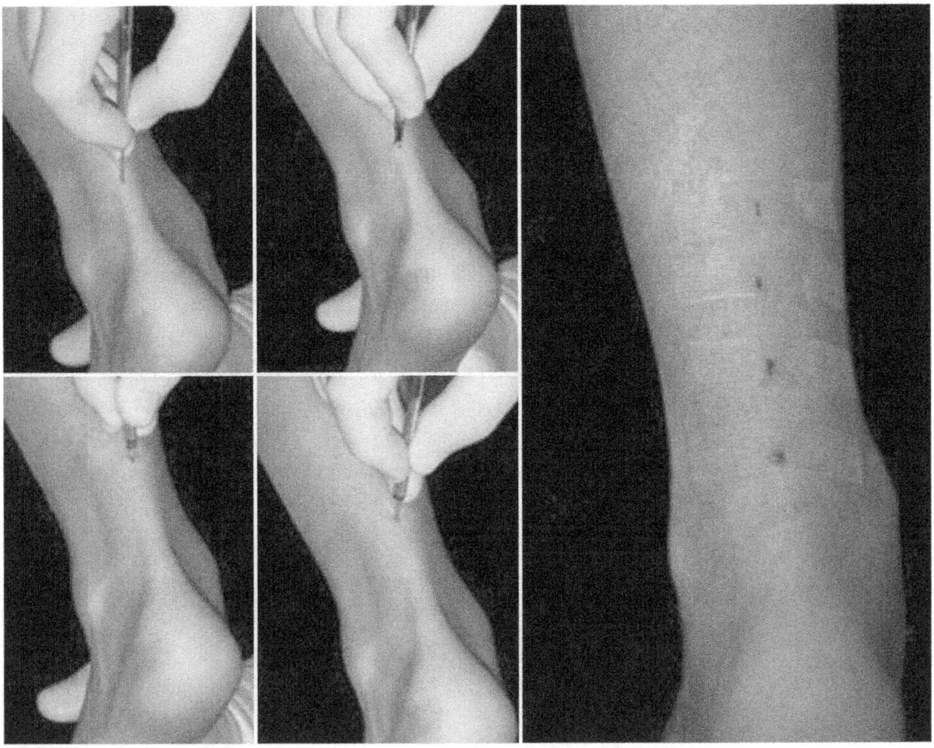

Fig. 1.6 Selective lengthening of a tendon can be performed by minimally invasive techniques, provided tendon has a sufficiently long subcutaneous path. The incisions should be at lest 2 cm apart. A lateral is perfomed through of is perfomed through one, and a medial is perfomed through through the other, progresively and forcibly stretching the tendon, observing how it slides on itself withinits s heath

appropriately placed incision allows to introduce sharp or blunt instruments to perform a percutaneous debridement. It is at times necessary to perform a simultaneous tendon lengthening.

1.3.5 Capsulotomy

A capsulotomy is performed with a scalpel blade, starting from the interior of the joint. The capsule is approached directly with the scalpel blade, applying adequate counter pressure to tension it. When the capsulotomy is performed, the range of motion will increase.

1.4 PercutaneousB oneS urgery

1.4.1 Exostosectomy

An exostosectomy is performed using a bur of a diameter proportional to the size of the exostosis. The incision and the general procedure should follow the principles outilined above, after producing a subcutaneous working area in which the bone be removed is deep, and the periosteum and fibrous tissue covering the exostosis are superficial to the burr.

An exostosectomy should be performed taking care not to produce bone tunnels, with speeds from 2,000 to 8,000 rpm, and applying gentle pressure on the bone to be removed. At the same time, gentle fanning motion are performed, using as a pivot point skin incision. After the procedure, the burr is removed, and gentle pressure is applied: a bone slurry willbe e xtruded(Figs. 1.7aa nd b).

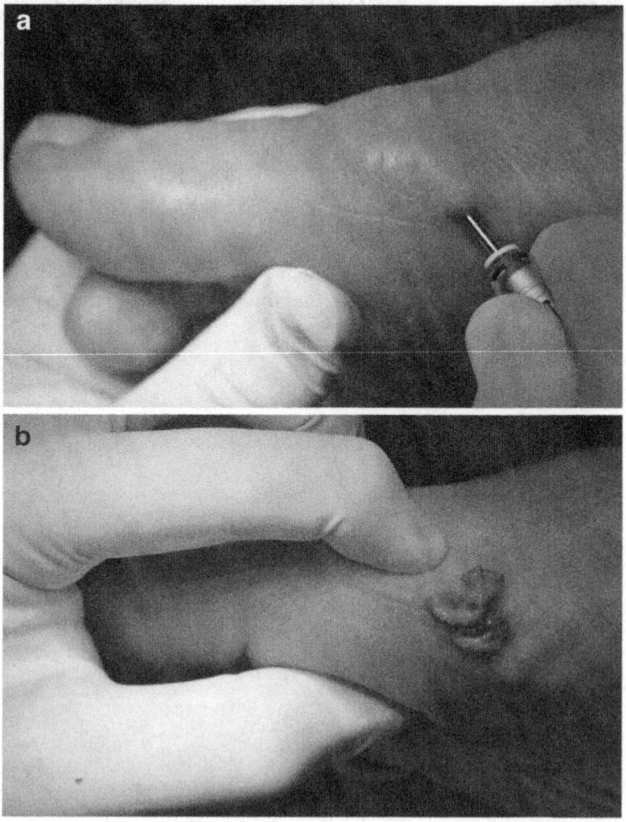

Fig.1.7 (**a, b**) After an exostosectomy, the burr is removed, and gentle pressure is applied: a bone slurryw illbe e xtruded

1.4.2 Osteotomies

The general principles should be followed, and the knife blade should be directed to the bone to be osteotomized, in the same direction of the osteotomy. Having reached the bone, the knife will be exchanged for a rasp, which will lie on the surface of the bone to be osteotomzed. The periosteum is gently removed, a side cutting burr is introduced. The address AYH (About your Health-2009) begins cutting designed to operate with the engine. As the burr starts its action, it may move from the planned osteotomy site. In this instances,we recommend to maintain firm pressure and to use image intensifer control to make sure that the osteotomy is actually perfomed as planned. Once a sufficiently deep notch in the cortical bone is produced, the surgeon can no longer change the direction of the osteotomy: if the surgeon tries to, the side-cutting bur will break. To advance the osteotomy, the surgeon should use a twisting motion of the hand, on the pivot point on the skin incision. This allows more precise and progressive osteotomies, and the technique can beus edt ode signa ppropriatew edges.

References

1. Bycura BM. *Bycura on Minimal Incision Surgery*. Weissman SD, ed. New York, NY: B.M. Bycura;1986:24–25 .
2. De Prado M, Ripoll PL, Golanó P. *Cirugía Percutánea del Pie*. Barcelona, Spain: Elsevier-Masson;2003.
3. De Prado M, Ripoll PL, Golanó P. *Minimally Invasive Foot Surgery*. Barcelona, Spain: AYH; 2009.
4. Gorman B, Plon M. *Minimal Incision Surgery and Laser Surgery in Podiatry*. Warminster, PA: JackB.Gorman;1983.
5. Hymes L. *Forefoot Minimum Incision Surgery in Podiatric Medicine*. New York, NY: Futura Publishing;1977.
6. Maffulli N. Minimally invasive orthopaedic surgery. *Orthop Clin North Am*. 2009; 40:491–498.
7. PerroneM A. *Podiatric Nail and Bone Surgery with Rotary Air Motor*. Canton, OH: 1972.
8. Schilero J. Minimal incisión podiatric surgery-principles and applications. *J Am Podiatr Med Assoc*.1985;75:568–574.
9. Van Enoo R, Cane E. Minimal incision surgery, a plastic technique of a cover-up? *Clin Podiatr Med Surg*.1986;3:321–335.

Computer-Assisted Surgery (CAS) in Foot and Ankle Surgery

2

Martinus Richter

2.1 Introduction

Foot and ankle surgery at the end of the twentieth century was characterized by the use of sophisticated computerized preoperative and postoperative diagnostic and planning procedures.[13,39] However, intraoperative computerized tools that assist surgeons during their struggle for the planned optimal operative result are lacking. This results in an intraoperative "black box" without optimal visualization, guidance and biomechanical assessment.[39] In the future, this intraoperative "black box" will be opened, and we shall have more intraoperative tools to achieve the planned result.[39] Intraoperative three-dimensional imaging (ISO-C-3D/ARCADIS-3D), Computer Assisted Surgery (CAS) and Intraoperative Pedography are three possible innovations to realize the planned procedure intraoperatively.[48,49]

2.2 Part 1: CAS Guided Retrograde Drilling in Talar Osteochondral Lesions (OCD)

The goal in the management of stages I and II osteochondral defects of the talus is revascularisation of the lesion.[7] A debridement of the chondral part is required,[3,62] limited to loose cartilage or cartilage with poor quality.[3,59,62] Subchondral drilling of the lesion allows revascularisation. Retrograde drilling leaves the chondral surface intact, and may therefore be advantageous compared with antegrade drillings.[16] Arthroscopically guided drillings are limited to those lesion that can be accessed arthroscopically.[59] In the remaining cases, open procedures are undertaken.[54] Based on these principles, CT based Computer Assisted Surgery (CAS) guided retrograde drilling of osteochondral lesions has been described with promising results.[16,52] Computed tomography (CT)- and fluoroscopy-based navigation

M. Richter
Department for Trauma, Orthopaedic and Foot Surgery, Coburg Clinical Center and Hospital Hildburghausen, Coburg and Hildburghausen, Germany
e-mail: info@foot-trauma.org

N. Maffulli and M. Easley (eds.), *Minimally Invasive Surgery of the Foot and Ankle*,
DOI: 10.1007/978-1-84996-417-3_2, © Springer-Verlag London Limited 2011

systems in current use are of limited flexibility.[38] On of the drawbacks of fluoroscopy are lack of three-dimensional imaging intraoperatively. CT-based navigation still requires intra-operative cumbersome registration, extra preoperative planning, and imaging with use of further technical resources.[43] In addition to the current method of arthroscopic evaluation and treatment, we earlier introduced an alternative technique of using 3D-imaging with ISO-C-3D (Siemens Medical Inc., Munich, Germany) based CAS guided retrograde drilling of the lesion.[43] This method was feasible, accurate and showed good clinical outcome.[39,43] However, the technical equipment of the earlier 3D-imaging devices (model ISO-C-3D, Siemens Medical Inc., Munich, Germany) and CAS devices (Model Surgigate, Medivision Inc., Oberdorf, Switzerland & Northern Digital Inc., Waterloo, Ontario, Canada; Medivision later sold and renamed Praxim Inc., Grenoble, France) was cumbersone and error-prone.[39,43] These devices were further developed for easier and faster handling, and were less prone to error. We introduce a 3D-imaging based CAS guided retrograde drilling with a combination of these modern devices (model ARCADIS-3D, Siemens Medical Inc., Munich, Germany, and model Navivision, Brainlab Inc., Heimstetten, Germany).

2.2.1 ClinicalE xample

An OCD stage II according to Berndt and Harty and stage IIa according Hepple/Winson at the talus was diagnosed (Fig. 2.1a–c)[7,21,46] at imaging, and the diagnosis confirmed at arthroscopy (Fig. 2.2).[46] The cartilage was intact but softer than the surrounding cartilage. In the procedure, a Dynamic Reference Base (DRB) was fixed to the talar head through a small incision (Fig. 2.5a),[46] and an intraoperative image acquisition with ARCADIS followed (Figs. 2.3a–f).[46] The 2D-images were obtained to show the poor visibility of the OCD lesion on 2D images.[11,43] Retrograde drilling was planned with a starting point at the lateral talar process, and an endpoint in the area of subchondral sclerosis beneath the intact cartilage (Fig. 2.4).[46] The drilling was performed with a 4.5 mm drill (Figs. 2.5a and b).[46] The subchondral sclerosis is removed during the drilling as part of the drilling floor. After the drilling, a 1 mm titanium Kirschner wire was inserted in the drill hole (Fig. 2.6),[46]a nd 2D- and 3D ARCADIS imaging was performed (Fig. 2.7).[46] Then, the Kirschner wire was removed and autologous cancellous bone graft harvested from the ipsilateral distal tibia was inserted. Arthroscopy confirmed the intact and stabilized cartilage after drilling and bone grafting. The time needed for the entire procedure was 45 min. The radiation contamination is comparable to 104 pulsed digital fluoroscopic images or 42 s pulsed fluoroscopic imaging. Figures 2.8a and b[46] show MRI images at 2 year-follow-up with intact cartilagea nda ni ncorporatedbone gr aft.

2.2.2 Results

Fifty-two patients with symptomatic talar OCD Stadium I and II were included in a clinical follow-up study. Time needed for preparation, including the placement of the DRB, scanning time and preparation of the trajectories was 7 min 32 s (4–30 min). In 50 patients

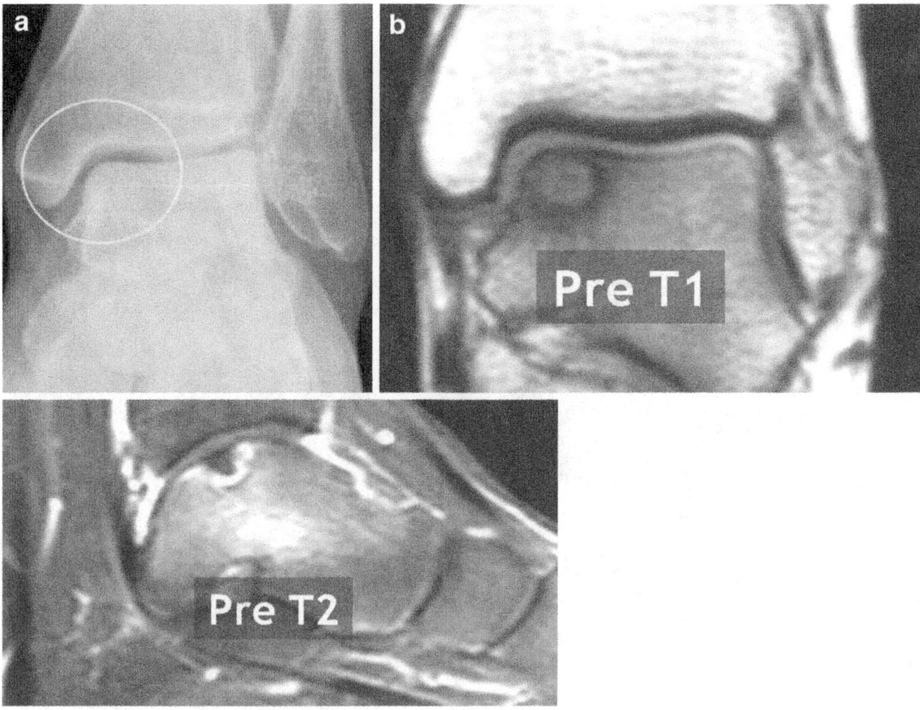

Fig. 2.1 Radiograph and MRI images of an osteochondrosis dissecans (OCD) tali at the medial talar shoulder (Berndt and Harty Stage II, Hepple and Winson stage IIa; (**a**), anteroposterior radiograph; (**b**), coronal T1 reconstruction; (**c**), parasagittal T2 reconstruction)[7,21]

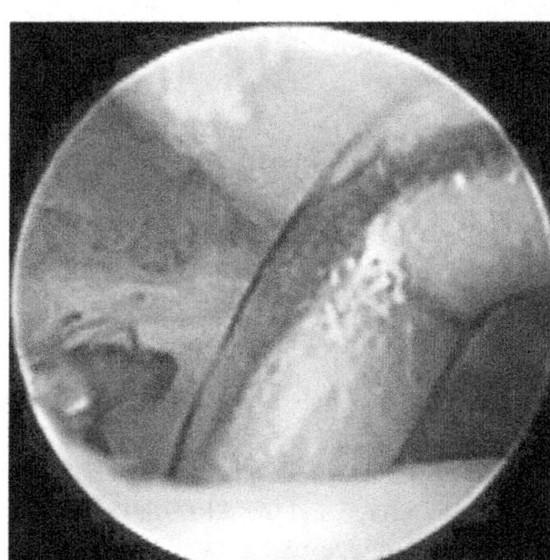

Fig. 2. 2 Arthroscopic image before drilling showinginta ctbuts oftc artilage

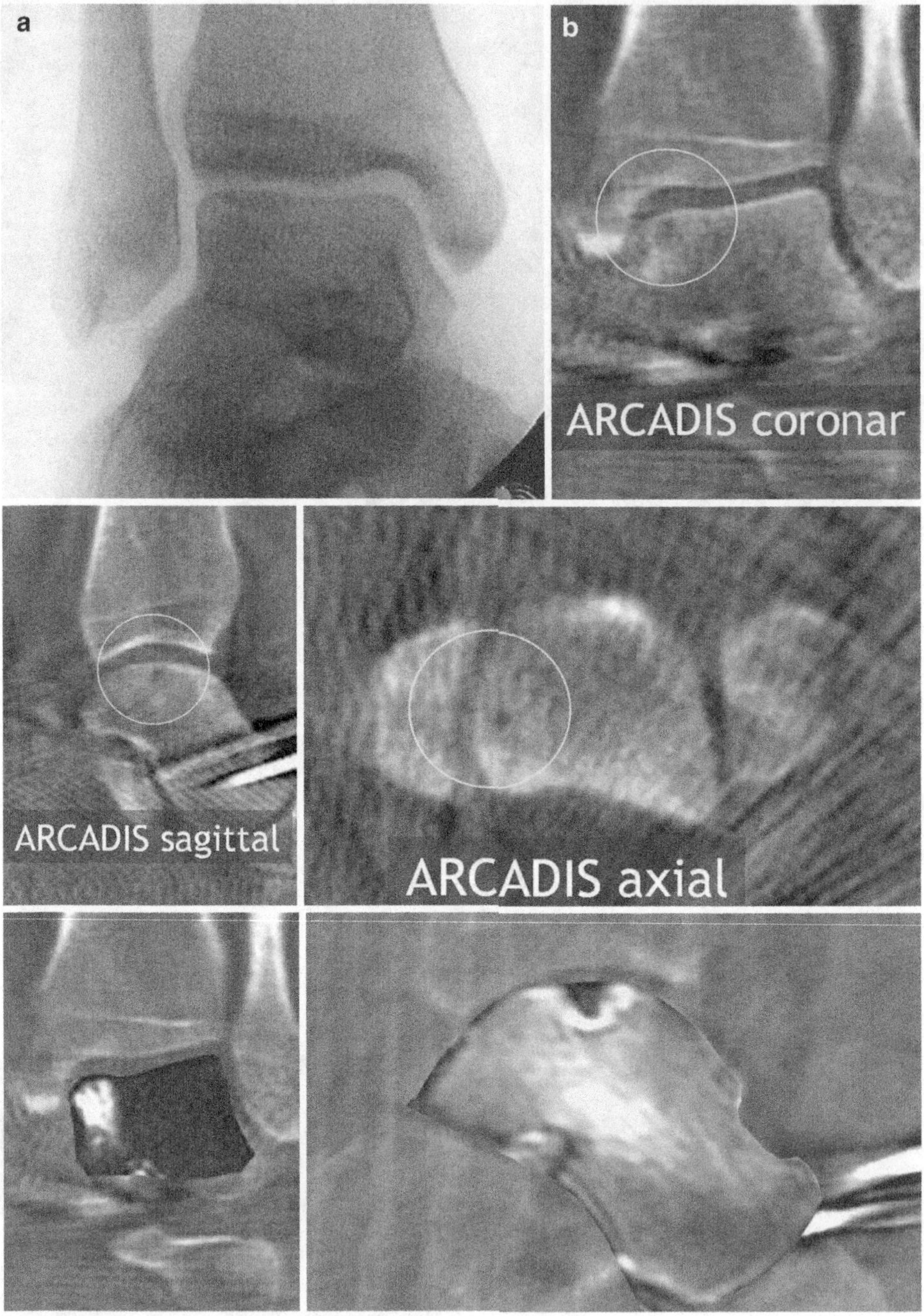

Fig. 2.3 Intraoperative image acquisition with ARCADIS-3D. (**a**) Shows a 2D-image without sufficient visibility of the OCD lesion. (**b–d**) Show the reformations of the 3D-dataset from the ARCADIS scan with good visibility of the OCD lesion. (**e**) and (**f**) show an optional image fusion of the MRI image and the ARCADIS 3D-reformation for better visualization ((**e**), fusion of coronal MRI T2 image of the talar body with a coronal ARCADIS 3D reformation; (**f**), fusion of parasagittal MRI T1 image of the talar body with a parasagittal ARCADIS 3D reformation)

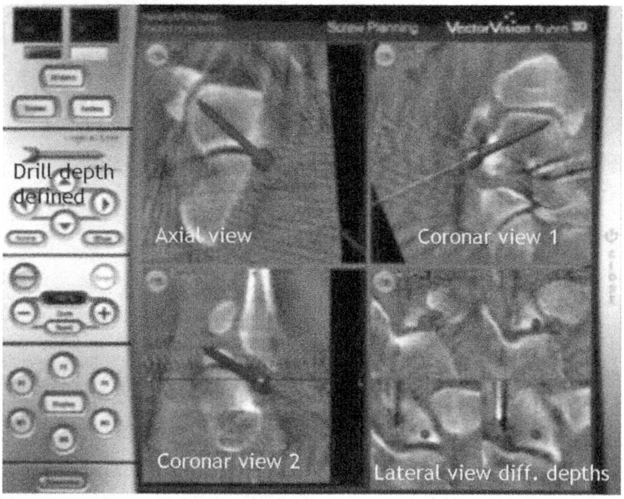

Fig. 2.4 Planning of the drilling with the Vectorvision fluoro 3D software. A virtual screw with the planned length and diameter of the drill (here 4.5 mm diameter) is placed digitally by the surgeon on the screen of the CAS device

(96%), the drilling was judged to be correct at 3D imaging. In the remaining two patients (4%), the drilling ended in the caudal portion of the lesion. A perforation of the cartilage was never evident at arthroscopy. Forty-eight (92%) patients were followed up after 12 (range 6–36) months. Three patients (6%) had been received bone cartilage transplantation (OATS) due to recurrent symptoms. These patients were excluded from follow-up. At follow up, the Visual-Analogue-Scale Foot and Ankle showed a mean of 93 points (range 86–100), and the SF 36 (standardized to 100-point-maximum) showed a mean of 90 points (range 79–100).[26,50]

2.2.3 Discussion

Several options are available for the operative management of osteochondritis dissecans stage I and II at the posterior medial talar shoulder (Berndt and Harty).[3,19,59,62] One such option is retrograde drilling.[3,19,59,62] An open procedure requires an extensile approach, including osteotomy of the medial malleolus.[54] Minimal invasive techniques have been developed with fluoroscopically based aiming devices.[3,59,62] Arthroscopy-based techniques require an arthroscopically *detectable* and *reachable* lesion; this might be problematic in lesions at the postero-medial talar shoulder.[3,59,62] To date, a thorough inspection of the entire joint is possible given the improved features of the arthroscopes (smaller diameter, better image quality). However, the identification of the exact location and size of early stage defects is still problematic, even for experienced arthroscopists with modern equipment.[60] The use of CT-based Computer Assisted Surgery (CAS) guided retrograde drilling was introduced for these patients.[5,16,24,52] This method requires preoperative CT data that are transferred to the navigation system. Preoperative data are then synchronized with the intraoperative site in a matching process. This process of synchronization causes the main problems in CT-based CAS in the foot.[38,43] The major issue lies in the difficult bony

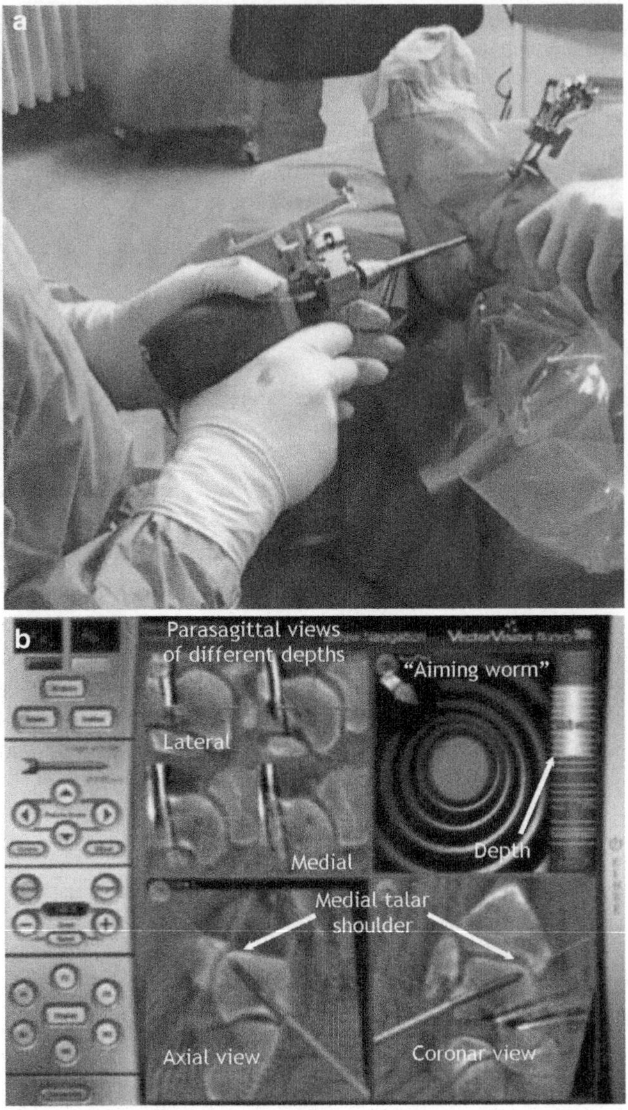

Fig.2. 5 Retrogradedr illing with starting point at the lateral talar process and visualization on the screen in real time. (**a**) shows the operative site, and (**b**)t he screen of the CAS device with an axial view, a coronal view, four parasagittal views at different depths, the "aiming" worm, and a display for the planned and achieved depth. The "aiming" worm contains a red point and a virtual worm leading to that point. This visualization prompted the surgeon to hit the red point, which results in correct direction and length of the drilling

architecture of the foot with 28 bones and more than 30 joints. Given these anatomic conditions, the foot does not remain in the same position in the period between preoperative CT and registration. This makes the registration in the foot much more difficult than in other body regions such as the spine or the pelvis, which has bigger bones, and a lower number of bones.[38] Two novel CAS methods without necessary registration were designed, the C-arm based CAS and the ISO-3-D.[38,39,43] In both, the C-arm and ISO-3-D based CAS, data are collected intraoperatively. The DRBs (Dynamic Reference Base) are fixed to the bones before the procedure, which makes matching unnecessary. Both methods combine the accuracy of the CT based CAS without the stumbling block "matching."[38,39,43] The C-arm based CAS provides only two-dimensional images. This is problematic for the

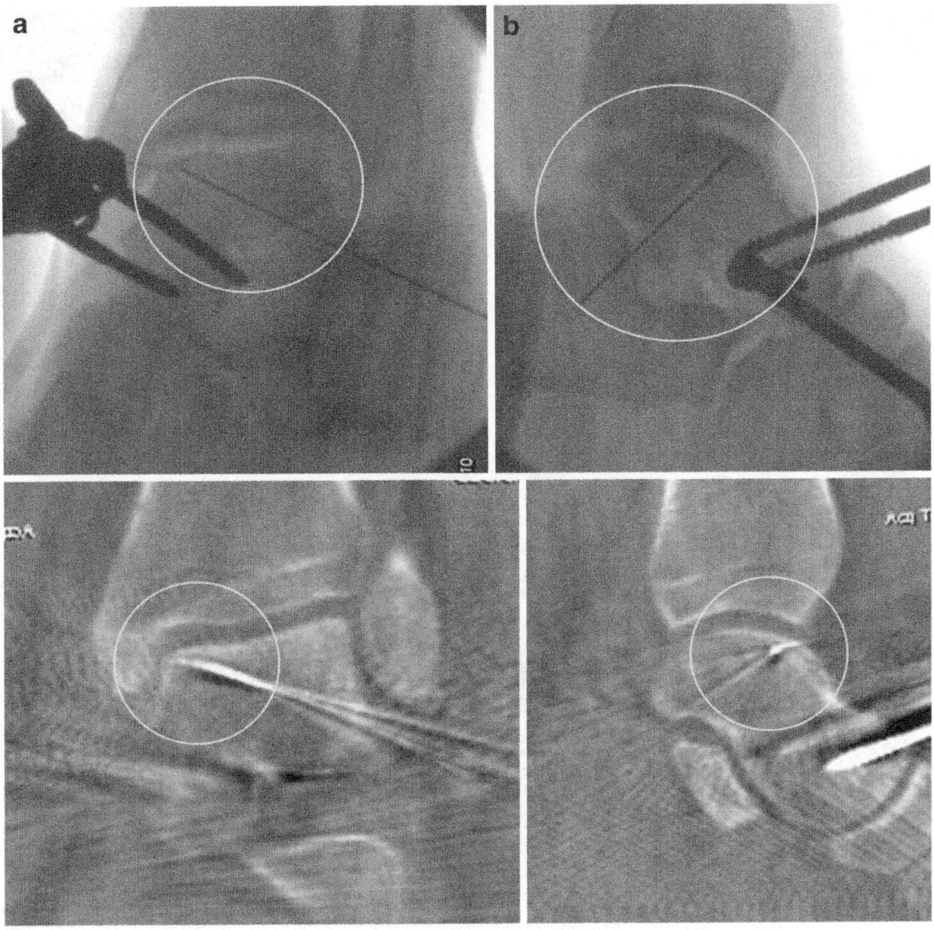

Fig. 2.6 Control of accuracy of the drilling with a second 2D- and 3D-ARCADIS scan after insertion of a Kirschner wire in the drillhole, showing the exact course of the drilling as planned preoperatively. The black areas around the Kirschner wire are artifacts, and are not equivalent to the diameter of the drilling ((**a**), 2D anteroposterior view; (**b**), 2D lateral view; (**c**), 3D coronal reconstruction; (**d**),3D pa rasagittalr econstruction)

three-dimensional aiming necessary for retrograde drilling in osteochondral lesions of the talus.[11,43] For this purpose, the ISO-3-D based CAS guided drilling is more favorable.[11,43] In vivo and in vitro, the 3D-imaging based method is clearly superior to the 2D-imanging based method.[11,43] However, the handling of this system was very complex. The devices were further developed for easier and faster handling less prone to error. The present ARCADIS-3D based CAS worked without problems in the patient shown. We choose a 4.5 mm drill because this was the thickest drill that was available for navigation at the time of the surgery (2004). Studies suggest that drill bit deflection interferes with the precision of the system. The precision is decreased when using small diameter and longer drill bits.[25] At present, we use a 5 mm drill, the thickest available for the Brainlab system.

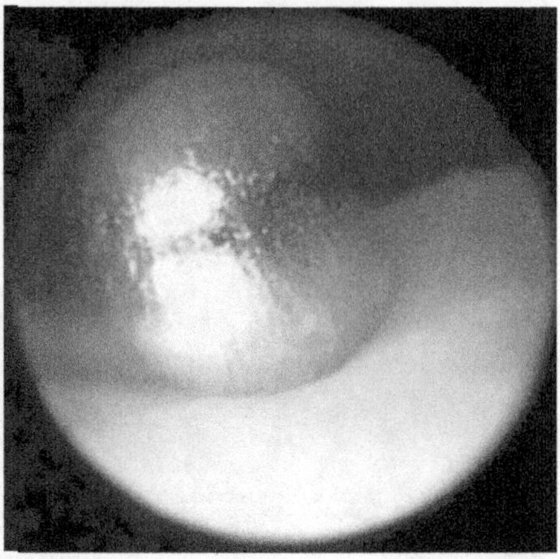

Fig. 2.7 Arthroscopic control after drilling and autologous cancellous bone grafting, showingi ntacta nds tablec artilages urface

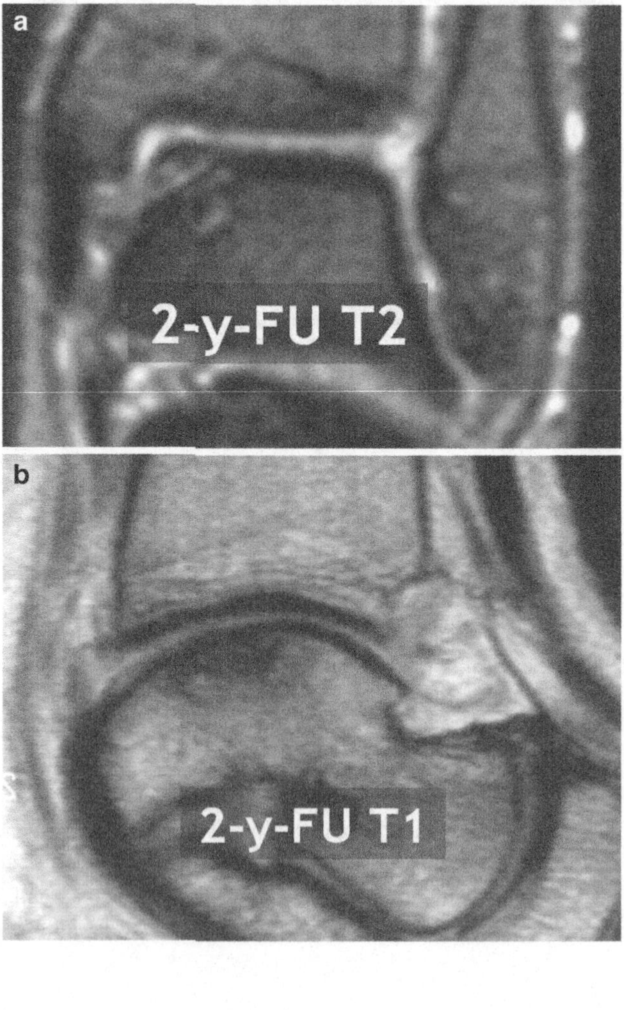

Fig. 2.8 MRIfollow -up ((**a**), coronal reconstruction; (**b**),pa rasagittal reconstruction)

Another important issue is the device costs: these are much higher for the ARCADIS-3D based CAS (€500,000) than for arthroscopy systems. These huge device costs for the ARCADIS-3D based CAS will prevent standard use for retrograde drilling in osteochondral lesions of the talus alone despite the advantages. However, the ARCADIS-3D based CAS is also useful for other body regions such as the spine and the pelvis.[23,31,34] Furthermore, the ARCADIS-3D alone is a valuable tool for intraoperative three-dimensional visualization.[29,42,51] Radiation protection for patient and personnel is another important topic. The radiation of an ARCADIS-3D based CAS guided drilling procedure is higher compared with arthroscopically based drilling. However, the ARCADIS-3D based CAS procedures produce less radiation than all conventional C-arm based procedures and CT based CAS.[17]

In conclusion, the advantages of this technique are real time intraoperative three-dimensional imaging for the use of navigation without the need for anatomical registration (matching) and an immediate intraoperative control of surgical management. Accuracy is confirmed with immediate intraoperative three-dimensional imaging. Our results indicate that ARCADIS-3D based Computer Assisted Surgery (CAS) guided retrograde drilling is a good alternative to arthroscopically guided or 2D-imaging based CAS guided drilling of OCD lesions of the talus

2.3 Part 2: CAS Guided Correction Arthrodeses at Foot and Ankle

Ankle, hindfoot and midfoot deformities are common.[1,4,8,20,22,33,37,45,57,67,68] The biomechanical consequences of these deformities frequently lead to clinical symptoms like pain and gait disturbances.[2,12,28,33,35,53,55,56,63,66,67] Corrective osteotomy and joint fusion (arthrodesis) is useful for these peri-articular deformities.[32,33,37,55,64,67] The correction of the deformities is challenging, since nonunion and remaining deformity with symptoms is frequent.[32,33,37,55,64,67] Preoperative planning of a correction is standard, and during the operative procedure the goal is to achieve the planned correction.[32,33,37,55,64,67] Preoperative imaging with radiographs and computer tomography (CT) allows accurate planning of the correction, and accuracy is enhanced using computerized planning systems.[13] However, during the procedure the realization of the planned correction is difficult, as the correction process is performed without guidance by a conventional C-arm.[32,33,37,39,64,67] In other fields of orthopedic surgery such as spine, hip and knee surgery, Computer Assisted Surgery (CAS) is helpful and more accurate than the conventional methods without navigation.[9,10,14,18,27,30,36,40,44,58,65] For the foot, a system for C-arm based CAS guided correction was developed, since CT-based CAS did not work successfully in experimental settings.[38] This system showed then sufficient feasibility and accuracy in the first clinical cases.[39,41] The method is in routine use in the author's institution. The first 118 cases were analyzed regarding how CAS affected the time spent, the accuracy of the procedure, and what problems occurred with the use of the CAS in each case.

2.3.1 Methods

2.3.1.1 Devices

Two different navigation systems with wireless Dynamic Reference Bases (DRB) were used (Models VectorVision and Navivision, Brainlab Inc., Kirchheim-Heimstetten, Germany). Before September 1, 2006, a VectorVision system with VectorVision Trauma software (Brainlab Inc., Kirchheim-Heimstetten, Germany) was used. The system was connected with a modified C-arm (Model Exposcope, Instrumentarium Imaging Ziehm Inc., Nuernberg, Germany). The accuracy of the correction was checked with intraoperative three-dimensional imaging with ISO-C-3D (Siemens Medical Inc., Munich, Germany). ISO-C-3 is a motorized mobile C-arm that provides fluoroscopic images during a 190° orbital rotation, resulting in a 119 mm data cube.[42] Multiplanar and two-dimensional reconstructions can be obtained from these 3D data sets.[42]

From September 1, 2006, a Navivision with VectorVision Trauma software (Brainlab Inc., Kirchheim-Heimstetten, Germany) was used. This system was built in an ARCADIS-3D (Siemens Medical Inc. Germany), which is a further development from the ISO-C-3D (Siemens Medical Inc., Munich, Germany). The accuracy of the correction was checked with ARCADIS-3D with a comparable function such as ISO-C-3D (see paragraph 'Evaluation').

The two navigation systems were not compared since the functions including the software was identical. The principal difference was the hardware: the Navivision is built in the ARCADIS-3D, whereas the Vectorvision is not built in the ISO-C-3D.

2.3.1.2 CAS-Procedure

One DRB was fixed to each of the two bones or fragments that had been planned for correction in relation to each other (Fig. 2.9).[47] Calibration images, anteroposterior and lateral digital radiographic images were obtained (Figs. 2.10a–c).[47] Before September 1, 2006, a modified C-arm was used and the data was transferred to the navigation device. From September 1, 2006, the images were obtained with the ARCADIS-3D without data transfer, since the navigation system is built in the ARCADIS-3D. A verification process with a DRB-equipped pointer followed (Fig. 2.11).[47] The correction was then planned and performed. For the planning, a manual selection of the bone for navigation and a definition of the bone axis were performed. This step was performed by the surgeon using the sterile draped touch screen of the navigation system (Fig. 2.12).[47] During the correction, the angle motion and translational motion between the bones or fragments in all degrees of freedom were displayed on the screen of the navigation system (Fig. 2.13).[47] Furthermore, virtual radiographs with the moving bones or fragments were displayed on the screen (Fig. 2.14).[47] The C-arm/ARCADIS-3D was not used during the correction process. After correction,

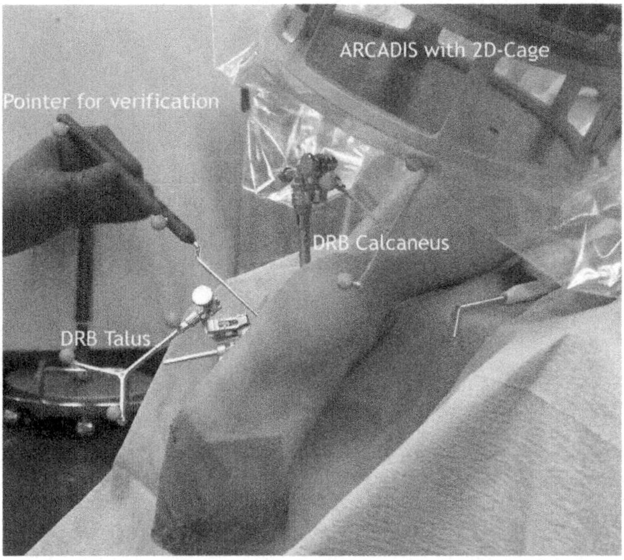

Fig. 2.9 Correction arthrodesis of the subtalar joint. The patient is prone position, and a posterolateral approach was used. Two autologous tricortical bone blocks and autologous cancellous bone was obtained from the posterior pelvic rim. Two 7.3 mm cancellous screws with short threads (Synthes, Umkirch, Germany) were inserted. The image shows the DRBs fixed to talus and calcaneus the ARCADIS-3D with 2D-navigation cage. The pointer for verification later used for verificationis s hown(s eeFig. 2.11)

retention was performed with 2.0 mm Kirschner wires. Internal fixation with screws, plates or intramedullary nails followed. For ankle or subtalar fusions, the drillings for the screws were CAS guided (Fig. 2.14a–c).[47] For the combined ankle and subtalar fusions, the guide wire for the nail reamer was inserted with CAS guidance. The accuracy of the correction and implant position was then checked with intraoperative three-dimensional imaging withI SO-C-3D/ARCADIS-3D(Figs. 2.15a a ndb) .

The times for the different CAS steps were measured with a stopwatch by a medical student or student nurse who attended the cases. The time for preparation was measured with the starting point when the first DRB fixation was started and the endpoint when the current values for angles and translation were displayed on the screen of the CAS device. The period includes fixation of the two DRBs, 2D-image acquisition, verification of the accuracy with the DRB-equipped pointer, definition of the two bones including the bone axes, and reading of the current angles and values on the screen of the CAS device. The time of the correction process was measured with the starting point when the surgeon started to move the bones for the definite correction, and the endpoint when this correction process was ended and before the correction was fixed with Kirschner wires (see above). This time period did not include the additional surgical maneuvers described below.

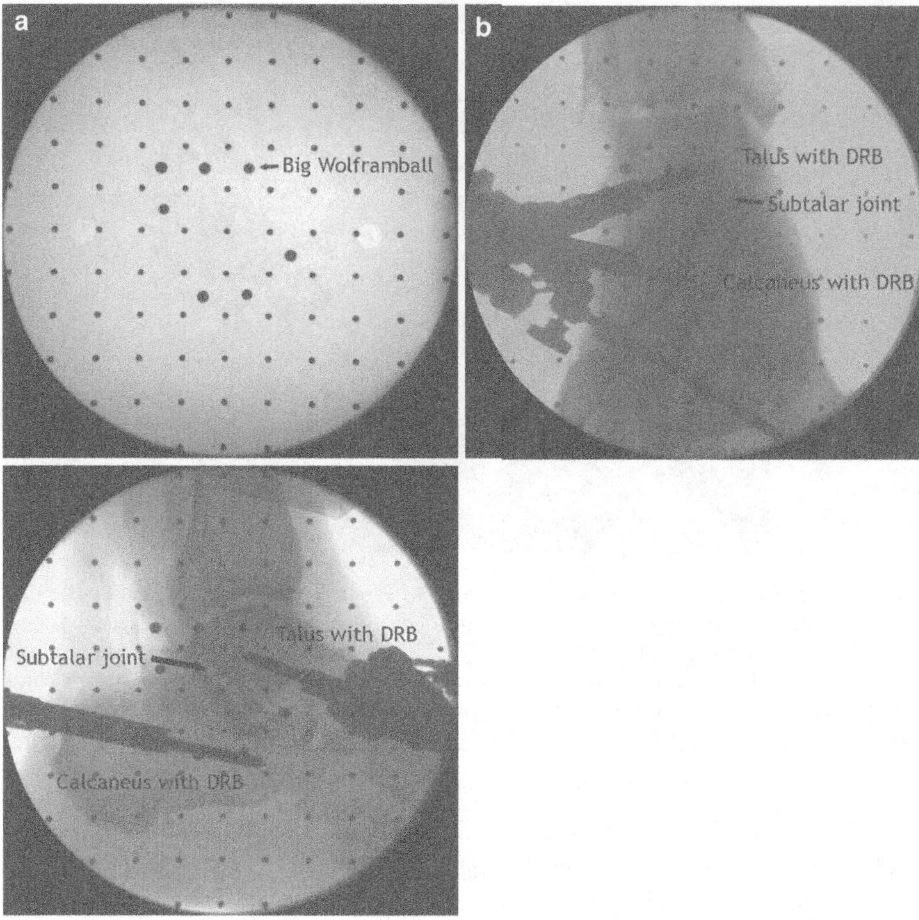

Fig. 2.10 Same patient as Fig. 2.9. 2D-Image Acquisition. First, an empty image showing the all seven large Wolfram balls of the 2D-navigation cage is acquired (**a**). This allows later exact placement of the foot, regardless of the visibility of the seven large Wolfram balls. This is a very important step, since the navigation system needs at least five clearly visible large Wolfram balls for exact verification. This is typically not the case when the foot with the DRBs is correctly placed for the anteroposterior (**b**) and the lateral (**c**)vi ews

2.3.1.3
Additional Surgical Maneuvers

No external distraction devices for correction means were used. No osteotomies with CAS guidance were performed. After the two bones were equipped with DRBs, the remaining articolar cartilage was removed. The bones were moved with CAS guidance in relation to each other until the planned position was achieved. Osteotomies were performed only in the tarsometatarsal joint of the first ray to achieve sufficient area of bone contact at the fusion site. In none of the patients hindfoot osteotomies were performed to achieve the

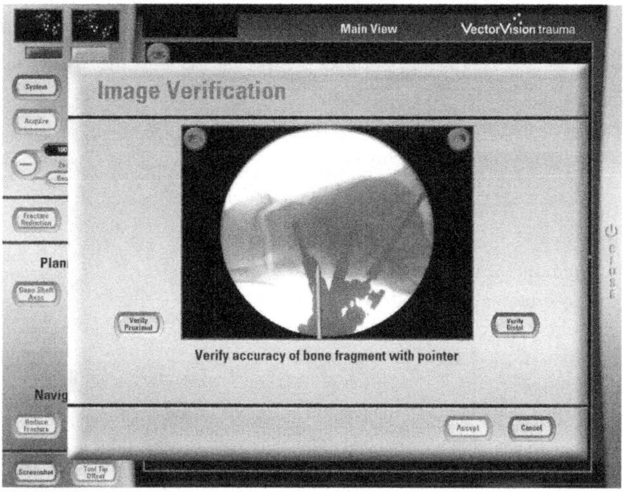

Fig. 2. 11 Same patient as in Figs. 2.9a nd 2.10. Verification with the Pointer. The pointer is placed at the base of the proximal DRB (see Fig. 2.9). This position is exactly shown on the screen which proves an exact verification

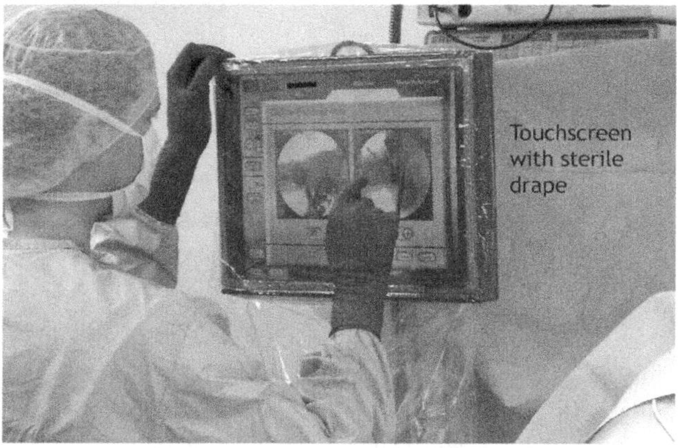

Fig. 2. 12 Same patient as in Figs. 2.9–2.11.Thi s ist he definition of the bone axis of the talus and calcaneus, and the definition of the bones by outlining them digitally on the sterile draped touch screen. These steps have to be performed before the bone position is altered, for example by opening the joint and removing the remaining cartilage

planned position. However, soft tissue releases were frequently performed in patients operated without CAS.[32,33,37,55,64,67] After the correct positions of the bone were achieved, the remaining gaps or defects were filled with cancellous bone and/or tricortical bone blocks from the pelvic rim.

2.3.1.4 Study Setting

A clinical study was performed in a university hospital level I trauma center before September 1, 2006, and in a university teaching hospital level II trauma center from September 1, 2006. The surgical staff involved in the study consisted of qualified and experienced orthopedic trauma surgeons, interns, residents, and fellows. The surgical

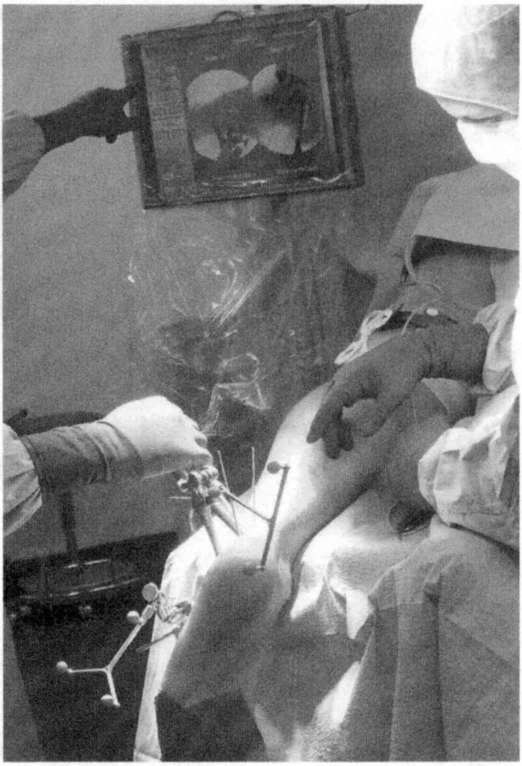

Fig.2. 13 Same patient as in Figs. 2.9–2.12.C ASgui dedc orrectionof calcaneus in relation to the talus. Both bones, the angles and translations between the bones are shown in an anteroposterior and lateral virtual fluoroscopic view on the screen in real time. Real fluoroscopy is not needed during this correction process. Insertion of the bone grafts and later transfixation of the subtalar joint with two 2.0 mm Kirschner wires is performed under permanent monitoring of the angles and translations

procedures were exclusively performed by the first author. The assessment of the deformity and the planning was performed on the basis of the clinical finding, radiographs with full bearing and computer tomography (CT). Pathological angles and translation, for example a talocalcaneal angle, were identified on the standing radiographs and CT, and the amount of correction was defined. The preoperative angles or translations, the planned correction, and the amount of correction was then drawn with lines, angles and translations on the corresponding CT images using a terminal and software of the institutional Picture Archiving Communication System (PACS). These images served as the baseline for the plannedc orrection.

2.3.1.5 Results

One hundred and eighteen patients were included (correction arthrodeses at ankle, n = 24; subtalar joint, n = 28; ankle and subtalar joint, n = 19; midfoot/tarsometatarsal (TMT) joint, n = 28, others, n = 19). The average time needed for preparation was 5 min and 45 s (4–30 min), and the correction process took 27 s (12–240). The CAS system encountered

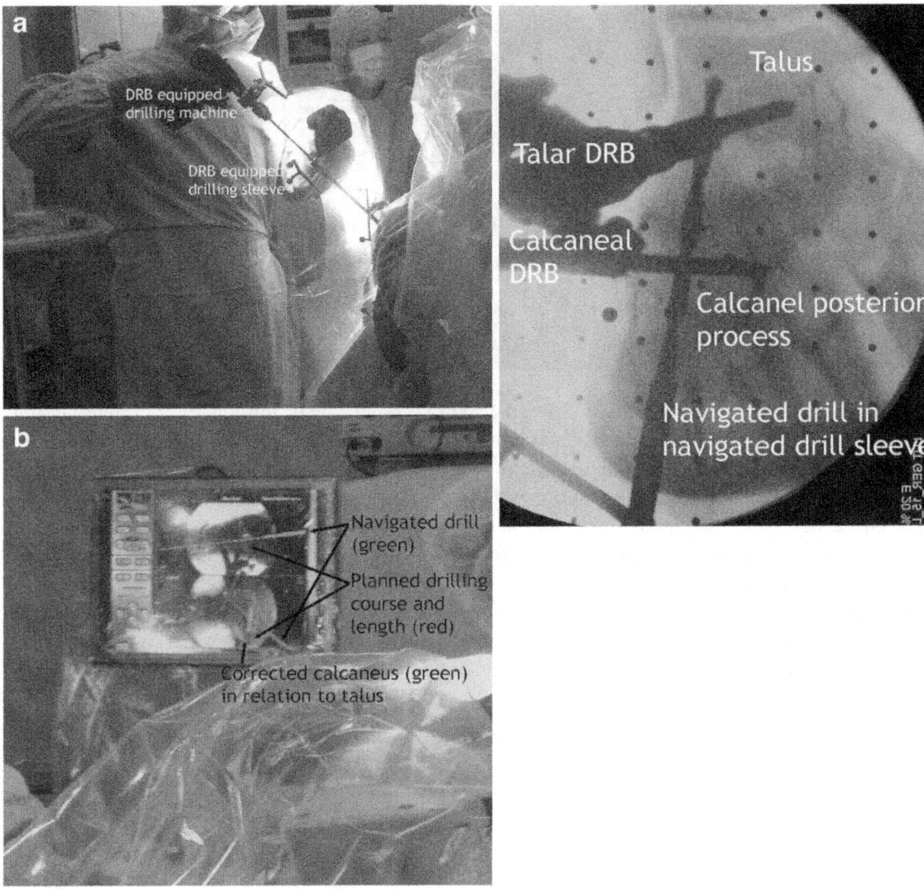

Fig. 2.14 Same case as Figs. 2.9–2.13. CAS guided drilling with a 5.0 mm drill with a navigated drilling machine and a navigated drill sleeve was used (**a**). In (**b**), the real time view of the planned drilling direction is shown, including depth (red), and the actual drilling direction including depth (green). The images with the altered/corrected position of the calcaneus are used, not the images with the earlier position of the calcaneus, and not the images of the actual calcaneus position. (**c**) Shows a fluoroscopic image obtained during the firstdr illing

malfunctions in four procedures (3%) in which the verification process was not successful, i.e., the system did not consider the bones in the correct position. In the remaining cases, all the achieved angles/translations were within a maximum deviation of 2°/mm when compared to the planned correction ($p < 0.05$).

One hundred and two (86%) patients completed follow-up after 9.2 (6–36) months. In all cases fusion, was registered. The scores were AOFAS 82 (46–100, maximum possible hindfoot score for ankle fusion 92, subtalar fusion 94, ankle and subtalar fusion 86), Visual-Analogue-Scale Foot and Ankle 79 (43–100).

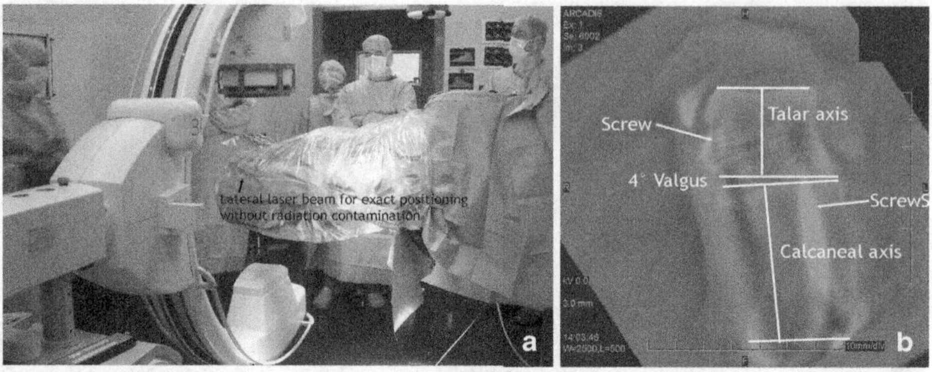

Fig. 2.15 Same patient as in Figs. 2.9–2.14. Three-dimensional intraoperative imaging with ARCADIS-3D for analysis of implant and bone position after screw fixation is complete. The table with the legs is totally draped with a sterile plastic bag and the ARCADIS-3D is placed with laser aiming devices for correct anteroposterior and lateral positing without radiation contamination (**a**). The entire staff leaves the area with radiation contamination before the scan. (**b**) Shows the analysis on a paracoronal reconstruction through the posterior facet with measurement of the achieved axis between talus and calcaneus. Here, 4° of valgisation in the frontal/coronal plane was planned and achieved. No other abnormality was observed and considered for correction, including, for example, talo-calcaneal axis, talo-metatarsal-1-axis in the dorsoplantar view and the lateral view, congruity of the talo-navicular-joint, and calcaneal inclination/pitch angle

2.3.1.6 Discussion

The CAS guided correction showed great accuracy. Despite pre-operative planning, correction is sometimes limited by soft tissues and other restraints.[33,37,55,64,67] Still, the surgeon involved in this study was always able to achieve the pre-operative planning goals intraoperatively. Some of the complex deformities involved in this study had bony abnormalities which were not correctable with the CAS system, and not exactly measureable with the ISO-C-3D/ARCADIS-3D system (e.g., widening of the lateral wall of the calcaneus). These components of the deformities were assessed, but they were not measured with a pre-operative CT. After the correction, they were assessed with an intraoperative ISO-C-3D/ARCADIS-3D scan (data not shown). A measurement of these components, for example the widening of the lateral wall of the calcaneus, has not been performed in any other study to our knowledge. We are aware of the problems in measuring angles on images.[15,33,37,41,56,64] To avoid these problems, we measured the angles and translations digitally on the computer that was involved in obtaining the images, either pre-operative CT or intraoperative ISO-C-3D/ARCADIS-3D. The accuracy of the correction achieved was measured by a co-investigator, who was not involved in the planning and the surgical procedures, with images that were obtained intraoperatively, and a re-evaluation of the "remaining" accuracy at a later stage is in process. In the follow-up until now, we have observed the similar problems as in cases without CAS. During the study, we have especially observed a loss of correction. For example, in one patient necessitating subtalar arthrodeses with correction of a decreased talocalcanel angle in the lateral radiographs, the data at a 3 months follow-up differed in comparison with the intraoperative measurement taken (data not shown).

The time spent was less in cases, mostly more than 10 min spent for preparation. The correction process itself was very fast, especially regarding the problems with the conventional C-arm based correction.[33,41] In our experience, the correction without CAS guidance needs more time because the necessary frequent C-arm checks.[61] However, no data from other groups are available about the time spent of in correction process in comparable cases.

We could not isolate data from the literature regarding measurements of the difference between the pre-operatively planned versus the achieved corrected angles and translations with conventional correction or without.[15,33,37,56,64] Even in previous data from conventional arthrodeses of the subtalar joint, we could not determine the difference, as the planned correction was not recorded.[61] Rammelt et al. indirectly reported a difference between the planned and the achieved correction in correction arthrodeses of the subtalar joint.[37] They described that the measurements of the unaffected side were used as a template for the planning of the correction.[37] These measurements, i.e., the planned corrections, were achieved 38.5–61.8% of the times for the different measurements.[37] In our study, the planned correction was achieved on an average of 75–100% (mean, 95.0%), of the time for all types of correction arthrodeses, and 87.5–100% (mean, 98.6%) of the time for correction arthrodeses of the subtalar joint. Regarding the higher percentages in our study, a sufficient comparison of the conventional correction without CAS and CAS guided correction in one single randomized controlled study is available. We observed that, in patients with a higher amount of planned correction, the deviation of the achieved correction in percent from the planned correction is higher than in patients with small amounts of planned correction.

Based on our results, CAS is helpful in complex three-dimensional corrections, and in drillings.[38,39,41] The clinical relevance of CAS-based methods might be high in those cases, because the improved accuracy may lead to an improved clinical outcome, i.e., complex corrections in ankle, hind- and midfoot deformities.[2,6,12,28,33,35,53,56,63,66,67]

In conclusion, C-arm based CAS guided correction of posttraumatic deformities of the ankle and hindfoot provides a very high accuracy and a fast correction process.[41] The clinical relevance of these methods is high in these patients, as high accuracy may lead to an optimized clinical outcome.[2,6,12,28,33,35,53,56,63,66,67] Further studies, including clinical outcome assessment, will show whether patients will benefit from the high accuracy provided with this method.

For the future, the integration of the different computerized systems will improve the handling and clinical feasibility. An integration of pre-operative pedography, planning software, CAS, ISO-C-3D/ARCADIS-3D and Intraoperative Pedography (IP) in one Integrated Computer System for Operative Procedures (ICOP) will be favorable.[39] Within this type of ICOP, pre-operative computerized planning will include pre-operative radiographic, CT, MRI and pedography data. Pre-operative computerized planning results will be transferred to the CAS device. The CAS-system will be guided by biomechanical assessment with IP that allows not only morphological, but also biomechanical based CAS. The intraoperative three-dimensional imaging (ISO-C-3D/ARCADIS-3D) data and the IP-data will be matched with the data from the planning software to allow immediate improvements of reduction, correction and or drilling/implant position in the same procedure.[39]

References

1. Adelaar RS. The treatment of complex fractures of the talus. *Orthop Clin North Am.* 1989;20:691–707.
2. Adelaar RS, Kyles MK. Surgical correction of resistant talipes equinovarus: observations and analysis - preliminary report. *Foot Ankle.* 1981; 2:126–137.
3. Alexander AH, Lichtman DM. Surgical treatment of transchondral talar-dome fractures (osteochondritis dissecans). Long-term follow-up. *J Bone Joint Surg Am.* 1980; 62:646–652.
4. Amon K. Luxationsfraktur der kuneonavikularen Gelenklinie. Klinik, Pathomechanismus und Therapiekonzept einer sehr seltenen Fussverletzung. *Unfallchirurg.* 1990; 93:431–434.
5. Bale RJ, Hoser C, Rosenberger R, Rieger M, Benedetto KP, Fink C. Osteochondral lesions of the talus: computer-assisted retrograde drilling–feasibility and accuracy in initial experiences. *Radiology.* 2001;218: 278–282.
6. Bechtold JE, Powless SH. The application of computer graphics in foot and ankle surgical planning and reconstruction. *Clin Podiatr Med Surg.* 1 993;10:551–562.
7. Berndt AL, Harty M. Transchondral fractures (osteochondritis dissecans) of the talus. *Am J Orthop.* 1959;41 -A:988–1020.
8. Brutscher R. Frakturen und Luxationen des Mittel- und Vorfusses. *Orthopäde.* 1991;20:67–75.
9. Chauhan SK, Clark GW, Lloyd S, Scott RG, Breidahl W, Sikorski JM. Computer-assisted total knee replacement. A controlled cadaver study using a multi-parameter quantitative CT assessment of alignment (the Perth CT Protocol). *J Bone Joint Surg Br.* 2004; 86:818–823.
10. Chauhan SK, Scott RG, Breidahl W, Beaver RJ. Computer-assisted knee arthroplasty versus a conventional jig-based technique. A randomised, prospective trial. *J Bone Joint Surg Br.* 2004;86:372–377.
11. Citak M, Haasper C, Behrends M, Kupka T, Kendoff D, Hufner T, Matthies HK, Krettek C. [A web-based e-learning tool in academic teaching of trauma surgery. First experiences and evaluation results]. *Unfallchirurg.* 2007; 110:367–372.
12. Coetzee JC, Hansen ST. Surgical management of severe deformity resulting from posterior tibial tendon dysfunction. *Foot Ankle Int.* 2001; 22:944–949.
13. Dahlen C, Zwipp H. Computer-assistierte OP-Planung 3D-Software für den PC. *Unfallchirurg.* 2001;104:466–479.
14. DiGioia AM III, Blendea S, Jaramaz B. Computer-assisted orthopaedic surgery: minimally invasive hip and knee reconstruction. *Orthop Clin North Am.* 2004; 35:183–189.
15. Easley ME, Trnka HJ, Schon LC, Myerson MS. Isolated subtalar arthrodesis. *J Bone Joint Surg Am.* 2000;82: 613–624.
16. Fink C, Rosenberger RE, Bale RJ, Rieger M, Hackl W, Benedetto KP, Kunzel KH, Hoser C. Computer-assisted retrograde drilling of osteochondral lesions of the talus. *Orthopade.* 2001;30:59–65.
17. Gebhard F, Kraus M, Schneider E, Arand M, Kinzl L, Hebecker A, Batz L. Radiation dose in OR - a comparison of computer assisted procedures. *Unfallchirurg.* 2003; 106:492–497.
18. Haaker RG, Stockheim M, Kamp M, Proff G, Breitenfelder J, Ottersbach A. Computer-assisted navigation increases precision of component placement in total knee arthroplasty. *Clin Orthop Relat Res.* 2005; 433:152–159.
19. Hankemeier S, Muller EJ, Kaminski A, Muhr G. Ten year-results on bone marrowstimulating therapy in the treatment of osteochondritis dissecans of the talus. *Unfallchirurg.* 2003;106:461–466.
20. Hansen STJ. *Functional Reconstruction of the Foot and Ankle.* Philadelphia, PA/Baltimore, MA/NewYork: Lippincott Williams & Wilkins; 2000.
21. Hepple S, Winson IG, Glew D. Osteochondral lesions of the talus: a revised classification. *Foot Ankle Int.* 1999; 20:789–793.

22. Hildebrand KA, Buckley RE, Mohtadi NG, Faris P. Functional outcome measures after displaced intra-articular calcaneal fractures. *J Bone Joint Surg Br.* 1996; 78:119–123.
23. Holly LT, Foley KT. Three-dimensional fluoroscopy-guided percutaneous thoracolumbar pedicle screw placement. Technical note. *J Neurosurg.* 2003; 99:324–329.
24. Hoser C, Bichler O, Bale R, Rosenberger R, Rieger M, Kovacs P, Lang T, Fink C. A computer assisted surgical technique for retrograde autologous osteochondral grafting in talar osteochondritis dissecans (OCD): a cadaveric study. *Knee Surg Sports Traumatol Arthrosc.* 2003;12:65–71.
25. Hufner T, Geerling J, Oldag G, Richter M, Kfuri M Jr, Pohlemann T, Krettek C. Accuracy study of computer-assisted drilling: the effect of bone density, drill bit characteristics, and use of a mechanical guide. *J Orthop Trauma.* 2005; 19:317–322.
26. Jenkinson C, Coulter A, Wright L. Short form 36 (SF36) health survey questionnaire: normative data for adults of working age [see comments]. *BMJ.* 1993; 306:1437–1440.
27. Jolles BM, Genoud P, Hoffmeyer P. Computer-assisted cup placement techniques in total hip arthroplasty improve accuracy of placement. *Clin Orthop Relat Res.* 2004; 426:174–179.
28. Koczewski P, Shadi M, Napiontek M. Foot lengthening using the Ilizarov device: the transverse tarsal joint resection versus osteotomy. *J Pediatr Orthop B.* 2002; 11:68–72.
29. Kotsianos D, Rock C, Euler E, Wirth S, Linsenmaier U, Brandl R, Mutschler W, Pfeifer KJ. [3-D imaging with a mobile surgical image enhancement equipment (ISO-C-3D). Initial examples of fracture diagnosis of peripheral joints in comparison with spiral CT and conventional radiography]. *Unfallchirurg.* 2001; 104:834–838.
30. Langdown AJ, Auld J, Bruce WJ. Computer-assisted knee arthroplasty versus a conventional jig-based technique. *J Bone Joint Surg Br.* 2005; 87:588–589.
31. Langlotz F, Bachler R, Berlemann U, Nolte LP, Ganz R. Computer assistance for pelvic osteotomies. *Clin Orthop.* 1998; 354:92–102.
32. Madezo P, de Cussac JB, Gouin F, Bainvel JV, Passuti N. [Combined tibio-talar and subtalar arthrodesis by retrograde nail in hindfoot rheumatoid arthritis]. *Rev Chir Orthop Reparatrice Appar Mot.* 1998;84: 646–652.
33. Marti RK, de Heus JA, Roolker W, Poolman RW, Besselaar PP. Subtalar arthrodesis with correction of deformity after fractures of the os calcis. *J Bone Joint Surg Br.* 1999; 81:611–616.
34. Merloz P, Tonetti J, Pittet L, Coulomb M, Lavallee S, Troccaz J, Cinquin P, Sautot P. Computer-assisted spine surgery. *Comput Aided Surg.* 1998; 3:297–305.
35. Mosier-LaClair S, Pomeroy G, Manoli A. Operative treatment of the difficult stage 2 adult acquired flatfoot deformity. *Foot Ankle Clin.* 2001; 6:95–119.
36. Nogler M. Navigated minimal invasive total hip arthroplasty. *Surg Technol Int.* 2004;12: 259–262.
37. Rammelt S, Grass R, Zawadski T, Biewener A, Zwipp H. Foot function after subtalar distraction bone-block arthrodesis. A prospective study. *J Bone Joint Surg Br.* 2004; 86:659–668.
38. Richter M. Experimental comparison between Computer Assisted Surgery (CAS) based and C-Arm based correction of hind- and midfoot deformities. *Osteo Trauma Care.* 2003;11:29–34.
39. Richter M. Computer based systems in foot and ankle surgery at the beginning of the 21st century. *Fuss Sprungg.* 2006; 4:59–71.
40. Richter M, Amiot LP, Neller S, Kluger P, Puhl W. Computer-assisted surgery in posterior instrumentation of the cervical spine: an in-vitro feasibility study. *Eur Spine J.* 2000;9: S65–S70.
41. Richter M, Geerling J, Frink M, Zech S, Knobloch K, Dammann F, Hankemeier S, Krettek C. Computer Assisted Surgery Based (CAS) based correction of posttraumatic ankle and hindfoot deformities – Preliminary results. *Foot Ankle Surg.* 2006;12:113–119.
42. Richter M, Geerling J, Zech S, Goesling T, Krettek C. Intraoperative three-dimensional imaging with a motorized mobile C-Arm (SIREMOBIL ISO-C-3D) in foot and ankle trauma care: a preliminary report. *J Orthop Trauma.* 2005; 19:259–266.

43. Richter M, Geerling J, Zech S, Krettek C. ISO-C-3D based Computer Assisted Surgery (CAS) guided retrograde drilling in a osteochondrosis dissecans of the talus: a case report. *Foot.* 2005;15:107–113.
44. Richter M, Mattes T, Cakir B. Computer-assisted posterior instrumentation of the cervical and cervico-thoracic spine. *Eur Spine J.*2004; 13:50–59.
45. Richter M, Wippermann B, Krettek C, Schratt E, Hufner T, Thermann H. Fractures and fracture dislocations of the midfoot – occurrence, causes and long-term results. *Foot Ankle Int.* 2001;22:392–398.
46. Richter M, Zech S. 3D-Imaging (ARCADIS) based Computer Assisted Surgery (CAS) guided retrograde drilling in osteochondritis dissecans of the talus. *Foot Ankle Int.* 2008;29: 1243–1248.
47. Richter M, Zech S. Computer Assisted Surgery (CAS) guided arthrodesis of the foot and ankle: an analysis of accuracy in 100 cases. *Foot Ankle Int.*2008; 29:1235–1242.
48. Richter M, Zech S. Intraoperative 3D imaging in foot and ankle trauma. The first clinical experience with a second device generation (ARCADIS-3D). *J Orthop Trauma.* 2009;23: 213–220.
49. Richter M, Zech S. Is intraoperative pedography helpful in clinical use - preliminary results of 100 cases from a consecutive, prospective, randomized, controlled clinical study. *Foot Ankle Surg.*2009.doi:10.1016/ j.fas.2009.03.002.
50. Richter M, Zech S, Geerling J, Frink M, Knobloch K, Krettek C. A new foot and ankle outcome score: questionnaire based, subjective, Visual-Analogue-Scale, validated and computerized. *Foot Ankle Surg.*2006; 12:191–199.
51. Rock C, Linsenmaier U, Brandl R, Kotsianos D, Wirth S, Kaltschmidt R, Euler E, Mutschler W, Pfeifer KJ. [Introduction of a new mobile C-arm/CT combination equipment (ISO-C-3D). Initial results of 3-D sectional imaging]. *Unfallchirurg.*2001; 104:827–833.
52. Rosenberger RE, Bale RJ, Fink C, Rieger M, Reichkendler M, Hackl W, Benedetto KP, Kunzel KH, Hoser C. [Computer-assisted drilling of the lower extremity. Technique and indications]. *Unfallchirurg.*20 02;105:353–358.
53. Sammarco GJ, Conti SF. Surgical treatment of neuroarthropathic foot deformity. *Foot Ankle Int.*1998;19:102 –109.
54. Seil R, Rupp S, Pape D, Dienst M, Kohn D. [Approach to open treatment of osteochondral lesions of the talus]. *Orthopade.*2001; 30:47–52.
55. Stephens HM, Sanders R. Calcaneal malunions: results of a prognostic computed tomography classification system. *Foot Ankle Int.*1996; 17:395–401.
56. Stephens HM, Walling AK, Solmen JD, Tankson CJ. Subtalar repositional arthrodesis for adult acquired flatfoot. *Clin Orthop.*1999; 365:69–73.
57. Suren EG, Zwipp H. Luxationsfrakturen im Chopart- und Lisfranc-Gelenk. *Unfallchirurg.* 1989;92:130–139.
58. Swank ML. Computer-assisted surgery in total knee arthroplasty:recent advances. *Surg Technol Int.*2004; 12:209–213.
59. Taranow WS, Bisignani GA, Towers JD, Conti SF. Retrograde drilling of osteochondral lesions of the medial talar dome. *Foot Ankle Int.*1999; 20:474–480.
60. ThermannH . *Neue Techniken in der Fußchirurgie.* Darmstadt, Germany: Steinkopff; 2004.
61. Thermann H, Hufner T, Schratt HE, Held C, Tscherne H. Subtalar fusion after conservative or operative treatment of intraarticular calcaneus fracture. *Unfallchirurg.*1999; 102:13–22.
62. Tol JL, Struijs PA, Bossuyt PM, Verhagen RA, van Dijk CN. Treatment strategies in osteochondral defects of the talar dome: a systematic review. *Foot Ankle Int.*2000; 21:119–126.

63. Toolan BC, Sangeorzan BJ, Hansen ST Jr. Complex reconstruction for the treatment of dorsolateral peritalar subluxation of the foot. Early results after distraction arthrodesis of the calcaneocuboid joint in conjunction with stabilization of, and transfer of the flexor digitorum longus tendon to, the midfoot to treat acquired pes planovalgus in adults. *J Bone Joint Surg Am.* 1999;81:1545–1560.
64. Trnka HJ, Easley ME, Lam PW, Anderson CD, Schon LC, Myerson MS. Subtalar distraction bone block arthrodesis. *J Bone Joint Surg Br.*2001; 83:849–854.
65. Victor J, Hoste D. Image-based computer-assisted total knee arthroplasty leads to lower variability in coronal alignment. *Clin Orthop Relat Res.*2004; 428:131–139.
66. Wei SY, Sullivan RJ, Davidson RS. Talo-navicular arthrodesis for residual midfoot deformities of a previously corrected clubfoot. *Foot Ankle Int.*2000; 21:482–485.
67. ZwippH . *Chirurgie des Fusses.* Wien, New York/Berlin, Heidelberg: Springer; 1994.
68. Zwipp H, Dahlen C, Randt T, Gavlik JM. Komplextrauma des Fusses. *Orthopäde.* 1997;26: 1046–1056.

Tendoscopy

3

Maayke Nadine van Sterkenburg, Peter Albert Johannes de Leeuw, and Cornelis Nicolaas van Dijk

3.1 Introduction

In contrast to arthroscopy, which has become the preferred technique to treat intra-articular ankle pathology, extra-articular problems of the ankle have traditionally demanded open surgery. Open ankle surgery has been associated with complications such as injury to the sural nerve or superficial peroneal nerve, infection, scarring, and stiffness of the ankle joint.[1–3] The percentage of complications reported with open surgery for posterior ankle impingement (removal of os trigonum, scar tissue, hypertrophic posterior talar process, or ossicle) varies between 15% and 24%.[1–4] The incidence of these complications has stimulated the development of extra-articular endoscopic techniques. Endoscopic surgery offers the advantages related to any minimally invasive procedure, such as fewer wound infections, less blood loss, smaller wounds and less morbidity. Aftertreatment is functional, and surgery is performed on an outpatient basis.[5]

Tendoscopy can be performed for the treatment and diagnosis of various pathologic conditions of the peroneal tendons, the posterior tibial tendon, and the Achilles tendon. In this chapter, we describe these procedures and their indications.

3.2 Tendoscopy of the Peroneal Tendons

3.2.1 Introduction

Pathology of the peroneal tendons is most often seen with, and secondary to chronic lateral ankle instability. These disorders frequently cause chronic ankle pain in runners and ballet

M.N.va nSte rkenburg(✉)
Department of Orthopaedic Surgery, Academic Medical Center, University of Amsterdam, 22700 1100D E, Amsterdam, TheN etherlands
e-mail:m.n.va nsterkenburg@amc.uva.nl

N. Maffulli and M. Easley (eds.), *Minimally Invasive Surgery of the Foot and Ankle*,
DOI: 10.1007/978-1-84996-417-3_3, © Springer-Verlag London Limited 2011

dancers.[6] Post-traumatic lateral ankle pain is seen frequently, but peroneal tendon pathology is not always recognized as a cause of these symptoms. In a study by Dombek and co-workers, only 60% of peroneal tendon disorders were accurately diagnosed at the first clinical evaluation.[7] Because the peroneal tendons act as lateral ankle stabilizers, in chronic instability of the ankle more strain is put on these tendons, resulting in hypertrophic tendinopathy, tenosynovitis, and ultimately in tendon tears.[8]

Pathology consists of tenosynovitis, tendon dislocation or subluxation, and (subtotal) rupture or snapping of one or both of the peroneal tendons. It accounts for the majority of symptoms at the posterolateral aspect of the ankle.[9,10] Other causes of posterolateral ankle pain are rheumatoid synovitis, bony spurs, calcifications or ossicles, pathology to the posterior talofibular ligament (PTFL), or disorders of the posterior compartment of the subtalar joint. Posterior ankle impingement can present as posterolateral ankle pain. On clinical examination, there is recognizable tenderness over the tendons on palpation. Swelling, tendon dislocation and signs of tenosynovitis can be found.

The diagnosis of peroneal tendon pathology can be difficult in a patient with lateral ankle pain. A detailed history should include the presence of associated conditions such as rheumatoid arthritis, psoriasis, hyperparathyroidism, diabetic neuropathy, calcaneal fracture, fluoroquinolone use, and local steroid injections. These can all increase the prevalence of peroneal tendon dysfunction.[11] A diagnostic differentiation must be made with fatigue fractures or fractures of the fibula, posterior impingement of the ankle, and lesions of the lateral ligament complex.

Additional investigations such as MRI and ultrasonography may be helpful in confirming the diagnosis in (partial) tears of the tendon of peroneus brevis or longus.[12] Post-traumatic or post-surgical adhesions and irregularities of the posterior aspect of the fibula (peroneal groove) can also be responsible for symptoms in this region.

The primary indication of treating pathology of the peroneal tendons is pain. Conservative management should be attempted first. This includes activity modification, footwear changes, temporary immobilization, and corticosteroid injections. Also, lateral heel wedges can take the strain off the peroneal tendons which may allow healing. Failure of these conservative measures may be an indication for surgery. We therefore developed a safe and reliable endoscopic technique which we describe in detail here.[13,14]

3.2.2 Surgical Technique

Anatomically, the peroneus brevis tendon is situated dorsomedially to the peroneus longus tendon from its proximal aspect up to the fibular tip, where it is relatively flat. Just distally to this lateral malleolus tip, the peroneus brevis tendon becomes rounder, and crosses the round peroneus longus tendon. The distal posterolateral part of the fibula forms a sliding channel for the two peroneal tendons. This malleolar groove is formed by a periosteal cushion of fibrocartilage that covers the bony groove. The tendons are held into position by the superior peroneal retinaculum.[8,15,16]

The patient is placed in the lateral decubitus position, with the operative side up. Before anaesthesia is administered, the patient is asked to actively evert the affected foot. In this way, the tendon can be palpated, and the location of the portals is drawn onto the skin. The surgery can be performed under local, regional, epidural or general anaesthesia. A support is placed under the affected leg making it possible to move the ankle freely. After exsanguination a tourniquet is inflated around the thigh of the affected leg.

A distal portal is made first, 2–2.5 cm distal to the posterior edge of the lateral malleolus. An incision is made through the skin, and the tendon sheath is penetrated with an arthroscopic shaft with a blunt trocar. After this, a 2.7 mm 30° arthroscope is introduced (Fig. 3.1a–f).

The inspection starts approximately 6 cm proximal from the posterior tip of the fibula, where a thin membrane splints the tendon compartment into two separate tendon chambers (Fig. 3.1f). More distally, the tendons lie in one compartment. A second portal is made 2–2.5 cm proximal to the posterior edge of the lateral malleolus under direct vision by placing a spinal needle, producing a portal directly over the tendons (Fig. 3.1g–j). Through the distal portal, a complete overview of both tendons can be obtained.

By rotating the arthroscope over and in between both tendons, the whole compartment can be inspected. When a total synovectomy of the tendon sheath is to be performed, it is advisable to produce a third portal more distal or more proximal than the portals described previously.

When a rupture of one of the tendons is seen (Fig. 3.2), endoscopic synovectomy is performed, and the rupture is repaired through a mini-open approach.

In patients with recurrent dislocation of the peroneal tendon, endoscopic fibular groove deepening can be performed through this approach. This is a time consuming procedure, because of the limited working area. Groove deepening is performed from within the tendon sheath with the risk of iatrogenic damage to the tendons. We therefore prefer an approach by the two hindfoot portal technique.[17]

At the end of the procedure, the portals are sutured to prevent sinus formation, and a compressive dressing is applied. Full weight bearing is allowed as tolerated and active range of motion exercises are advised starting immediately post surgery.

3.2.3 Results

We reported the results of peroneal tendoscopy in 23 patients operated on between 1995 and 2000, with a minimum follow up of 2 years.[16] Eleven patients were diagnosed with a longitudinal rupture of the peroneus brevis tendon; eight of these presented with pain and swelling over the posterior aspect of the lateral malleolus and three presented with a snapping sensation at the level of the lateral malleolus.

Ten patients had persisting symptoms after surgery for a fracture of the fibula, lateral ankle ligament reconstruction, or after operative repair of recurrent tendon dislocation. Surgery consisted of endoscopic tenosynovectomy, adhesiolysis, removal of an exostosis, and suturing a longitudinal rupture via a mini-open procedure. The two remaining patients underwent endoscopic groove deepening of the fibular groove for complaints of recurrent tendon dislocation.

No complications occurred, and complaints disappeared after surgery. Since then, we performed another 28 procedures mainly for adhesiolysis, and diagnosis and management of longitudinal ruptures. For recurrent peroneal tendon dislocation we treated another 12 patients by means of endoscopic groove deepening with good results at 1 year follow-up.

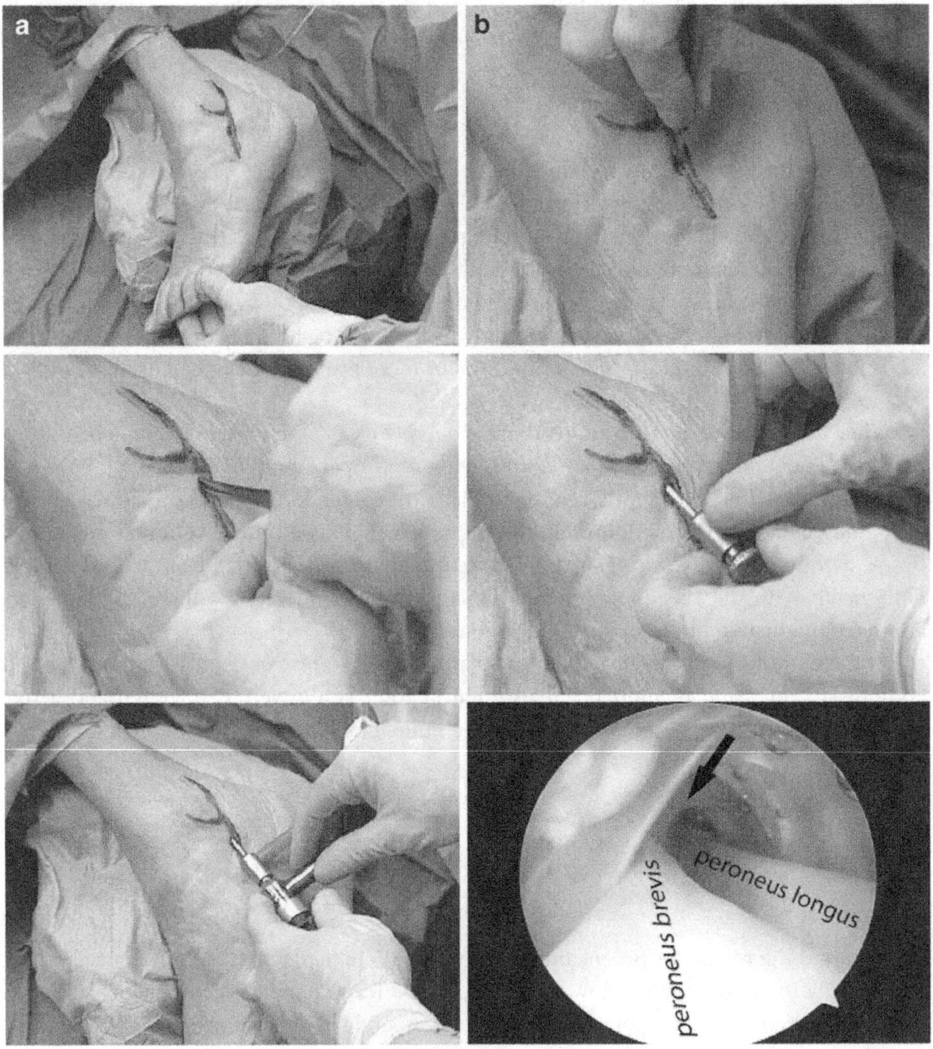

Fig. 3.1 Peroneal tendoscopy of the left ankle: (**a**) marking the anatomy of the peroneal tendons. (**b**) Incision of the skin for preparation of the distal portal. (**c**) Blunt dissection of peritendineum with mosquito clamp. (**d**) Introduction of arthroscopic shaft with a blunt trocar. (**e**) Introduction of 2.7 mm 30° arthroscope. (**f**) Arthroscopic view at introduction of the arthroscope looking from distal to proximal. An arrow indicates a thin membrane separating the two tendons proximally. (**g**) Placement of spinal needle under direct vision for preparation of the second portal. (**h**) Endoscopic view of needle looking from distal to proximal. (**i**) Incision for proximal portal. (**j**) Endoscopic view of the tip of the knife inside the tendon sheath. (*PB* peroneus brevis, *PL*pe roneusl ongus)

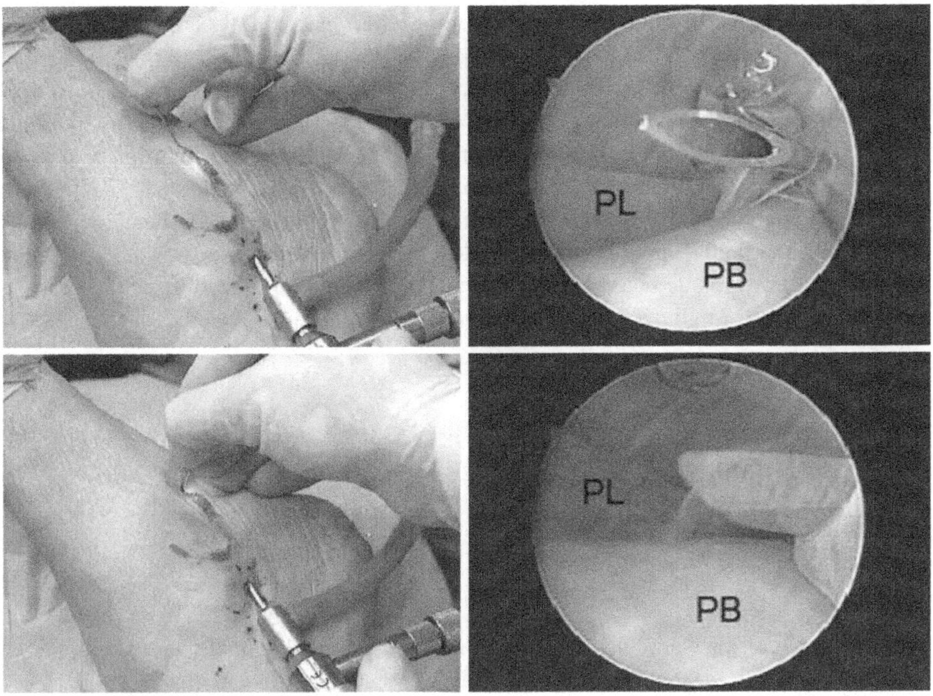

Fig. 3.1 (continued)

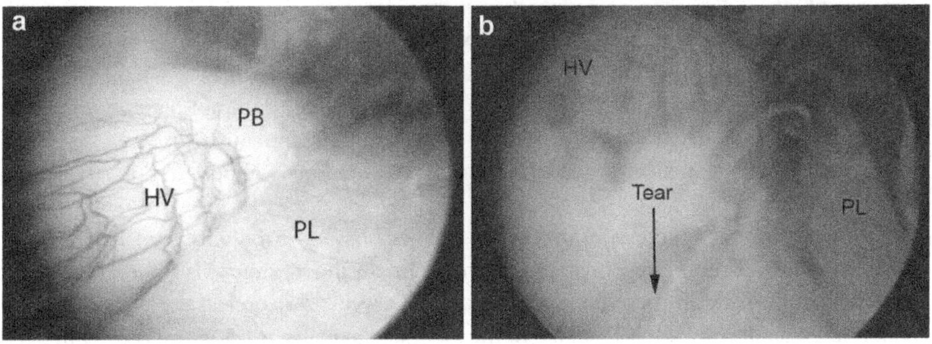

Fig. 3.2 Peroneal tendoscopy in a 38-year-old male patient with a longitudinal tear of the left peroneus brevis tendon. The arthroscope is introduced through the distal portal looking into a proximal direction. (**a**) Hypervascularisation of peroneus brevis tendon as an expression of chronic irritation. (**b**) Endoscopic view of a longitudinal tear of the peroneus brevis tendon (*HV* hypervascularisation, *PB* peroneus brevis tendon, *PL* peroneus longus tendon. The arrow indicates the tear.)

The technique uses the two traditional hindfoot portals and one additional superoposterolateral working portal.[4,17]

Lui and co-workers[18] described an endoscopic technique to reconstruct the superior peroneal retinaculum keeping the peroneal tendons in place when intact. In addition to the two portals described earlier, retinacular openings are made slightly larger than the skin openings of the portals. The lateral surface of the lateral malleolus where the retinaculum is stripped off is roughened with an arthroscopic burr or curette. Three holes are drilled through the portals with an interval of 1 cm, and three suture anchors are inserted into the fibular ridge. A needle is inserted through the portal and the retinaculum pierced in an "inside-out" manner. The sutures are pulled out and then retrieved at the surface of the retinaculum through the skin wounds. When the sutures are tightened the retinaculum can be pushed onto the fibular ridge. The authors describe two cases with good outcome, and a possible great advantage could be that patients with endoscopic reconstruction seem to have less subjective tightness as compared to those undergoing open procedures.

3.3 Tendoscopy of the Posterior Tibial Tendon

3.3.1 Introduction

In the absence of intra-articular ankle pathology, posteromedial ankle pain is most often caused by disorders of the posterior tibial tendon.

Inactivity of the posterior tibial tendon gives midtarsal instability and is the commonest cause of adult onset flatfoot deformity. The relative strength of this tendon is more than twice that of its primary antagonist, the peroneus brevis tendon. Without the activity of the posterior tibial tendon, there is no stability at the midtarsal joint, and the forward propulsive force of the gastrocnemius/soleus complex acts at the midfoot instead of at the midtarsal heads. Total dysfunction eventually leads to a flatfoot deformity.

These disorders can be divided in two groups: the younger group of patients with dysfunction of the tendon, caused by some form of systemic inflammatory disease (e.g., rheumatoid arthritis); and an older group of patients whose tendon dysfunction is mostly caused by chronic overuse.[19]

Following trauma, surgery, and fractures, adhesions and irregularity of the posterior aspect of the tibia can be responsible for symptoms in this region. Also, the vincula can become symptomatic in these circumstances.[20,22] The vincula connect the posterior tibial tendon to its tendon sheath.[21] Damage to the vincula can cause thickening, shortening and scarring of the distal free edge. In these patients, a painful local thickening can be palpated posterior and just proximal of the tip of the medial malleolus.

Most dysfunctions of the posterior tibial tendon evolve in a painful tenosynovitis. Tenosynovitis is also a common extra-articular manifestation of rheumatoid arthritis, where hindfoot problems are a significant cause of disability. Tenosynovitis in rheumatoid patients eventually leads to a ruptured tendon.[22]

Although the precise aetiology is unknown, the condition is classified on the basis of clinical and radiographic findings. In the early stage of dysfunction, patients complain of persisting ankle pain medially along the course of the tendon, in addition to fatigue and aching on the plantar medial aspect of the ankle. When a tenosynovitis is present, swelling is common. On clinical examination, valgus angulation of the hindfoot is frequently seen, with accompanying abduction of the forefoot, the "too-many-toes" sign.[23] This sign is positive when the examiner inspects the patient's foot from behind: in case of significant forefoot abduction, three or more toes are visible lateral to the calcaneus, where normally only one or two toes are seen.

Intra-articular lesions such as a posteromedial impingement syndrome, subtalar pathology, calcifications in the dorsal capsule of the ankle joint, loose bodies or osteochondral defects should be excluded. Entrapment of the posterior tibial nerve in the tarsal canal is commonly known as a tarsal tunnel syndrome. Clinical examination is normally sufficient to adequately differentiate these disorders from an isolated posterior tibia tendon disorder.

For additional investigation, magnetic resonance imaging (MRI) is the best method to assess a tendon rupture. Also, ultrasound imaging is known as a cost-effective and accurate to evaluate disorders of the tendon.[24]

Initially, conservative management is indicated, with rest, combined with nonsteroidal anti-inflammatory drugs (NSAIDS), and immobilization using a plaster cast or tape. There is no consensus whether to use corticosteroid injections; some cases of tendon rupture following corticosteroid injections have recently been described.[25]

After failure of 3–6 months of conservative management, surgery can be indicated.[26] This can be performed open or endoscopically. An open synovectomy is performed by sharp dissection of the inflamed synovium, while preserving blood supply to the tendon. Post-operative management consists of plaster cast immobilization for 3 weeks with the possible disadvantage of new formation of adhesions, followed by wearing a functional brace with controlled ankle movement for another 3 weeks, and physical therapy.[27]

Endoscopic synovectomy is our surgical modality of choice when access allows radical removal of inflamed synovium.[28] Several studies have been described previously in which endoscopic synovectomy was successfully performed, offering the advantages that are related to minimally invasive surgery.[15,16,22]

3.3.2 Surgical Technique

The procedure can be performed on an outpatient basis under local, regional or general anaesthesia. Patients are placed in the supine position. A tourniquet is placed around the upper leg. Before anaesthesia, the patient is asked to actively invert the foot, so that the posterior tibial tendon can be palpated and the portals can be marked (Fig. 3.3a). Access to the tendon can be obtained anywhere along the course of it.

We prefer to make the two main portals directly over the tendon 2–3 cm distal and 2–3 cm proximal to the posterior edge of the medial malleolus. The distal portal is made first: the incision is made through the skin, and the tendon sheath is penetrated by the arthroscopic shaft with a blunt trocar. A 2.7 mm 30° arthroscope is introduced, and the tendon sheath is filled with saline (Fig. 3.3b–f) Irrigation is performed using gravity flow.

Under direct vision, the proximal portal is made by introducing a spinal needle, and subsequently an incision is made into the tendon sheath (Fig. 3.3g–i). Instruments as a retrograde knife, a shaver system, blunt probes, and scissors can be used. For synovectomy in patients with rheumatoid arthritis, a 3.5 mm shaver can be used. The complete tendon sheath can be inspected by rotating the arthroscope around the tendon.

Synovectomy can be performed with a complete overview of the tendon from the distal portal, over the insertion of the navicular bone to approximately 6 cm above the tip of the medial malleolus.

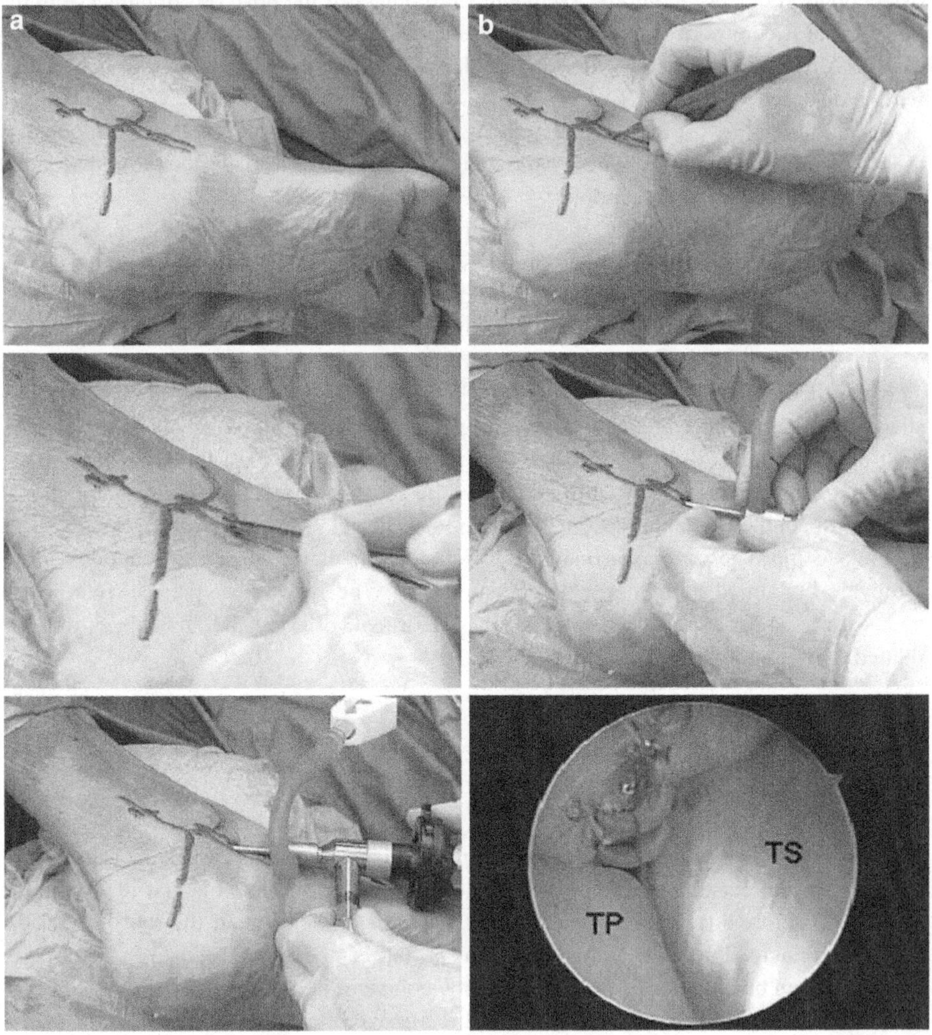

Fig. 3.3 (**a**) Marked anatomy of posterior tibial tendon of the left foot. (**b**) Skin incision for the distal portal. (**c**) Blunt dissection of the peritendineum with mosquito clamp. (**d**) Introduction of the arthroscopic shaft with a blunt trocar. (**e**) Introduction of a 2.7 mm 30° arthroscope. (**f**) Endoscopic view of the posterior tibial tendon at introduction of the arthroscope. (**g**) Placement of a spinal needle under direct vision to prepare a second proximal portal. (**h**) Endoscopic view of the needle looking from distal to proximal. (**i**) Blunt dissection of the proximal portal with mosquito clamp

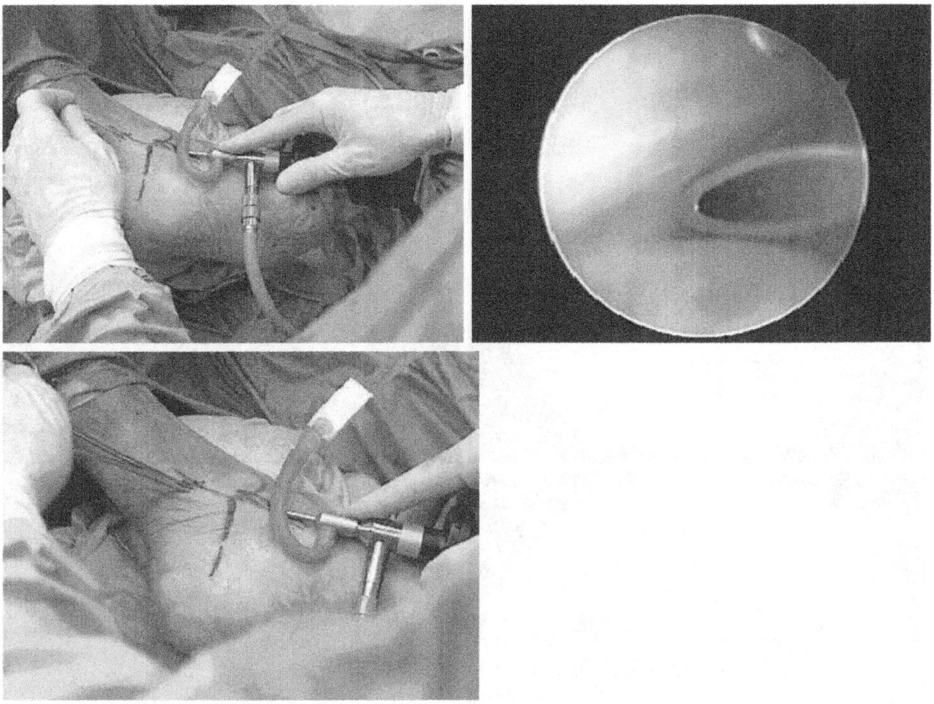

Fig. 3.3 (continued)

Special attention should be given to inspecting the tendon sheath, the posterior aspect of the medial malleolar surface, and the posterior ankle joint capsule. The tendon sheath between the posterior tibial tendon and the flexor digitorum longus is relatively thin: inspection of the correct tendon should always be checked. This can be accomplished by passively flexing and extending the toes; if the tendon sheath of the flexor digitorum longus tendon is entered, the tendon will move up and down.

When remaining in the posterior tibial tendon sheath, the neurovascular bundle is not in danger.

When a rupture of the posterior tibial tendon is seen (Fig. 3.4), endoscopic synovectomy is performed and the rupture is repaired through a mini-open approach. The advantage to start this procedure endoscopically over the standard open procedure is that localization of the problem is made easier by exploration of the endoscopically magnified tendon, and consequently the size of the incision for repair of the rupture can be minimized.

At the end of the procedure, the portals are sutured to prevent sinus formation.

Post-operative management consists of a pressure bandage and partial weight-bearing for 2–3 days. Active range of motion exercises are encouraged from the firstda y.

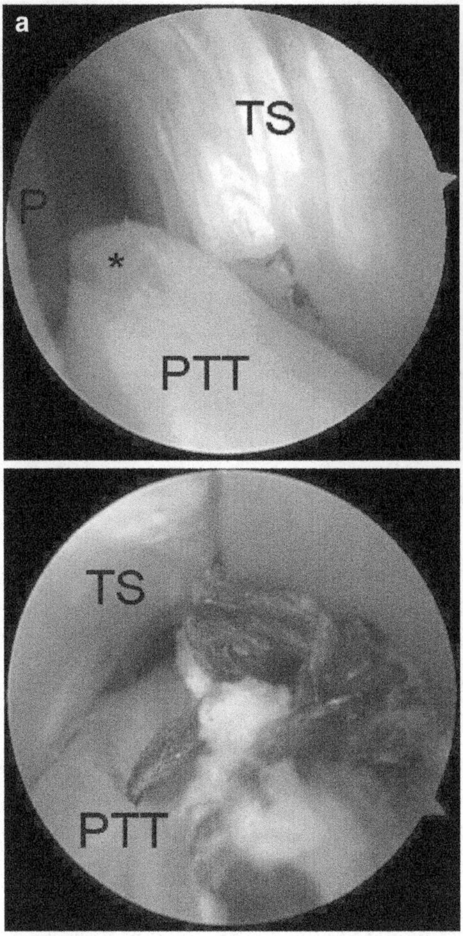

Fig. 3.4 Posterior tibial tendoscopy of the left foot in a 48-year-old female patient with pain over the posterior tibial tendon. The arthroscope is in the anterolateral portal looking proximally. (**a**) Superficial tear of the posterior tibial tendon (asterisk). (**b**) Rupture demonstrated with the arthroscopic probe. (**c**) Repair of the rupture through a mini open repair (*P* probe, *PTT* posterior tibial tendon, *TS*te ndons heath)

3.3.3 Results

In 1997, the senior author first described tendoscopy of the posterior tibial tendon to manage pathology of this tendon in an anatomic study.[22] From 1994 to 1997, 16 procedures were performed on 16 patients with a mean follow up of 1.1 years.[21] All had a history of persistent posteromedial ankle pain for at least 6 months, with pain on palpation of the posterior tibial tendon, positive resistance test results, and often local swelling. Five patients underwent a diagnostic procedure after surgery, in five a diagnostic procedure after a fracture was performed, a diagnostic procedure after trauma in one, chronic tenosynovitis in two, screw removal from the medial malleolus in one, and posterior ankle arthrotomy in two patients. No complications were observed.

Between 1997 and 2004, we performed 19 procedures in 17 patients.[21] Ten endoscopic synovectomies were performed in eight patients who had chronic tenosynovitis due to rheumatoid arthritis. All had a history of persistent posteromedial ankle pain, with pain on palpation of the posterior tibial tendon, positive resistance test results, and local swelling. All patients were first managed conservatively, and experienced temporary pain relief. All eight patients were diagnosed with synovitis without a tendon rupture by MRI or ultrasound. In three of these eight patients, the endoscopy was combined with an arthroscopic synovectomy of the ankle or a hallux valgus correction. In the other nine patients, tendoscopy of the posterior tibial tendon was performed for miscellaneous reasons. Patients were allowed full weight bearing after the operation, except for the patient who had hallux valgus correction. All were able to actively move the ankle post-operatively.

Johnson and Strom classified tenosynovitis of the posterior tibial tendon into three stages[29]: stage one tenosynovitis, where the tendon length is normal; stage two, elongated tendon with mobile hindfoot deformity; and stage three, elongated tendon with fixed hindfoot deformity. Myerson modified the classification by adding stage four: a valgus angulation of the talus and early degeneration of the ankle joint.[20] Chow[30] reported a case series of six patients with posterior tibial tendon synovitis who underwent an endoscopic synovectomy for stage 1 posterior tibial tendon insufficiency. All patients reported good results.

Lui and co-workers[27] described an endoscopic assisted posterior tibial tendon reconstruction for stage 2 posterior tibial tendon insufficiency, when the posterior tibial tendon has become permanently elongated but the flatfoot deformity still is flexible. The endoscopic technique used is similar to the one described above. Additionally, a portal is made close to the insertion of the anterior tibial tendon, of which the medial half is cut and stripped to the insertion with a tendon stripper. The tendon is then retrieved through the distal portal, and the graft is transferred to the posterior tibial tendon. The construction is augmented by side-to-side anastomosis with the flexor digitorum longus tendon, which is supplemented by a subtalar arthroereisis with a bioabsorbable implant. Thus far only one case was described, with a good clinical outcome.

3.4 Achilles Tendoscopy

3.4.1 Introduction

Pathology of the Achilles tendon can be divided into non-insertional and insertional problems.[31,32] The first type can present as local degeneration of the tendon that can be combined with paratendinopathy. Insertional problems are related to abnormalities at the insertion of the Achilles tendon, including the posterior aspect of the calcaneus and the retrocalcaneal bursa. This chapter will describe the management of non-insertional tendinopathy. These can be divided into three entities: tendinopathy, paratendinopathy, and a combination of both. General symptoms include painful swelling typically 2–7 cm proximal to the insertion, and stiffness especially when getting up after a period of rest.

Patients with tendinopathy can present with three patterns: diffuse thickening of the tendon, local degeneration of the tendon which is mechanically intact, or insufficiency of the tendon with a partial tear. In paratendinopathy, there is local thickening of the paratenon. Clinically, a differentiation between tendinopathy and paratendinopathy can be made. Maffulli and co-workers describe the Royal London Hospital test, which is found to be positive in patients with isolated tendinopathy of the main body of the tendon: the portion of the tendon originally found to be tender on palpation shows little or no pain with the ankle in maximum dorsiflexion.[33,34] In paratendinopathy, the area of swelling does not move with dorsiflexion and plantarflexion of the ankle, where it does in tendinopathy.[34,35,36] Paratendinopathy can be acute or chronic. Often, the pain is more prominent on the medial side in patients with chronic tendinopathy.[37] This might be due to a hyperpronation abnormality of the foot placing greater forces on the medial part of the Achilles tendon, degeneration of the soleus tendon, or involvement of the plantaris tendon in the process.[36] This tendon is the distal part of a biarticular plantaris muscle and is absent in 6–8% of the population.[38,39] It inserts distally on the calcaneus at the medial side of the Achilles tendon, and proximally on the lateral femoral condyle. Simultaneous knee and ankle movements result in a different pull of soleus and plantaris tendons at the level of the combined tendinopathy and paratendinopathy. In a healthy patient, the plantaris tendon can glide in relation to the Achilles tendon. When chronic paratendinopathy is present, the plantaris tendon is more or less fixed to the Achilles tendon at the level of the nodule. Separate movement of both tendons is restricted as a consequence and therefore might provide an explanation for the medial pain.[36]

Differential diagnoses are pathology of the tendons of the peroneus longus and brevis, intra-articular pathology of the ankle joint and subtalar joint, degenerative changes of the posterior tibial tendon, and tendinopathy of the flexor hallucis longus muscle must be ruled out. MRI and ultrasound can be used to differentiate between the various forms of tendinopathy.[40]

We normally initiate conservative management. Modification of the activity level of the patient is advised together with avoidance of strenuous activities in case of paratendinopathy. Shoe modifications and inlays can be given. Physical therapy includes an extensive eccentric exercise program, which can be combined with icing and NSAIDs.[41–45] Shockwave treatment, a night splint, and cast immobilization are alternative conservative methods. Sclerosing injections of neovascularisation and accompanying nerves around the Achilles tendon have initially shown promising results, and is based on the observation that neovascularisation is seen in the vast majority of patients with Achilles tendinopathy but not in pain free normal tendons.[46–52]

If these conservative measures fail, surgery must be considered. The percentage of patients requiring surgery is around 25%.[33,53,54] The technique used for operative management of tendinopathy depends on the stage of the disease. Local degeneration and thickening are usually treated by excision and curettage. An insufficient Achilles tendon due to extensive degeneration can be reconstructed. Isolated paratendinopathy can be treated by excision of the diseased paratenon.

Open surgery produces a guarded prognosis, and is associated with a higher risk of complications than endoscopy.[1–3] Open techniques are also associated with an extensive rehabilitation period of 4–12 months. Therefore, recently minimally invasive techniques were developed. Percutaneous needling of the tendon has been described, but until now no results have been published. Testa and co-workers described a minimally invasive technique consisting of percutaneous longitudinal tenotomise,[55,56] which was later optimized by adding ultrasound control. Eighty-three percent of patients reported symptomatic benefit at the time of their best outcome; however, the median time to return to sports was 6.5 months.[57]

In combined tendinopathy and paratendinopathy, the question is whether both pathologies contribute to the complaints. An anatomic cadaver study described degenerative changes of the Achilles tendon in as much as 34% of subjects with no complaints.[58] Khan and co-workers only found abnormal morphology in 65% (37 of 57) of symptomatic tendons, but also in 32% (9 of 28) of asymptomatic Achilles tendons assessed by ultrasound.[59] Therefore, it is questionable whether degeneration of the tendon itself is the main cause of the pain. The authors therefore focus mainly on management of the paratendinopathy leaving the tendinopathy untouched. The current approach is an endoscopic release or resection of the plantaris tendon at the level of the nodule and removal of the local paratendinopathy tissue at the level of the painful nodule.

3.4.2 Surgical Technique

Local, epidural, spinal and general anaesthesia can be used for this procedure, which can be performed on an outpatient basis. The patient is in prone position. A tourniquet is placed around the thigh of the affected leg, and a bolster is placed under the foot. Because the surgeon needs to be able to obtain full plantar and dorsiflexion, the foot is placed right over the end of the table (Fig. 3.5).

The authors mostly use a 2.7 mm arthroscope for endoscopy of a combined tendinopathy and paratendinopathy. This small-diameter short arthroscope yields an excellent picture comparable to the standard 4 mm arthroscope; however, it cannot deliver the same amount of irrigation fluid per time as the 4 mm sheath. This is important in procedures in which a large diameter shaver is used (e.g., in endoscopic calcaneoplasty). When a 4 mm arthroscope is used, gravity inflow of irrigation fluid is usually sufficient. A pressurized bag or pump device sometimes is used with the 2.7 mm arthroscope.

The distal portal is located on the lateral border of the Achilles tendon, 2–3 cm distal to the pathologic nodule. The proximal portal is located medial to the border of the Achilles tendon, 2–4 cm above the nodule. When the portals are placed this way, it is usually possible to visualize and work around the whole surface of the tendon, over a length of approximately 10 cm (Fig. 3.6).

The distal portal is made first. After making the skin incision, the mosquito clamp is introduced, followed by the blunt 2.7 mm trocar in a craniomedial direction. With this blunt trocar the paratenon is approached, and is blindly released from the tendon by moving around it. Subsequently, the 2.7 mm 30° arthroscope is introduced. To minimize the risk of iatrogenic damage, the arthroscope should be kept on the tendon. At this moment, it can be

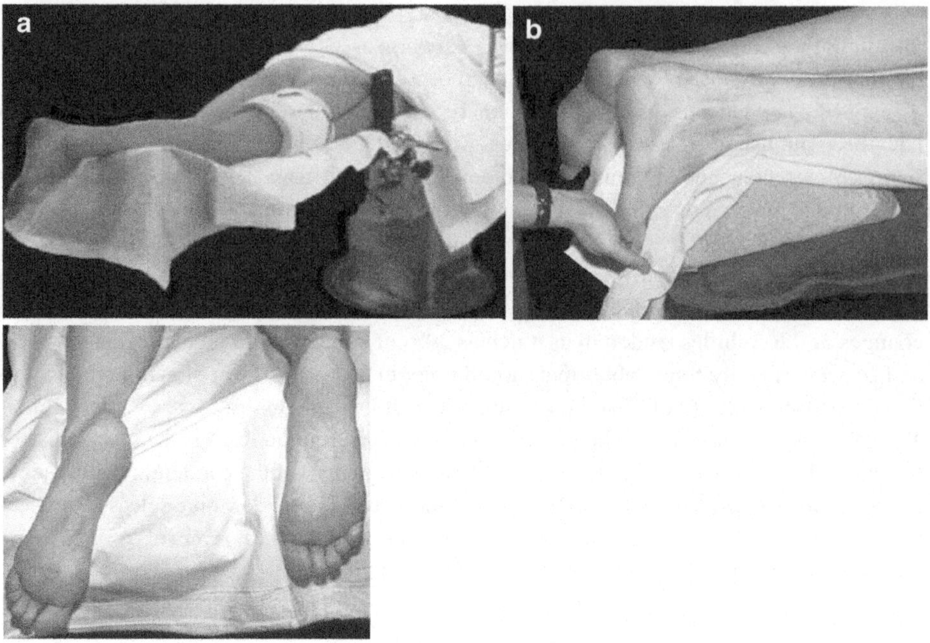

Fig. 3.5 Positioning of a patient for tendoscopy of the Achilles tendon. (**a**) The patient is placed prone. (**b**, **c**) The affected right leg is placed on a bolster and right over the end of the table. (**c**) The other foot is positioned so that the surgeon has sufficientw orkinga rea

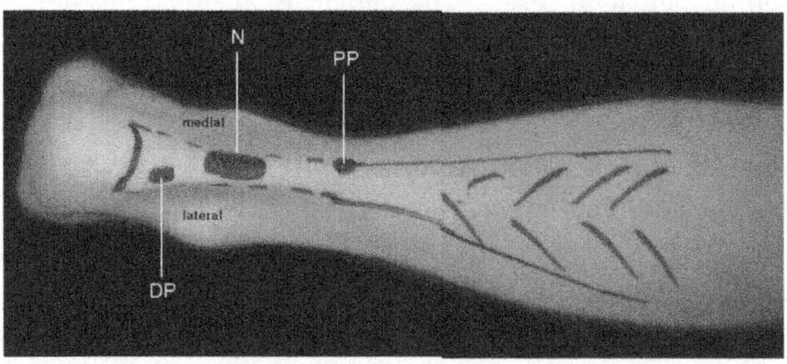

Fig. 3.6 Posterior aspect of the right foot and ankle. Anatomy and portals marked before surgery (*DP* distal portal, *N* nodule, *PP*pr oximalpor tal)

confirmed whether the surgeon is in the right layer between paratenon and Achilles tendon. If not, now it can be identified and a further release can be performed (Fig. 3.7a–c).

The proximal portal is made by introducing a spinal needle, followed by a mosquito clamp and probe. The plantaris tendon can be identified at the anteromedial border of the Achilles tendon (Fig. 3.7a). In a typical case of local paratendinopathy, the plantaris tendon, the Achilles tendon, and the paratenon are tight together in the process. Removal of the local thickened paratenon on the anteromedial side of the Achilles tendon at the level of the nodule, and release of the plantaris tendon (Fig. 3.7e) are the goals of this procedure. In

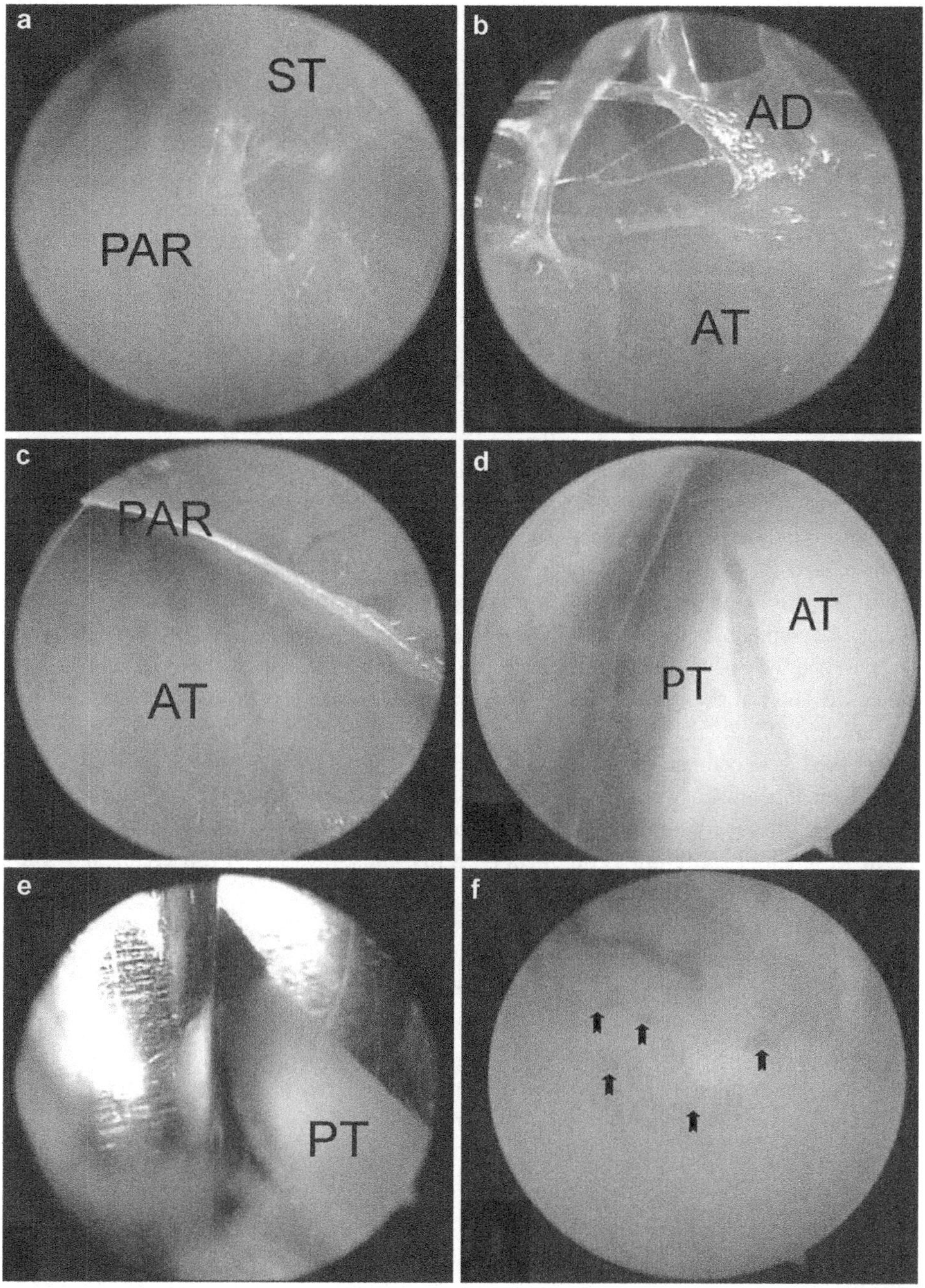

Fig. 3.7 Tendoscopy of the right Achilles tendon in a 52-year old female patient with combined tendinopathy and paratendinopathy. The 2.7 mm arthroscope is introduced through the distal portal looking proximally. (**a**) Adhesions of the paratenon (PAR) to the subcutaneous tissue (ST) overlying the Achilles tendon. (**b**) Removal of adhesions (AD) of the paratenon to the Achilles tendon (AT), looking from distal to proximal. (**c**) Paratenon released from the Achilles tendon. (**d**) Plantaris tendon (PT) running medial to the Achilles tendon (AT). (**e**) Release of the plantaris tendon. (**f**) Neovascularisation (*arrows*)be forer emovalbybone cutters haver

cases where the fibrotic paratenon is firmly attached to the lateral or posterior border of the tendon, a release in these areas is performed. Neovessels (Fig. 3.7f) accompanied by small nerve fibres can be found in this area and are removed with a 2.7 mm bonecutter shaver.

Changing portals can be helpful. At the end of the procedure it must be possible to move the arthroscope over the complete symptomatic area of the Achilles tendon.

After the procedure, the portals are sutured.

Aftercare consists of a compressive dressing for 2–3 days. Patients are encouraged to actively perform range of motion exercises. Full weight-bearing is allowed as tolerated. Initially, the foot must be elevated when not walking.

3.4.3 Results

The senior author earlier described the results of 20 patients treated with an endoscopic release for non-insertional tendinopathy combined with a paratendinopathy.[35] All patients had had complaints for more than 2 years, and underwent conservative treatment for their complaints before the indication for surgery was set. The results were analyzed with a follow up of 2–7 years with a mean of 6 years. Sixteen patients were assessed at follow up, which included completing of subjective outcome scores. The Foot and Ankle Outcome Score (FAOS) and the Short Form general health survey with 36 questions (SF-36) were utilized. There were no complications. Most patients were able to resume their sporting activities after 4–8 weeks. All patients had significant pain relief. The results of the subjective outcome scores used were comparable to a cohort of people without Achilles tendon complaints.

Maquirriain and co-workers reported the outcome of seven patients who underwent an endoscopic release for chronic Achilles tendinopathy, with similar results. The mean score of this group improved from 39 preoperatively to 89 post-operatively (on a scale of 0–100), and there were no complications.[60]

Patellar tendinopathy has a histological picture similar to that of Achilles tendinopathy. Recently, Wilberg and co-workers have developed an arthroscopic technique for patellar tendinopathy.[61] Part of their technique is comparable to Achilles tendoscopy; the main goal is to shave the area with neovessels and accompanying nerves on the posterior aspect of the patellar tendon, whereas this is one of the goals for endoscopic management of Achilles tendinopathy. A pilot study showed good clinical results in 13/15 tendons (6/8 elite athletes); all satisfied patients were back to their previous sport activity level.

3.5 Conclusions

The results of endoscopic surgery of tendons around the ankle seem promising. More experience must be acquired by different orthopaedic surgeons. Also, accurately designed studies need to be performed, to optimize techniques and ultimately be able to offer patients these minimally invasive treatments with its great advantages.

References

1. Abramowitz Y, Wollstein R, Barzilay Y et al. Outcome of resection of a symptomatic os trigonum. *J Bone Joint Surg Am.*2003; 85-A:1051–1057.
2. Hamilton WG, Geppert MJ, Thompson FM. Pain in the posterior aspect of the ankle in dancers. Differential diagnosis and operative treatment. *J Bone Joint Surg Am.* 1996;78: 1491–1500.
3. Marotta JJ, Micheli LJ. Os trigonum impingement in dancers. *Am J Sports Med.* 1992;20: 533–536.
4. van Dijk CN, Scholten PE, Krips R. A 2-portal endoscopic approach for diagnosis and treatment of posterior ankle pathology. *Arthroscopy.*2000; 16:871–876.
5. vanD ijkC N.H indfoote ndoscopy. *Sports Med Arthrosc Rev.*2000; 8:365–371.
6. Bassett FH III, Billys JB, Gates HS III. A simple surgical approach to the posteromedial ankle. *Am J Sports Med.*1993; 21:144–146.
7. Dombek MF, Lamm BM, Saltrick K, Mendicino RW, Catanzariti AR. Peroneal tendon tears: a retrospective review. *J Foot Ankle Surg.*2003; 42:250–258.
8. Scholten PE, van Dijk CN. Tendoscopy of the peroneal tendons. *Foot Ankle Clin.* 2006;11:415–420,vii.
9. Roggatz J, Urban A. The calcareous peritendinitis of the long peroneal tendon. *Arch Orthop Trauma Surg.*1980; 96:161–164.
10. Schweitzer GJ. Stenosing peroneal tenovaginitis. Case reports. *S Afr Med J.* 1982;61:521–523.
11. Heckman DS, Reddy S, Pedowitz D, Wapner KL, Parekh SG. Operative treatment for peroneal tendon disorders. *J Bone Joint Surg Am.*2008; 90:404–418.
12. Yao L, Tong DJ, Cracchiolo A, Seeger LL. MR findings in peroneal tendonopathy. *J Comput Assist Tomogr.*1995; 19:460–464.
13. Scholten PE, van Dijk CN. Endoscopic calcaneoplasty. *Foot Ankle Clin.* 2006;11: 439–446,viii.
14. van Dijk CN, van Dyk GE, Scholten PE, Kort NP. Endoscopic calcaneoplasty. *Am J Sports Med.*2001;29:185 –189.
15. van Dijk CN, Scholten PE, Kort N. Tendoscopy (tendon sheath endoscopy) for overuse tendon injuries. *Oper Techn Sports Med.*1997; 5:170–178.
16. van Dijk CN, Kort N. Tendoscopy of the peroneal tendons. *Arthroscopy.*1998; 14:471–478.
17. de Leeuw PAJ, Golano P, van Dijk CN. A 3-portal endoscopic groove deepening technique for recurrent peroneal tendon dislocation. *Techn Foot Ankle Surg.*2008; 7:250–256.
18. Lui TH. Endoscopic peroneal retinaculum reconstruction. *Knee Surg Sports Traumatol Arthrosc.*2006;14:478–481.
19. Myerson MS. Adult acquired flatfoot deformity: treatment of dysfunction of the posterior tibial tendon. *Instr Course Lect.*1997; 46:393–405.
20. Bulstra GH, Olsthoorn PG, Niek van DC. Tendoscopy of the posterior tibial tendon. *Foot Ankle Clin.*2006;1 1:421–427,vi ii.
21. van Dijk CN, Kort N, Scholten PE. Tendoscopy of the posterior tibial tendon. *Arthroscopy.* 1997;13:692–698.
22. Michelson J, Easley M, Wigley FM, Hellmann D. Posterior tibial tendon dysfunction in rheumatoid arthritis. *Foot Ankle Int.*1995; 16:156–161.
23. Trnka HJ. Dysfunction of the tendon of tibialis posterior. *J Bone Joint Surg Br.* 2004;86: 939–946.
24. Miller SD, Van HM, Boruta PM, Wu KK, Katcherian DA. Ultrasound in the diagnosis of posterior tibial tendon pathology. *Foot Ankle Int.*1996; 17:555–558.
25. Porter DA, Baxter DE, Clanton TO, Klootwyk TE. Posterior tibial tendon tears in young competitive athletes: two case reports. *Foot Ankle Int.*1998; 19:627–630.

26. Lui TH. Endoscopic assisted posterior tibial tendon reconstruction for stage 2 posterior tibial tendon insufficiency. *Knee Surg Sports Traumatol Arthrosc.*2007; 15:1228–1234.
27. Bare AA, Haddad SL. Tenosynovitis of the posterior tibial tendon. *Foot Ankle Clin.* 2001;6:37–66.
28. Paus AC. Arthroscopic synovectomy. When, which diseases and which joints. *Z Rheumatol.* 1996;55:394–400.
29. Johnson KA, Strom DE. Tibialis posterior tendon dysfunction. *Clin Orthop Relat Res.* 1989;196–206.
30. Chow HT, Chan KB, Lui TH. Tendoscopic debridement for stage I posterior tibial tendon dysfunction. *Knee Surg Sports Traumatol Arthrosc.*2005; 13:695–698.
31. Clain MR, Baxter DE. Achilles tendinitis. *Foot Ankle.*1992; 13:482–487.
32. Saltzman CL, Tearse DS. Achilles tendon injuries. *J Am Acad Orthop Surg.* 1998;6: 316–325.
33. Maffulli N, Walley G, Sayana MK, Longo UG, Denaro V. Eccentric calf muscle training in athletic patients with Achilles tendinopathy. *Disabil Rehabil.*2008; 30:1–8.
34. Maffulli N, Kenward MG, Testa V, Capasso G, Regine R, King JB. Clinical diagnosis of Achilles tendinopathy with tendinosis. *Clin J Sport Med.*2003; 13:11–15.
35. Steenstra F, van Dijk CN. Achilles tendoscopy. *Foot Ankle Clin.*2006; 11:429–438,vi ii.
36. Williams JG. Achilles tendon lesions in sport. *Sports Med.*1993; 16:216–220.
37. Segesser B, Goesele A, Renggli P. [The Achilles tendon in sports]. *Orthopade.* 1995;24:252–267.
38. Gruber, W. *Beobachtungen aus der Menschlichen und Vergleichenden Anatomie*. Berlin, Germany: A Hirschwald; 1879.
39. Schwalbe G, Pfitzner W. Varietäten-Statistik und Anthropologie. *DeutscheMed Wchnschr.* 1894;XXV:459.
40. KoR .,Porte rM . *Interactive Foot and Ankle 2.* London: Primal Pictures; 2000.
41. Mafi N, Lorentzon R, Alfredson H. Superior short-term results with eccentric calf muscle training compared to concentric training in a randomized prospective multicenter study on patients with chronic Achilles tendinosis. *Knee Surg Sports Traumatol Arthrosc.* 2001;9:42–47.
42. Norregaard J, Larsen CC, Bieler T, Langberg H. Eccentric exercise in treatment of Achilles tendinopathy. *Scand J Med Sci Sports.*2007; 17:133–138.
43. Ohberg L, Lorentzon R, Alfredson H. Eccentric training in patients with chronic Achilles tendinosis: normalised tendon structure and decreased thickness at follow up. *Br J Sports Med.*2004;38:8–1 1.
44. Woodley BL, Newsham-West RJ, Baxter GD. Chronic tendinopathy: effectiveness of eccentric exercise. *Br J Sports Med.*2007; 41:188–198.
45. Silbernagel KG, Thomee R, Thomee P, Karlsson J. Eccentric overload training for patients with chronic Achilles tendon pain–a randomised controlled study with reliability testing of the evaluation methods. *Scand J Med Sci Sports.*2001; 11:197–206.
46. Alfredson H, Ohberg L. Increased intratendinous vascularity in the early period after sclerosing injection treatment in Achilles tendinosis: a healing response? *Knee Surg Sports Traumatol Arthrosc.*2006;14: 399–401.
47. Alfredson H, Ohberg L, Zeisig E, Lorentzon R. Treatment of midportion Achilles tendinosis: similar clinical results with US and CD-guided surgery outside the tendon and sclerosing polidocanol injections. *Knee Surg Sports Traumatol Arthrosc.*2007; 15:1504–1509.
48. Alfredson H, Lorentzon R. Sclerosing polidocanol injections of small vessels to treat the chronic painful tendon. *Cardiovasc Hematol Agents Med Chem.*2007; 5:97–100.
49. Andersson G, Danielson P, Alfredson H, Forsgren S. Nerve-related characteristics of ventral paratendinous tissue in chronic Achilles tendinosis. *Knee Surg Sports Traumatol Arthrosc.* 2007;15:1272–1279.
50. Ohberg L, Alfredson H. Ultrasound guided sclerosis of neovessels in painful chronic Achilles tendinosis: pilot study of a new treatment. *Br J Sports Med.*2002; 36:173–175.

51. Willberg L, Sunding K, Ohberg L, Forssblad M, Fahlstrom M, Alfredson H. Sclerosing injections to treat midportion Achilles tendinosis: a randomised controlled study evaluating two different concentrations of Polidocanol. *Knee Surg Sports Traumatol Arthrosc.* 2008;16: 859–864.
52. Lind B, Ohberg L, Alfredson H. Sclerosing polidocanol injections in mid-portion Achilles tendinosis: remaining good clinical results and decreased tendon thickness at 2-year follow-up. *Knee Surg Sports Traumatol Arthrosc.*2006; 14:1327–1332.
53. Kvist M. Achilles tendon injuries in athletes. *Ann Chir Gynaecol.*1991; 80:188–201.
54. Maffulli N. Augmented repair of acute Achilles tendon ruptures using gastrocnemius-soleus fascia. *Int Orthop.*2005; 29:134.
55. Maffulli N, Testa V, Capasso G, Bifulco G, Binfield PM. Results of percutaneous longitudinal tenotomy for Achilles tendinopathy in middle- and long-distance runners. *Am J Sports Med.* 1997;25:835–840.
56. Testa V, Maffulli N, Capasso G, Bifulco G. Percutaneous longitudinal tenotomy in chronic Achilles tendonitis. *Bull Hosp Jt Dis.*1996; 54:241–244.
57. Testa V, Capasso G, Benazzo F, Maffulli N. Management of Achilles tendinopathy by ultrasound-guided percutaneous tenotomy. *Med Sci Sports Exerc.*2002; 34:573–580.
58. Kannus P, Jozsa L. Histopathological changes preceding spontaneous rupture of a tendon. A controlled study of 891 patients. *J Bone Joint Surg Am.*1991; 73:1507–1525.
59. Khan KM, Forster BB, Robinson J et al. Are ultrasound and magnetic resonance imaging of value in assessment of Achilles tendon disorders? A two year prospective study. *Br J Sports Med.*2003;37:149 –153.
60. Maquirriain J, Ayerza M, Costa-Paz M, Muscolo DL. Endoscopic surgery in chronic achilles tendinopathies: a preliminary report. *Arthroscopy.*2002; 18:298–303.
61. Willberg L, Sunding K, Ohberg L, Forssblad M, Alfredson H. Treatment of Jumper's knee: promising short-term results in a pilot study using a new arthroscopic approach based on imaging findings. *Knee Surg Sports Traumatol Arthrosc.*2007; 15:676–681.

Part II

Hallux

Arthroscopy of the First MetatarsophalangealJ oint

4

Tun Hing Lui

4.1 Introduction

Arthroscopy of the first metatarsophalangeal joint (MTP-1) was originally described by Watanabe[1] in 1972. Advancements in small joint instrumentation and arthroscopic technique have expanded the application of arthroscopy in the management of the first metatarsophalangeal joint pathology. Although the use of the arthroscopy in the MTP-1 has not been as popular as in the knee or the shoulder, its value continues to grow in the management of various pathologies from traumatic to degenerative and reconstruction.

4.2 Anatomy/Pathoanatomy

The MTP-1 is composed of the first metatarsal head and neck, proximal phalangeal base, medial and lateral sesamoids. It has two compartments: metatarsophalangeal and metatarso-sesamoid compartments. The metatarsophalangeal compartment composes of the oval, concave proximal phalanx articular surface and the convex metatarsal head articular surface. The proximal phalanx articular surface is smaller than the corresponding articular surface of the metatarsal head. The metatarso-sesamoid compartment composes of the articular surfaces of the sesamoid bones and the plantar articular surface which is separated into two sloped surfaces by a small crista.

The articular surface of each sesamoid is convex in the coronal plane and concave in the sagittal plane and fits well with the corresponding trochlear surface. The dorsomedial aspect of the joint contains a sizable synovial fold with the average width of 7 mm covering 29% of the joint. At the level of the MTP-1, the distribution of the cutaneous nerve is highly variable, but usually the dorsomedial and dorsolateral cutaneous branches originate

T.H.Lui
Department of Orthopaedics and Traumatology, North District Hospital,
9PoK inR oad,SheungS hui, NT HongK ongS AR, China
e-mail:luithde rek@yahoo.co.uk

N. Maffulli and M. Easley (eds.), *Minimally Invasive Surgery of the Foot and Ankle*,
DOI: 10.1007/978-1-84996-417-3_4, © Springer-Verlag London Limited 2011

from the medial dorsal cutaneous branch of the superficial peroneal nerve and the deep peroneal nerve, respectively.

The plantarmedial and plantarlateral branches originate from the medial plantar nerve. The dorsomedial cutaneous nerve is in proximity of the dorsomedial portal and is on average 13.1 mm medial to the extensor hallucis longus tendon[2] but has been reported to be 2–5 mm from it.[3] The plantarmedial hallucal nerve is on average 10.6 mm plantar to the midline, which is the location for the medial portal.[4] Given the variations of the nerves in the foot, all the arthroscopic portals should be handled with care assuming that a nerve is located directly underneath.

4.3 Arthroscopic Technique

4.3.1 Positioning

We undertake arthroscopy of the MTP-1 with the patient supine and both hips abducted so that the surgeon will have a 360° access to the forefoot. I prefer to sit at the lateral side of the operated foot with the monitor at the end of the bed. Plantar portals, if needed, can be approached with the surgeon sitting between the patient's legs.

4.3.2 Traction

Manual traction is usually sufficient to visualize the metatarsal head and the base of the proximal phalanx. We do not routinely use the finger trap traction. Joint distraction, while opening the space between the articular facets, makes the intra-articular gutters obliterated and decreases the maneuverability of the arthroscope and instruments. However, it may be useful in the access to some osteochondral lesions and in arthroscopy-assisted arthrodesis which requires passing instruments between the joint facets. The finger trap traction can be attached to a 3–5 kg weight, or the limb can be suspended from a pole so that it is just off the operating table.

4.3.3 Instruments

Either 1.9 or 2.7 mm 30° small joint arthroscopy is used for most arthroscopic visualization of the MTP-1. The 1.9 mm arthroscope is used in tight joints or when no traction is applied, but should be handled with care due to its fragility. A long 2.7 or 4 mm 30° arthroscope which provides wider field of view and easier orientation is helpful in periarticular endoscopy, such as in endoscopic distal soft tissue release and gouty tophi excision. Gravity driven inflow is usually adequate, and an arthroscopic pump is generally not required.

4.3.4 Portals

The dorsomedial portal is at the level of joint line just medial to the extensor hallucis longus tendon joint. The dorsolateral portal is at the same level but just lateral to the extensor hallucis longus tendon. The dorsomedial and dorsolateral hallucal nerves can be directly beneath or send off a branch in close proximity to the dorsal portals. The medial portal is through the thick medial capsule at the level of joint line at the equator of the joint, and is away from neurovascular structures.[2] The plantar medial portal[7] described for the instrumentation in the metatarso-sesamoid compartment is located 4 cm proximal to the joint line between the abductor hallucis tendon and the medial head of the flexor hallucis brevis (Fig. 4.1).

An easy way to introduce instruments through the medial portal without traction is firstly introducing the instrument to the adjacent dorsal capsular gutter and then "swapped" into the metatarsophalangeal compartment (Fig. 4.2).

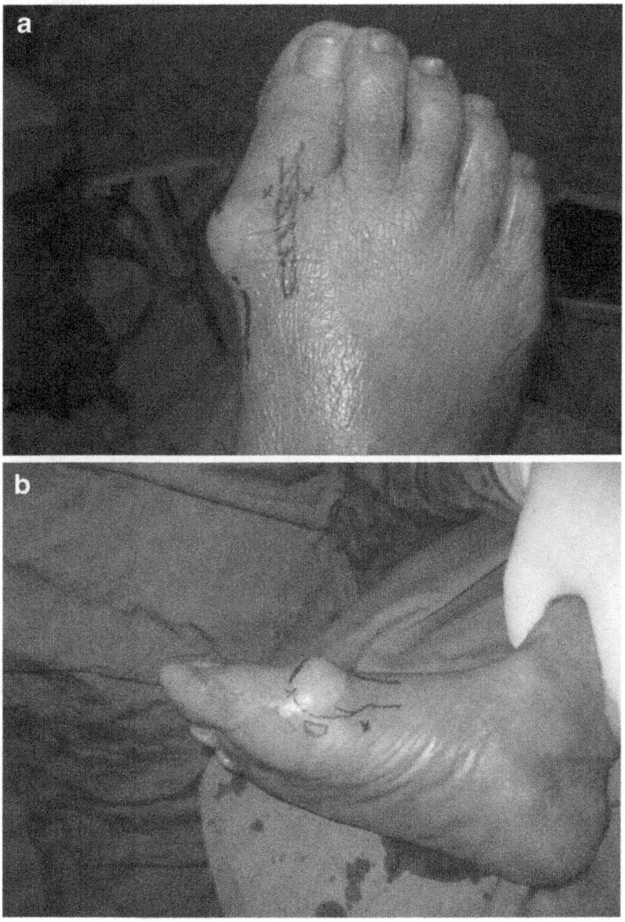

Fig.4.1 (**a**) Dorsolateral and dorsomedial portals at the lateral and medial aspects of the tendon of extensor hallucis longus (**b**)M edial portal and proximal medial portal

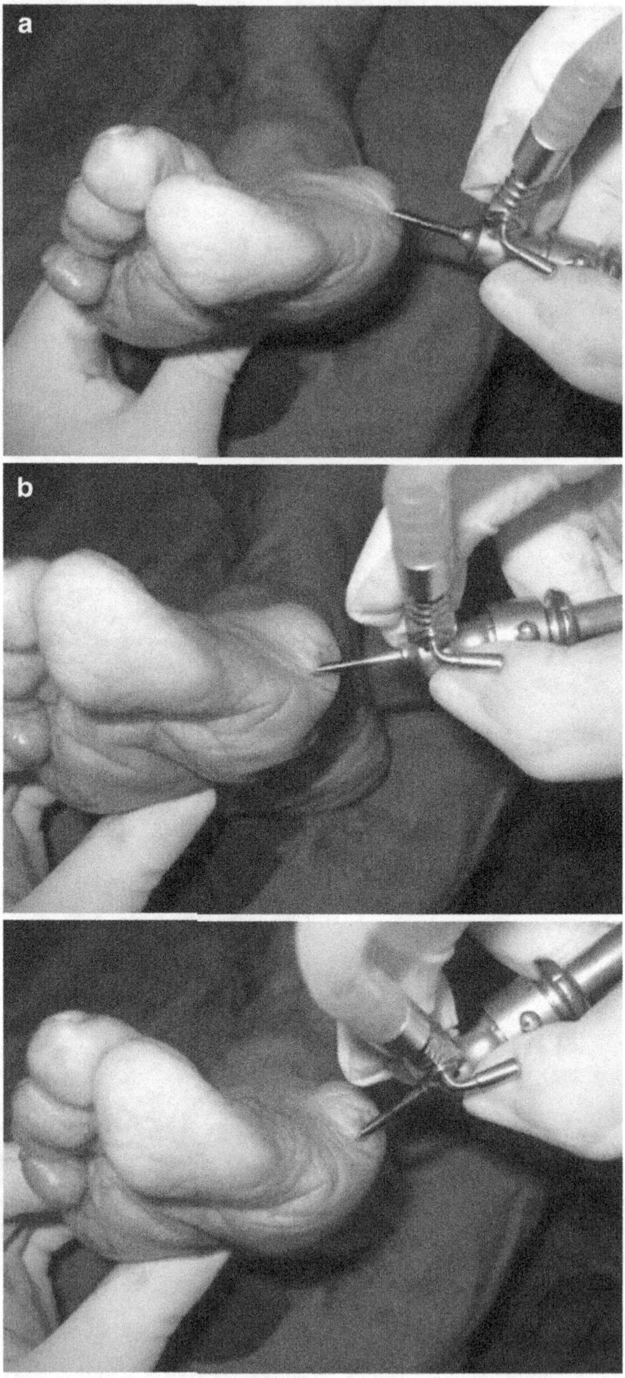

Fig.4. 2 (**a**) The cannula and trocar is inserted into the dorsal capsular gutter. (**b**) The cannula and trocar are swapped into the metatarsophalangeal compartment for arthroscopy of the metatarsophalangeal compartment. (**c**)The cannula and trocar are swapped into the metatarso-sesamoid compartment for arthroscopy of the metatarso-sesamoid compartment

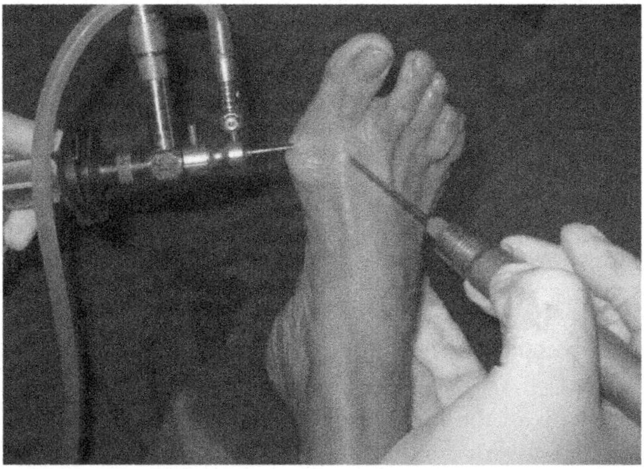

Fig. 4.3 Metatarso-phalangeal compartment arthroscopy with the dorsolateral and middleporta ls

We use the dorsolateral and medial portals for arthroscopy of the metatarso-phalangeal compartment because of the wider distance between the portals can reduce crowding of the instruments(Fig. 4.3).

The proximal medial portal is in line with the medial portal but is just proximal to the medial eminence. This portal is used for the medial exostectomy.[5,6] The toe web portal and the plantar portal[5,6] are required for the endoscopic lateral release of the hallux valgus correction. The toe web portal is just dorsal to the first web space. The plantar portal is approximately 4–5 cm proximal to the web space produced using an inside-out technique with a Wissinger rod from the toe web portal passing underneath the intermetatarsal ligament. The toe web portal is relatively safe from the neurovascular structures but the plantar portal is in the vicinity of the branches from the medial plantar nerve.

The 2.0 mm probe is used to palpate the cartilage surface to detect softening, crevices, delamination, or osteochondral lesions. Loose bodies are removed with small straight hemostats which are preferable over the graspers due to the suction effect pulling the loose body to the jaws when opened. At times, a tight joint may require manual manipulation to enhance visualization such as plantarflexion to open the metatarso-sesamoid compartment.

4.4 ArthroscopicE xamination

The joint line is identified by a puckering with straight traction of great toe and by direct palpation.

The dorsolateral portal is established at the previously described location by making a longitudinal 3 mm incision followed by blunt dissection with a curved hemostat. The medial portal placement can be assisted by arthroscopic localization with a 21 gauge needle. Through the dorsolateral portal, the medial gutter, distal part of the sesamoid apparatus and the plantar plate, the middle and distal part of the lateral gutter, the medial part of the dorsal gutter and the middle and distal part of the articular surfaces of the metatarso-phalangeal compartment can be examined. Through the medial portal, the metatarso-sesamoid compartment (except the most lateral part of the compartment especially in case of severe hallux vallgus deformity), the lateral and dorsal gutters and the lateral and central part of the articular surfaces of metatarso-phalangeal compartment can be examined.

4.5 ArthroscopicS ynovectomy

Synovitis of the first metatarso-phalangeal joint (Fig. 4.4) can arise from metabolic, e.g., gouty arthritis; inflammatory, e.g., rheumatoid arthritis; infective causes, and can be associated with abnormal mechanical stress, e.g., hallux valgus. The management of synovitis should be according to the underlying cause. Arthroscopic synovectomy is indicated once conservative treatment fails to control the disease. However, it should be supplemented with appropriate medical treatment if indicated e.g., in case of rheumatoid arthritis.

4.5.1 Technique

Arthroscopic synovectomy can usually be performed with the dorsolateral and the medial portals. If complete synovectomy of the metatarso-sesamoid compartment, a portal 4 cm proximal to the joint and between the abductor hallucis and flexor hallucis brevis tendons can be made to complete the synovectomy around the sesamoid bones (Fig. 4.5).

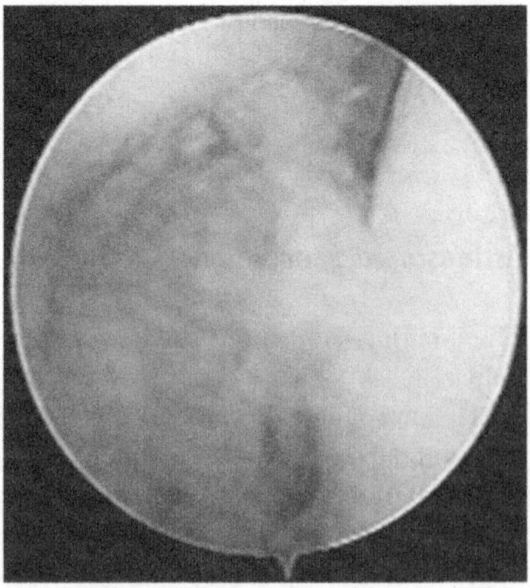

Fig.4. 4 Synovitis of the first metatarso-phalangealj oint

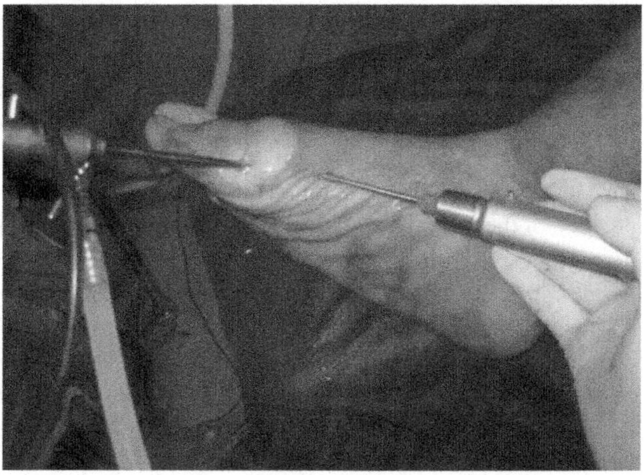

Fig.4.5 Metatarso-sesamoid compartment arthroscopy with medial and plantar medialporta ls

Alternatively, the synovectomy of the metarso-sesamoid compartment can be performed together with the endoscopic distal soft tissue procedure through the medial and the toe web portal in patients with first metatarso-phalangeal synovitis associated with hallux valgus.[6,8] Visualization of the, occasional enlarged, dorsomedial synovial fold is easier performed through the dorsolateral portal. Thorough debridement of the inflamed synovial tissue which is usually a major pain generator can be performed with a 3.0 full-radius shaver.[9] Traction is typically not required for a synovectomy. Suction is kept at minimum given the limited inflow from the small arthroscopic cannula.

4.5.1.1 Endoscopic Resection of Gouty Tophus Around the First Metatarso-phalangeal Joint

Gouty arthritis is one of the commonest type of arthritides faced by orthopedic surgeon. The commonest joint involved is the first metatarso-phalangeal joint. Tophi formation around the first metatarso-phalangeal joint will affect shoewear. Moreover, ulceration of the tophus will lead to persistent discharge and chronic ulceration which will take a long time to heal. Secondary infection is common. Wound breakdown, skin necrosis and impaired healing are common after open resection of the tophus. Minimally invasive decompression of the tophus minimizes wound complications.[10] However, this is mainly a blind percutaneous procedure, and the completeness of the resection cannot be ascertained. Also, protection of the digital nerve is difficult. The endoscopic approach[11] allows resection of the tophus under direct visualization and arthroscopic examination of the first metatarso-phalangeal joint.[11,12] In addition to the advantage of minimization of wound complication, this can ensure complete resection without damage to the normal tissue.

The patient is supine with a thigh tourniquet. Two portals are established at the proximal and distal ends of the gouty tophus. A tunnel is produced between the two portals with the cannula and trocar. The two portals are switched as the visualization and working portals and the tophaceous materials are removed under arthroscopic visualization starting from the tunnel and proceed to the periphery of the tophus. The pockets of tophaceous materials are removed until the pseudo-capsule is reached. Great care is performed to avoid injury to the dorsomedial hallucal nerve superficial to the pseudocapsule (Fig. 4.6). After adequate decompression of the tophus, the overlying skin will be loose enough to allow free mobilization of the portals to plantar and dorsal directions to remove the plantar and dorsal extension of the tophus. Moreover, the distal portal can be mobilized to the position of the medial portal of first metatarso-phalangeal joint and the intra-articular condition can be examined with a 1.9 mm 30° arthroscope. If synovitis or tophaceous material is present, a dorsolateral portal is established to complete the debridement. The use of warm irrigation fluid is recommended to increase the solubility of the urate thus preventing clogging of the system.[10] Post-surgical gout attacks can be prevented by pre-surgical control of serum uric acid and prophylactic perioperative administration of colchicine.

Post-operatively, the patient is allowed to weight bearing walking with wooden baseds andal.

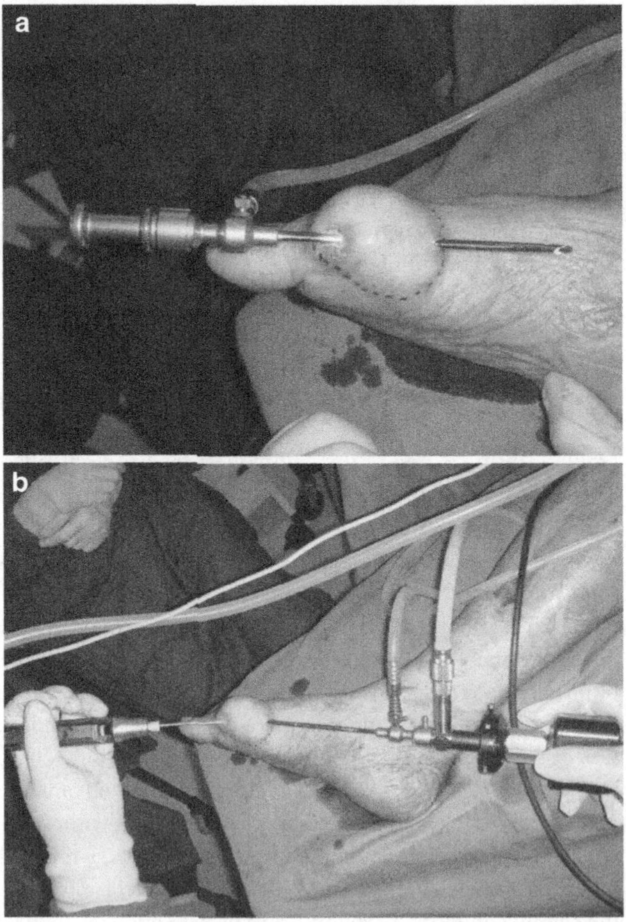

Fig.4. 6 (**a**) Cannula and trocar pass through the proximal and distal portals. (**b**) Endoscopic resection of goutyt ohpus

4.5.1.2
Endoscopic Distal Soft Tissue Procedure for Hallux valgus Correction

Endoscopic distal soft tissue procedure employs the same principle of open procedure.[5,6] The lateral soft tissue release is performed through the toe web and plantar portals. The medial exostectomy and medial capsular plication are performed through the proximal and distal bunion portals. The distal bunion portal is the same as the medial portal of first metatarso-phalangeal arthroscopy, and the proximal portal is at the proximal pole of the bunion. The reduction of the sesamoid apparatus can be assessed arthroscopically through the toe web and distal bunion portals. The intermetatarsal space is then closed up manually and held with a positioning screw bridging the two metatarsals. This endoscopic approach is indicated in hallux valgus with incongruent metatarso-phalangeal joint and no significant bony abnormality e.g., severe hallux valgus interphalangeus or abnormal distal metatarsal articular angle. However, it is contra-indicated if the intermetatarsal angle cannot be closed up manually e.g., presence of os intermetatarsium. First metatarso-phalangeal arthrosis, deformity secondary to neuromuscular condition are other contra-indications of this procedure. It has the advantages of better assessment of the sesamoid reduction, better cosmetic result and avoids the need of metatarsal osteotomy. This approach will be discussed in another chapter.

4.6
Arthroscopic Dorsal Cheilectomy for Dorsal Impingement Syndrome

Dorsal impingement syndrome of the first metatarso-phalangeal joint is due to impingement of the dorsal osteophytes during dorsiflexion. Dorsal cheilectomy is indicated when conservative treatment has failed.[13] Dorsomedial and dorsolateral portals are made at the medial and lateral corner of the dorsal osteophytes, which is further away from the tendon of extensor hallucis longus than the usual dorsal portals described above. This can avoid the crowding of the instruments. The two portals can be interchanged as the visualization and instrumentation portals and the dorsal impinging bony prominence can be removed with arthroscopic burr under arthroscopic visualization. Stripping of the dorsal capsule from the phalangeal and metatarsal insertions can improve the "working space" for bone shaving. Small osteophytes can be easily removed with a bone cutting shaver, and the round-tip abrader is reserved for large osteophytes or unusually hard bone. For an arthroscopic cheilectomy, the dorsal metatarsal head including a small amount of articular cartilage is decompressed until 50–70° of dorsiflexion is achieved. If there is any question regarding the amount of the decompression, fluoroscopy can be utilized. The prominent osteophyte on the proximal phalangeal base should be evaluated and adequately decompressed(Fig. 4.7).

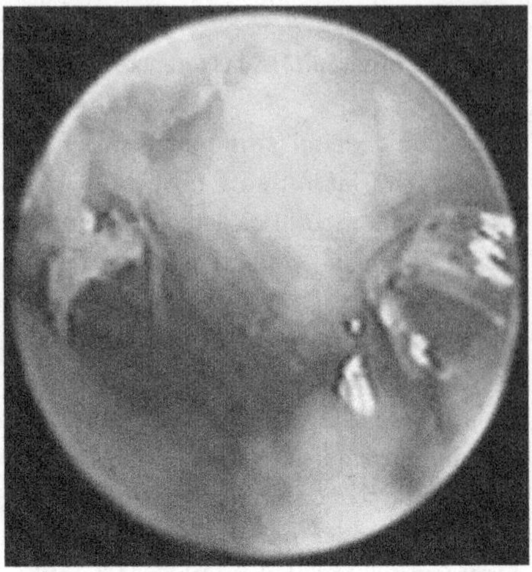

Fig. 4.7 Dorsal cheilectomy of the phalangealba se

4.7 Osteoarthritis

Mild to moderate osteoarthritis of the MTP-1 with pain, arising mainly from synovitis is an appropriate indication for arthroscopic management, especially when the arthrodesis or arthroplasty is not yet indicated. However, patients with advanced osteoarthritis with mid-range pain have not shown a lasting benefit from arthroscopic debridement. Large osteophytes (>5 mm) may obliterate the dorsal joint space. This can be addressed arthroscopically by firstly stripping the dorsal capsule with a small periosteal elevator through the dorsal portals to increase the working space. Moreover, the placement of the dorsal portals at the dorsomedial and the dorsolateral corners of the joint allows debridement of the osteophytes in the dorsal, medial and lateral gutters. For example, the medial osteophytes can be debrided with the dorsolateral portal as visualization portal and the dorsomedial portals as the instrumentation portals. If adequate debridement is not possible arthroscopically, it can be converted to open debridement.

Arthroscopic assisted arthrodesis[14,15] has been described for end stage disease (Fig. 4.8) without gross deformity or bone loss. It is contraindicated in patients with marked bone deformity or if shortening of the first ray is required, as in correction of deformity of the forefoot in rheumatoid patients. Dorsolateral and medial portals are used, and continuous traction with a finger trap is usually not required. Residual cartilage is debrided using curettes, shavers, or abraders. The preserved subchondral bone is microfractured using small chondral picks.

The position of fusion is in 15° of valgus and 20° of dorsiflexion. If the positioning of the joint is affected by contracted capsular structure, the capsule can be released through the corresponding portal wound. If the positioning is affect by bony impingement, the impinging bone can be removed with the 2 mm Isham straight flute burr through the corresponding portal. Provisional fixation is made with a Kirschner wire, and the position

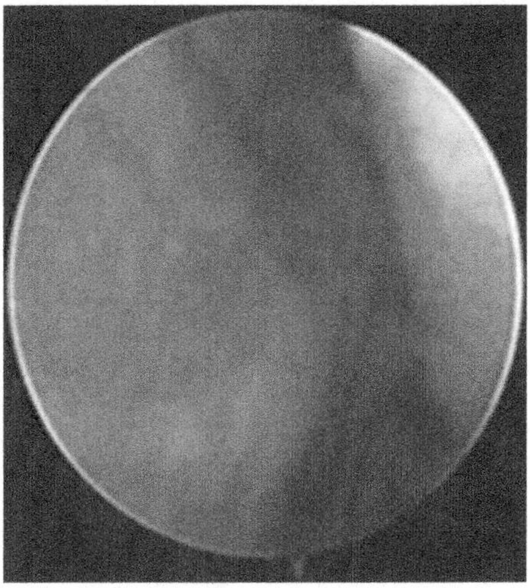

Fig. 4.8 Advanced degeneration of the first metatarso-phalangealjoi nt

confirmed with fluoroscopy. When the foot is placed flat on a metal tray, the interphalangeal joint should be slightly elevated from the surface. Crossed 4.0 mm cannulated screws are inserted under fluoroscopicgui dance.

4.8 Chondral and Osteochondral Lesions

Chondral and osteochondral lesions have been successfully managed arthroscopically with the benefits of less pain, stiffness, and reduced rehabilitation time. In patients with cartilage lesions, the aims are to remove the source of pain, stimulate fibrocartilage production, and eliminate mechanical symptoms. Partial thickness cartilage injury can be treated with the radiofrequency probe to provide smooth edges. We recommend microfracture technique using a small joint microfracture probe or a Kirschner wire for a full thickness cartilage loss or an osteochondral defect. For osteochondral lesions in situ, the overlying cartilage may look deceptively normal but with careful palpation with a probe, the lesion can be identified. A curette can be used to remove the osteochondral fragments, but the 2.0 mm probe is less traumatic to the surrounding tissue. Softened cartilage can be easily penetrated and cut with the tip of the probe. The probe can then be used as a hook to pull the fragment loose. The fragment can be debrided with a shaver or removed with hemostats. The defect is further debrided until fresh subchondral surface is reached (Fig. 4.9). Microfracture is then performed (Fig. 4.10). The joint is mobilized through the range of motion, and any potential area that can produce mechanical catching are smoothened with a radiofrequency probe. The corresponding kissing lesion that can present on the proximal phalangeal base should be managed concurrently.[16]

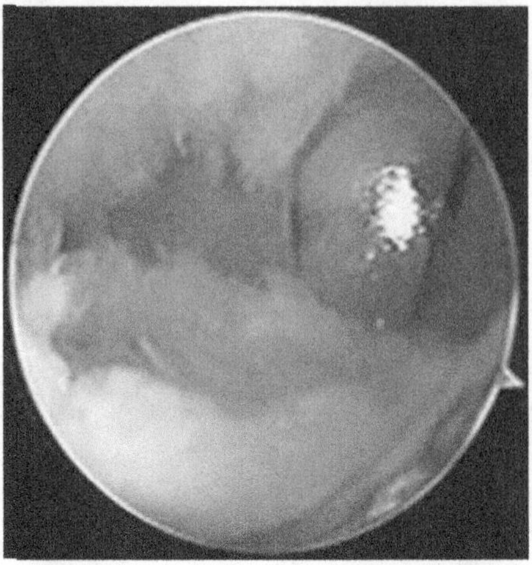

Fig.4. 9 Debridement of the osteochondral lesion of metatatarsalhe ad

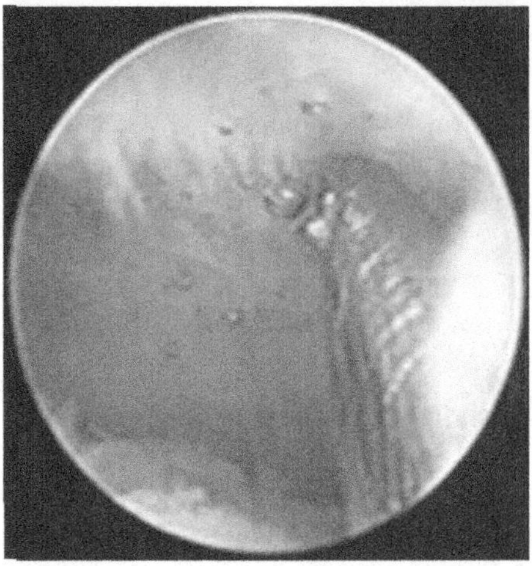

Fig.4. 10 Microfracture of the osteochondral lesion

4.9 Arthroscopic Sesamoidectomy for Sesamoid Pathology

First metatarso-phalangeal sesamoidectomy is well-established for sesamoiditis, osteochondritis resistant to conservative management, infection secondary to diabetic neuropathy, and in non-union of sesamoid fractures. Open surgical procedure uses a standard medial arthrotomy approach, opening up the capsule and retracting it plantarward until the articular surface of the sesamoid can be visualized. The potential complications of open surgical approach included the risk of damage to the lateral digital nerve, which is just at the lateral side of fibular sesamoid. Excessive soft tissue dissection during open procedure may result in post-operative stiffness. Moreover, deformities such as hallux varus and cock-up deformity may result from open procedure, because of the disruption of ligamentous and tendinous structures around the sesamoids. The use of arthroscopy may decrease surgical morbidity and complications associated with open procedures. Arthroscopy also provides thorough assessment of the intra-articular status of the metatarso-phalangeal joint.

Arthroscopic medial bipartite sesamoidectomy[17] had been described for the management of bipartite medial sesamoid. Arthroscopic lateral sesamoidectomy[18] has also been described for the management of chronic osteomyelitis of the lateral sesamoid bone.

The medial sesamoid has been removed using the dorsolateral portal for visualization and the medial portal for instrumentation. The lateral sesamoid can be removed using the medial and plantar medial portals. The toe web and plantar portals may be needed in case of severe hallux valgus. The sesamoid can be excised in piecemeal with a pituitary rongeur or a 2.0 mm round abrader. The ligamentous attachments are preserved.

4.10 Arthroscopic Assisted Plantar Plate Tenodesis for First Metatarso-phalangeal Instability

Injuries to the first metatarso-phalangeal can range from a mild sprain to a frank dislocation. Late complication can occur depending the types and severity of the injury, the initial treatment and rehabilitation. The commonest late complications are joint stiffness and pain with athletic activity. Other complications include arthrofibrosis, different types of deformity e.g., hallux valgus, cock up deformity, and chronic instability. Plantar plate repair and abductor hallucis transfer are the treatment of choice for plantar plate insufficiency. However, the procedure requires extensive soft tissue dissection. Plantar plate tenodesis is first described as an arthroscopic assisted technique for correction of lesser toe deformity. It stabilizes the plantar plate by connecting the plantar plate to the long extensor tendon with a figure-of-eight of suture. The pull of the extensor tendon will redirect plantarly to stabilize the plantar plate. This technique can also be used to stabilize the plantar plate in instability of the first metatarso-phalangeal joint. This technique is feasible if the plantar plate is disrupted at the metatarsal side or the inter-sesamoid ligament is torn, because the figure of eight construct of the suture can close up the inter-sesamoid distance and the plantar plate is shifted proximally to its proximal insertion. It is not feasible if the plantar plate is disrupted at its phalangeal insertion. Plantar plate tenodesis[19] has the advantage of accurate arthroscopic examination of the first metatarso-phalangeal joint and assessment of status of the plantar plate before plantar plate reconstruction. Plantar plate tenodesis is performed through the arthroscopic portal wounds if the phalangeal insertion of the plantar plate is intact. This minimizes the degree of soft tissue dissection.

4.10.1 Technique

Arthroscopy of the first metatarso-phalangeal joint is performed through the dorsomedial and dorsolateral portals. After examination of the joint, plantar plate tenodesis is performed through the portal wounds. A PDS 1 suture is passed through the lateral part of the plantar plate and the plantar skin with a straight eyed needle through the dorsolateral portal. The suture is then retrieved from the plantar surface of the plantar plate through the medial side of the metatarsal to the proximal dorsal wound at the mid shaft of the metatarsal using of a curved hemostat. The other limb of the suture is passed from the dorsolateral portal to the dorsomedial portal deep inside the joint. It is then passed through the medial part of the plantar plate via the dorsomedial portal. The suture is then retrieved through the lateral side of the metatarsal to the proximal wound. The suture is anchored to the tendon of extensor hallucis longus. Then, a figure of eight configuration of the suture, connecting the plantar plate to the tendon of extensor digitorum longus, is constructed.

4.11 Arthroscopic Release for First Metatarso-phalangeal Arthrofibrosis

Arthrofibrosis of the first metarso-phalangeal joint occurs in patients following bunion surgery or trauma to the hallux. In patients with functional limitation who do not respond to conservative management, surgery is indicated. Patient should be carefully evaluated clinically and radiographically to plan the surgical strategy. First ray deformity, e.g., hallux elevatus, and first metatarso-phalangeal joint osteoarthrosis should be managed accordingly. In patient with first metatarso-phalangeal joint arthrofibrosis, surgical soft tissue release is indicated. However, open release has a high chance of recurrence. Early post-operative vigorous mobilization is allowed after arthroscopic release[20] because of the minimal wound pain.

4.11.1 Technique

The patient is supine with a thigh pneumatic tourniquet. No traction of the joint is applied. A 1.9 mm 30° arthroscope is used. First, the dorsolateral and dorsomedial portals are using as the visualization and working portals for the dorsal gutter. The dorsal portals should be placed in the dorsomedial and dorsolateral corners of the joint as in arthroscopic dorsal cheilectomy (Fig. 4.11). At the initial portal placement, the trocar should be used to free up the dorsal fibrotic tissue by sweeping it back and forth. The fibrosis in the dorsal gutter is cleared up, and the dorsal capsule can be stripped from the metatarsal head using and arthroscopic shaver and a small periosteal elevator. This produces an intra-articular working space for the subsequent procedures.

Secondly, the lateral gutter of the joint is cleared with the dorsomedial portal as the visualization portal and the dorsolateral portal as the working portal (Fig. 4.12). Fibrous bands at the lateral gutter can then be debrided. Beware not to strip the lateral capsule from the metatarsal head because of the potential risk of hallux varus deformity.

After clearance of the lateral gutter, the medial gutter is visualized through the dorsolateral portal. Medial gutter fibrosis can be cleared using an arthroscopic shaver through the dorsomedial portal. The medial capsule can be stripped from the metatarsal head in case of over-plication of the medial capsule during bunion surgery.

Finally, the metatarso-sesamoid compartment can be visualized through the medial portal. The fibrous adhesions of the compartment can be debrided through the plantar medial

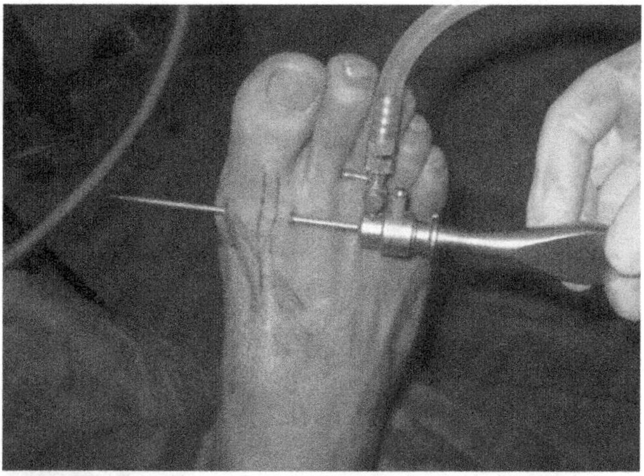

Fig.4. 11 Thedors alport als should be at the dorsomedial and dorsolateral corners of thejoint

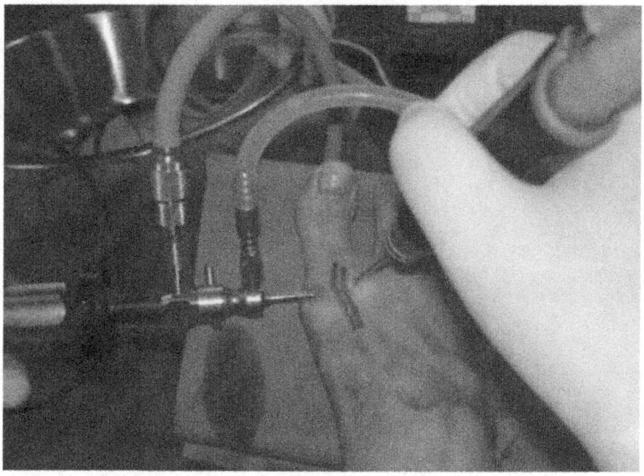

Fig.4. 12 Thela teralgutt er of the joint is cleared with the dorsomedial portal as the visualization portal and the dorsolateral portal asthe w orkingporta l

portal. Manipulation to achieve maximum range of motion is usually performed after the release. After release of the dorsal capsule and clearance of the medial and lateral gutters, the first metatarso-phalangeal joint can be plantarflexed to allow easier instrumentation.

The circumference of the joint can then be released arthroscopically without excessive soft tissue dissection. Active and passive mobilization of the first metatarso-phalangeal joint is started on the first post-operative day.

4.12 Arthroscopic Assisted Reduction and Fixation of Intra-articular Fracture of the First Metatarsal Head

In case of intra-articular fracture of the metatarsal head, first metatarso-phalangeal arthroscopy can assist the reduction of the intra-articular fragment (Fig. 4.13) and the fracture can be stabilized with percutaneous screw fixation(Fig. 4.14).

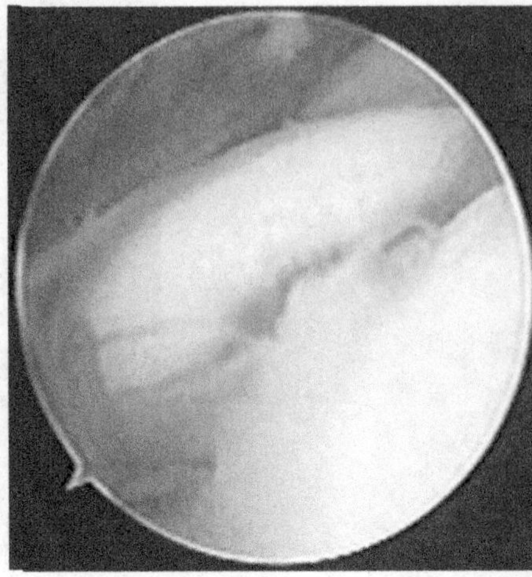

Fig.4. 13 Intra-articular fracture of the metatarsal head

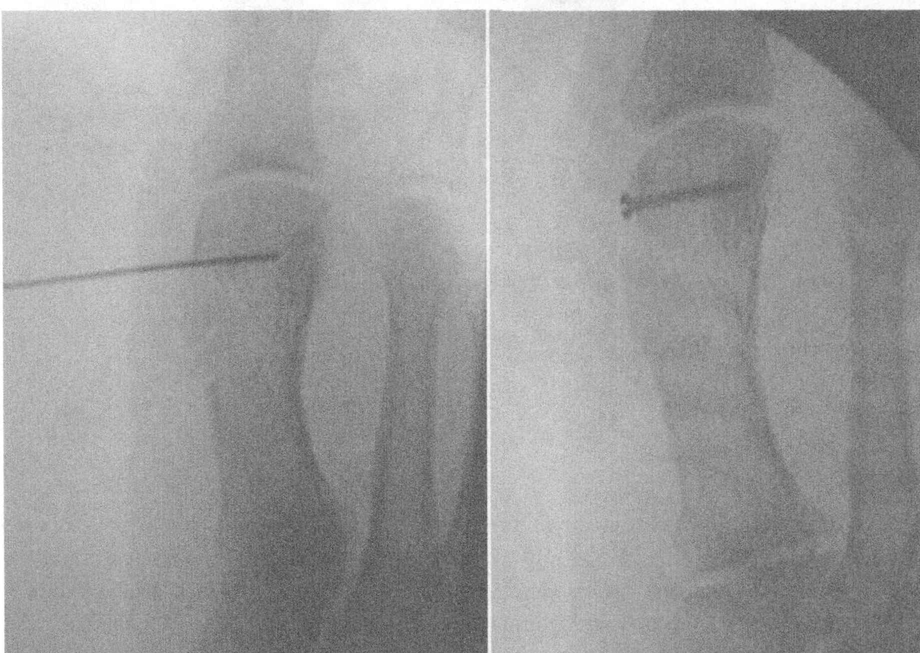

Fig.4. 14 Percutaneouss crewfi xation

References

1. Watanabe M. *Selfox-Arthroscope (Wantantabe No. 24 arthroscope)*. Tokyo, Japan: Teishin Hospital;1972.
2. Solan MC, Lemon M, Bendall SP. The surgical anatomy of the dorsomedial cutaneous nerve of the hallux. *J Bone Joint Surg Br.*2001; 83:250–252.

3. Ferkel R. Great-toe arthroscopy. In: Whipple T, ed. *Arthroscopic Surgery: The Foot & Ankle*. Philadelphia, PA: Lippincott-Raven; 1996:255–272.
4. Phisitkul P, et al. The surgical anatomy of the plantarmedial hallucal nerve in relation to the medial approach of the first metatarsophalangeal joint. *Foot Ankle Int.*I npr ess.
5. Lui TH, Ng S, Chan KB New technique: endoscopic distal soft tissue procedure in hallux valgus. *Arthroscopy*.2005; 21:1403.e1–1403.e7.
6. Lui TH, et al. Arthroscopy-assisted correction of hallux valgus deformity. *Arthroscopy*. 2008;24:875–880.
7. van Dijk CN, Veenstra KM, Nuesch BC. Arthroscopic surgery of the metatarsophalangeal first joint. *Arthroscopy*.1998; 14:851–855.
8. Lui TH. First metatarsophalangeal joint arthroscopy in patients with hallux valgus. *Arthroscopy*. 2008;24:1122–1129.
9. Lidtke RH, George J. Anatomy, biomechanics, and surgical approach to synovial folds within the joints of the foot. *J Am Podiatr Med Assoc*.2004; 94:519–527.
10. Lee SS, et al. The soft-tissue shaving procedure for deformity management of chronic tophaceous gout. *Ann Plast Surg*.2003; 51:372–375.
11. Lui TH. Endoscopic resection of the gouty tophi of the first metatarsophalangeal joint. *Arch Orthop Trauma Surg*.2008; 128:521–523.
12. Wang CC, et al. Arthroscopic elimination of monosodium urate deposition of the first metatarsophalangeal joint reduces the recurrence of gout. *Arthroscopy*.2009; 25:153–158.
13. Iqbal MJ, Chana GS. Arthroscopic cheilectomy for hallux rigidus. *Arthroscopy*. 1998;14: 307–310.
14. Carro LP, Vallina BB. Arthroscopic-assisted first metatarsophalangeal joint arthrodesis. *Arthroscopy*.1999; 15:215–217.
15. Stroud CC. Arthroscopic arthrodesis of the ankle, subtalar, and first metatarsophalangeal joint. *Foot Ankle Clin*.2002; 7:135–146.
16. Bartlett DH. Arthroscopic management of osteochondritis dissecans of the first metatarsal head. *Arthroscopy*.1988; 4:51–54.
17. Perez Carro L, Echevarria Llata JI, Martinez Agueros JA. Arthroscopic medial bipartite sesamoidectomy of the great toe. *Arthroscopy*.1999; 15:321–323.
18. Chan PK, Lui TH. Arthroscopic fibular sesamoidectomy in the management of the sesamoid osteomyelitis. *Knee Surg Sports Traumatol Arthrosc*.20 06;14:664–667.
19. Lui TH. Stabilization of first metatarsophalangeal instability with plantar plate tenodesis. *J Foot Ankle Surg*.I npr ess.
20. Lui TH. Arthroscopic release of first metatarsophalangeal arthrofibrosis. *Arthroscopy*. 2006;22:906e 1–4.

Minimally Invasive Management of Hallux Rigidus

5

Mariano de Prado, Pedro-Luis Ripoll, and Pau Golanó

5.1 Introduction

Hallux rigidus is the clinical expression of osteoarthritis of the metatarsophalangeal joint of the hallux. Hallux rigidus presents with limited joint mobility, especially in extension, and pain, with osteophytes on the dorsal aspect of the head of the first metatarsal (Fig. 5.1) and of the base of the proximal phalanx of the hallux. It has a prevalence of 2% of the population between 30 and 60 years of age.[8,16]

Davies-Colley,[4] in 1887, first described the condition, calling it hallux flexus, and a few months later, Cotterill[3] referred to it as hallux rigidus, a term that seems more accurate and which is now widespread.

5.2 Pathogenesis

5.2.1 Intrinsic Causes

The presence of a relatively long first toe, secondary to a long first metatarsal (plus index) or a foot that, despite having a formula index or index plus minus, has a large phalanx of the hallux, will impose abnormal strain to the metatarsophalangeal joint of the hallux.

Another factor is a relatively flattened shape of the head of the first metatarsal. This alters the normal mobility of this joint, favoring degenerative joint disease. Flattening of the first metatarsal head changes the angle of incidence of the first metatarsal to the ground, which impacts the lower half of the metatarsophalangeal joint during walking. Also, the upper half of the metatarsophalangeal joint will be subjected to abnormal contact with the articular surface of the proximal phalanx of the hallux.

M. de Prado (✉)
Department of Orthopaedics, Hospital USP San Carlos, Murcia, España
e-mail: de prado@hospitalsancarlos.net

N. Maffulli and M. Easley (eds.), *Minimally Invasive Surgery of the Foot and Ankle*,
DOI: 10.1007/978-1-84996-417-3_5,

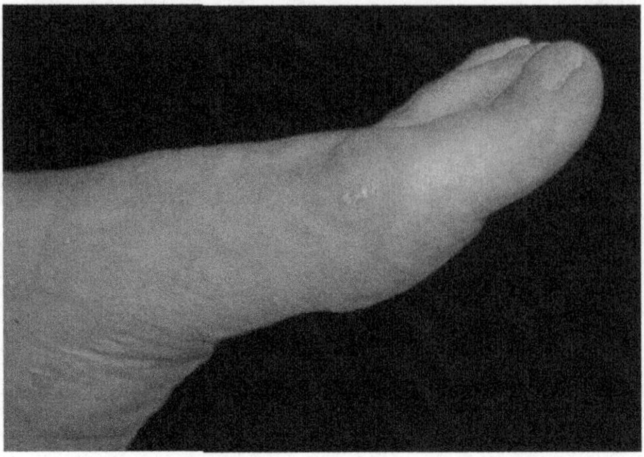

Fig. 5.1 Halluxrigidus presents with visible osteophytes on the dorsal aspect of the head of the first metatarsal

Osteochondritis of the head of the first metatarsal, by producing a cartilage lesion, promotes early osteoarthritis.

Pronation of the foot can also be associated with hallux rigidus.

Systemic diseases that cause arthritis localized to the metatarsophalangeal joint are gout and rheumatoid arthritis.

5.2.2 ExtrinsicC auses

Repetitive microtrauma to the hallux from sporting endeavors or work promote the development of hallux rigidus. Osteochondral fractures of the metatarsal head or base of the proximal phalanx, with irreversible damage to the cartilage, with use of inappropriate footwear are also associated with the condition.

5.3 Clinical

Patients normally report pain and decreased mobility of the first metatarsophalangeal joint during gait, especially in the push off, with a progressive dorsal deformity. This limits normal activities, and produces skin irritation. Often patients use flat shoes with a stiff sole. In more advanced stages, the mobility of first metatarsophalangeal joint is very limited, and exostoses develop both dorsally and medially. The patient will walk with the foot externally rotated and the forefoot supinated to compensate for the lack of mobility.

The metatarsophalangeal joint of the hallux is larger than normal, both dorsally and medially, with local limited inflammation and possibly bursitis. The interphalangeal joint

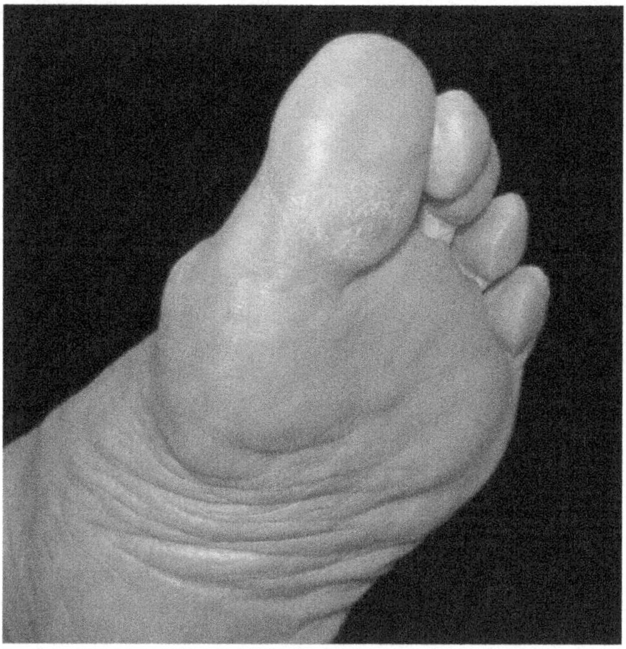

Fig. 5.2 Theinte rphalangeal joint may be in hyperextension, with a plantar callus at the base of thedis talpha lanx

may be in hyperextension, with a plantar callus at the base of the distal phalanx (Fig. 5.2) and another on the head of the fifthm etatarsal.

Palpation elicits dorsal tenderness, with crepitus. Flexion is painful, and the rubbing of the dorsal osteophytes with the sheath of the extensor tendons of the hallux may cause mechanical synovitis. Clinically, two distinct stages can be identified:[1]

- Stage 1 (hallux dolorosus). The metatarsophalangeal joint pain is virtually the only symptom, sometimes accompanied by discomfort in the lateral aspect of the foot. Pain is elicited on extension of the metatarsophalangeal joint, which shows limited range of motion.
- Stage 2 (hallux limitus). Mobility is almost blocked. There are callosities of the fifth metatarsal head and the base of the proximal phalanx of the hallux. The patient walks with external rotation of the foot, to avoid dorsiflexion of the first metatarsophalangeal joint.

5.4 Imaging and Further Investigations

Radiographs of both feet should include weight-bearing dorsoplantar and lateral views, and oblique views.[7] Radiographs show arthritis with osteophytes, sclerosis, subchondral cysts, etc. Regnault described three radiographic stages:

- Stage 1. Slight narrowing of the joint with small osteophytes over the lateral and dorsal aspect of the first metatarsal head and dorsal. (Fig. 5.3).
- Stage 2. Osteophytes develop on both sides of the joint. The metatarsal head is flattened, with lateral subchondral sclerosis (Fig. 5.4).
- Stage 3. Total loss of joint space, with florid osteophytes and irregularities of the articular surface, alternating with areas of intense sclerosis (Fig. 5.5).

Other complementary studies are not usually needed to confirm the diagnosis and start treatment, as radiography is sufficiently indicative.[17] We do not recommend any other investigations, but in some patients in whom there may be suspicion of associated injuries, magnetic resonance imaging (MRI), computed tomography (CT), and bone scans can be used.

5.4.1 Surgery

In patients with marked pain and an active life, and in whom conservative management (rocker bottom shoes, insoles, steroid injections) has not provided sufficient relief of symptoms and functional impairment, surgery should considered.

Contraindications for surgery are vascular problems and local infection.

In the remaining part of this chapter, we describe our minimally invasive technique.[5,6,12]

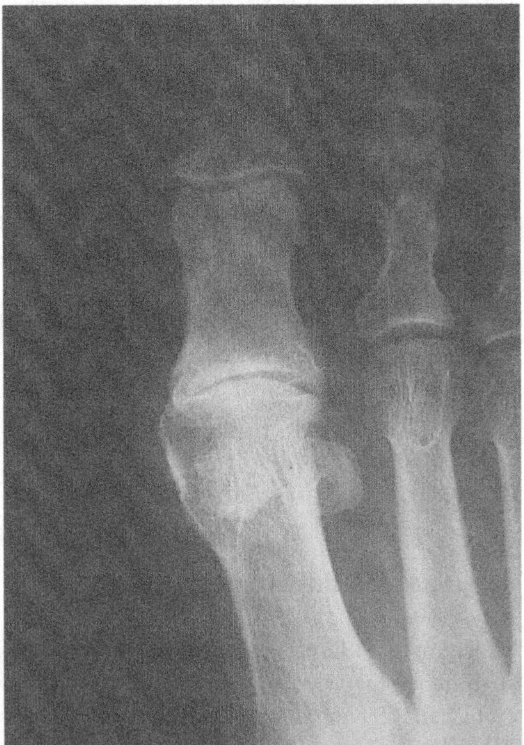

Fig.5.3 Slight narrowing of the joint with small osteophytes over the lateral aspect of the first metatarsal head. Small osteophytes are also seen dorsally

Fig.5.4 Osteophytes develop on both sides of the joint. The metatarsal head is flattened, with lateral subchondral sclerosis

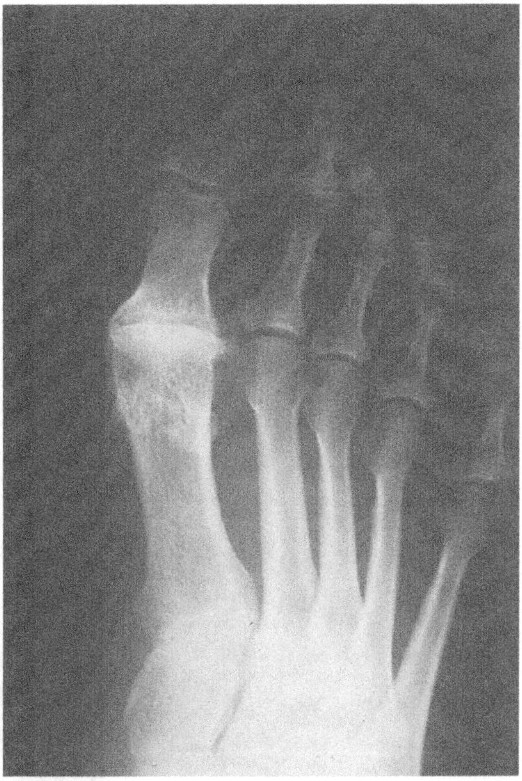

5.4.2 Instruments

- Completege nerali nstruments et.
- BeaverN o.64s calpel.
- Long Shannon No. 44 burrs, 3.1 Xmas Tree and 4.1 Wedge burrs, and Brophy Burr.

5.4.3 Anesthesia

We use a peripheral ankle block, but some patients may prefer general anesthesia.

5.4.4 Cheilectomy

A 0.5 cm incision is made in the dorsal medial forefoot, just behind the metatarsal neck and under the dorsal digital nerve with Beaver blade 64 (Figs. 5.6 and 5.7). The incision is deepened, accommodating the blade on the medial exostosis at the level of its dorsal aspect,

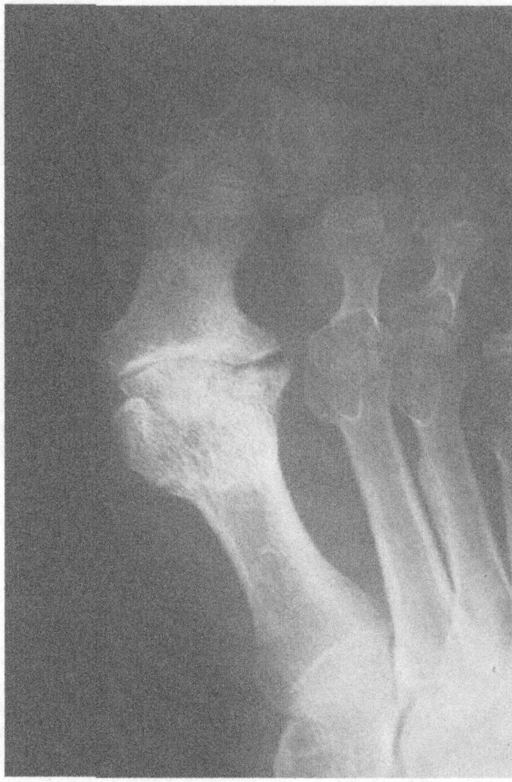

Fig.5. 5 Total loss of joint space, with florid osteophytes and irregularities of the articular surface, alternating with areasof i ntenses clerosis

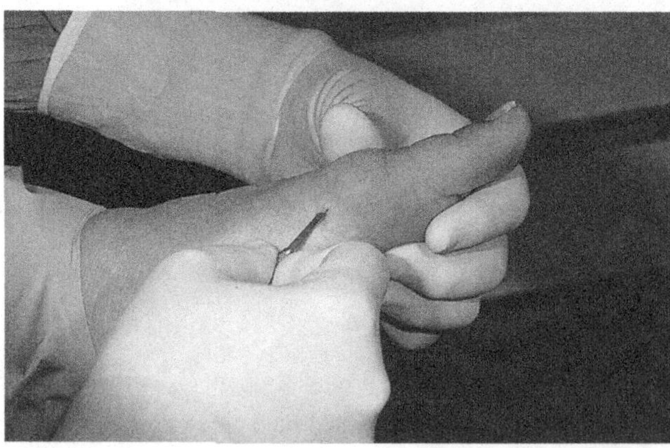

Fig.5. 6 Ape rcutaneous cheilectomy procedure starts with a 0.5 cm incision in the dorsal medial forefoot, just behind the metatarsal neck and under the dorsal digital nervew ithB eaverbl ade64

and goes under the capsule covering the exostosis, both medially and dorsally. A rasp is introduced to remove the fibrous remains of the exostosis, and to produce a working space between the dorsal and medial exostosis below and above the joint capsule. We introduce the small triangular bur to abrade the exostosis (Fig. 5.8). One should be very aggressive to the dorsal exostosis. In some patients, it is necessary to proceed with the exostosectomy to the dorsal base of the proximal phalanx. At times, it can be difficult to reach the lateral portion of the dorsal exostosis. In these instances, a new 0.5-cm incision, also at the level of the metatarsophalangeal joint, should be produced, parallel to the tendon of the extensor

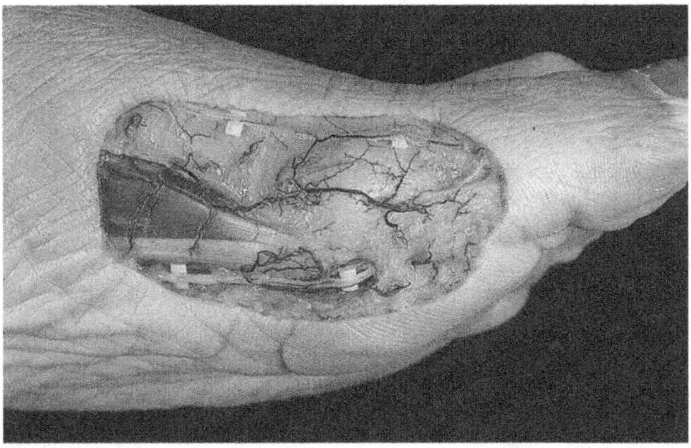

Fig. 5.7 Theinc isionis deepened, accommodating the blade on the medial exostosis at the level of its dorsal aspect, and goes under the capsule covering the exostosis, both medially anddors ally

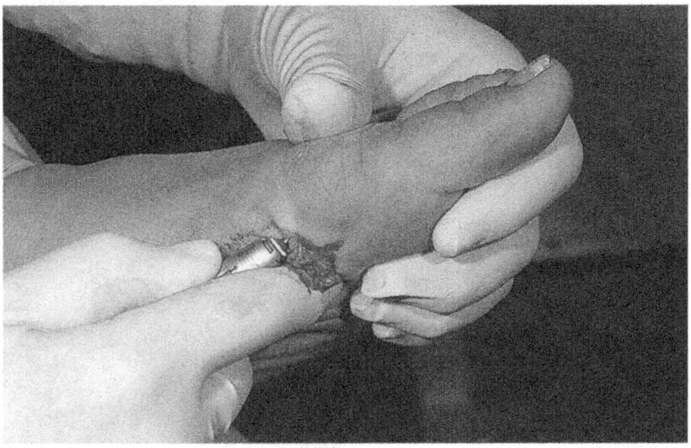

Fig. 5.8 As malltria ngular burrtoa bradethe e xostosis

hallucis longus. In this case, the joint capsule and the insertion of abductor tendon at the base of the proximal phalanx should be spared not to destabilize the joint.

On completion of the cheilectomy on the metatarsal head and the base of the phalanx, very thorough cleaning of the bone residues (mush or fragments produced by the bone abrasion) must be performed. Removal of the residues from the intermetatarsal space is more difficult, as pressure cannot easily be applied, and much greater use must be made of the DPR® rasps in order to extract the bone detritus.

5.4.5 Distal First Metatarsal Osteotomy

A long Shannon 44 burr is used on the medial aspect of the metatarsal neck, angled 45° from dorsal distal to plantar proximal, starting just proximal to the articular surface of the metatarsal head, and ending immediately above the sesamoid (Figs. 5.9 and 5.10). The cutting should start on the medial cortex, and the osteotomy should proceed severing the dorsal cortex, then the lateral cortex. In this way, a dorsal closing wedge is designed, and the plantarc ortexunde rgoesm anualos teoclasis(Figs. 5.11a nd 5.12).

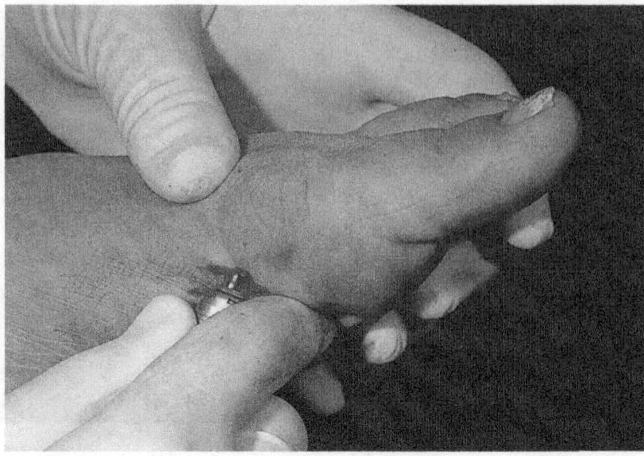

Fig. 5.9 A long Shannon 44 burr is used on the medial aspect of the metatarsal neck, angled 45° from dorsal distal to plantar proximal, starting just proximal to the articular surface of the metatarsal head, and ending immediately above the sesamoid

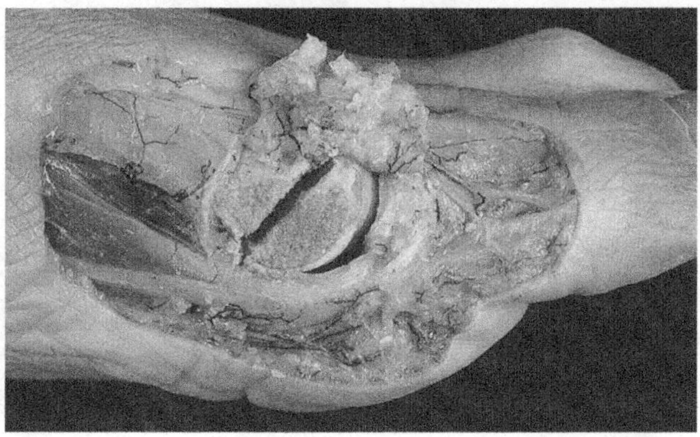

Fig. 5.10 A long Shannon 44 burr is used on the medial aspect of the metatarsal neck starting just proximal to the articular surface of the metatarsal head, and ending immediately above the sesamoid

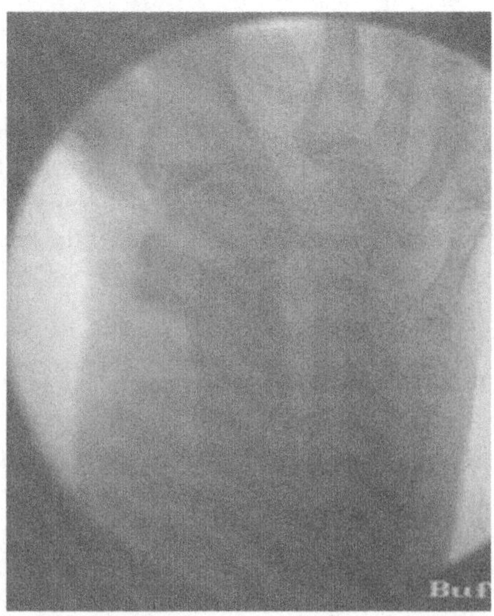

Fig. 5.11 The osteotomy is started on the medial cortex, and the cut is continued on the dorsal cortex followed by the lateral cortex. Before completing the osteotomy of the plantar surface of the metatarsal, a wedge with a dorsal base should be cut; this is performed by passing the long Shannon No. 44 repeatedly over the bone surface of the proximal side of the osteotomy

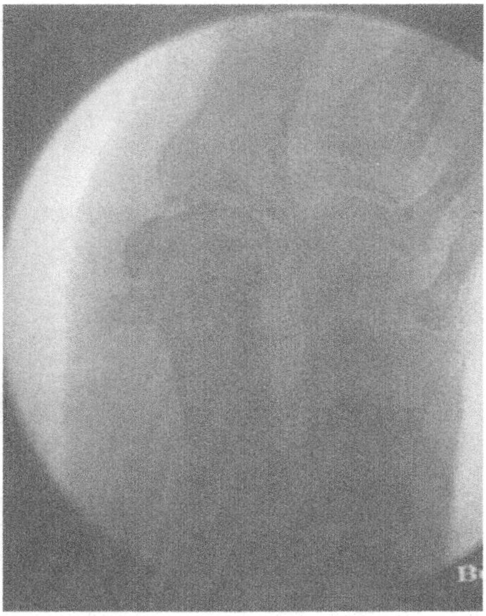

Fig.5.12 After creating a wedge of the desired size , the osteotomy of the plantar cortex is completed by osteoclasis or with the motorized cuttingins trument

5.4.6 Osteotomy of the Base of the Proximal Phalanx

The base of the proximal phalanx is approached medial to the tendon of the extensor hallucis longus, producing a working space in the usual fashion. A long Shannon 44 strawberry bur rests on the medial aspect of the base of the phalanx, and the osteotomy is started (Figs. 5.13 and 5.14), sparing the last few millimeters of bone from the plantar aspect of the phalanx. The osteotomy is completed on both the lateral and dorsal aspects, designing a dorsal closing wedge. The osteotomy is completed by osteoclasis. This completes the plantar osteotomy once achieved the wedge in the right way. The three entry portals used are sutured in a routine fashion (Figs. 5.15 and 5.16). A bandage similar to that used in hallux valgus will aim to keep the first ray in dorsiflexion

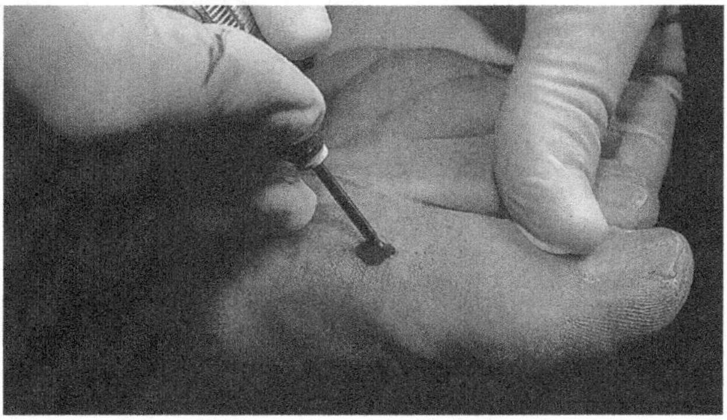

Fig.5.13 The base of the proximal phalanx is approached medial to the tendon of the extensor hallucis longus, producing a working space in the usual fashion. A long Shannon 44 strawberry burr rests on the medial aspect of the base of the phalanx, and the osteotomyis s tarted

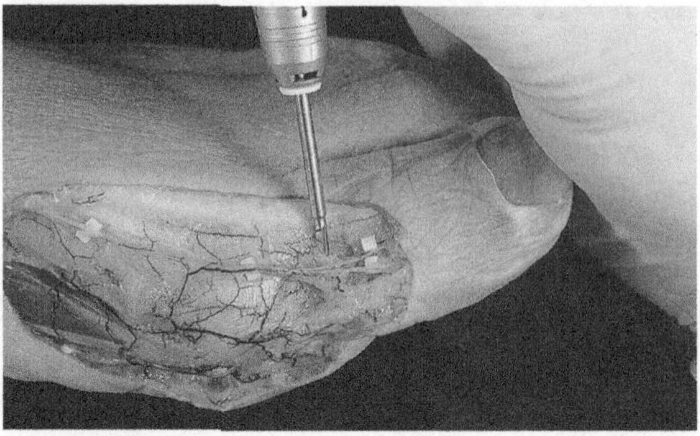

Fig.5. 14 The base of the proximal phalanx is approached medial to the tendon of the extensor hallucis longus, producing a working space in the usual fashion. A long Shannon 44 strawberry burr rests on the medial aspect of the base of the phalanx, and the osteotomyi ss tarted

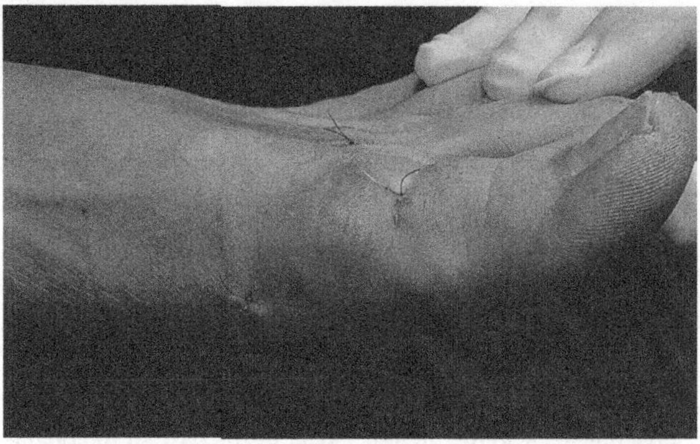

Fig.5. 15 Thethre ee ntry portals used are sutured in a routinef ashion

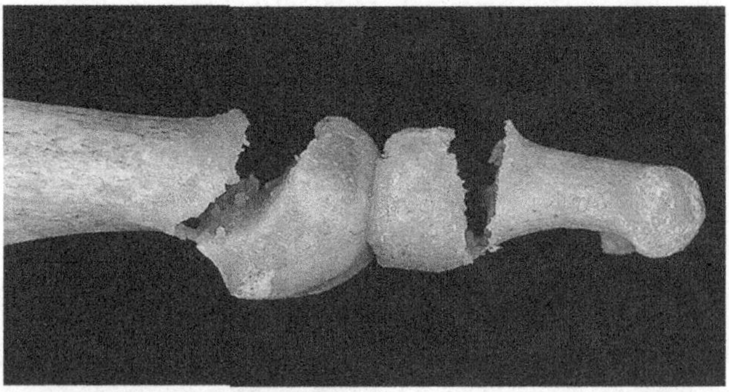

Fig.5. 16 Patientsa re reviewed 7 days after surgery, when the stitches removed. A 3-mm toe separator is placed between the hallux and the second toe, aiming to close the wedge in the proximal phalanx

5.4.7 PostoperativeC are

Weight bearing is allowed with a stiff-soled boot. Patients are reviewed 7 days after surgery, when the stitches removed. A 3-mm toe separator is placed between the hallux and the second toe, aiming to close the wedge in the proximal phalanx. Patients are instructed to change the bandage every day, and are reviewed at 3 weeks, when new radiographs are taken. If the closing wedges continue to stay closed, gentle mobilization is initiated, and the bandages are kept until the sixth postoperative week. Normal walking is usually restored after 2 months, and sports and physical activity are allowed 4–6 months postoperatively(Figs. 5.17a,ba ndc).

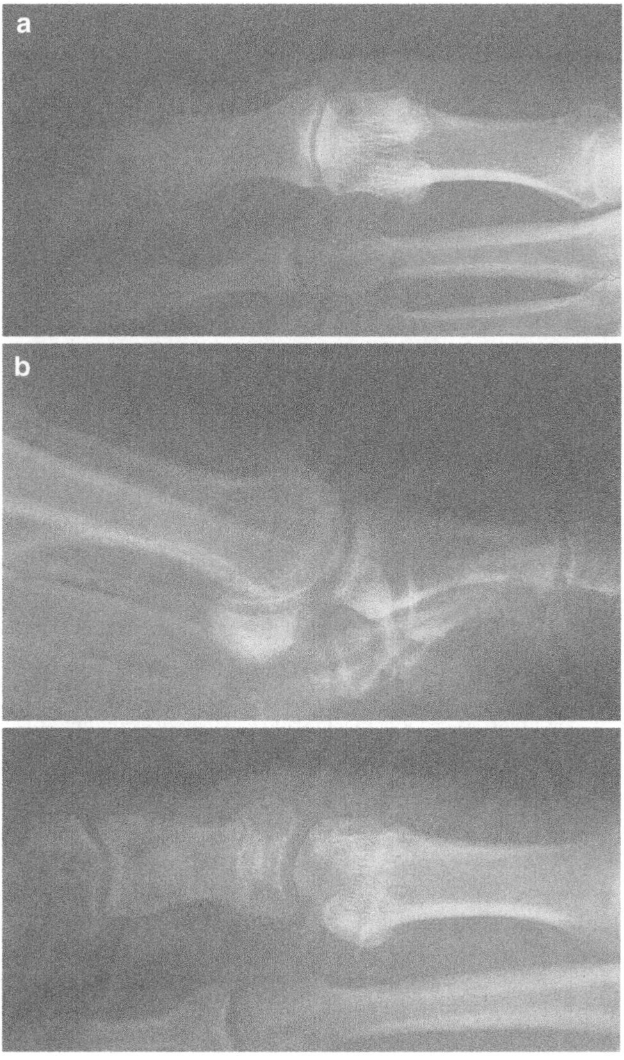

Fig.5. 17 Patientsa re instructed to change the bandage every day, and are reviewed at 3 weeks, when new radiographs are taken. If the closing wedges continue to stay closed, gentle mobilization is initiated, and the bandages are kept until the sixth post-operativew eek

5.5 Surgicall ndications

5.5.1 Cheilectomy

A cheilectomy on its own is indicated in elderly patients with little pain and no functional limitation on their usual activities.

5.5.2 Cheilectomy Plus Metatarsal Osteotomy and the Phalanx

It is indicated in young patients or those with marked pain and functional limitations to their usual activities.[2,9,13,14,15]

5.5.3 MetatarsophalangealA rthrodesis

In our hands, it is indicated after failure of previous surgery.[10,11]

References

1. Beeson P, Phillips C, Corr S, Ribbans W. Classification systems for hallux rigidus: a review of the literature. *Foot Ankle Int.*A pril2008; 29:407–414.
2. Bonney G, Macnab I. Hallux valgus and hallux rigidus: a critical survey of operative results. *J Bone Joint Surg (Br).*1952; 34:366–385.
3. Cotterill JM. Stiffness of the great toe in adolescents. *BMJ.*1888; 1:1158.
4. Davies-Colley MR. Contraction of the metatarsophalangeal joint of the great toe. *BMJ.* 1887;1:728.
5. De Prado M, Ripoll PL, Golanó P. *Cirugía percutánea Del Pie.* Barcelona, Spain: Elsevier (masson);2003.
6. De Prado M, Ripoll PL, Golanó P. *Minimally Invasive Foot Surgery.* Barcelona, Spain: AYH; 2009.
7. DuVries HL. Hallux rigidus (hallux limitus). In: DuVries HL, ed. *Surgery of the Foot.* St. Louis, MO: Mosby; 1959:392–399.
8. Easley ME, Anderson RB. Hallux rigidus in the adult and adolescent. In: Adelaar RS, ed. *Disorders of the Great Toe.* Rosemont, IL: American Academy of Orthopaedic Surgeons; 1997:23–32.
9. Haddad SL. The use of osteotomies in the treatment of hallux limitus and hallux rigidus. *Foot Ankle Clin.*2000; 5:629–662.
10. Keiserman LS, Sammarco VJ, Sammarco GJ. Surgical treatment of the hallux rigidus. *Foot Ankle Clin.*M arch2005; 10:75–96.

11. Mann RA, Coughlin MJ, DuVries HL. Hallux rigidus: a review of the literature and a method of treatment. *Clin Orthop.* 1979; 142:57–63.
12. Mesa-Ramos M, Mesa-Ramos F, Carpintero P. Evaluation of the treatment of hallux rigidus by percutaneous surgery. *Acta Orthop Belg.* A pril2008; 74:222–226.
13. Moberg E. A simple operation for hallux rigidus. *Clin Orthop.* 1979; 142:55–56.
14. Pittman SR, Burns DE. The Wilson bunion procedure modified for improved clinical results. *J Foot Surg.* 1984;23: 314–320.
15. Waterann H. Die arthritis deformans Grosszehen-Grundgelenkes. *Orthop Chir.* 1927;48: 346–355.
16. Yee G, Lau J. Current concepts review: hallux rigidus. *Foot Ankle Int.* June 2008;29: 637–646.
17. Zgonis T, Jolly GP, Garbalosa JC, Cindric T, Godhania V, York S. The value of radiographic parameters in the surgical treatment of hallux rigidus. *J Foot Ankle Surg.* May–June 2005;44:184–189.

Percutaneous First Metatarso-Phalangeal JointF usion

6

Thomas Bauer

6.1 Introduction

Fusion of the first metatarso-phalangeal (MTP1) joint is a useful procedure in forefoot surgery, and is still considered the gold standard for the management of severe painful hallux rigidus. Normal walking and running are possible after MTP1 fusion, as the interphalangeal (IP) joint develops compensatory hypermobility in dorsi-flexion.[1,2] The main difficulty in this procedure is the 3D positioning of the arthrodesis that should be adapted to global foot anatomy, daily activity and shoe wearing habits of each patient.[3–7] Another non specific difficulty is linked to the primary stability of the fusion depending on both technique for fusion site preparation and type of internal fixation.[6–13] Several open or arthroscopically assisted procedures for MTP1 arthrodesis have been described, with fusion rates from 90% to 100%. The authors present a percutaneous procedure for MTP1 fusion with details on the surgical technique, first results and discussion of the benefits and indications.

6.2 Operative Technique

Instruments: Surgical tools for percutaneous MTP1 fusion are identical to those used for all percutaneous forefoot surgical procedures including a conic burr, a Beaver® blade, elevators, rasps, low speed and high torque drill and a fluoroscope. We normally internally fix the fusion with cannulated 3.0 mm compression screws, but other percutaneous fixation systems can be used.

Patient set up: The patient is supine, under regional or local anaesthesia, with the foot free over the end of the table to allow antero-posterio and lateral fluoroscopic control.

T. Bauer
Ambroise Paré Hospital, West Paris University Department of Orthopaedic Surgery, 9 av Charles de Gaulle 92100 Boulogne, France
e-mail:thoma s.bauer@apr.aphp.fr

N. Maffulli and M. Easley (eds.), *Minimally Invasive Surgery of the Foot and Ankle*, DOI: 10.1007/978-1-84996-417-3_6, © Springer-Verlag London Limited 2011

Portals: Percutaneous MTP1 fusion is performed with one main portal and two accessory portals (Fig. 6.1). The main portal is medial at the MTP1 joint line level, and is used for the preparation of bony areas. Two accessory portals can be useful in some patients: one proximal medial and plantar portal at the level of the first metatarsal head, and one distal lateral and dorsal portal at the level of the first phalanx (P1) basis. The accessory proximal medial portal is used for dorsal and medial osteophytes removal and the accessory distal lateral portal is used for dorsal and lateral osteophytes removal and for lateral MTP1 joint capsule and ligaments release.

Method of fusion site preparing: The procedure begins with the removal of metatarsal or phalangeal osteophytes. The resection is performed through the two accessory portals with the large conic burr after periosteal peeling off with the elevators to create a working area and avoid soft tissue damages. Bone debris is carefully evacuated with rasps, and the resection site is abundantly cleaned with normal saline. The quantity and quality of osteophytes removal must be assessed under fluoroscopic control; this resection must be adapted to patient's symptoms (dorsal and medial osteophytes often create impingement with shoes but lateral osteophytes are rarely symptomatic). Excessive resection with risk of bone loss (most often on the first metatarsal head) must be avoided not to interfere with the stability of the arthrodesis.

Preparation of the site of arthrodesis is a most important step, and is performed through the principal medial portal (Fig. 6.2). The conic burr is placed in the MTP1 joint with

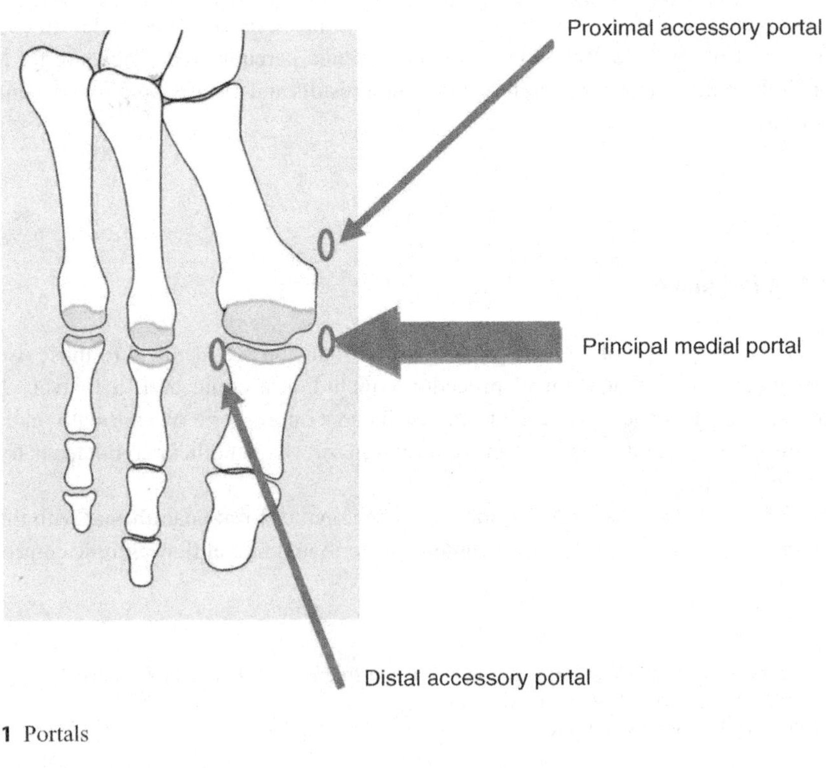

Fig. 6.1 Portals

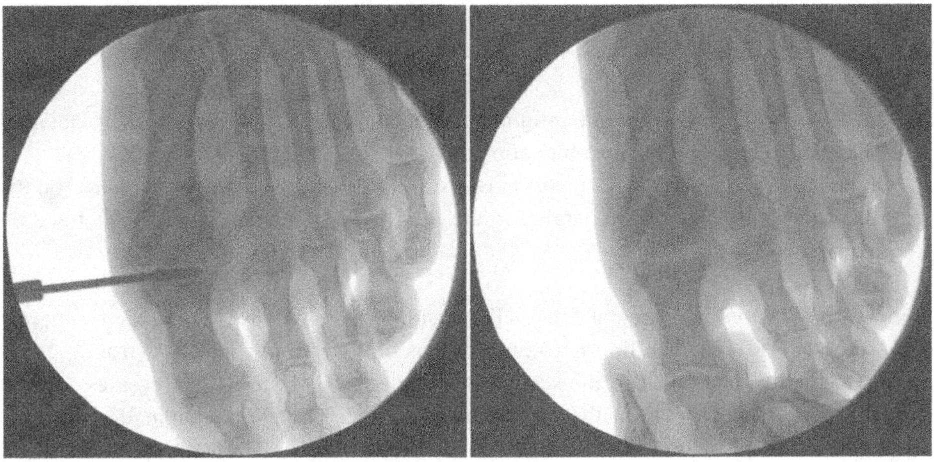

Fig.6.2 Preparationofthe bone s urfaces

traction on the hallux. Cartilage resection and bony areas preparation are performed with the burr under fluoroscopic control to assess both quantity and quality of bone resection. In this technique the fusion site is prepared by cutting two flat and parallel surfaces. The preparation of this area is the most difficult step of this procedure and the main risk is to have an asymmetrical resection. Some pitfalls must be avoided:

- Excessive metatarsal bone resection: the bone of the proximal phalanx is more dense than the bone of the metatarsal head, and the burr will tend to remove the weakest bone, on the metatarsal side. The risk is to obtain an excessive bone resection on the metatarsal head with first metatarsal shortening, loss of primary stability, metatarsus elevatus positioning of the arthrodesis with an increased risk of transfer metatarsalgia. It is thus important to control the burr and press more on the proximal phalanx than on the metatarsal head and assess the progression of the resection with fluoroscopic control.
- Excessive dorsal resection: it is often more difficult to reach the plantar part of the MTP1 joint than the dorsal part, and again the burr will tend to remove the bone easiest to reach, on the dorsal portion of the joint. The risk is to obtain an asymmetrical V-shaped bone resection from excessive dorsal resection with loss of primary stability and positioning of the arthrodesis with excessive dorsal flexion of P1. Bone preparation with the burr must be performed with continuous gentle traction on the hallux to open the MTP1 joint, to facilitate the access on the plantar part, to control bone resection and have parallel cuts on lateral fluoroscopic view.

After bone resection, the bone debris are evacuated with rasps and the arthrodesis site is abundantly washed with normal saline to avoid prolonged inflammation.

MTP1 arthrodesis positioning: Contact between P1 and M1 is obtained by pressure in the axis of the first ray and the position is maintained with an oblique Kirschner wire.

The positioning of the arthrodesis is assessed clinically and under fluoroscopic control:

- On AP view (Fig. 6.3): first ray alignment or slight valgus, first ray length, metatarso-phalangeal bone contact, no subluxation.
- On lateral view (Fig. 6.4): P1 position is assessed using a flat metal tray applied on the sole of the foot. P1 must be parallel to the floor plane with good bone contact and no plantar-flexion.

Arthrodesis fixation: the percutaneous MTP1 fusion is fixed with two cannulated compression screws (Fig. 6.5). The first Kirschner wire is oblique from P1 to M1 (from medial-distal to lateral-proximal), and the second is oblique from M1 to P1 and crosses the first Kirschner wire at the level of the first metatarsal head. The two cannulated screws are inserted and compression is obtained alternately on each screw. The stability of the MTP1 arthrodesis in dorsal and plantar flexion is then controlled and all the portals are closed (Fig. 6.6).

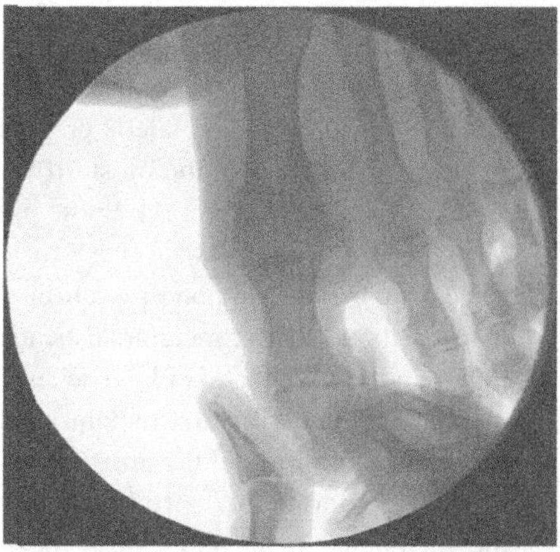

Fig. 6.3 Arthrodesis positioning on antero-posterior view

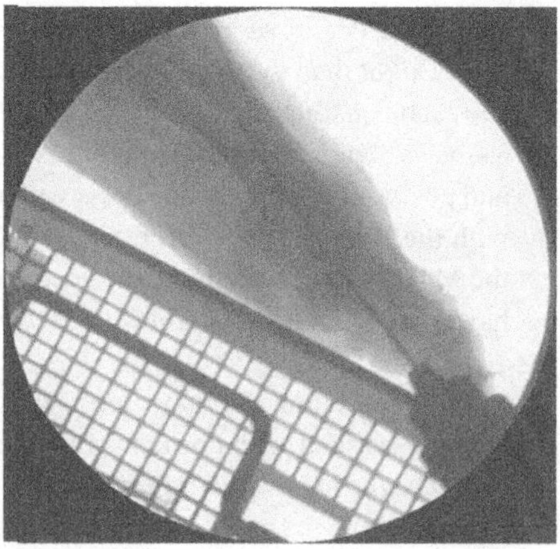

Fig. 6.4 Arthrodesis positioning on lateral view

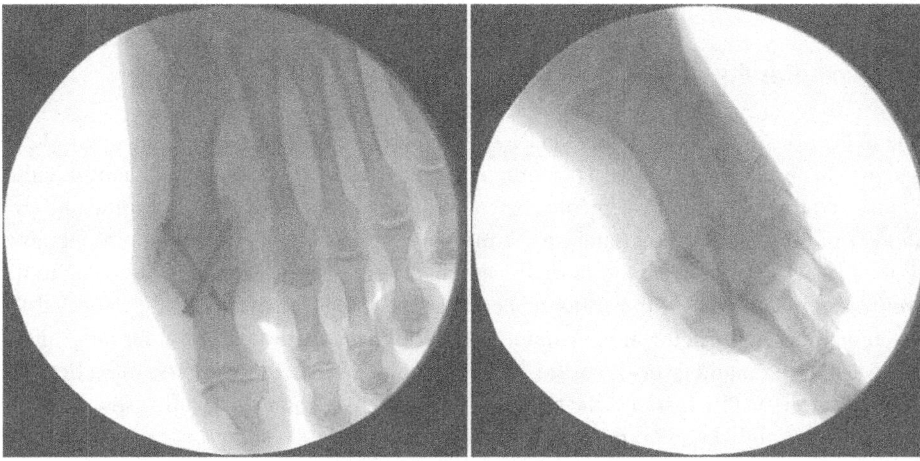

Fig.6. 5 Arthrodesisfi xation

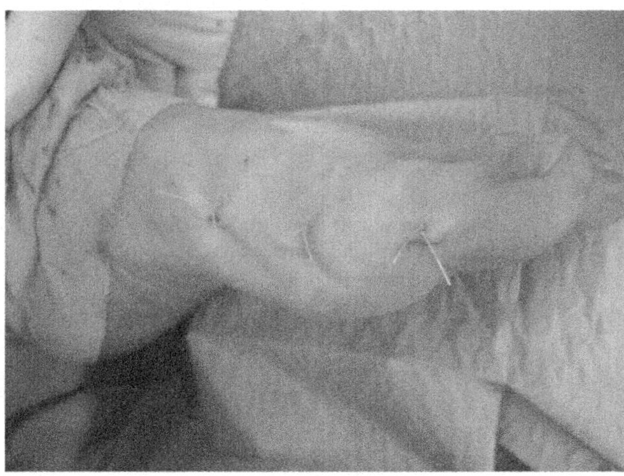

Fig.6. 6 Post-operativev iew afters kins uture

6.3 Post-OperativeC are

Percutaneous MTP1 fusion is performed in outpatients. The first dressing is changed after 10 days, and then a less bulky dressing is applied with a cohesive bandage. Immediate full weight bearing is authorized with a post-operative shoe with a flat and rigid insole. Radiographs are taken after 10 days and 1 month. Normal shoes are worn after 1 month according to clinical and radiographic findings.

6.4 Indications:R esults

The indications for percutaneous MTP1 fusion are basically the same as for open MTP1 fusion. This procedure is mainly performed for the treatment of severe and painful hallux rigidus and functional improvement is better and faster achieved in case of painful and stiff hallux rigidus with a compensatory hypermobility of the IP joint. Without a pre-operative IP joint hypermobility return to normal walking and shoe wearing can be slow due to the progressive adaptation of the IP joint. Percutaneous MTP1 fusion can be performed for severe hallux valgus deformity, symptomatic hallux varus, complex forefoot deformities (in case of rheumatoid arthritis) or for failed previous forefoot surgery. The main limit for a percutaneous MTP1 fusion is the presence of an extensive bone loss with a short first ray and indication for a bone graft.

Thirty-two percutaneous MTP1 joint fusions were analyzed in a prospective continuous series including 30 patients with an average age of 66. The indications for MTP1 joint fusion were symptomatic hallux rigidus or hallux rigido-valgus in most of the cases. All the patients underwent the same percutaneous procedure, in 1-day surgery for 26 cases. Clinical results were assessed with the functional AOFAS forefoot scoring system pre-operatively and at the latest follow-up. Radiographic analysis focused on the positioning and quality of bone fusion of the procedure. No patient was lost at a mean follow up of 18 months. The functional AOFAS score improved in all patients from a mean 36/100 pre-operatively to a mean 80/100 post-operatively ($p = 0.02$). Thirty patients were satisfied or very satisfied with the final outcome of the procedure, one patient was disappointed, and one was not satisfied. For the satisfied or very satisfied patients, normal shoe wearing was achieved after a mean 50 days. At plain radiography, fusion was obtained in 31 cases on 32. Post-operative mean dorsal flexion of the MTP1 joint fusion was 21° (range 15° to 35°).

6.5 Discussion

Percutaneous MTP1 fusion is a simple and quick procedure which can achieve functional results comparable to those obtained with open MTP1 fusion with more than 90% of patients satisfied.[7,13–17]

In open MTP1 fusion, the method of bone preparing requires a large approach with a risk of post-operative prolonged pain and swelling or wound healing difficulties.[6,7] One of the benefits of the percutaneous MTP1 fusion is the decreased morbidity, with few patients reporting pain and scar problems, and the procedure can be performed on an outpatient basis with immediate full weight bearing.

Bone preparation is a crucial step of this procedure, and requires experience in percutaneous forefoot surgery. In this technique, bone cuts are flat and any mistake on the preparation will have an impact on the positioning of the arthrodesis. Bone resection with the burr must be controlled to avoid any bone loss or asymmetrical resection that would affect primary stability and bone contact of the arthrodesis. A cup-and-cone configuration of bone preparation is more sound than flat bone cuts either for biomechanical reasons and for the arthrodesis positioning that is simpler without first ray shortening.[10,13] However, this method of preparing the fusion site cannot be undertaken percutaneously.

Arthrodesis positioning is perhaps the most critical of all the technical considerations. It is not only a problem of alignment of the hallux in terms of valgus/varus, dorsal flexion/plantar flexion or medial rotation/lateral rotation, but also a question of metatarsus varus, metatarsal length, hindfoot positioning (valgus flatfoot, pes cavus), forefoot symptoms (metatarsalgias, lesser toes deformities) and shoe wear habits (flat shoes or high heel shoes).[3–7] Arthrodesis positioning is easy to perform percutaneously, and the various stages of the procedures can be followed clinically and with fluoroscopy. A flat metallic tray to reproduce the effect of weight bearing is useful to judge accurately the appropriate position of the hallux.[6,7]

The fixation with cannulated compression crossed screws is a very simple technique but is not biomechanically the most stable technique. It is therefore important to assess with accuracy the position of the screws.[7]

6.6 Conclusion

Percutaneous MTP1 fusion is a simple procedure providing comparable results to fusions performed with open techniques. Post-operative care is simplified, with immediate full weight bearing on rigid flat shoes and quick return to normal walking. Bone preparation is an important step and requires an experience in percutaneous forefoot surgery. Arthrodesis positioning and fixation with this percutaneous procedure are simple to verify clinically radiolographically. The indications for percutaneous MTP1 fusion are those of the open procedure, and only severe bone loss or osteoporosis can be, in our hands, relative contraindicationst ous et hist echnique.

References

1. Mann RA, Oates JC. Arthrodesis of the first metatarsophalangeal joint. *Foot Ankle.* 1980;1:159–166.
2. DeFrino PF, Brodsky JW, Pollo F et al. First metatarsophalangeal arthrodesis: a clinical, pedobarographic and gait analysis study. *Foot Ankle Int.*2002; 23:496–502.
3. Conti SF, Dhawan S. Arthrodesis of the first metatarsophalangeal and interphalangeal joints of the foot. *Foot Ankle Clin N Am.*1996; 1:33–53.
4. Harper MC. Positioning of the hallux for first metatarsophalangeal joint arthrodesis. *Foot Ankle Int.*1997;18 :827.
5. Alexander IJ. Hallux metatarsophalangeal joint arthrodesis. In: Kitaoka HB, ed. *Masters Techniques in Foot and Ankle Surgery.* 2nd ed. Philadelphia, PA: Lippincott Williams and Wilkins;2002: 45–60.

6. Kelikian AS. Technical considerations in hallux metatarsophalangeal arthrodesis. *Foot Ankle Clin N Am.*2005; 10:167–190.
7. Womack JW, Ishikawa SN. First metatarsophalangeal arthrodesis. *Foot Ankle Clin N Am.* 2009;14:43–50.
8. Chana GS, Andrew TA, Cotterill CP. A simple method of arthrodesis of the first metatarsophalangeal joint. *J Bone Joint Surg (Br).*1984; 66:703–705.
9. Wu KK. Fusion of the metatarsophalangeal joint of the great toe with Herbert screws. *Foot Ankle.*1993;14:165–169.
10. Curtis MJ, Myerson M, Jinnah RH et al. Arthrodesis of the first metatarsophalangeal joint: a biomechanical study of internal fixation techniques. *Foot Ankle Int.*1993; 14:395–399.
11. Rongstad DJ, Miller GJ, Vadergriend RA et al. A biomechanical comparison of four fixation methods of first metatarsophalangeal joint arthrodesis. *Foot Ankle Int.*1994; 15:415–419.
12. Watson AD, Kelikian AS. Cost-effectiveness comparison of three methods of internal fixation for arthrodesis of the first metatarsophalangeal joint. *Foot Ankle Int.*1998; 19:304–310.
13. Goucher NR, Coughlin MJ. Hallux metatarsophalangeal joint arthrodesis using dome-shaped reamers and dorsal plate fixation: a prospective study. *Foot Ankle Int.*2006; 27:869–876.
14. Coughlin MJ, Shurnas PS. Hallux rigidus: grading and long-term results of operative treatment. *J Bone Joint Surg (Am).*2003; 85A:2072–2088.
15. Flavin R, Stephens MM. Arthrodesis of the first metatarsophalangeal joint using a dorsal titanium contoured plate. *Foot Ankle Int.*2004; 25:783–787.
16. Brodsky JW, Passmore RN, Pollo FE et al. Functional outcome of arthrodesis of the first metatarsophalangeal joint using parallel screw fixation. *Foot Ankle Int.*2005; 26:140–146.
17. Yee G, Lau J. Current concepts review: hallux rigidus. *Foot Ankle Int.*2008; 29:637–646.

The Reverdin-Isham Procedure for the Correction of Hallux valgus

7

A Distal Metatarsal Osteotomy Procedure Using Minimall nvasive Technique

Stephen A. Ishama nd Orlando E. Nunez

Hallux valgus is perhaps one of the most challenging of all forefoot deformities facing the surgeon today. More than 150 procedures have been developed during the last century to correct hallux valgus deformity. The first metatarso-phalangeal joint supports 125% of the weight of a walking person during the propulsive phase of gait, and must perform this function thousands of times a day for a lifetime.

The minimally invasive Reverdin-Isham procedure is highly effective in a wide range of bunion deformities. The definition, cause, and classification of hallux valgus, the Reverdin-Isham procedure with its preoperative criteria, the techniques of operation, post-operative management, and the advantages and disadvantages are presented.

7.1 Definition

Hallux valgus is a combination of a transverse and frontal plane deformity of the hallux on the first metatarso-phalangeal head. This frequent deformity exists with progressive abduction and pronation of the first phalanx, abduction, pronation, and elevation of the first metatarsal with lateral capsule retraction of this joint. This results in the hallux being laterally deviated toward the lesser digits, and rotated into pronation with its dorsal surface

S.A.Is ham(✉)
SanFra nciscoH ospital,Sa natorioS anF rancisco, MexicoD F, Mexico
ema il:dris ham@frontier.com

N. Maffulli and M. Easley (eds.), *Minimally Invasive Surgery of the Foot and Ankle*,
DOI: 10.1007/978-1-84996-417-3_7, © Springer-Verlag London Limited 2011

more medially. Most bunions, mild, moderate, or severe, contain some combination of these deformities. These deformities involve both soft tissue and osseous components, producing, respectively, positional and structural deformities.

7.2 Etiology

The primary cause of hallux valgus is a congenitally abnormal foot structure, which is exposed to abnormal pronatory forces resulting in hypermobility of the joints of the foot and an overdependence on soft tissues for stability during weight bearing, especially during the last phase of the propulsive stage of gait. The severity of hallux valgus is proportional to the severity of the abnormal pronatory forces present.

Other causes of hallux valgus deformities are systemic disease, such as gouty or rheumatoid arthritis, neurologic disorders, and trauma causing permanent osseous or soft-tissue damage to the first metatarso-phalangeal joint. The progression and severity of hallux valgus increase when more than one cause is present. Footwear, although not a primary cause, can aggravate the symptoms of the deformity.

7.3 Classification

Appropriate classification of the deformities enables the surgeon to select or modify a procedure to achieve the best results for a given patient. To classify the severity of a hallux valgus deformity, we use the following measurements: hallux abductus angle, distal articular set angle, proximal articular set angle, first intermetatarsal angle, and first metatarso-phalangeal joint position.

7.3.1 HalluxA bductusA ngle

The hallux abductus angle (HA angle) is formed by the bisection of the longitudinal axis of the first proximal phalanx and the longitudinal axis of the first metatarsal. The normal angle formed by these lines is between 5° and 15°.

7.3.2 Distal Articular Set Angle

The distal articular set angle (DASA) is formed by the bisection of the longitudinal axis of the proximal phalanx and the line drawn perpendicular to the articular surface of the base of the proximal phalanx.

7.3.3
Proximal Articular Set Angle

The proximal articular set angle (PASA) is formed by the bisection of the longitudinal axis of the first metatarsal and the active cartilage of the head of the first metatarsal (DMMA).

7.3.4
FirstI ntermetatarsalA ngle

The first intermetatarsal angle is formed by the bisection of the line of the longitudinal axis of the first and second metatarsals. Normal range is between 6° and 8°.

7.3.5
First Metatarso-Phalangeal Joint Position

Thefi rst metatarso-phalangeal joint (MTPJ) position has three components:

- Congruous – The articular surface of the first MTPJ is parallel or equal.
- Deviated – The articular surface of the first MTPJ is unequal. The lines of intersection fall outside the joint.
- Subluxed – The articular surface of the first MTPJ is unequal with lines of intersection intersecting inside of the MTPJ.

The presence of a deviated or subluxed joint position is evidence of the presence of increasedpos itionalde formity(Fig. 7.1).

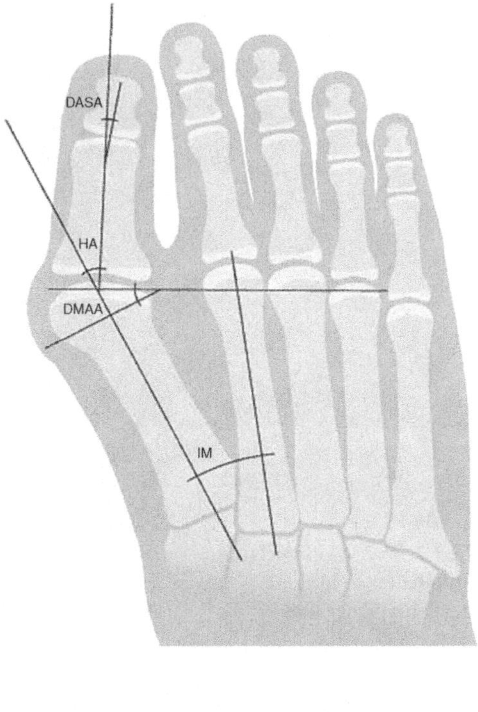

Fig.7.1 The presence of a deviated or subluxed joint position is evidence of the presenceofinc reasedpos itionalde formity

7.4 Classification of Hallux valgus

Hallux valgus deformity is classified into three classes: mild, moderate, and severe.

7.4.1 MildH alluxv algus

In these patients, there is a hallux abductus angle of 5–20°, and a first intermetatarsal angle of 6° to 8°. The MTPJ surface is generally congruous (Fig. 7.2).

7.4.2 ModerateH alluxv algus

Patients with moderate hallux valgus exhibit a hallux abductus angle between 20° and 40°, and a first intermetatarsal angle of 8° and 15°. The first MTPJ is generally deviated (Fig. 7.3).

7.4.3 SevereH alluxv algus

Deformities of severe hallux valgus contain a hallux abductus angle of 40° or greater. The first intermetatarsal angle is 15° or greater. The MTPJ is usually subluxed (Fig. 7.4).

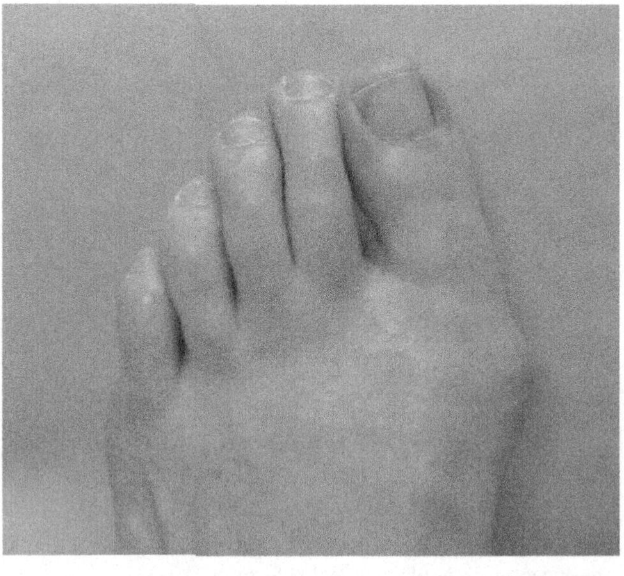

Fig.7. 2 The MTPJ surface in mild hallux valgus is generallyc ongruous

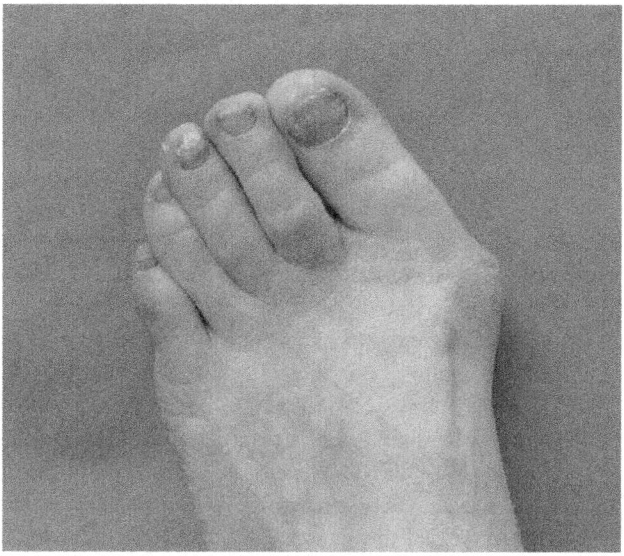

Fig. 7.3 The first MTPJ is generally deviated in moderate hallux valgus

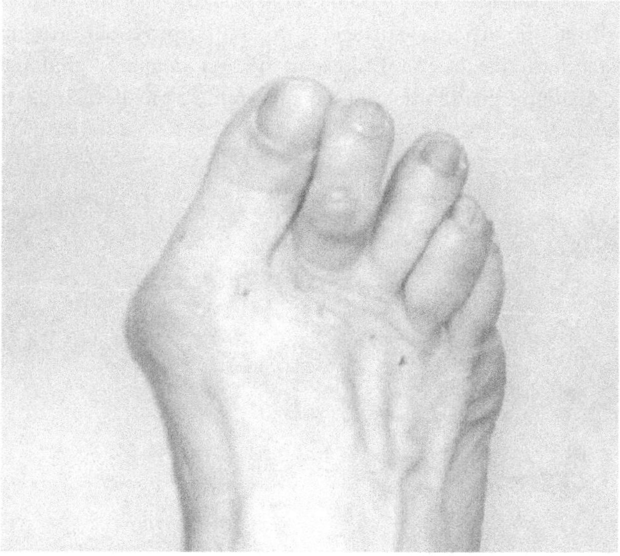

Fig. 7.4 The MTPJ is usually subluxed in severe hallux valgus

7.5 Reverdin-Isham Procedure

Prior to 1985, minimal incision hallux valgus corrective procedures available to the surgeon, with the exception of a Wilson bunionectomy, although highly effective, were a compromise and failed to take into consideration the importance of the proximal articular set angle. An increased proximal articular set angle in the HAV deformity results in instability of the MTPJ and increased structural and positional forces that increase the first intermetatarsal angle and the hallux abductus angles. From a structural view point, a joint that is straight on a metatarsal bone is more stable than one that is set at an angle. This confirms the importance of the PASA (DMMA) in producing a hallux valgus deformity, and the need to reduce it in hallux valgus corrective surgery.

In the early 1980s, Isham perfected the hallux valgus corrective procedure using minimally invasive surgery. Using minimal incision techniques, Reverdin bunionectomies were performed. These minimal incision Reverdin bunionectomies proved to be superior to previously used procedures in the correction of the involved structural positional components of HAV disorders. As with large incision Reverdin bunionectomy procedures, in which a medial wedge osteotomy was performed through the first metatarsal head dorsal to plantar perpendicular to the weight-bearing surface of the first metatarsal, degenerative joint disease resulted when the osteotomy was placed through the articular surface on the plantar aspect of the head of the first metatarsal. The osteotomy interfered with the normal function of the sesamoid bones, resulting in decreased range of motion at the MTPJ.

The author modified the Reverdin osteotomy with the Isham osteotomy by performing the medial wedge osteotomy in the head of the first metatarsal at an angle from dorsal distal, just proximal to the articular surface on the dorsal aspect of the head, to plantar proximal to a point just proximal to the articular surface on the plantar aspect of the first metatarsal head (Fig. 7.5a,b). This placement of the Isham osteotomy preserves and repositions the articular surface, corrects the proximal articular set angle, and redirects and stabilizes the structural forces at the first metatarso-phalangeal head. The placement of the osteotomy inside the joint capsule in the cancellous bone of the first metatarsal head was

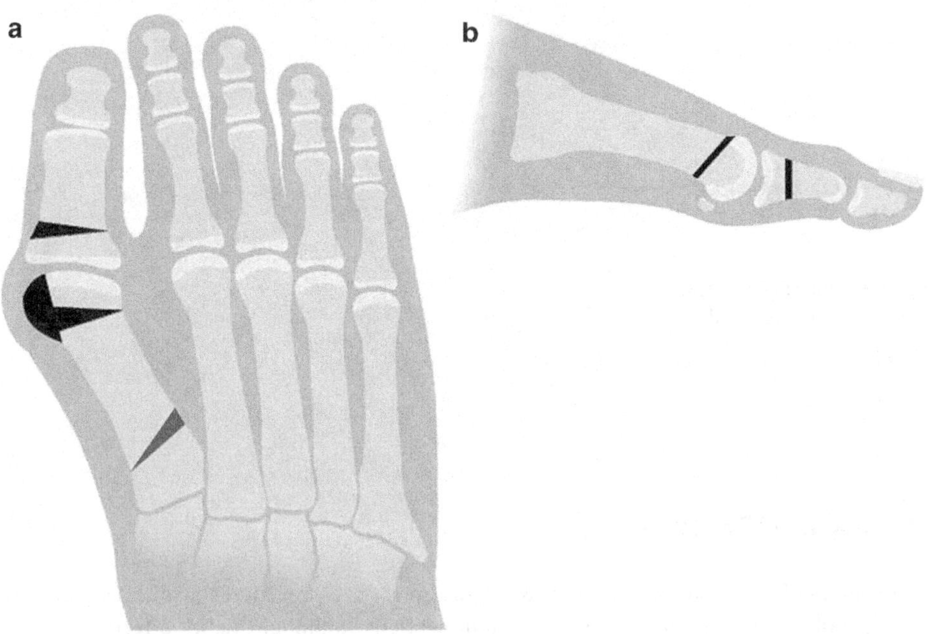

Fig. 7.5 The Isham modification of Reverdin osteotomy starts by undertaking a medial wedge osteotomy in the head of the first metatarsal from dorsal distal, just proximal to the articular surface on the dorsal aspect of the head, to plantar proximal to a point just proximal to the articular surface on the plantar aspect of the firstm etatarsalhe ad

highly stable, and eliminated the need for internal fixation. As hoped, the post operative management proved to be the same as is needed for the minimal incision Silver-Akin procedure or modified McBride-Akin. No increased pain or disability was noted. Marked improvement of short and long term results were immediately apparent.

7.6
PreoperativeC riteria

This procedure is directed at the structural correction of the deformities of HAV that are manifested at the metatarsal head. Specific criteria for the Reverdin-Isham procedure are;

- As ymptomaticm edialbuni onde formity
- good range of motion for the first MTPJ; no pain, no crepitus, and no degenerative changes
- congruousde viatedj oint
- An intermetatarsal angle of 20° or less for straight foot and 16° or less for an adducted foot
- Ani ncreasedP ASA
- normalD ASA
- HA angle measurements that are from slightly too highly abnormal
- hallux axial rotation that is mild or absent
- Relative metatarsal protrusion that is normal to positive

If the DASA is abnormal, then the Reverdin-Isham procedure should be combined with an Akin procedure. A plantarflexed first metatarsal may or may not be present. Another procedure to correct a plantarflexed metatarsal is not needed.

7.7
Operative Technique

The Reverdin-Isham procedure is performed by combining several minimally invasive procedures. The first being an exostectomy of the dorsal medial aspect of the first metatarsal head, a distal metatarsal osteotomy, a Reverdin-Isham, an adductor release, and finally an Akin phalangeal osteotomy.

7.8
Minimallyl nvasive Technique

A 0.5–1 cm longitudinal incision is made on the plantar medial aspect of the first metatarsal head. The incision is carried deep through subcutaneous tissue to expose the capsule of the first MTPJ. A capsulotomy is performed, and the dorsal medial aspect of the head is freed of the capsule and ligamentous attachments. The medial eminence is then resected using a bone reducing Burr 3.1 wedge (Vilex, 111 Moffitt Street, McMinnville, TN 37110, USA). The dorsal eminence and the tibial sesamoid is palpated and identified through the skin. A bone cutting instrument (e.g., Isham Straight Flute, Burr, Vilex, 111 Moffitt Street, McMinnville, TN 37110, USA) is inserted into the incision, and an angular medial wedge osteotomy is performed from dorsal distal to plantar proximal in the metaphyseal portion of the head of the first metatarsal. Care must be taken to preserve the lateral cortex and the articular surface of the halluxal sesamoids and the dorsal articular surface of the head. The use of a fluoroscope facilitates placement of the osteotomy and indicates the amount of bone to be removed. The hallux is then rotated into adductus, and the osteotomy is compressed and closed. Remaining osseous structures are rasped smooth.

Attention is then directed to the lateral aspect of the first MTPJ, where a 0.5 cm oblique incision is made over the first MTPJ. The incision is deepened, a lateral capsulotomy and an adducto hallucis tenotomy is performed (Fig. 7.6). Skin edges are approximated using 4–0 nonabsorbable suture. If indicated by an increased distal articular set angle, an Akin procedure is performed. An Akin procedure is indicated in most patients. The wound is dressed, and a position is maintained with a sterile splint dressing of the surgeon's choice.

7.9 PostoperativeM anagement

The patient is given a surgical shoe and discharged. The patient is allowed to increase weight bearing as tolerated. Postoperative pain, as with most ambulatory procedures, may require minimal amounts of pain control medication. Many patients take none.

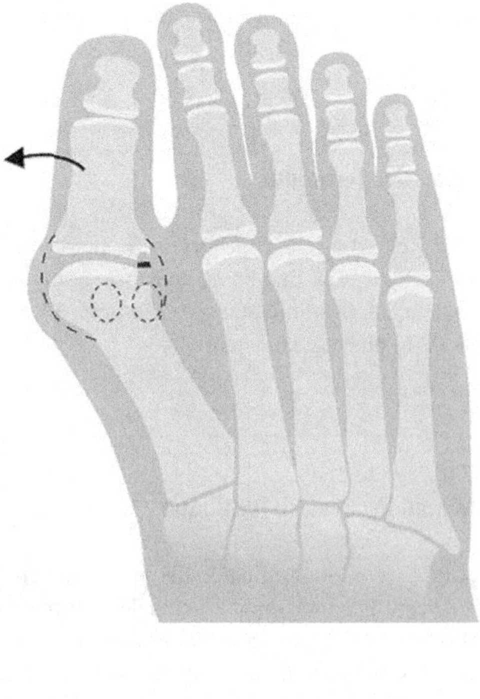

Fig.7. 6 The lateral aspect of the first MTPJ, where a 0.5 cm oblique incision is made over the first MTPJ. The incision is deepened, a lateral capsulotomy and a tenotomy of the adductor hallucis is performed

The dressing is changed on day 2 or 3 after surgery, and the sutures are removed at this time. A splint dressing is reapplied. The second dressing change occurs 1 week after surgery, and a removable splint dressing is applied and changed daily by the patient. Bathing is then permitted. The patient is allowed to ambulate in the self surgical shoe or a supportive athletic-type shoe until normal shoes can be worn. Postoperative radiographs are taken on the first redressing and again 3–4 weeks after surgery for evaluation of healing. It should be noted that, as with an Austin-type bunionectomy, a minimal amount of bony callous formation is expected.

7.10 PostoperativeB andaging

Minimal incision procedures, by design, are very atraumatic, with a minimal amount of soft-tissue disruption. A second metatarsal, for example, has seven tendons passing over the MTPJ. These tendons pass over the dorsal, medial, plantar, and lateral aspects of the MTPJ. The head of the second metatarsal is also stabilized by a strong intermetatarsal ligament, attached to the third, fourth, and fifth metatarsals. A properly performed osteotomy at the proximal aspect of the metatarsal head does not disrupt these soft-tissue structures. These structures, during the initial postoperative healing phase of the first 3–6 weeks, contract and stabilize the osteotomy site. We call this contracture of the soft tissues "intrinsic fixation." Although internal fixation is not required, external splinting is required to enable the patient to bear weight.

Postoperative splint dressings in minimal incision foot surgery should stabilize the surgical site in its corrected position, be a comfort to the patient that is easy to apply, and maintain a sterile barrier.

Postoperative dressings are presented in two phases. The first phase represents the type of dressing used during the first postoperative week. These dressings are applied by the surgeon. The second phase of the dressings consists of splint dressings used for the following 4 weeks. Figure 7.7a,b,c depict phase one dressing, and Fig. 7.8 depicts phase two dressing. The phase two dressings are initially applied by the surgeon and are changed daily by the patients after they have been instructed in their application. Bathing is permitted on a daily basis after the firstpos toperativew eek.

7.11 Advantages of the Reverdin-Isham Procedure

- Good healing as the osteotomy is performed in metaphyseal bone.
- Minimal fixation (internal or external) is required because the procedure is intracapsular and compressed by the retrograde force of the hallux.
- It provides biplane correction of the structural deformity with improved positions of sesamoids.

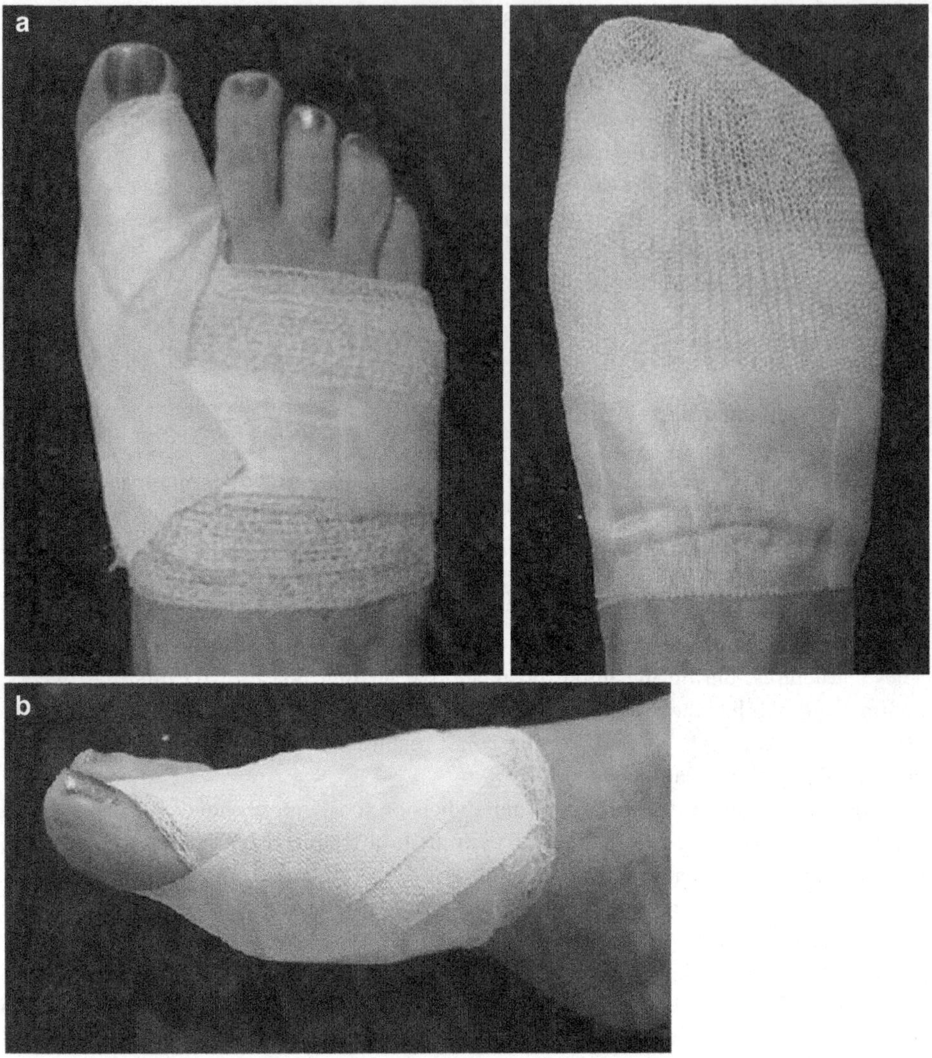

Fig.7. 7 Postoperative dressings are presented in two phases: phase one dressing

- It involves minimal amount of postoperative disability, similar to the minimal incision Silver-Akinpr ocedure.
- It can be performed on children prior to epiphyseal closure because the epiphysis is located at the metatarsal base.
- It can be performed in the presence of uncontrollable pronatory forces.
- The average reduction of the intermetatarsal angle of 7° has been noted, especially when the procedure is performed with the Akin procedure.

Fig. 7.8 Postoperativedr essingsa re presented in two phases: phase two dressing

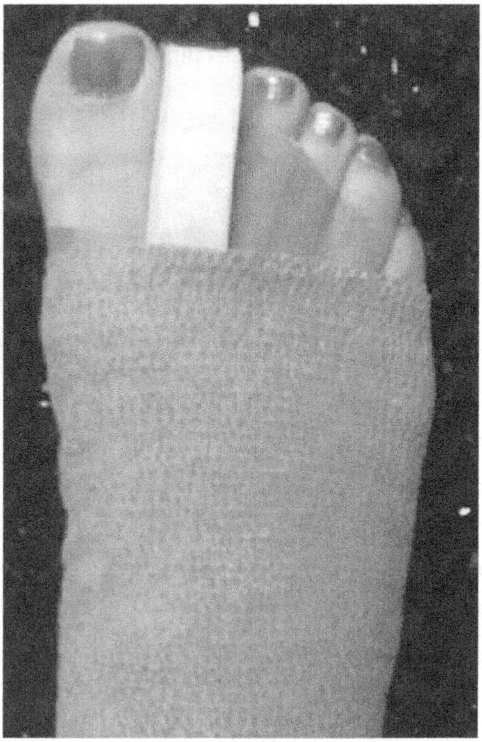

7.12 Disadvantages of the Reverdin-Isham Procedure

- The sagittal plane deformity may not be corrected, however, with reduction of the first intermetatarsal angle; relative sagittal place correction is noted. With a modified Reverdin-Isham, in which the head is slid laterally, the sagittal plane correction is obtained when indicated.
- An average shortening of the first metatarsal of 5 mm should be expected. If poor healing at the osteotomy site occurs, greater shortening of the firstm etatarsali spos sible.

7.13 Summary

The Reverdin-Isham procedure is a distal metatarsal osteotomy procedure that has stood the test of time. If the IMA needs to be corrected, the Reverdin-Isham procedure will involve an osteotomy of the lateral cortex, allowing the metatarsal head to be shifted laterally, directly reducing the intermetatarsal angle. Another option is a closing wedge osteotomy of the first metatarsal base. Using one or more of these modifications, the surgeonc anc orrects evereha lluxva lgusde formities.

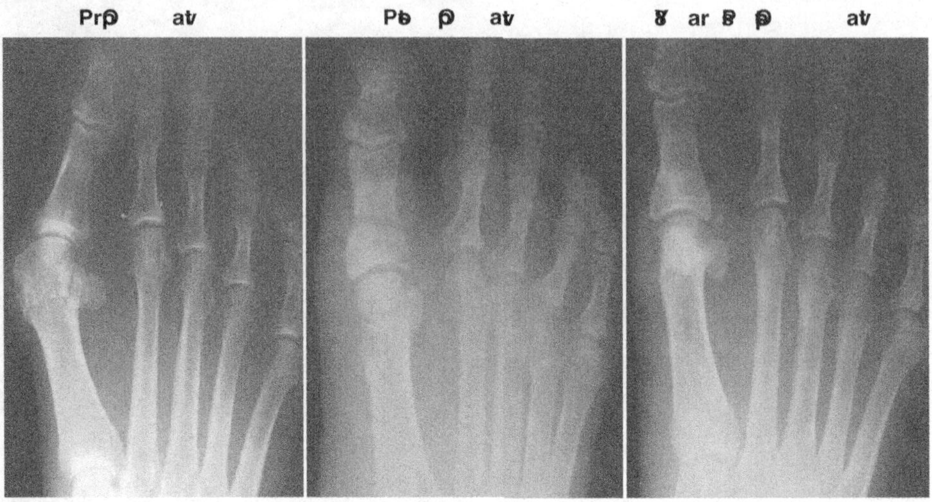

Fig. 7.9 X-ray example of the Reverdin-Isham and associate procedures pre operatively, post operatively and eight years post operatively

References

1. Akin OF. The treatment of hallux valgus: A new operative procedure and its results. *Med Sentinal.*1925;33 :678–679.
2. Colloff B, Weitz EN. Proximal phalangeal osteotomy and hallux valgus. *Clin Orthop.* 1967;54:105.
3. Funk JF, Wells R. Bunionectomy with distal osteotomy. *Clin Orthop Rel Res.*J une1972.
4. GerbertJ . *Textbook of Bunion Surgery.* Mount Kisco, New York: Futura Publishing; 1981.
5. Gerbert J, Melillo T. A modified Akin procedure for the correction of hallux valgus. *J Am Podiatric Assoc.* 1971;61:132.
6. Gertbert J, Mercado OA, Sokoloff TH. The surgical treatment of hallux abducto-valgus and allied deformities. In: Fielding MD, ed. *Podiatric Medicine and Surgery: Monograph Series.* Mount Kisco, New York: Futura Publishing; 1973.
7. Isham SA. The Reverdin-Isham procedure for the correction of hallux valgus. *Curr Podiatric Med.*J une1985: 11–13.
8. Kelikian H. *Hallux Valgus, Allied Deformities of the Forefoot and Metatarsalgia.* Philadelphia, PA: W.B. Saunders Co; 1965.
9. Maffulli N. Minimally invasive surgery in orthopedic surgery. *Orthop Clin North Am.* October 2009;40:441–568.
10. Peabody CW. Surgical cure of hallux valgus. *J Bone Joint Surg.*1931; 13A:273.
11. PodiatricsSino- AmericanC onferenceO nFoot D isorders.O ctober1987,B eijing,C hina.

Arthroscopic Assisted Correction of Hallux valgusDe formity

8

Tun Hing Lui

8.1 Introduction

Endoscopic assisted distal soft-tissue correction for hallux valgus deformity follows the same principle of the open procedure.[1–3] This approach is indicated with symptomatic hallux valgus with an incongruent metatarsophalangeal joint and no significant bony abnormality (e.g., severe hallux valgus interphalangeus or abnormal distal metatarsal articular angle). It is contraindicated if the intermetatarsal angle cannot be corrected manually (e.g., presence of os intermetatarseum). Sometimes, the correction may be obstructed by the dislocated fibular sesamoid bone in the web space. This is not a contraindication of the procedure, since the sesamoid can be reduced after lateral release and the intermetatarsal space can then be closed up. Osteoarthritis of the first metatarso-phalangeal joint and deformity resulting from neuromuscular conditions are other contraindications.

Endoscopic assisted distal soft-tissue correction for hallux valgus deformity has the advantages of better assessment of sesamoid reduction, and avoids the need for metatarsal osteotomy. The potential complications are similar to those of the open procedure, including recurrence of deformity, digital nerve injury, and implant failure.

8.2 Technique of Endoscopic Distal Soft Tissue Procedure

The patient is supine with an ipsilateral thigh tourniquet on the spread leg table. We use a 2.7 mm 30° arthroscope, an arthroscopic shaver and burr, retrograde knife and straight needle. The procedure has four steps. The first is lateral soft tissue release, the second is medial bunionectomy, and the third is reduction of the 1,2 intermetatarsal angle and fixation of the 1,2 metatarsals. The final step is plication of medial capsule.

T.H.Lui
Department of Orthopaedics and Traumatology, North District Hospital, 9 Po Kin Road, Sheung Shui, NT, Hong Kong SAR, China
e-mail:luithde rek@yahoo.co.uk

N. Maffulli and M. Easley (eds.), *Minimally Invasive Surgery of the Foot and Ankle*,
DOI: 10.1007/978-1-84996-417-3_8,

8.2.1 Lateral Soft Tissue Release

There are two approaches of the lateral soft tissue release: ligament sacrifying[1–3] and ligament preserving[4] approaches. The difference is whether the intermetatarsal ligament is cut or not.

8.2.1.1 Ligament Sacrifying Approach

For the lateral release, two portals are made, the plantar portal and the toe web portal. The toe web portal is established by a stab incision over the dorsum of the first web space, followed by blunt dissection of the subcutaneous tissue using a haemostat until the plantar surface of the intermetatarsal ligament is felt (sensation of hitting a wash board). The 2.7 mm arthroscopic cannula together with the trocar are passed through the toe web portal, and advanced proximally underneath the ligament. The plantar aponeurosis is then reached and pierced by the trocar. There should be minimal resistance before the plantar aponeurosis is reached. The trocar should be advanced gently to avoid injury to the plantar neurovascular structures, especially the medial digital nerve to the second toe. The plantar portal should be just proximal to the penetration point of the plantar aponeurosis to maximize the "working length" of the portal tract.

To have adequate working length, the plantar portal should be at the level of the tarso-metatarsal joint (Fig. 8.1). If the plantar portal is too distal, there will be inadequate working length. The cannula and the trocar are retrieved, and only the trocar is reinserted into the toe web portal and exits through the plantar portal. The arthroscopic cannula is then introduced through the plantar portal and exited through the toe web portal along the trocar (Fig. 8.2).

The trocar is then removed, and a 2.7 mm 30° arthroscope is introduced. The retrograde knife is then passed through the toe web portal under arthroscopic guidance until it reaches the proximal edge of the intermetatarsal ligament, the proximal edge of which is relatively

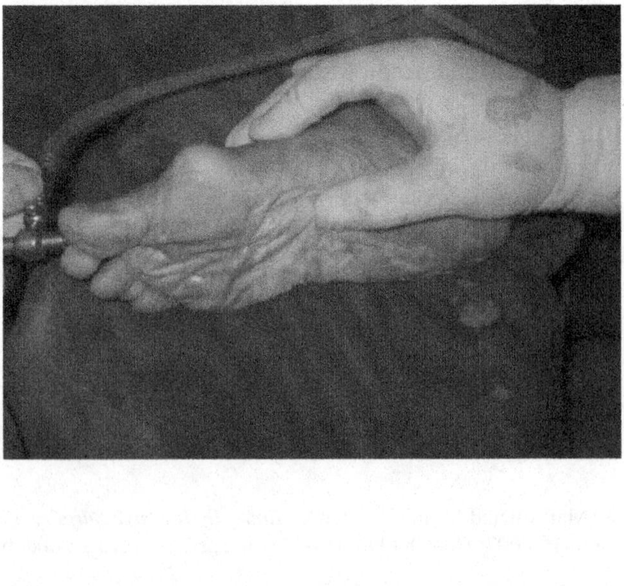

Fig. 8.1 The plantar portal is established immediate after the trocar has passed through the plantar aponeurosis at the level of tarso-metatarsal joint

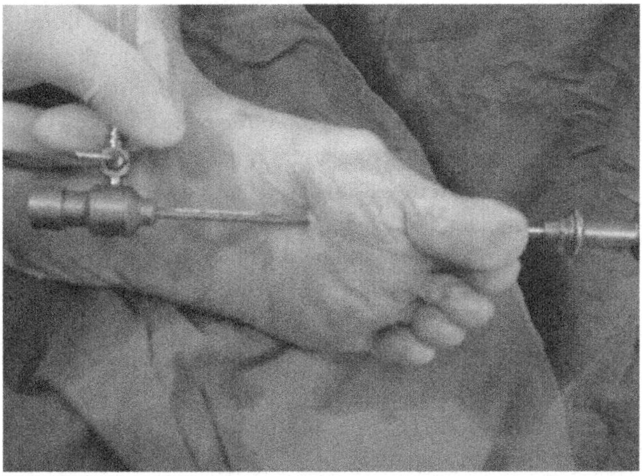

Fig. 8.2 The trocar is used as a guide rod for the introduction of the cannula throughthe pla ntarpor tal

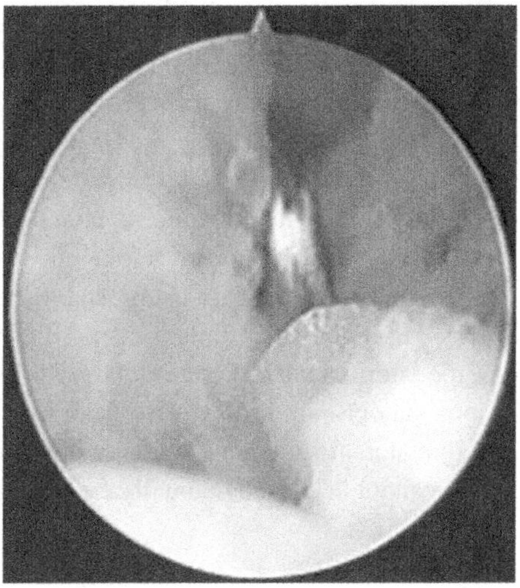

Fig. 8.3 Release of the intermetatarsal ligament byre trogradeknife

easy to identify by probing with the retrograde knife. The ligament is then released using the retrograde knife (Fig. 8.3).

After the ligament is released, the arthroscope is moved slightly dorsally through the cut ends of the ligament, and is turned 90° towards the hallux to visualise the insertion of the tendon of adductor hallucis (Fig. 8.4).

The insertion is released with the retrograde knife, and the fibular sesamoid bone can then been seen. The lateral capsule release is started a bit proximal to the fibular sesamoid bone and at the midpoint of metatarsal neck to avoid injury to the lateral digital nerve to the hallux. The release is progressed distally just dorsal to the fibular sesamoid bone to the base of proximal phalanx. This can release the metatarsal sesamoidal suspensory ligament and preserve the metatarso-phalangeal collateral ligament. To ensure that the phalangeal insertional band is released, the retrograde knife should be shifted slightly laterally when it hits the base of the proximal phalanx and finished the release of the band. This is important for the reduction of the sesamoid bones to the corresponding metatarsal grooves. However, it should be kept in mind that sudden "give way" after the release of the band may lead to accidental extension of the toe web portal wound.

After completion of the lateral release, the hallux valgus deformity and the sesamoid apparatus can be reduced by abducting and supinating the proximal phalanx. The lateral part of the metatarso-phalangeal joint and metatarso-sesamoid compartment can be examined by the arthroscope through the toe web portal (Fig. 8.5). During the lateral release, the instruments should be kept away from the fat tissue plantar to the intermetatarsal ligament to minimize the risk of injury to the digital nerve.

8.2.1.2 Ligament Preserving Approach

It is similar to the standard procedure except that the arthroscope is passed just dorsal to the intermetatarsal ligament. The intermetatarsal ligament is left intact, and only the insertion of the tendon of the adductor hallucis and the lateral capsular structures are released. This is technically more difficult, and may not have a protective role to the neurovascular structure.[4]

The degree of correction of the deformity can be checked by abducting and supinating the hallux and closing the intermetatarsal space manually. In case of total dislocation of the fibular sesamoid, it is useful to plantar flex the first metatarso-phalangeal joint to relax the plantar capsule and pass a haemostat through the toe web portal into the metarsosesamoid interval to reduce the fibular sesamoid. The correction can usually be maintained by closing the intermetatarsal space alone if the lateral release is adequate (Fig. 8.6). If the correction is suboptimal, it may arise from inadequate lateral release, inadequate closure of the intermetatarsal space or excessive pronation of the first metatarsal. If the intermetatarsal space cannot be closed manually even after adequate lateral soft tissue release, a metatarsal

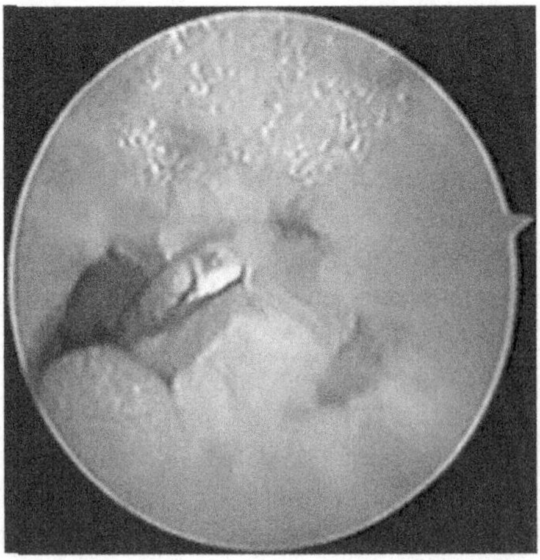

Fig.8. 4 The tendon of adductor hallucis insertioni sr eleased

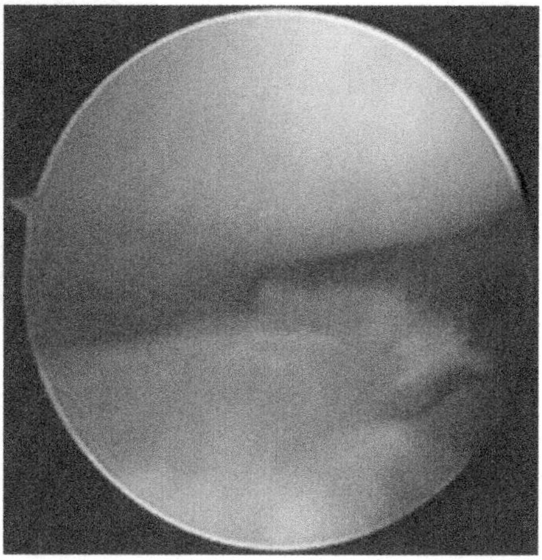

Fig. 8.5 Reduction of the fibular sesamoid to the corresponding metatarsal groove can be assessedthroughthe toe w ebpor tal

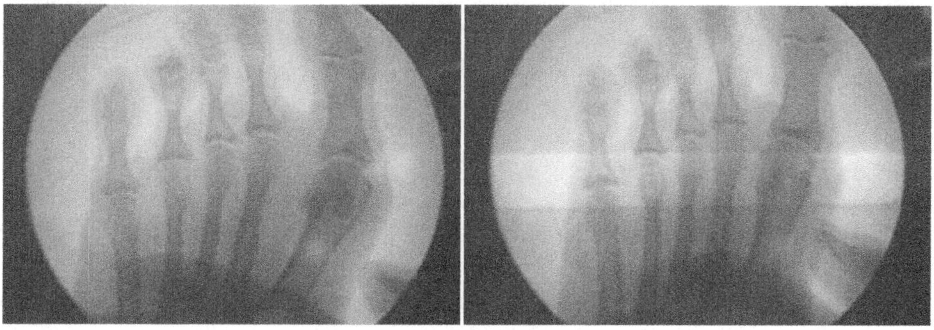

Fig. 8.6 After adequate lateral release, the sesamoid bones and the metatarso-phalangeal joint can be reduced by closure of the intermetatarsal space

osteotomy is indicated. In case of excessive metatarsal pronation, derotation of the metatarsal is needed before insertion of the positioning screw.

8.2.2
MedialE xostectomy

It relies on two portals on the medial aspect of the foot. The distal bunion portal is located at the mid-point of the medial side of the first metatarso-phalangeal joint, as the medial portal of the first metatarso-phalangeal arthroscopy. The proximal portal is at the level of the proximal pole of the bunion. They can be both viewing and working portals, depending on the stage of the procedure (Fig. 8.7). The first metatarso-phalangeal joint is examined through the distal bunion portal using a 1.9 mm arthroscope. An arthroscopic synovectomy is performed through the dorsolateral portal if synovitis is present and the patient complained of first metatarso-phalangeal joint pain with joint line tenderness.[3,5]

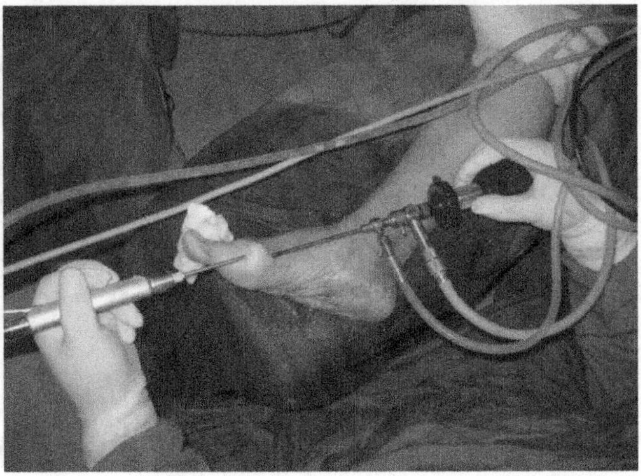

Fig. 8.7 Mediale xostectomy through the proximal and distalbuni onpor tals

The medial capsule is first stripped from the bony bunion using a small periosteal elevator through the proximal and distal portals. The bony prominence can be removed using arthroscopic burr under direct arthroscopic visualization, removing more bone dorsally. The adequacy of the exostectomy can be checked with fluroscopy.

8.2.3 Reduction and Fixation of Intermetatarsal Angle

A 2 mm bone tunnel of the neck of the first metatarsal is made through the proximal bunion portal. A long small catheter is passed through the bone tunnel, and the tip is caught with a haemostat through the toe web portal. The needle is removed, and the tip of the cannula is retrieved through the toe web portal and a double-stranded PDS 1 suture is passed from the proximal bunion portal to the toe web portal through the angiocath cannula to the toe web portal. The suture is then wrapped around the second metatarsal neck using an aneurysmal needle through the toe web portal. The suture is retrieved to the proximal bunion portal with a haemostat. The suture should be deep to the extensor tendons of both hallux and second toe and dorsal nerve and superficial to the dorsal capsule of the first metatarsophalangeal joint (Fig. 8.8). The first intermetatarsal space is closed manually and held with

Fig. 8.8 (**a**) A long angiocath is passed through the bone tunnel and the tip is caught by a haemostat through the toe web portal. (**b**) The needle is removed and the tip of the cannula is retrieved through the toe web portal. (**c**) A double-stranded PDS 1 suture is passed from the proximal bunion portal to the toe web portal through the angiocath cannula to the toe web portal. (**d**, **e**, **f**) The suture is then wrapped around the second metatarsal neck using an aneurysmal needle through the toe web portal. (**g**, **h**) The suture is retrieved from the proximal bunion portal with a haemostat. The suture should be deep to the extensor tendons of both hallux and second toe and dorsal nerve, and superficial to the dorsal capsule of the firstm etatarso-phalangealj oint

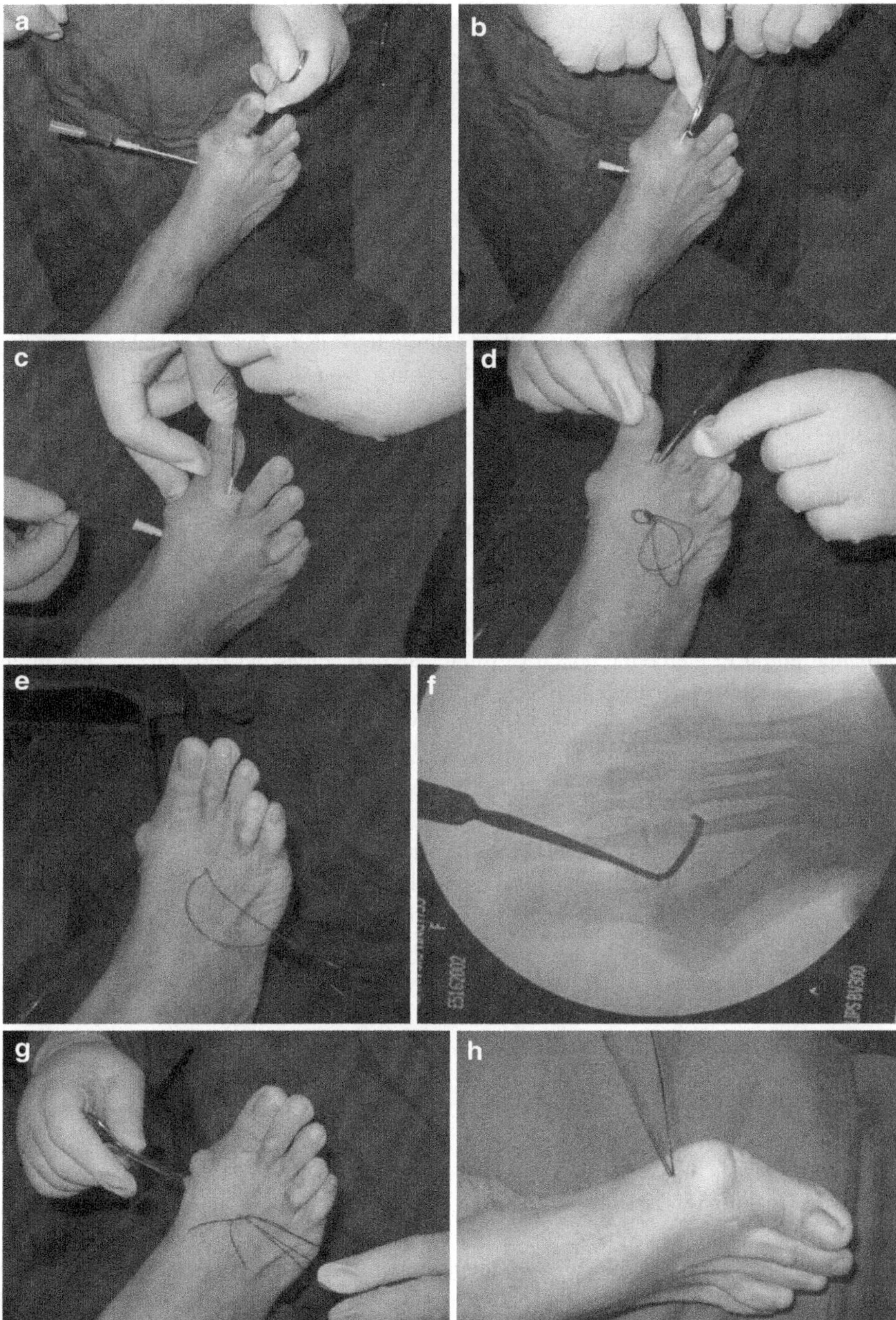
a
b
c
d
e
f
g
h

a 4.0 mm cannulated positioning screw bridging the bases of the two metatarsals.[6] The intermetatarsal sutures are then tied.

8.2.4 Plication of the Medial Capsule

The PDS-1 sutures with a cutting-tip curved eyed needle are prepared to plicate the medial capsule. The aim of medial capsular plication is to anchor the distal plantar corner of medial capsule to the proximal dorsal corner, to provide adduction and supination force to proximal phalanx.[1] The needle is introduced through the distal bunion portal to pierce the plantar capsular flap and come out through the skin in an inside out fashion. Then, the skin is retracted with a skin hook, and the surface of the capsule is cleared with a haemostat until the suture is seen. The suture is retrieved at the surface of the capsule, making sure that the digital nerve is not entrapped. The suture is then passed through the plantar capsular flap again under direct visualization to avoid trapping the digital nerve, through the joint lastly, and finally above the the dorsal capsule and through the skin, in an outside in fashion.

The suture is retrieved from the joint through the distal bunion portal. The suture is passed to the proximal portal deep to the capsule. The needle is introduced through the proximal portal to pierce the dorsal capsular flap and comes out through the skin in an inside out fashion. The sutures are retrieved at the surface of the capsule, as described above(Fig. 8.9).

The medial capsular suture should be inserted before tying the intermetatarsal space. The medial capsular suture is tied with the hallux held in the reduced position, and should be tied after tying the intermetatarsal suture.

Post-operatively, the foot is put in a bulky dressing for 2 weeks, when the dressing is changed to a light dressing, and active toe mobilization is allowed with a dynamic hallux valgus splint (Fig. 8.10). The screw transfixing the first and second metatarsal is removed under local anesthesia 8 weeks after the operation.

8.3 AdjunctP rocedures

8.3.1 Derotation of the First Metatarsal

If the apparent sesamoid subluxation in the dorsoplantar radiograph arises from excessive pronation of the first metatarsal rather than true sesamoid subluxation, it can be detected using sesamoid view preoperatively. The sesamoid bones are seated into the corresponding groove of the metatarsal head, and the sesamoid grooves are facing plantarlaterally in sesamoid view. Intra-operatively, excessive metatarsal pronation should be suspected if the reduction of a sesamoid is suboptimal even after complete lateral soft tissue release.

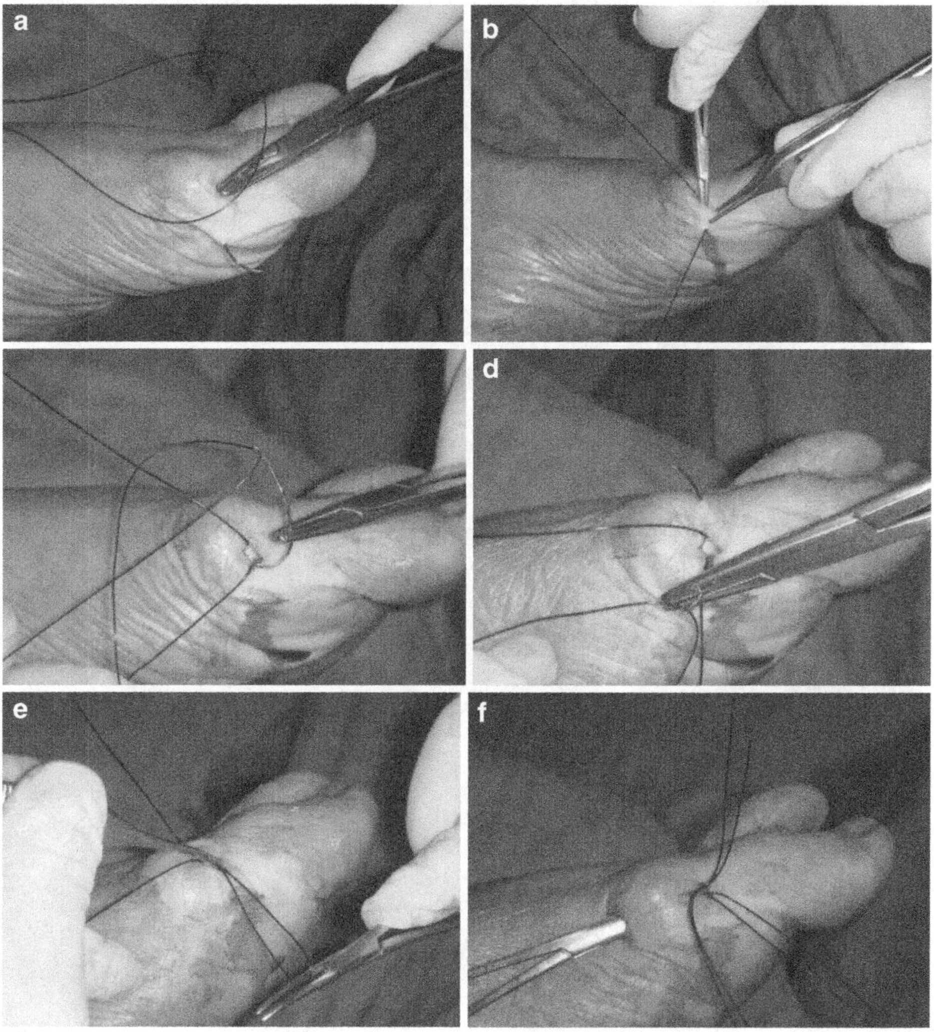

Fig. 8.9 (**a**) The needle is introduced through the distal bunion portal to pierce the plantar capsular flap and come out through the skin in an inside out fashion. (**b**) The surface of the capsule is cleared with a haemostat until the suture is seen. The suture is retrieved at the surface of the capsule, making sure that the digital nerve is not entrapped. (**c**, **d**) The suture is then passed through the plantar capsular flap again under direct visualization to avoid trapping the digital nerve, through the joint lastly, and finally above the dorsal capsule and through the skin in an outside in fashion. (**e**) The suture is retrieved from the joint through the distal bunion portal. (**f**) The suture is passed to proximal portal deep to the capsule. (**g**, **h**) The needle is introduced through the proximal portal to pierce the dorsal capsular flap and come out through the skin in an inside out fashion. (**i**) The sutures are retrieved at the surface of the capsule and deep to the extensor tendon and digital nerve. (**j**) The hallux valgus deformity can be corrected by tensioning the medial capsular plication suture

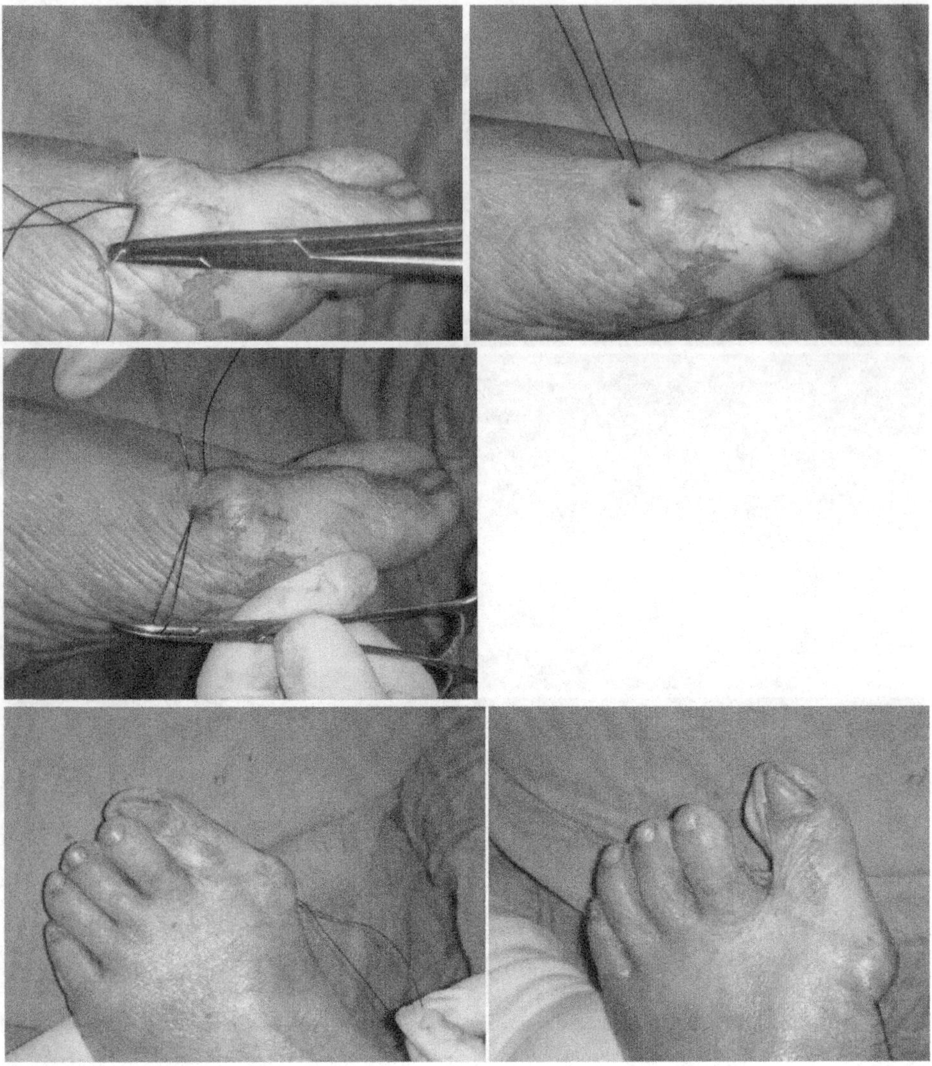

Fig. 8.9 (continued)

Arthroscopic examination of the metatarso-sesamoid compartment through the distal bunion portal and the toe web portal will show that the sesamoid bones seated in the corresponding grooves. In a study of metatarso-phalangeal arthroscopy in patients with hallux valgus, there was a high chance of cartilage degeneration of the metatarso-sesamoid compartment because of the joint incongruity as a result of sesamoid subluxation. If there is no cartilage degeneration of the metatarso-sesamoid compartment, metatarsal pronation should be suspected. The first metatarsal is de-rotated with a Kirschner wire before insertion of the proximal fixation screw (Fig. 8.11).[3]

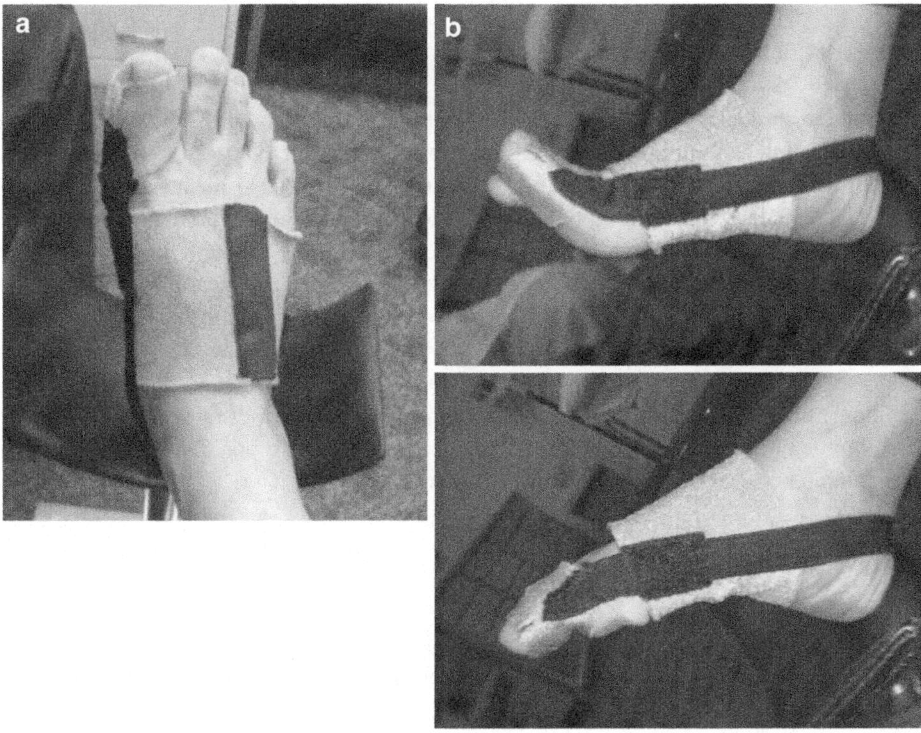

Fig. 8.10 Dynamic hallux valgus splint can help to maintain the correction and allow active hallux dorsiflexion and plantarflexion

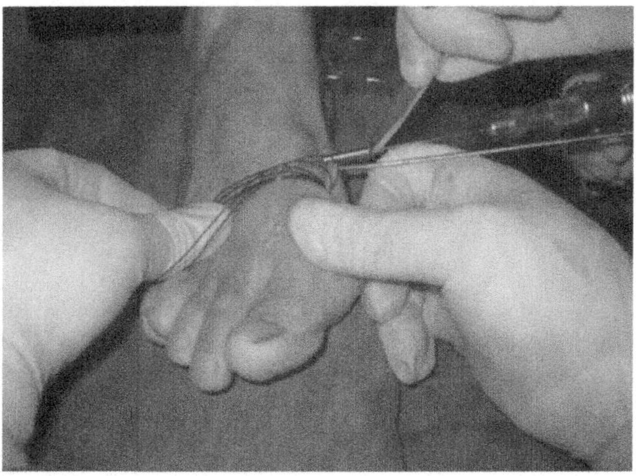

Fig. 8.11 Thefi rst metatarsal is supinated and plantarflexed, and the intermetatarsal space is closed by the surgeons right hand while the assistant is insertingthe guide w ire

8.3.1.1 Arthroscopic First Tarso-metatarsal (Lapidus) Arthrodesis

A Lapidus arthrodesis is indicated in patients with hypermobility of the medial cuneiform metatarsal joint. Stability of the first ray may be restored after surgical correction of the hallux valgus deformity despite leaving the capsule of the first tarso-metatarsal joint undisturbed.[7] Preoperatively, we establish the need for the arthroscopic Lapidus procedure by performing the relocation drawer test.[2] We perform the drawer test with the hallux valgus deformity reduced manually. We believe that first tarso-metatarsal arthrodesis is indicated only if the first tarso-metatarsal joint hypermobility persists during the relocation drawer test. The open procedure has been criticized for its prolonged healing and high nonunion rate, as well as the tendency for dorsal angulation of the first metatarsal. Arthroscopic Lapidus arthrodesis[8] has the advantage of more thorough preparation of the fusion site with minimal bone removal and better control of the arthrodesis position with less chance of malunion because of preservation of soft tissue around the joint.

8.3.1.2 Technique

With the patient supine and a pneumatic thigh tourniquet and no distraction, the first tarso-metatarsal is located and arthroscopy (Fig. 8.12) is performed through the plantar medial and dorsomedial portals at the plantar medial and dorsomedial corners of the joint which can be located with a G21 needle.

The instruments used are 2.7 mm 30° arthroscope, small periosteal elevator, arthroscopic osteotome and arthroscopic awl. The articular cartilage is removed using an arthroscopic osteotome and a small periosteal elevator, leaving the subchondral bone intact. Micro-fracture of the subchondral bone is then performed by means of arthroscopic awls (Fig. 8.13). The intermetatarsal angle is closed manually, and the first metatarsal is held in plantarflexion

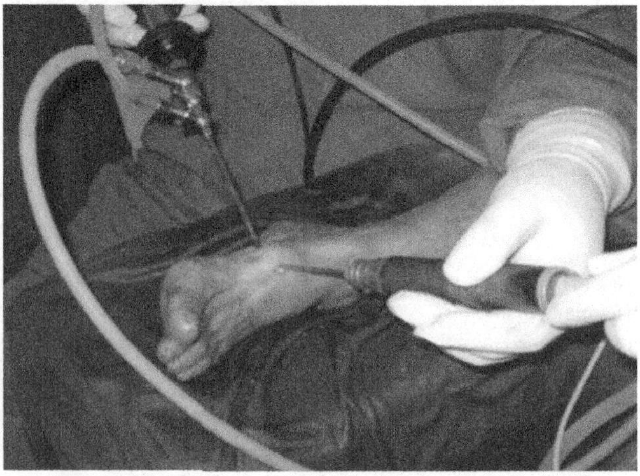

Fig.8. 12 Firstta rso-metatarsala rthroscopy

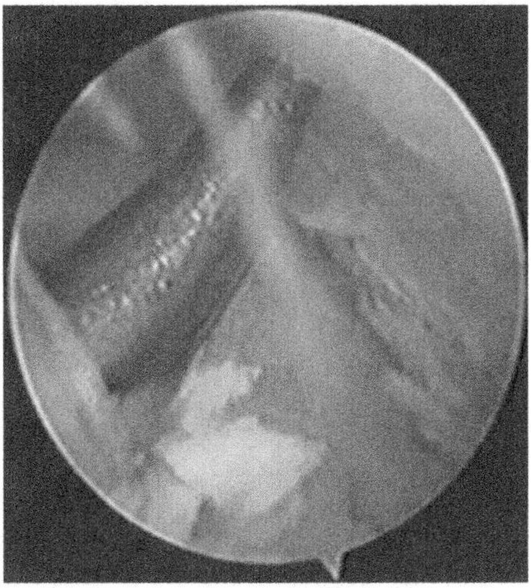

Fig. 8. 13 Micro-fracture of the subchondral bone witha rthroscopica wl

via dorsiflexion of the first metatarso-phalangeal joint. A 4.0 mm cannulated screw is inserted from a proximal dorsal direction to a distal plantar direction across the joint. Finally, a 4.0 mm positioning screw is inserted from the first metatarsal base to the second metatarsal base. The patient is given an ankle foot orthosis (AFO) and kept non weight bearing. The positioning screw is removed 12 weeks later.

8.3.2 Endoscopic Assisted Lengthening of the Extensor Hallucis longus Tendon

Extensor hallucis longus contracture can occur in patients with severe deformity with long duration. Endoscopic Z-lengthening of the tendon[9] is indicated if there is hyperextension deformity of the interphalangeal joint at times associated metatarso-phalangeal joint after correction of the hallux valgus deformity. It should be used in caution as active extension of the hallux will be markedly impaired after the procedure.

8.3.2.1 Technique

Along the course of the extensor hallucis longus tendon at the foot dorsum, two portals are established. At the distal portal, at the level of the metatarsal neck, the medial half of the extensor hallucis longus tendon is cut and stripped proximally with a tendon stripper to the proximal portal at the level of the navicular bone. The lateral half of the tendon is cut at the proximal portal. Stay stitches are applied to the tendon ends. With the ankle in plantar flexion and the hallux kept in a position similar to the lesser toes, the stay stitches are sutured to the opposing tendon segments. The potential advantage of the procedure is less scarring around the extensor tendon, and better hallux motion is expected. The tendon repair is less secure as compared with the open procedure, and the risk of rupture of the repair is greater.

References

1. Lui TH, Dr Ng S, Dr Chan KB. New technique: endoscopic distal soft tissue procedure in hallux valgus. *Arthroscopy.*21: 1403.e1–1403.e7.
2. Lui TH. Current concepts: foot and ankle arthroscopy and endoscopy: indications of new technique. *Arthroscopy.*2007; 23:889–902.
3. Lui TH, Chan KB, Chow HT, Ma CM, Chan PK, Ngai WK. Arthroscopy-assisted correction of hallux valgus deformity. *Arthroscopy.*2008; 24:875–880.
4. Lui TH, Chan KB, Chan LK. Lateral release of endoscopic distal soft tissue procedure in treatment of hallux valgus: a cadaveric study. *Arthroscopy.*2010; 26:1111–1116.
5. Lui TH. First metatarsophalangeal arthroscopy in patients with hallux valgus. *Arthroscopy.* 2008;14:1122–1129.
6. Friscia DA. Distal soft tissue correction for hallux valgus with proximal screw fixation of the first metatarsal. *Foot Ankle Clin.*2000; 5:581–589.
7. Coughlin MJ, Jones CP, Viladot R, Glano P, Grebing BR, Kennedy MJ. Hallux valgus and first ray mobility: a cadeveric study. *Foot Ankle Int.*2004; 25:537–44.
8. Lui TH, Chan KB, Ng S. Technical note: arthroscopic lapidus arthrodesis. *Arthroscopy.* 2005;21:1516.e1–1516.e4.
9. Dr Lui TH. Arthroscopically assisted Z-lengthening of the extensor hallucis longus tendon. *Arch Ortho Trauma Surg.*2007; 127:855–857.

Minimally Invasive Hallux valgus Correction 9

Francesco Oliva, UmileGiuseppe Longo, and Nicola Maffulli

9.1 Introduction

There is an increasing concern among orthopaedists towards the potentials of minimally invasive procedures. Applied to foot surgery, minimally invasive surgery (MIS) can be accomplished is shorter time respect of a conventional surgery, together with less distress and problems to the soft tissues. In addition, the operation can be done bilaterally, it allows use of distal anaesthetics blocks and early weight-bearing.[1]

In 1986, Van Enoo defined the minimum-incision surgery as an operation done through the smallest incision required for a proper procedure, and the percutaneous surgery as that performed within the smallest possible working incision in a closed fashion.[2,3]

A percutaneous MIS requires the use of dedicated instruments and frequently a fluoroscopy. Lui and other colleagues from Hong Kong have described arthroscopic and endoscopic assisted correction of hallux valgus deformities.[4,5] Morton Polokoff, a podiatric physician, in 1945 tried to use fine chisels, rasps and spears to perform subdermal surgery. Years later, Leonard Britton accomplished the first osteotomy on bunion deformities with percutaneous exposure of the first metatarsal, a closing wedge osteotomy, and the Akin procedure.

North American podiatrists started to adopt MIS of the foot in 1970.[7] The technique percutaneous surgery for hallux valgus correction that we use derives from that described by Lamprecht-Kramer-Bösch in 1982.[8–10] These authors based the procedure on the subcapital metatarsal linear osteotomy of Hohmann.[11] In 1991, Isham described a minimally invasive distal metatarsal osteotomy without implantation.[12] The results of recent French studies showed that patients treated with minimally invasive surgery for hallux valgus needed less hospitalization time and recovered earlier.[13]

Minimum incision techniques, by allowing limb safety with reduced damage of soft tissue or bones trauma should be a first choice indication to patients at high risk of ulceration.[14–17]

N. Maffulli (✉)
Centre for Sports and Exercise Medicine, Queen Mary University of London, Barts and The London School of Medicine and Dentistry, Mile End Hospital, London, England, UK
e-mail: n.maffulli@qmul.ac.uk

N. Maffulli and M. Easley (eds.), *Minimally Invasive Surgery of the Foot and Ankle*,
DOI: 10.1007/978-1-84996-417-3_9,

Recurrence of the deformity is the most frequent complication related to the use of MIS to foot deformity correction. Recurrence can arise from inadequate correction, or incorrect application of the technique, or incorrect estimation of the healing time of the osteotomy.[13,18,19] European orthopedic foot surgeons[18,20,21] seem to show more interest in minimally invasive surgery than their North American counterparts.[19]

9.1.1 Indications

We have considered minimally invasive procedures to correct hallux valgus deformity when the hallux valgus angle (HVA) is up to 40°, and the intermetatarsal angle (IMA) is up to 20°. In the presence of congruency of the metatarso-phalangeal joint, the procedure has been indicated in patients showing significant increase of the distal metatarsal articular angle (DMAA), and in patients with mild degenerative arthritis of the metatarso-phalangeal joint (Fig. 9.1a–b). We do not recommend this approach in patients with severe deformity with IMA greater that 20°, severe degenerative disease or stiffness of the metatarso-phalangeal joint and when metatarso-cuneiform or the metatarso-phalangeal joint are highly unstable.[21]

According other authors, percutaneous surgical correction of hallux valgus is indicated in patients with painful primary mild–to–moderate hallux valgus with IMA between 10° and 20° and HVA of less than 40°, in juvenile hallux valgus deformities with an increased distal metatarsal articular angle and some hallux valgus interphalangeous deformity. The technique is not indicated in hallux rigidus and in patients in whom a Keller's procedure unsuccessful.[22,23] Giannini et al. apply MIS to correction of mild to moderate deformities with a HVA up to 40°, and an IMA up to 20°.[24]

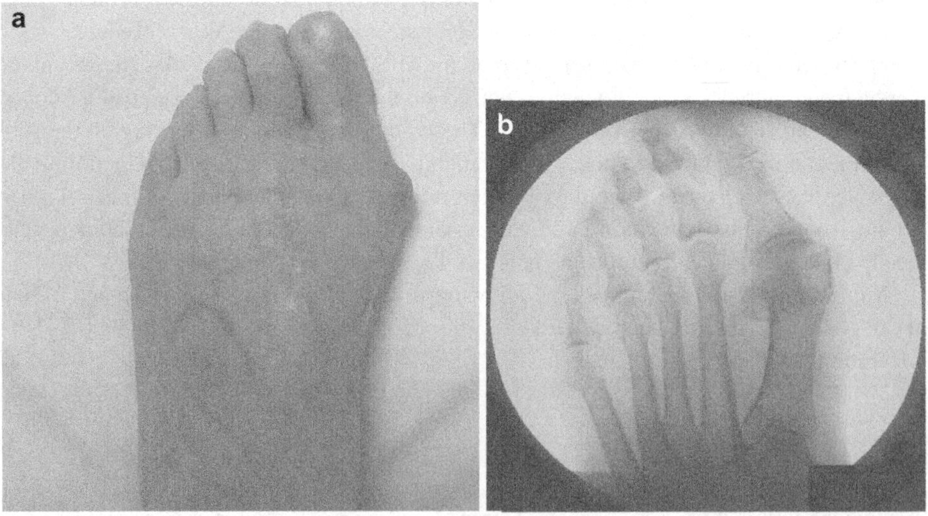

Fig. 9.1 (**a**) Clinical view of a left hallux valgus with a second toe deformity. (**b**) Intraoperative antero-posteriorr adiograph

9.2 Surgical Technique

With the patient supine with the desired anaesthesia, a calf tourniquet is applied. The foot is exsanguinated and prepared in the usual fashion. Soft tissue release, though not necessary given the large lateral shift of the metatarsal head, can be undertaken through a stab wound if desired. If there is stiffness of the metatarso-phalangeal joint, we perform a manual stretch of the adductor hallucis to force the hallux into some varus before incising the skin. A 2 cm medial incision is made just proximal to the bunion. The incision is deepened through skin and subcutaneous tissue, until the medial aspect of the first metatarsal is exposed. The soft tissues are retracted plantarly and dorsally. A linear osteotomy is performed with a standard 5 × 2 × 0.4 mm blade saw (STRYKER, USA) (Fig. 9.2a). A small osteotome is used to mobilize the head of the first metatarsal. A 2 mm Kirschner wire is inserted from the medial portion of the tip of the hallux, close to the nail. The wire is advanced in the soft tissues of the hallux, in a distal to proximal direction parallel to longitudinal axis if the hallux. The head of the metatarsal is displaced laterally, and the Kirschner wire penetrates the medullary canal of the first metatarsal (Fig. 9.2b).

If required, a slight varus position of the toe (up to 10°) can be forced after stabilization of the Kirschner wire (Fig. 9.3a–b). The operation ends with a standard skin suture. The protruding Kirschner wire is bent and cut. Recently, we have added a second Kirschner wire inserted in a proximal–to-distal and medial–to-lateral directions from the shaft of the first metatarsal towards the head. This second wire provides stability to the osteotomy by preventing dorsal translation of the metatarsal head in the post-operative stages. This second Kirschner wire is removed 2 weeks from the operation (Fig. 9.3c–d).

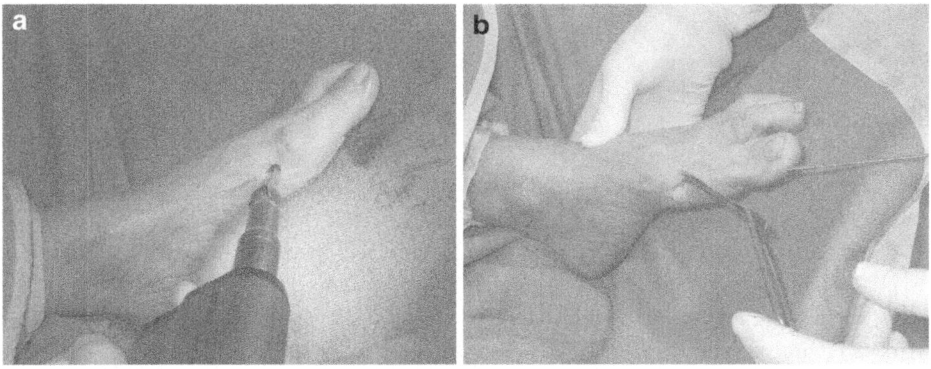

Fig. 9.2 Surgical technique. (**a**) Skin incision. The size of the incision is 2 cm, sufficient for insertion of the saw blade. The metatarsal osteotomy is performed using a standard oscillating saw. (**b**) Insertion of the Kirschner wire in the soft tissues of the hallux along the longitudinal axis, in a distal to proximal direction. A grooved device has been inserted at the the osteotomy site. The Kirschner wire will be guided through the device groove

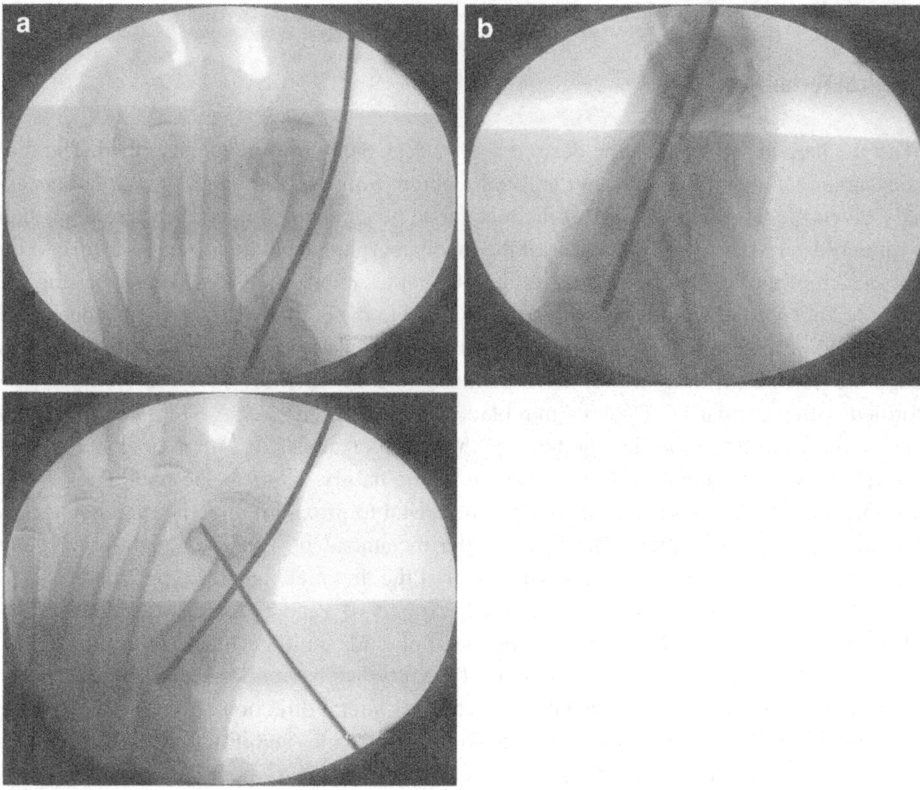

Fig. 9.3 (**a**) Intraoperative fluoroscopy: antero-posterior view. (**b**) Intraoperative fluoroscopy: lateral view. (**c**) Intraoperative fluoroscopy: the second Kirschner wire is inserted proximally to distally. (**d**) Plain radiographs showing an antero-posterior view of the left foot after 1 week after the procedure showing no displacement of the Kirschner wires

9.3 PostoperativeC are

The foot is kept with a compressive bandage, and plain radiographs of the foot (anteroposterior, lateral and oblique views) are taken.

Patients can walk immediately in a flat, rigid sole postoperative shoe, which allows not to put weight through the osteotomy, though in the beginning they are advised to walk for short times only, and to rest with the foot raised while supine or sitting. The longitudinal Kirscher wire remains in situ for 6 weeks from the date of surgery. At that time, it is removed in the outpatient department, and other plain radiographs are taken.[21]

At this point, patients are recommended to cycle and swim, and to wear comfortable plain shoes for 3–6 months, after which they can gradually return to their usual footwear. The patients have their next clinical and radiographic check in 3 months. Subsequent follow up varies depending on the patient.

Some authors prefer to remove the Kirschner wire 4 weeks after the operation, applying a corrective bandage around the hallux to be renewed once a week for the next 6 weeks. In this method, the bandage should apply a moderate hypercorrection to the hallux.[22]

9.4 Discussion

Recurrence of the deformity due to incorrect choice of technique is the most frequent complication of the type of surgery. Since the literature collects reports of only case series and there are not randomized studies that compare conventional open with mini invasive surgical techniques applied to hallux valgus, we do not have adequately powered level one evidence studies.[25]

In Weil's work there are descriptions of tendon, vascular and nerves injuries from minimal incision surgeries.[26]

De Prado recorded such rates as 0.2% of infections and 1% of phlebitis. He also described shortening of the first metatarsal in 100% of cases, osteotomy displacement in 3%, and delayed union in 8%. Soft tissue complications occurred, especially skin complications related to portal placement. There were also neuro-vascular complications. Portal and skin complications were mainly burns (3%). Nervous complications related to nerves were transient in 12% of cases, and permanent in 0.5%. Vascular complications were bleeding and hematomas, with no records of ischemic complications. Other type of complications recorded were reduced mobility (4%) and persistent pain (3%).[12]

Magna and colleagues observed that 49% of patients with dorsiflexion presented plantar displacement subsequent to surgery, while recurrence of the deformity occurred in three of the 118 ft.[22] The clinical significance of these morphological features are unclear.

Weimberg and colleagues performed a study of 301 percutaneous non-internally fixed first metatarsal surgery for correction of hallux valgus. Their study showed a moderate metatarsal shortening of the metatarsal between 2.6 and 5.8 mm, 47 (15.6%) cases of malunions, 11 (3.7%) infections, seven stress fractures of the second metatarsal (2.3%), four (1.2%) delayed unions, and one (0.3%) hallux varus.[27]

Giannini, in a 4 years study on 190 patients treated with MIS, found only nine cases that were scored lower than 60 in the AOFAS satisfaction level scale. Portaluri in a retrospective clinical and radiographic evaluation of 182 Bosch procedures with a mean follow-up of 16.4 +/− 2.4 months reported eight superficial infections (4.4%), two ulcerations around the hallux pin site (1.1%), and two dorsal malunions (1.1%).[28]

Sanna and Ruiu, in a retrospective review of 52 ft that had percutaneous distal-first metatarsal osteotomies over a period of 31.5 months, found four (7.4%) superficial infections and three (5.8%) ulcerations by the hallux pin site, one (2%) recurrent deformity, one (2%) permanent anesthesia around the hallux, and one (2%) over lengthening of the first metatarsal.[29]

Pique-Vidal's prospective evaluation of 94 percutaneous, non-internally fixed first metatarsal and Akin osteotomy type, similar to the Bocsh procedure, reported four delayed unions (4.3%) but no infections, nonunions, or avascular necrosis.[30]

De Giorgi et. al. studied 27 consecutive patients receiving a Bosch technique, who were followed up for an average of 19 months (range 6 months to 5 years). The technique appeared give eary satisfactory results, but the radiographs taken during after a few years showed some loss of correction. However, the patients were clinically satisfied. Only one non union was recorded.[31]

Baieta and colleagues studied 98 percutaneous distal osteotomies of the first metatarsal, with an average follow up of 76.2 months, obtaining an AOFAS score of 89.9, with 96% of patients satisfied. Four superficial infections around the wire were reported, two recurrences of hallux valgus, one hallux rigidus, and five metatarsalgias.[32]

Among the 94 patient undergoing arthroscopy-assisted hallux valgus deformity corrections with percutaneous screw fixation, there were three symptomatic recurrences which required revision.[5]

Using MIS techniques, the osteotomy healing time is of the highest importance as it can interfere with the procedure's definitive outcome. Lopez and colleagues believe that the healing time should be shorter than healing time required in conventional surgery of the type. Their hypothesis is based on two reasons: (a) the percutaneous technique produces minimal injury to vessels and surrounding soft tissues (b) the bone detritus ("bone mush") at the osteotomy site acts as internal bone graft.[33]

In the interval between the removal of the proximal Kirschner wire, after 2 weeks, and the removal of the main Kirschner wire after 6 weeks, the foot is exposed to chances of superficial infection. However, this second wire allows better stability to the transverse osteotomy to prevent dorsal migration and/or angulation of the capital fragment (Fig. 9.4 a–c).

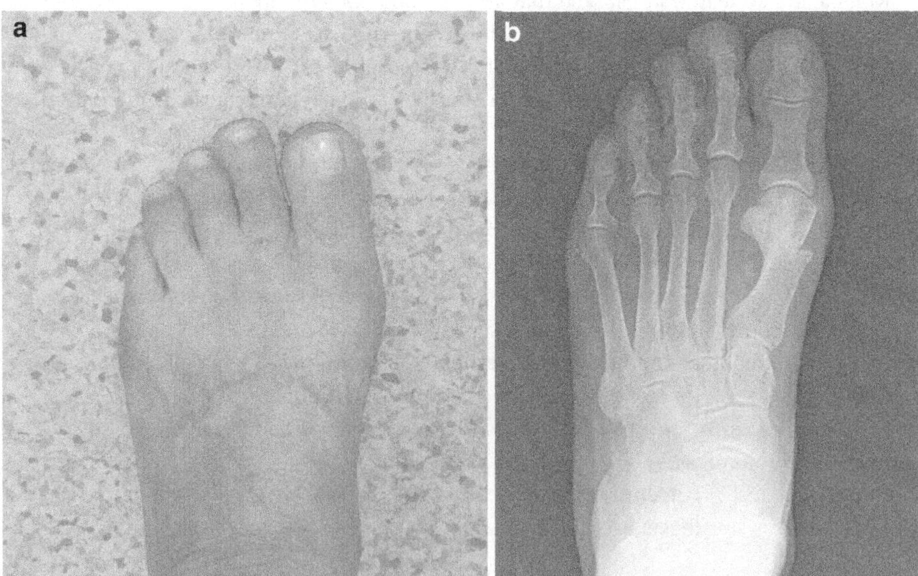

Fig. 9.4 (**a**) Clinical picture 12 months after the procedure. (**b**) and (**c**). Plain antero-posterior and lateral radiographs after 6 months showing healing of the osteotomy

Fig. 9.4 (continued)

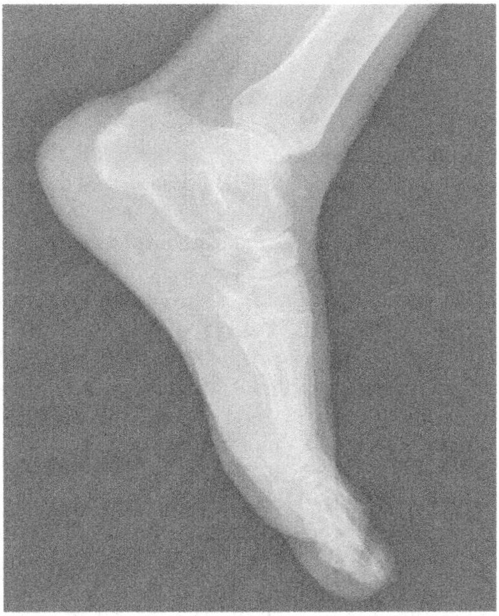

Provided that the indications are adequate and that sufficient experience has been matured with the used of dedicated instruments, MIS is a suitable surgical choice for the correction of mild to moderate hallux valgus deformities.[34] There is still need of randomized prospective clinical trials to enable valuable comparison of MIS applications with conventional open procedures.[35–37]

References

1. David C, Sammarco G, James G. Minimum incision surgery. *Foot Ankle Int.* 1992;13: 157–160.
2. Van Enoo RE, Cane EM. Minimal incision surgery: a plastic technique or a cover-up? *Clin Podiatr Med Surg.* 1986; 3:321–335.
3. David C, Sammarco G, James G. Minimum incision surgery. *Foot Ankle Int.* 1992;13: 157–160.
4. Lui TH, Ng S, Chan KB. Endoscopic distal soft tissue procedure in hallux valgus surgery. *Arthroscopy.* 2005; 21:1403.e1–1403.e7.
5. Lui TH, Chan KB, Chow HT et al. Arthroscopy-assisted correction of hallux valgus deformity. *Arthroscopy.* 2008A ug;24:875–880.
6. Hymes L. Introduction: brief history of the use of minimum incision surgery (MIS). In: Fielding MD, ed. *Forefoot Minimum Incision in Podiatric Medicine: A Handbook on Primary Corrective Procedures on the Human Foot Using Minimum Incisions with Minimum Trauma.* New York, NY: Futura Publishing; 1977:1–2.
7. De Lavigne C, Guillo S, Laffenêtre O, De Prado M. The treatment of hallux valgus with the mini-invasive technique. *Interact Surg.* 2007; 2:31–37.

8. Bösch P, Markowski H, Rannicher V. Technik und erste Ergebnisse der subkutanen distalen Metatarsale-I-Osteotomie. *Orthop Praxis.*1990; 26:51–56.
9. Hohmann G. Symptomatische oder physiologische Behandlung des Hallux valgus. *Münch Med Wochenschr.*1921; 68:1042–1045.
10. Lamprecht E, Kramer J. Die Metatarsale-I-Osteotomie nach Kramer zur Behandlung des Hallux valgus. *Orthop Prax.*1982; 28:635–645.
11. Bösch P, Wanke S, Legenstein R. Hallux valgus correction by the method of Bösch: a new technique with a seven-to-ten year follow-up. *Foot Ankle Clin.*2000; 5:485–498.
12. Isham SA. The Reverdin-Isham procedure for the correction of hallux abducto valgus. A distal metatarsal osteotomy procedure. *Clin Podiatr Med Surg.*1991; 8:81–94.
13. Leemrijse T, Valtin B, Besse JL. Hallux valgus surgery in 2005. Conventional, mini-invasive or percutaneous surgery? Uni- or bilateral? Hospitalisation or one-day surgery? *Rev Chir Orthop Reparatrice Appar Mot.*2008; 94:111–127.
14. Roukis TS. Central metatarsal head–neck osteotomies: indications and operative techniques. *Clin Podiatr Med Surg.*2005; 22:197–222.
15. Roukis TS. The Tailor's bunionette deformity: a field guide to surgical correction. *Clin Podiatr Med Surg.*2005; 22:223–245.
16. Weitzel S, Trnka H-J, Petroutsas J. Transverse medial slide osteotomy for bunionette deformity: long-term results. *Foot Ankle Int.*2007; 28:794–798.
17. Roukis TS, Schade VL. Minimum-incision metatarsal osteotomies. *Clin Podiatr Med Surg.* 2008;25:587–607.
18. De Prado M, Ripoll PL, Vaquero J, Golano P. Tratamiento quirurgico per cutaneo del hallux mediante osteotomias multiples. *Rev Orthop Traumatol.*2003; 47:406–416.
19. Kadakia AR, Smerek JP, Myerson MS. Radiographic results after percutaneous distal metatarsal osteotomy for correction of hallux valgus deformity. *Foot Ankle Int.*2007; 28:355–360.
20. De Prado M, Ripoll PL, Golano P. *Cirurgia percutanea Del Pie*. Barcelona, Spain: Masson; 2003.
21. Maffulli N, Oliva F, Coppola C et al. Minimally invasive hallux valgus correction: a technical note and a feasibility study. *J Surg Orthop Adv.*2005; 14:193–198.
22. Magnan B, Bortolazzi R, Samaila E et al. Percutaneous distal metatarsal osteotomy for correction of hallux valgus. Surgical technique. *J Bone Joint Surg Am.*2006; 88:135–148.
23. Magnan B, Samaila E, Viola G, Bortolazzi P. Minimally invasive retrocapital osteotomy of the first metatarsal in hallux valgus deformity. *Oper Orthop Traumatol.*2008; 20:89–96.
24. Giannini S, Vannini F, Faldini C et al. The minimally invasive hallux valgus correction (S.E.R.I.) *Interact Surg.*2007; 2:17–23.
25. Portaluri M. Hallux valgus correction by the method of Bosch: a clinical evaluation. *Foot Ankle Clin.*2000 ;5:499–511.
26. Weil LS. Minimal invasive surgery of the foot and ankle. *J Foot Ankle Surg.*2001; 40:61.
27. Weinberger BH, Fulp JM, Falstrom P et al. Retrospective evaluation of percutaneous bunionectomies and distal osteotomies without internal fixation. *Clin Podiatr Med Surg.* 1991;8:111–136.
28. Portaluri M. Hallux valgus correction by the method of Bosch: a clinical evaluation. *Foot Ankle Clin.*2000 ;5:499–511.
29. Sanna P, Ruiu GA. Percutaneous distal osteotomy of the first metatarsal (PDO) for the surgical treatment of hallux valgus. *Chir Organi Mov.*2005; 90:365–369.
30. Pique'-Vidal C. The effect of temperature elevation during discontinuous use of rotator burrs in the correction of hallux valgus. *J Foot Ankle Surg.*2005; 44:336–344.
31. De Giorgi S, Mascolo V, Losito A. The correction of hallux valgus by Bösch tecnique (PDO - Percutaneus Distal Osteotomy). *G.I.O.T.*2003; 29:161–164.
32. BaiettaD Perusi M,Cassini M. Hallux valgus surgical treatment with Bosch tecnique: clinical evaluation and surgical consideration after 5 years. *G.I.O.T.*2007; 33:107–113.

33. González López JJ, Rodríguez Sergio, Cadena Méndez L. Functional, esthetic and radiographic results of treatment of hallux valgus with minimally invasive surgery. *Acta Ortopédica Mexicana*.2005;19 :42–46.
34. Guillo S, Laffenêtre O, De Prado M. The treatment of hallux valgus with the mini-invasive technique. *Interact Surg*.2007; 2:31–37.
35. Maffulli N, Longo UG, Oliva F, Denaro V, Coppola C. Bosch osteotomy and scarf osteotomy for hallux valgus correction. *Orthop Clin North Am*. 2009 40:515–24.
36. Oliva F, Longo UG, Maffulli N. Minimally invasive hallux valgus correction.Orthop Clin *North Am*. 2009 40:525–30.
37. Maffulli N, Longo UG, Marinozzi A, Denaro V. Hallux valgus: effectiveness and safety of minimally invasive surgery. A systematic review. *Br Med Bull*. 2010. [Epub ahead of print] PubMedPM ID:20 710024.

Minimally Invasive Modified Wilson Osteotomy for the Treatment of Hallux valgus

10

Sheldon Nadal

10.1 Introduction

The modified Wilson osteotomy is a V-shaped osteotomy of the first metatarsal neck made in the sagittal plane with the apex of the V pointed proximally (Fig. 10.1). This osteotomy allows the head of the first metatarsal to be displaced laterally to reduce the intermetatarsal angle. The V-shape contributes stability. Best results are obtained when the procedure is performed on a foot with a mild to moderate hallux valgus deformity, a flexible first metatarsal phalangeal joint, and a mild to moderately increased metatarsus primus varus angle.

The procedure can be performed on an out-patient basis, under local anesthesia. Given the minimally invasive nature of the technique, patients can walk immediately after surgery and casts are not necessary. Most patients do not require crutches or medication stronger than a mild analgesic or non-steroidal anti-inflammatory.

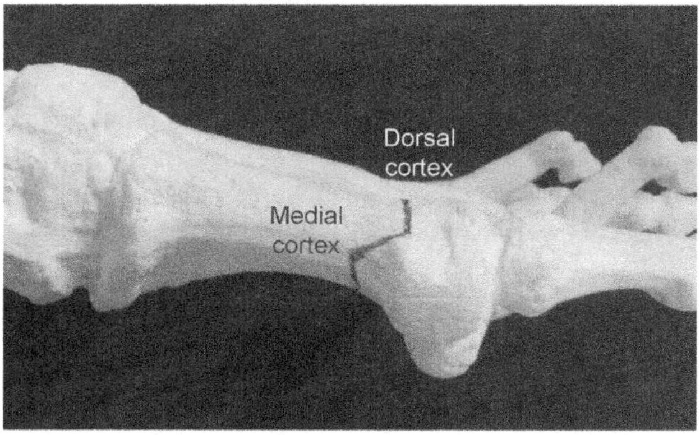

Fig.10.1 Themodifi ed Wilkson osteotomy, as viewed from a dorsal medial angle

S.N adal
586EglintonA venueEa st, Suite501 , Toronto, OntarioM 4P1P 2, Canadaa nd
Trustee, Academy of Ambulatory Foot and Ankle surgery,
Philadelphia, PA

N. Maffulli and M. Easley (eds.), *Minimally Invasive Surgery of the Foot and Ankle*,
DOI: 10.1007/978-1-84996-417-3_10, © Springer-Verlag London Limited 2011

10.2 History

The original Wilson osteotomy was described by J.N. Wilson in 1963 for patients with juvenile hallux valgus.[1] This was an oblique osteotomy, performed in the distal third of the first metatarsal, beginning just proximal to the medial bony eminence. The osteotomy was performed by Dr. Wilson using a 3/8 in. wide osteotome at 45° from distal medial to proximal lateral. The osteotomy was also combined with remodeling of the medial eminence of the first metatarsal head. The osteotomy was non-fixated and kept in a below knee plaster cast with the great toe over-corrected for 2 weeks. The over-correction was then reduced to a more neutral position and was followed by 6 weeks in a walking cast.

The idea of performing a minimally invasive Wilson osteotomy was originally suggested to Seymour Kessler, D.P.M., Abram Plon, D.P.M., and Marvin Arnold, D.P.M. by Lowell Weil Sr., D.P.M. of Chicago in the 1970s (Personal communication with Abe Plon, D.P.M, retired from private practice, Elkins Park, Pennsylvania, now deceased, by telephone June 20 2009).

Dr. Kessler performed an oblique osteotomy through a small dorsal incision using a Shannon 44 burr. The osteotomy was made from dorsal distal to plantar proximal, and relied on ground reactive forces to prevent the first metatarsal head from shifting plantarly and proximally (Personal communication with David Zuckerman, D.P.M., private practice, Woodbury, New Jersey, by telephone August 15 2009).

Doctors Plon and Arnold modified the osteotomy into a V-shaped osteotomy performed through a medial incision (Personal communication with Marvin Arnold, D.P.M., retired from private practice, West Palm Beach, Florida, by telephone August 25 2009). They first made a fail-safe hole at the neck of the first metatarsal running from medial to lateral, midway between the dorsal and plantar cortices. The dorsal arm of the V was then angled distally and superiorly from the fail-safe hole at approximately a 45° angle to the long axis of the first metatarsal. The plantar cut was made, beginning at the fail-safe hole, and angled plantarly at approximately a 90° angle to the long axis of the first metatarsal. The osteotomy was not fixated and the foot was taped firmly by the clinician for 3 weeks and an additional 3 weeks by the patient. The author angles the plantar cut so that it is perpendicular to the supporting surface or, on some occasions, aimed slightly more distal to reduce the chance of the head of the metatarsal slipping plantarly and proximally.

10.3 Anesthesia

The modified Wilson osteotomy was designed to be performed under local anesthesia, in an office based setting. This can be accomplished using an ankle block or by using a modified Mayo block adding local infiltration between the first and second metatarsal heads and at the medial aspect of the first metatarsal head and neck using a mixture of 1% lidocaine mixed with 0.5% bupivacaine in equal quantities. Epinephrine and an ankle tourniquet are not used, allowing bleeding at the surgical site. Bleeding will reduce the possibility of thermal necrosis during the bone cutting process.

10.4 Instrumentation

The following instruments may be used to perform the procedure.

1. Anum ber15bl ade
2. AL ockee levatoror s imilari nstrument[2](Fig. 10.2)

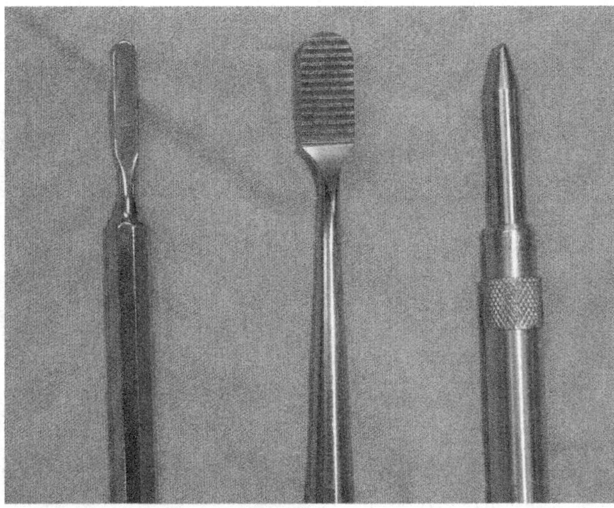

Fig.1 0.2 *Left* to *right*:L ocke elevator,r asp,e yem agnet

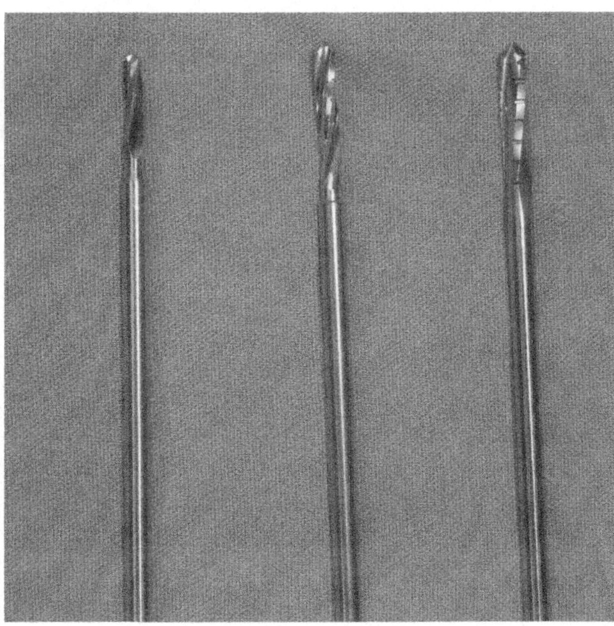

Fig.10. 3 *Left* to *right*:Shor t Shannon 44 burr, medium Shannon 44 burr, 3 mm wedgeb urr

3. Three medium Shannon 44 burrs, 2 mm in diameter[3](Fig. 10.3)
4. One short Shannon 44 burr, 2 mm in diameter[3](Fig. 10.3)
5. One3m mdi ameterw edgeb urr[3](Fig. 10.3)
6. One 7.5 in. Lewis nasal rasp, or similar instrument (Fig. 10.2)
7. Best results will be obtained by using some manner of intra-operative fluoroscopy. The author utilizes a XI-Scan unit, model 1000–1[4](Fig. 10.4)
8. A high torque, low speed drill such as the Osada PEDO[5] unit with the 2:7:1 reduction speedha ndpi ece(Fig. 10.5a,b)

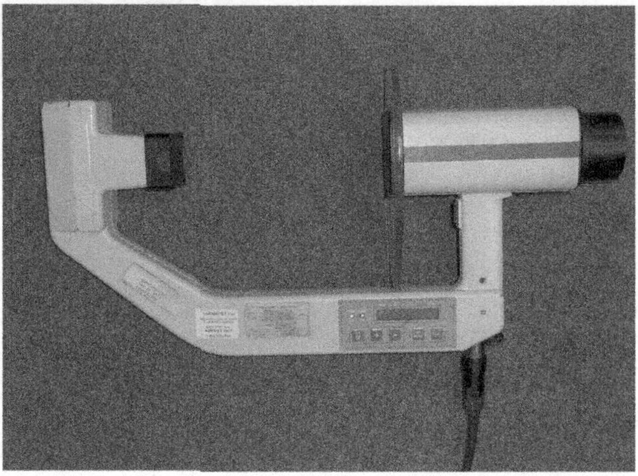

Fig.10. 4 Xi-Scanport able fluoroscope,m odel1000–1

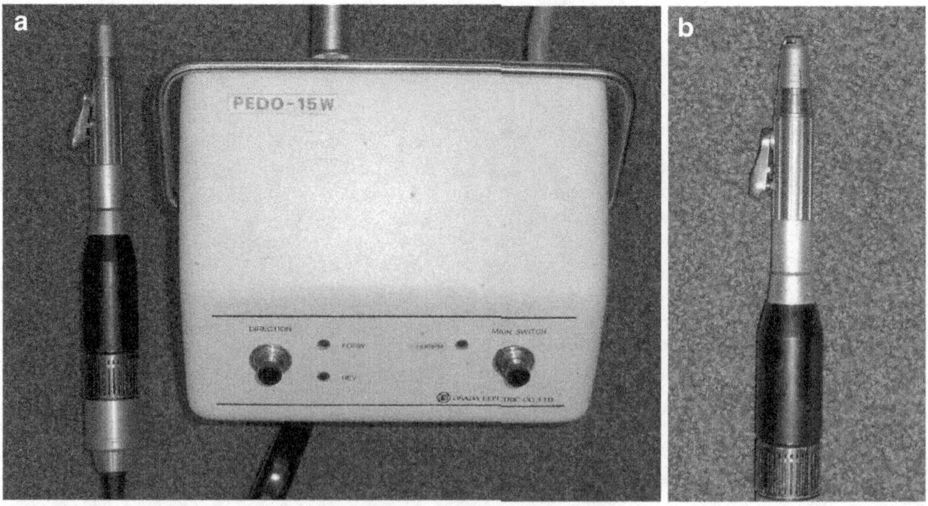

Fig.10. 5 (**a**) Osada PEDO drill. (**b**) Close up of Osada 2:7:1 reduction speed handpiece

10.5 Technique

The surgical site is prepped and draped in the usual sterile manner.

With the number 15 blade, a 5 mm longitudinal skin incision is made and then deepened to bone at the medial aspect of the first metatarsal (Fig. 10.6), just proximal to the medial eminence, midway between the dorsal and plantar cortices. At the incision, using a medium Shannon 44, a fail-safe hole is created (Fig. 10.7). The purpose of the fail-safe hole is to create a reference point from which the dorsal and plantar osteotomy cuts begin. The fail-safe hole is drilled from the medial cortex to and through the lateral cortex (Fig. 10.8), parallel to the supporting surface (Fig. 10.9) at a 90° angle to the long axis of the second metatarsal (Fig. 10.10a). This angle will allow the metatarsal head to shift laterally without undue shortening of the first metatarsal. The fail-safe hole can be angled slightly from proximal medial to distal lateral to further reduce shortening (Fig. 10.10b).

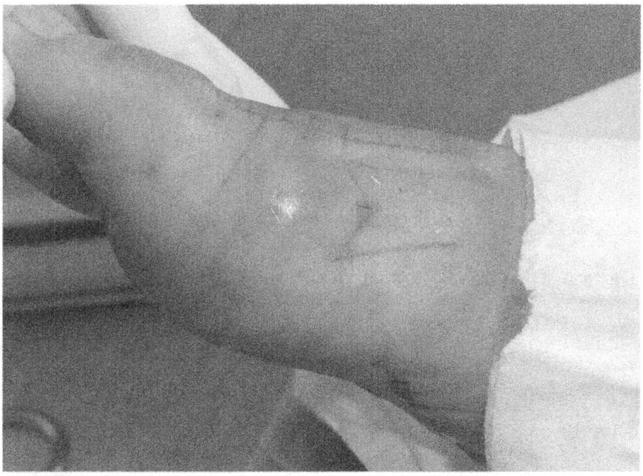

Fig.10.6 Skininc isionu sed to produce the fail-safe hole from which the modified Wilson osteotomy will be performed

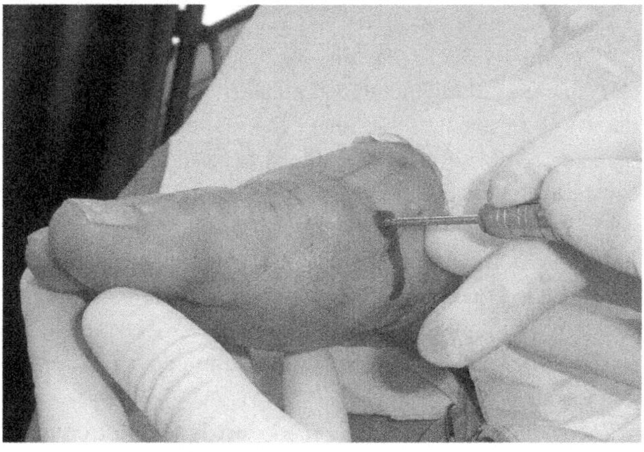

Fig.10.7 Creatingthe fail-safehol e

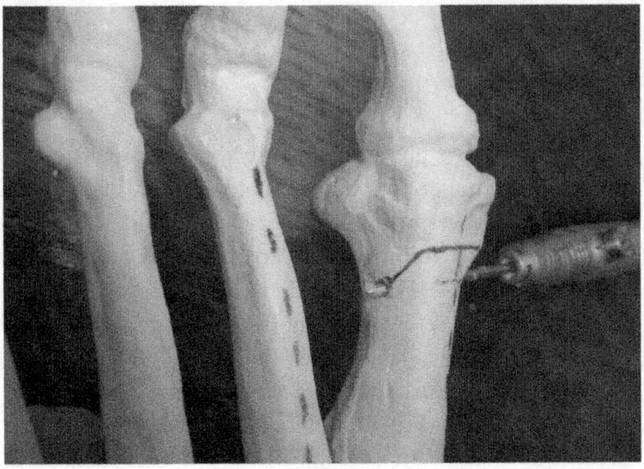

Fig. 10.8 The fail-safe hole is drilled from medial to lateral midway between the dorsal andpl antarc ortices

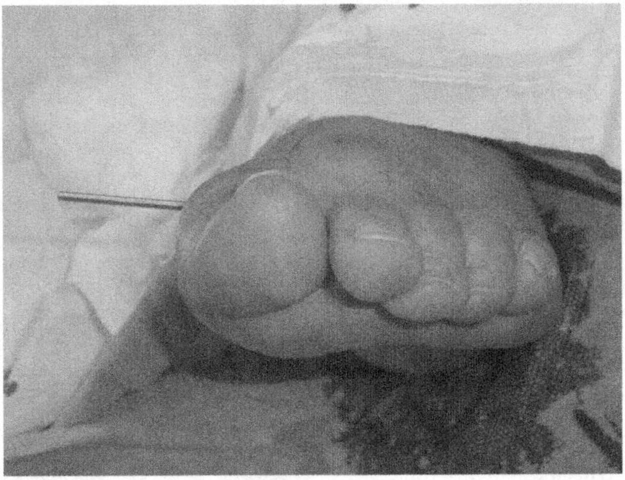

Fig. 10.9 The fail-safe hole is made parallel to the supporting surface. It may be angled slightly from dorsal medial to plantar lateral

In this instance, however, the surgeon may find it more difficult to displace the metatarsal head laterally.

The fail-safe hole may also be angled slightly from dorsal medial to plantar lateral to shift the head of the metatarsal plantarly as well as laterally to decrease the chance of producing excessive pressure under the second metatarsal head during midstance. Care must be taken not to shift the metatarsal head more than slightly plantarly, otherwise this may cause the hallux to elevate dorsally or cause excessive pressure under the tibial sesamoid.

A second longitudinal skin incision is now made 5 or 6 mm dorsal or plantar, according to the surgeon's preference, to the original skin incision and slightly posterior to it, and deepened to bone. This incision may be 2 or 3 mm longer than the first incision to facilitate the entry of the rasp later in the procedure. A Locke elevator is then inserted into the second incision and is used to separate the capsule from the medial eminence of the first metatarsalhe ad(Fig. 10.11).

A medium second Shannon 44 burr is then introduced into the fail-safe hole and the dorsal arm of the osteotomy is begun. The cutting surface of the Shannon follows a path

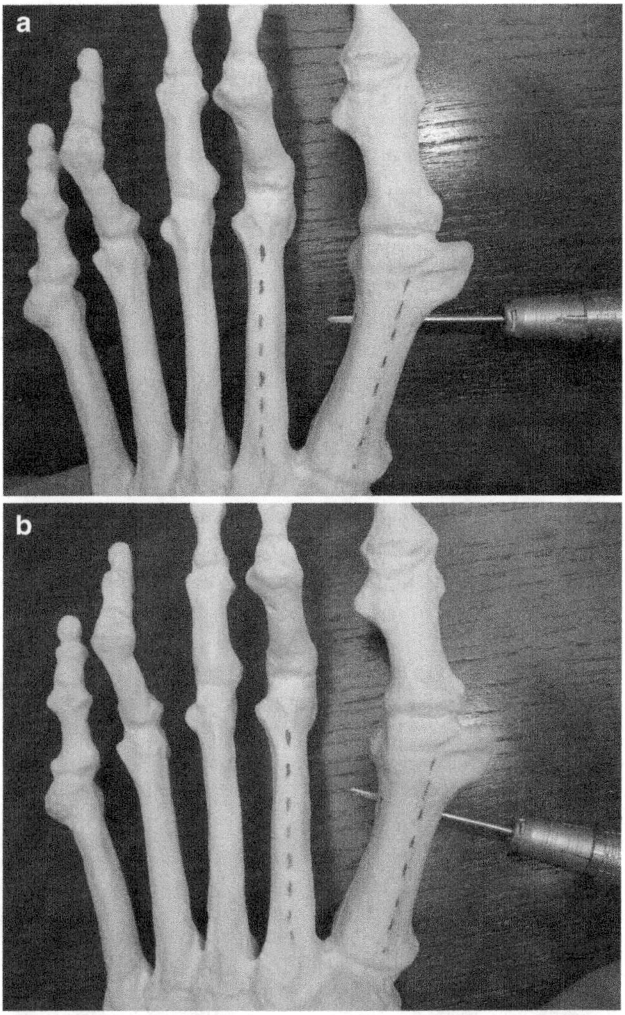

Fig.10. 10 (**a**) The fail-safe hole is drilled from medial to lateral at a 90° angle to the long axis of the second metatarsal. (**b**) The fail-safe hole may be angled slightly from proximal medial to distal lateral to further reduces hortening

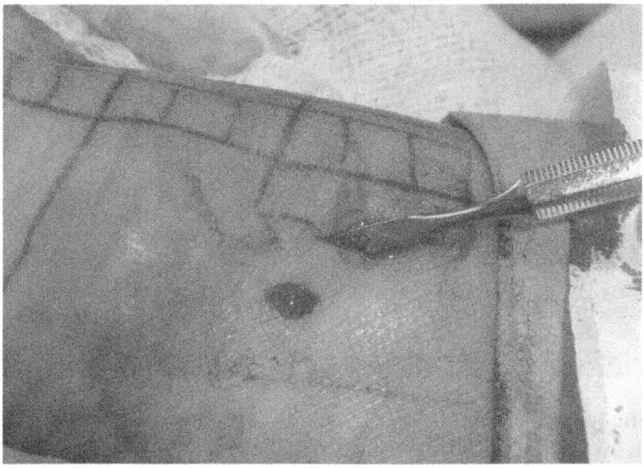

Fig.10. 11 ALoc ke elevator separates the capsule from the medial eminence of the firstme tatarsalhe ad

beginning at the lateral aspect of the neck of the metatarsal, midway between the dorsal and plantar surfaces (Fig. 10.8), and slowly cuts in a distal dorsal direction through the dorsal half of the lateral cortex until it reaches the dorsal lateral surface of the metatarsal neck, proximal to the articular cartilage (Fig. 10.12a). The cutting surface of the Shannon 44 burr then cuts through the dorsal cortex of the metatarsal from dorsal lateral to dorsal medial, parallel to the angle made by the fail-safe hole to the second metatarsal (Fig. 10.12b). The dorsal arm of the osteotomy is then completed as the burr cuts through the dorsal half of the medial cortex of the first metatarsal (Fig. 10.12c).

A third Shannon 44 is then inserted into the fail-safe hole to produce the plantar arm of the osteotomy. The cutting surface follows a path beginning at the lateral aspect of the first metatarsal, midway between the dorsal and plantar cortices (Fig. 10.13a), through the plantar half of the lateral cortex, toward the plantar lateral surface of the first metatarsal neck at an angle such that the plane of the osteotomy will be 90° to the supporting surface (Fig. 10.13b) or, according to the surgeon's discretion, angled slightly more distal. The cutting surface of the burr then goes from plantar lateral to plantar medial through the plantar cortex (Fig. 10.13c), again at an angle parallel to the fail-safe hole and perpendicular to the supporting surface. When making the plantar cut, the surgeon should take care to stay proximal to the crista and the sesamoid bones. The osteotomy is then carried through the

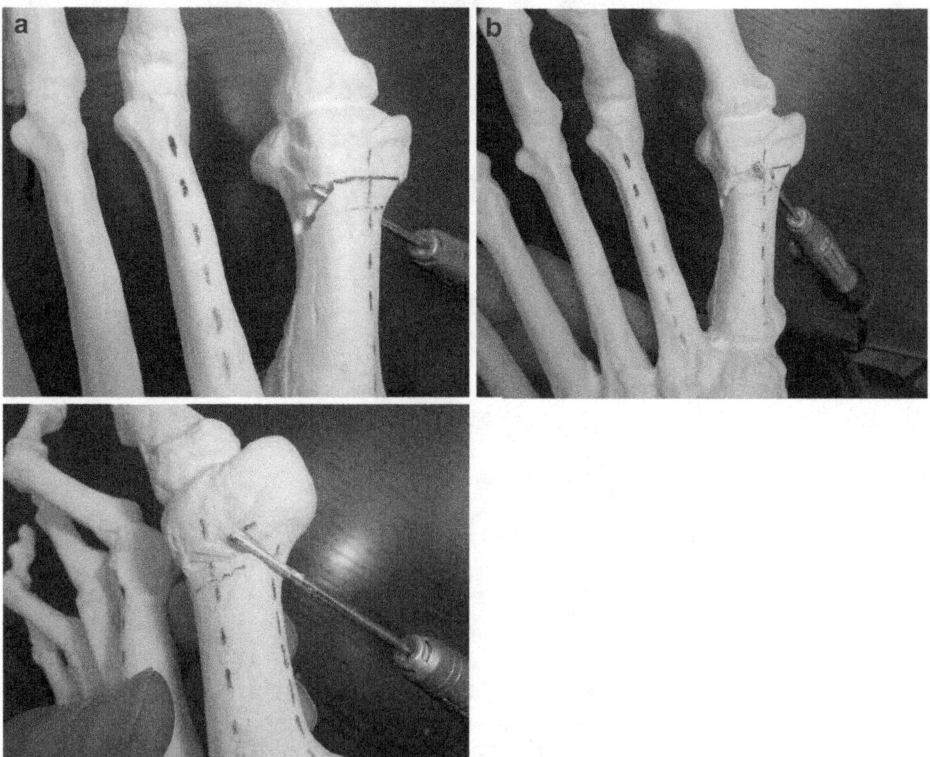

Fig. 10.12 (**a**, **b**, **c**) The dorsal arm of the osteotomy is created

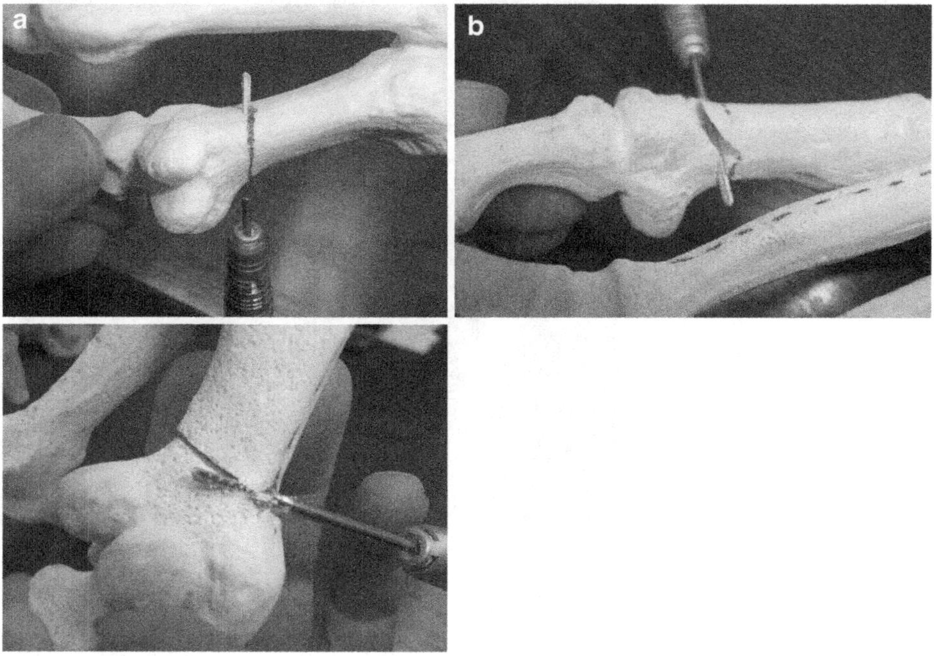

Fig. 10. 13 (**a**, **b**, **c**) The plantar arm of the osteotomy is created

plantar half of the medial cortex of the first metatarsal neck, thus completing the V-shaped osteotomy(Fig. 10.14).

The capital fragment is then distracted and displaced laterally. If necessary, a Locke elevator can be used to distract and displace the osteotomy. Once the metatarsal head has been shifted laterally, it then is impacted proximally against the metatarsal shaft (Fig. 10.15).

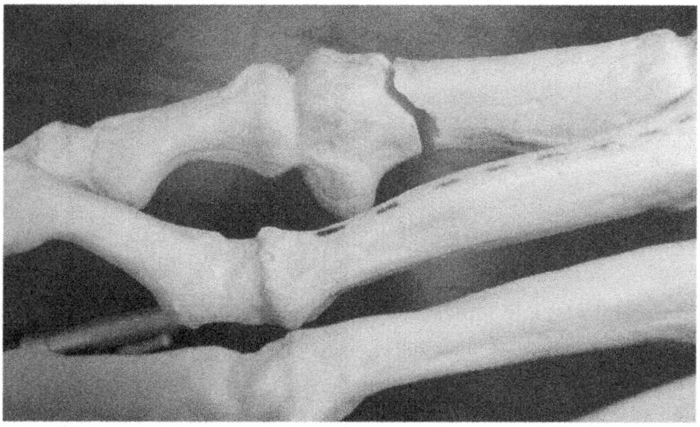

Fig. 10. 14 Thec ompleted osteotomy

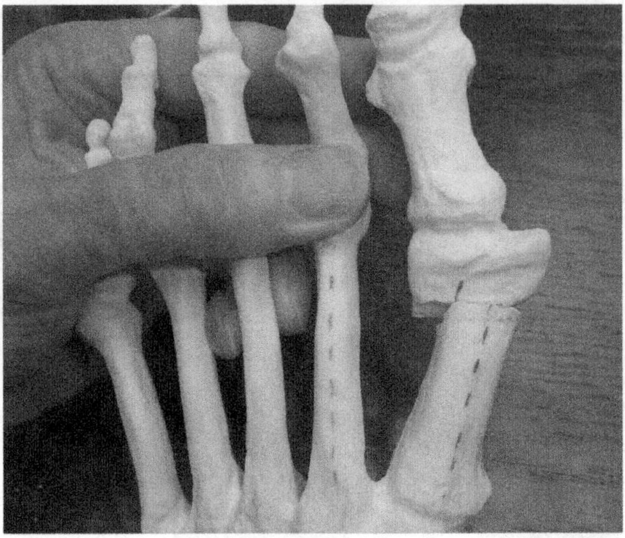

Fig.10.15 The head of the first metatarsal is displaced laterally and impacted againstt hem etatarsals haft

10.6 Remodeling the Medial Side of the First Metatarsal Head

It may be technically easier to remodel the metatarsal head prior to completing the metatarsal osteotomy, since the metatarsal head is more stable, but it is generally preferred to remodel the metatarsal head after the osteotomy is completed. The advantage of remodeling the head after performing the osteotomy is that less of the medial eminence will need to be removed after the head of the metatarsal has been displaced laterally (Fig. 10.16) and

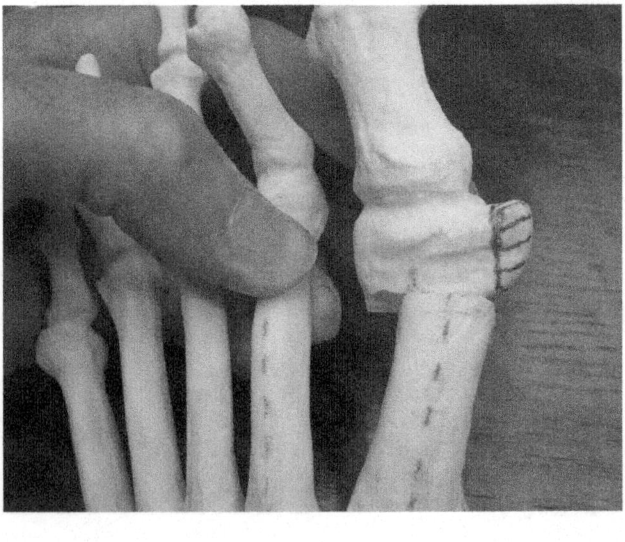

Fig.10.16 Mediale minence to be removed after lateral displacement of the metatarsalhe ad

the surgeon may be able to increase the lateral displacement of the metatarsal head and thus further reduce the intermetatarsal angle while still maintaining good bony apposition at the medial aspect of the osteotomy site.

The metatarsal head can be remodeled through the initial incision but the surgeon may find it easier to use the second more dorsal (or more plantar) incision to obtain a better angle of approach. This will also make it easier to remodel the medial aspect of the first metatarsal just proximal to the osteotomy site, if a palpable osseous prominence is present once the head has been displaced (Fig. 10.20).

A medium Shannon 44 burr is then introduced into the second incision, deep and under the capsule and a small amount of the bone is removed from the medial aspect of the metatarsal head (Fig. 10.17). This creates room to introduce the 3 mm wedge burr which is used to reduce the majority of the unwanted medial eminence. Care should be taken not to entangle the soft tissue around the rotating burrs. The rasp, or a similar instrument, may then be introduced to smooth any remaining bony projections. Subcapsular debris should then be removed using the rasp, with the teeth aimed toward the capsule. Bone paste and fragments are thus expressed. The surgeon may also choose to flush out any remaining debris with sterile saline solution.

If the surgeon deems it necessary, the osteotomy can be fixated percutaneously using Kirschner wires, although this may increase the chance of fracturing the dorsal ledge. A 0.45 gauge Kirschner wire is inserted proximal to the osteotomy site at the dorsal aspect of the shaft of the first metatarsal, carefully avoiding the Extensor Hallucis Longus tendon, and drilled in a distal and plantar direction into the head of the first metatarsal while holding the head firmly against the shaft of the metatarsal (Fig. 10.18a). A second Kirschner wire, 0.45 gauge for a lighter patient or 0.62 for a heavier patient, is then inserted into the medial aspect of the first metatarsal shaft, proximal to the osteotomy site, and drilled in a distal lateral direction into the head of the first metatarsal, again while holding the head in position against the shaft (Fig. 10.18b). Care should be taken not to introduce the Kirschner wires too close to the osteotomy in order to avoid fracturing the dorsal shelf during weight

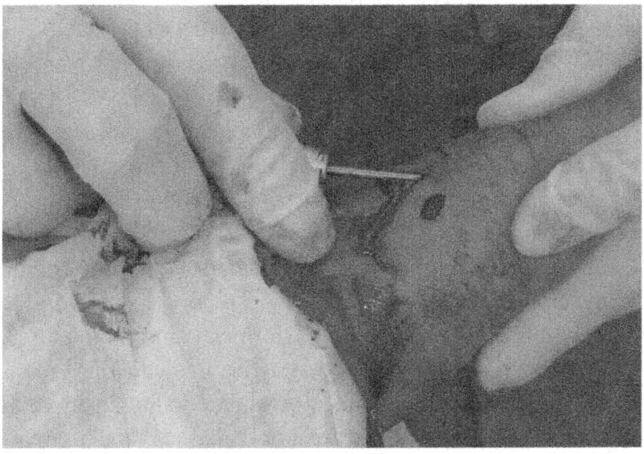

Fig.10.17 Reducingthe medial eminence of the first metatarsalhe ad

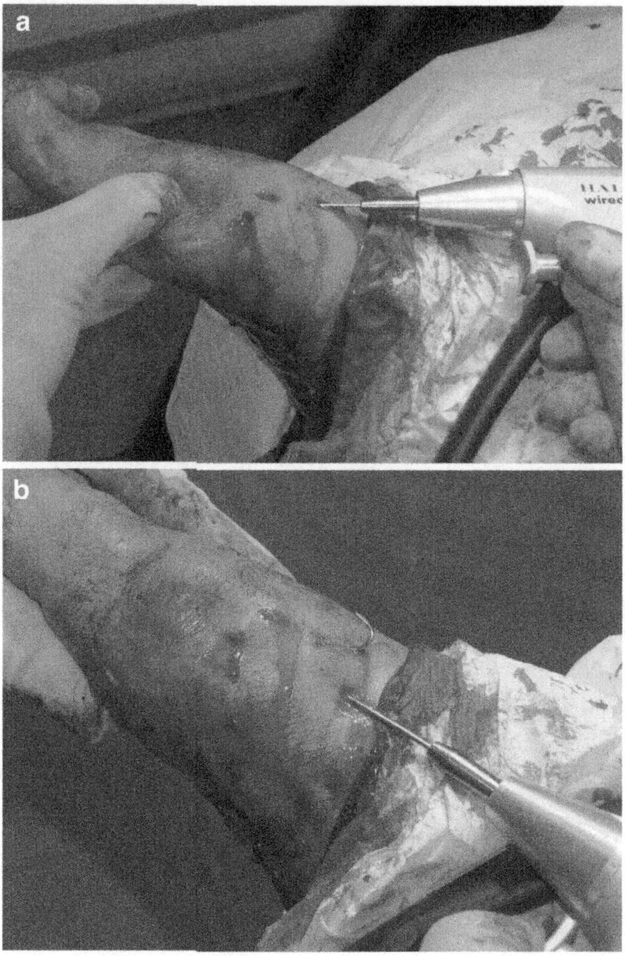

Fig.10. 18 Optional percutaneos fixation using Kirschner wires (**a**) The first Kirschner wire is introduced from proximal dorsal to distal plantar (**b**) The second Kirschner wire is introduced from proximal medial to distall ateral

bearing. The surgeon can reduce the chance of such a fracture, especially in a patient with reduced bone density, by incorporating a Dancer's pad made of 1/8 to 1/4 in. felt to the plantar surface of the postoperative dressing to reduce dorsiflexion pressure on the first metatarsalhe ad(Fig. 10.19).

If a palpable medial bony prominence is produced just proximal to the osteotomy site at the neck of the first metatarsal (Fig. 10.20), it can now be remodeled using a medium or short Shannon 44 through the second incision. The two incisions can then be closed using one or two nylon sutures. At this point, it is up to the discretion of the surgeon whether to use any combination of proximal phalanx osteotomy, adductor tenotomy, lateral capsulotomy, and Extensor Hallucis Longus tendon lengthening to further reduce the deformity. These procedures can also be performed using minimally invasive techniques.

The foot is then dressed with a sterile, non-adhering dressing such as Adaptic,[6] as well as 3 in. by 3in. gauze sponges, topical poviodine-iodine solution, and 2 in. conforming rolled stretch gauze (Fig. 10.21a). The proximal phalanx should be over-corrected in adduction to keep pressure on the medial portion of the osteotomy site. If percutaneous fixation is not used, the distal fragment should be taped into position firmly using one inch Durapore tape[7] (Fig. 10.21b).

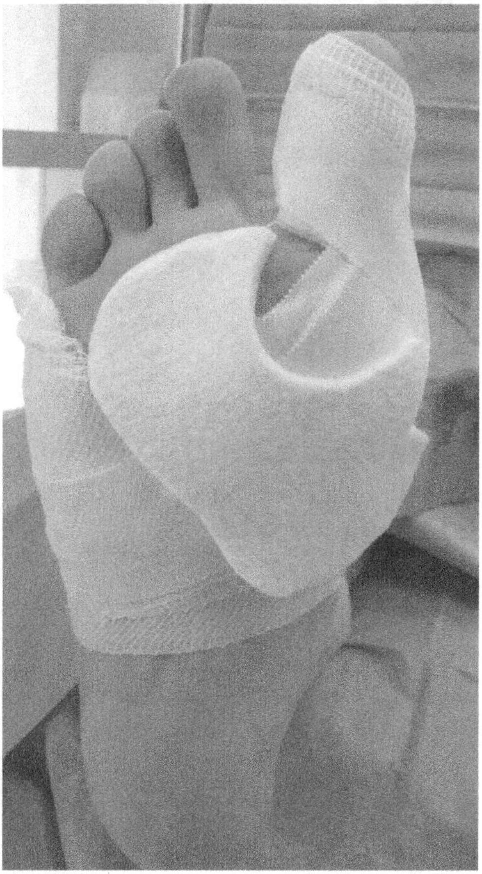

Fig. 10. 19 Felt Dancers pad which may be used to reduce dorsiflectory pressure on the firstme tatarsalhe ad

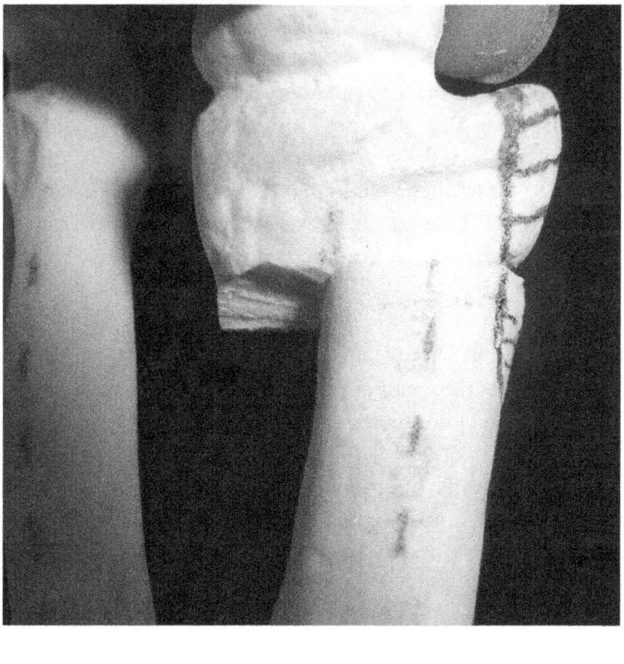

Fig. 10. 20 Medialos seous prominence just proximal to the metatarsal eminence. If the prominence is palpable, it should be reduced to avoid shoeirrita tion

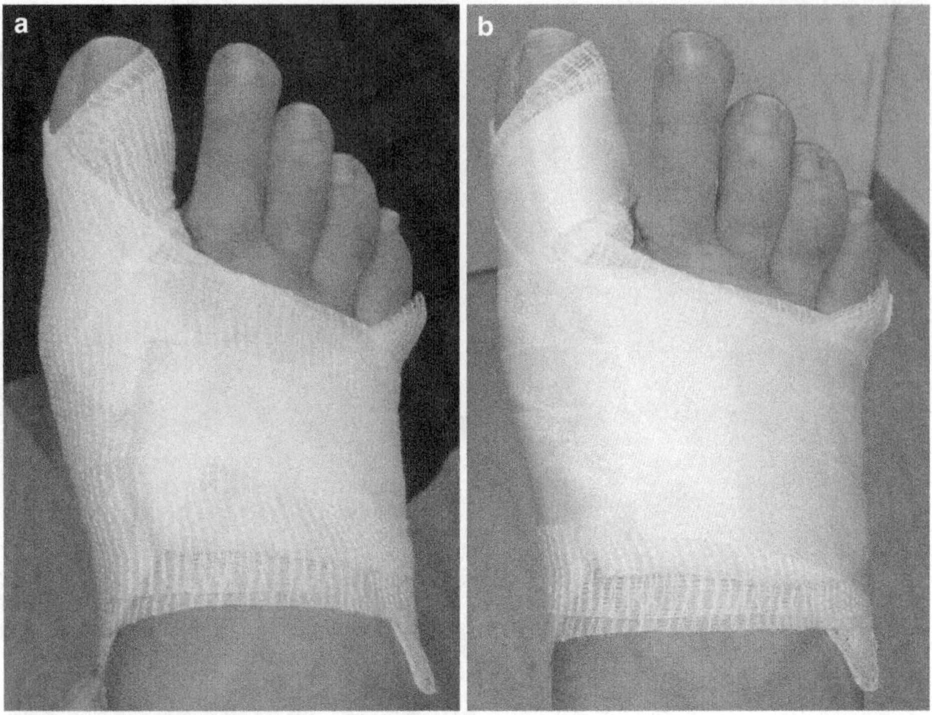

Fig. 10.21 (**a**) The foot is wrapped with 2 in. conforming rolled stretch gauze, with one 3 in. by 3 in. gauze sponge pads placed at the first and at the fifth metatarsal heads to protect the metatarsal heads from iriitation. (**b**) The dressing is reinforced with 1 in. Durapore tape

If percutaneous fixation is used, it is not necessary to tape the metatarsal head as firmly. Folded gauze 3in. by 3in. sponges should be placed just proximal and distal to the Kirschner wires (Fig. 10.22a) to avoid skin irritation from excessive pressure on the wires from the dressing or taping. The practitioner can then use one inch Durapore or 3 in. adhesive backed stretch tape to cover the dressing (Fig. 10.22b). The patient is given a surgical sandal to wear when walking for as long as the foot is taped.

The foot is taped for 6 weeks. If Kirschner wire fixation is not used, the foot should be taped firmly for 6 weeks. The taping does not have to be as firm for the first 3 weeks if Kirschner wires are in place. The foot should be taped firmly for 3 weeks after the wires have been removed.

The patient should be seen in 4 or 5 days post-operatively to change the dressing, rule out infection, and check the alignment of the osteotomy. If the alignment is incorrect, the Kirschner wires should be removed and the metatarsal head should be manipulated into place and firmly redressed. The patient is then seen 1 week later to change the dressing and to remove sutures. The patient is then seen 3 weeks post-operatively to change the dressing and to remove the Kirschner wires, if fixation was used. The patient should now begin passive range of motion exercises at the first metatarsal

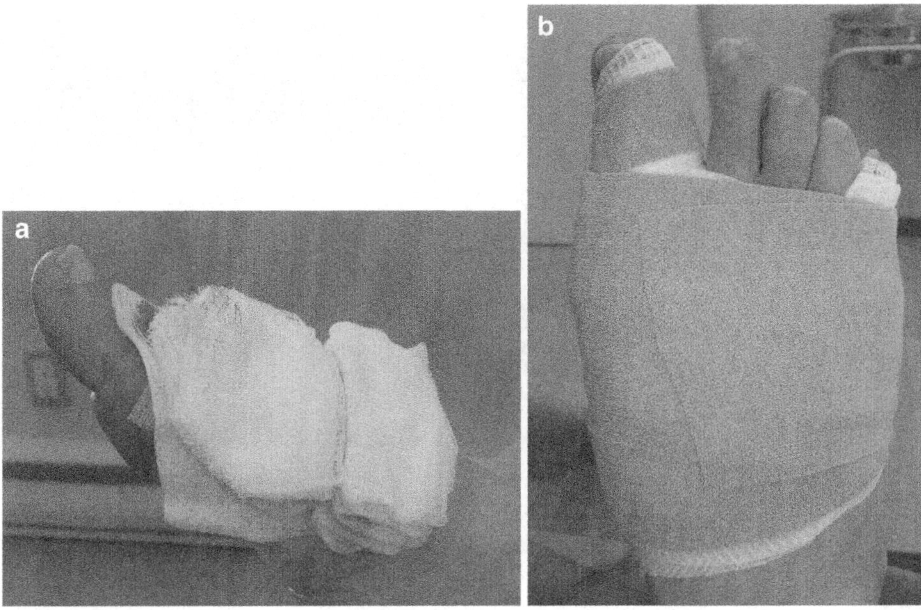

Fig. 10.22 (**a**) If Kirschner wires are used, gauzes are placed proximal and distal to the wires to avoid skin irritation. (**b**) The dressing is covered with 3 in. adhesive backed stretch tape

phalangeal joint using their contralateral hand (Fig. 10.23a, b). The patient can then be instructed on home taping of the foot for an additional 3 weeks, or the practitioner may choose to do this for the patient weekly in the office. The patient should be encouraged to walk to tolerance, but excessive walking should be avoided for 6 weeks following surgery.

Fig.10. 23 Thepa tient should begin range of motion exercises. Begin 3 weeks post-operatively and continue until there is adequate range of motion at the first metatarsal phalangeal joint. (**a**)Pla ntarflexion (**b**)P ost-operative dorsiflexion exercise

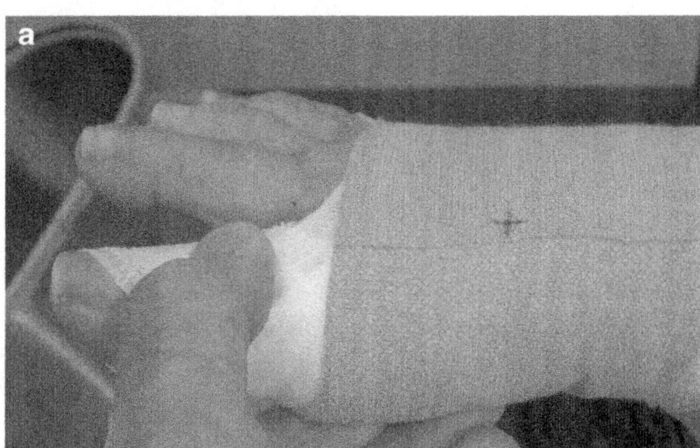

Fig. 10.23 (continued)

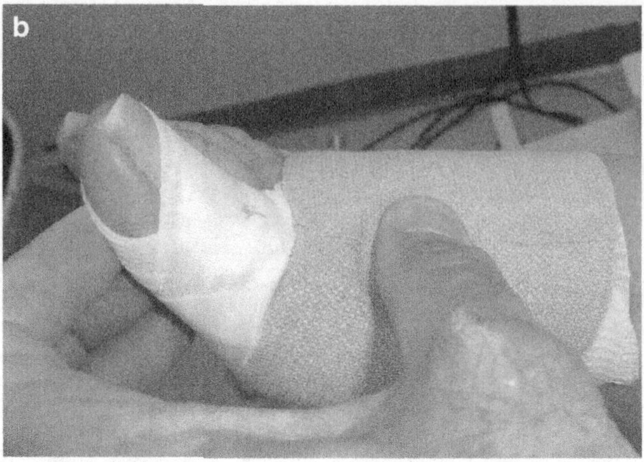

10.7 AdditionalS uggestions

When first performing this procedure, the surgeon may find it helpful to draw landmarks on the foot prior to surgery. These landmarks may include the plantar medial, dorsal medial and dorsal lateral cortices of the first metatarsal, the medial and dorsal aspect of the osteotomy itself, the first metatarsal phalangeal joint, and the Extensor Hallucis Longus tendon (Fig. 10.24). The surgeon may also choose to confirm the location of the initial skin incision for the fail-safe hole by placing a sterile, 7/8 in. needle at the proposed location of the incision and checking it under fluoroscopy.

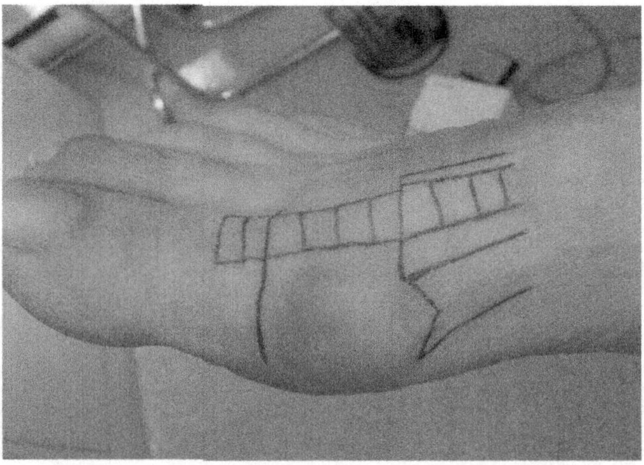

Fig.10. 24 Landmarksm aybe drawn prior to beginning surgery

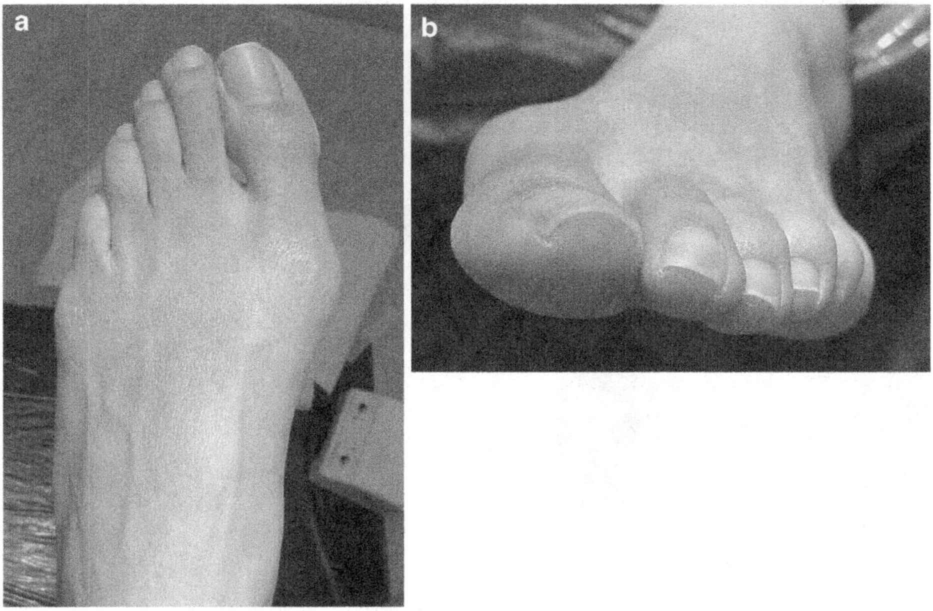

Fig. 10. 25 (**a**, **b**) Pre-operative photographs, firstp atient

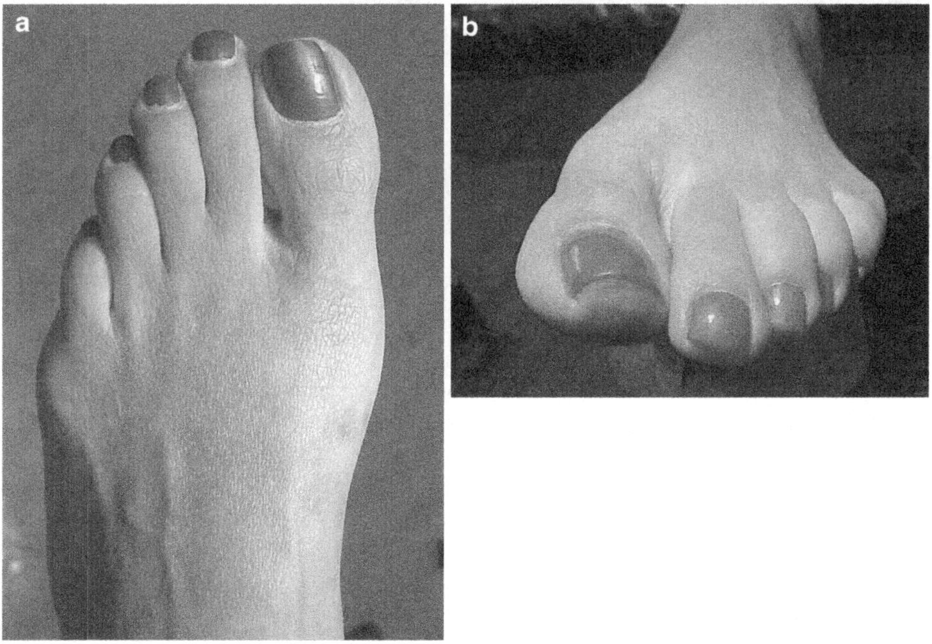

Fig. 10. 26 (**a**, **b**) Post-operative photographs, firstp atient

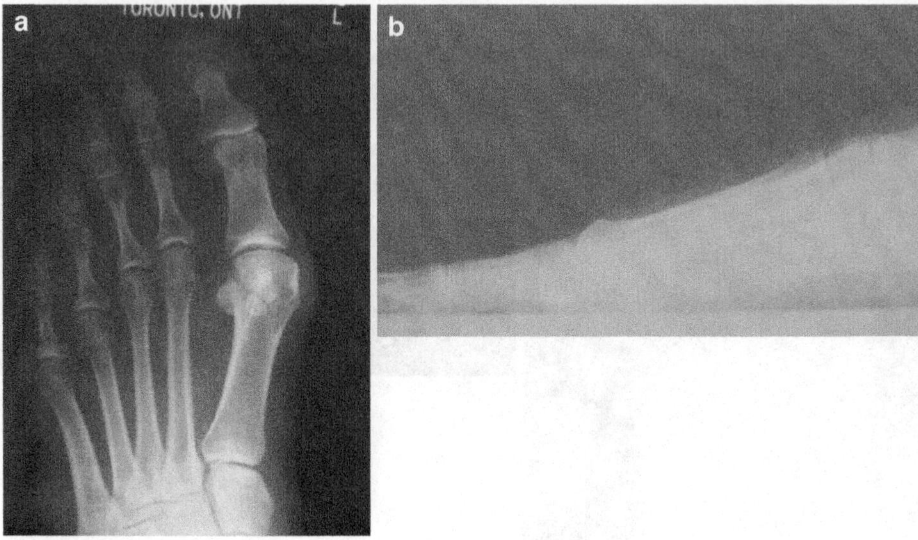

Fig.10.27 (**a**, **b**) Pre-operative radiographs, firstp atient

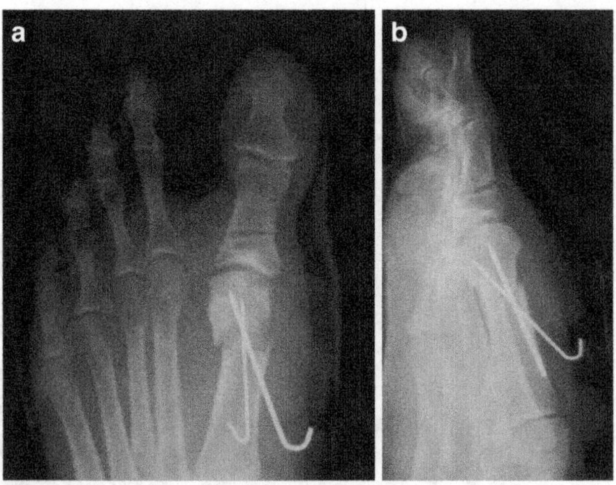

Fig.10.28 (**a**, **b**) Immediate Post-operative radiographs, firstpa tient

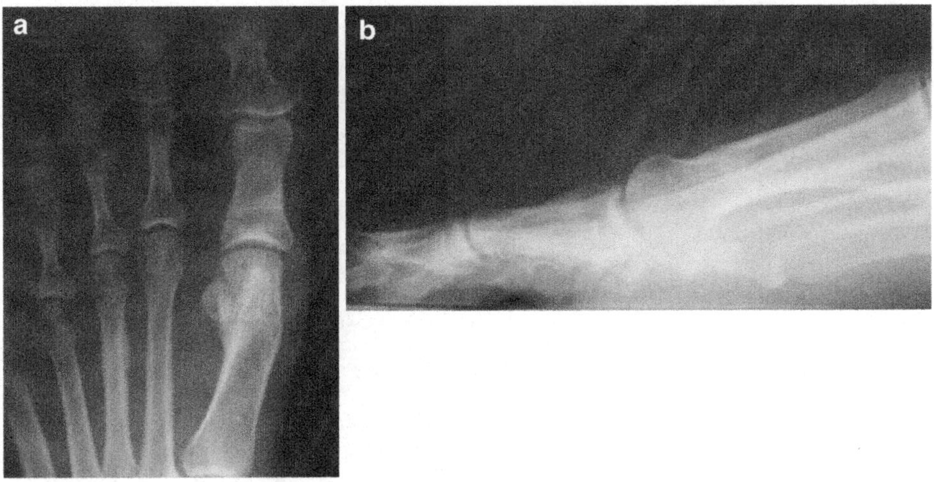

Fig. 10.29 (**a**, **b**) One year post-operative radiographs, firstp atient

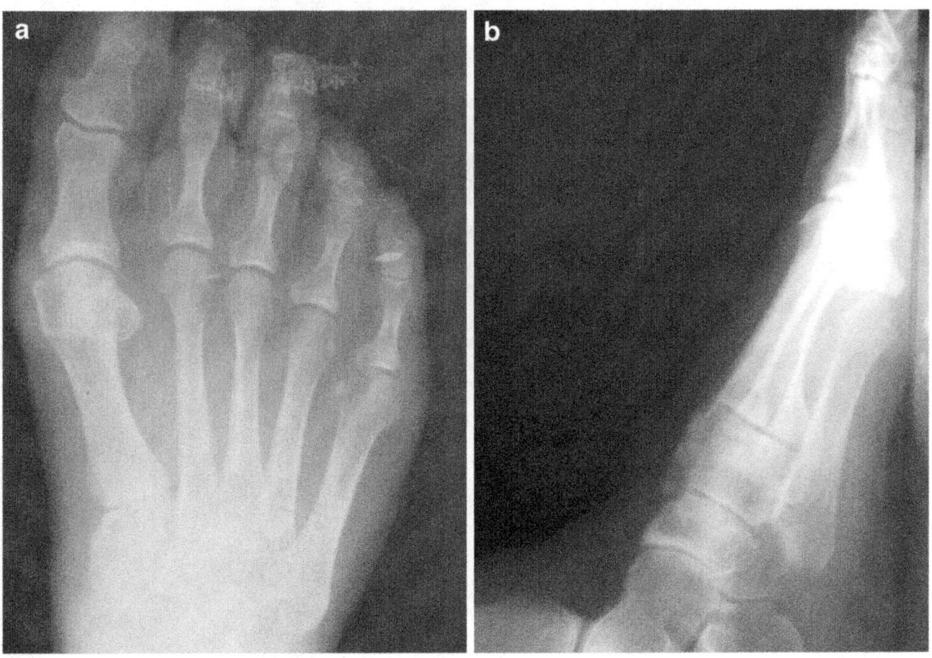

Fig. 10.30 (**a**, **b**)Pre -operativer adiographs,s econdpa tient

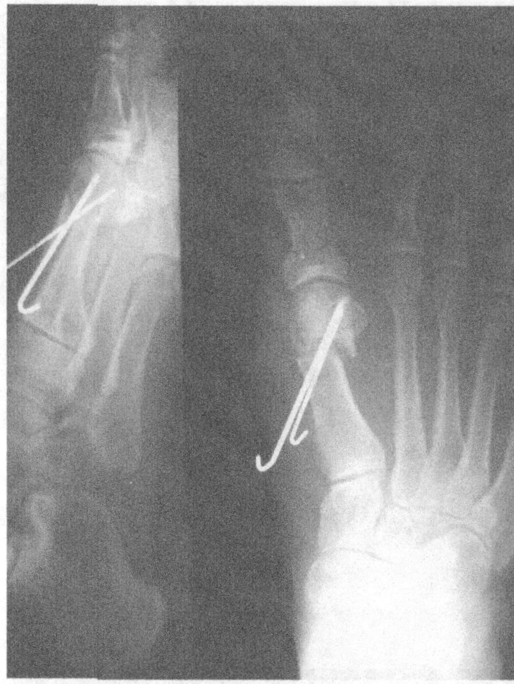

Fig.10. 31 Immediate post-operative radiographs,s econdpa tient

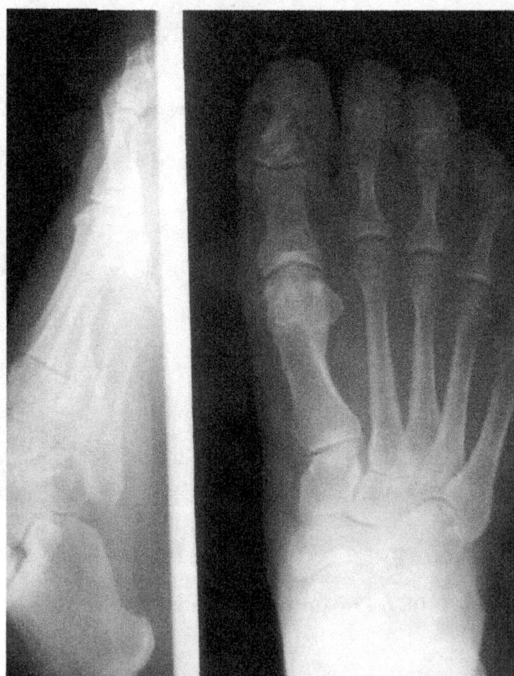

Fig.10. 32 Oneye arpos t-operative radiographs,s econdpa tient

When performing the osteotomy, to avoid thermal necrosis, the surgeon should avoid running the burrs at excessive speed, three Shannon 44 burrs should be used and the burrs should be sharp. Dull burrs should be discarded. Also, avoid applying undue pressure on the burrs to reduce the chance of burr breakage.

In case of burr breakage, if part of the fragment is protruding from the bone, the surgeon may use a hemostat or a needle driver to grasp the fragment, and pull it out, while using an unscrewing motion.

If the burr is unreachable inside a partially performed osteotomy, the surgeon should complete the osteotomy using another Shannon 44 burr to free up the burr fragment. An eye-magnet[2] (Fig. 10.2) can then be inserted into the osteotomy site, under fluoroscopy if available. In most instances, if the eye-magnet makes contact with the loose fragment, the surgeon will be able to remove it with little difficulty.

If the surgeon has difficulty shifting the metatarsal head laterally following the completion of the osteotomy, it may be necessary to again run the Shannon 44 inside the osteotomy to remove an additional small amount of bone.

It is not necessary to surgically revise the redundant skin in the area of the first metatarsal head. This will shrink on its own.

References

1. Wilson JN. Oblique displacement osteotomy for hallux valgus. *J Bone Joint Surg.* 1963;45B:552–556.
2. MiltexInc .,Y ork,P A.
3. VilexinT ennesseel nc.,M cMinnville,TN .
4. Xi-Tec, Inc., East Windsor, CT, company no longer in operation.
5. Osada,I nc.,Los Angeles,C A.
6. Johnson and Johnson Medical Limited, Gargrave, Skipton, UK.
7. 3MH ealthC are,St .P aul,M N.(**a, b**)

Part III

Lesser Toes

Percutaneous Surgery for Static Metatarsalgia

11

Thomas Bauer

11.1 Introduction

Metatarsalgias with plantar hyperkeratosis under the metatarsal heads of the lateral rays is very prevalent. Conservative management with insoles often provides a complete or partial relief of the symptoms. In case of failure of non-operative modalities, surgery can be indicated, and several metatarsal osteotomies have been described. Their aim is to shorten and to raise the metatarsals to decrease the pressure under the metatarsal heads of the lateral rays to provide relief of the symptoms.[1–12] The Weil osteotomy is the most popular distal metatarsal osteotomy and is still the gold standard treatment for metatarsalgia.[5] However, metatarso-phalangeal joint stiffness is a very frequent complication after Weil osteotomy, and difficulties with fixation or restoration of the distal metatarsal arch can be experienced. We present a percutaneous procedure for the treatment of metatarsalgias with details on the surgical technique, first results and discussion of the benefits and indications.[13–14]

11.2 Operative Technique

Instruments: The surgical tools required to perform a distal metatarsal mini-invasive osteotomy (DMMO) are those used for percutaneous forefoot procedures, including a straight burr, a Beaver® blade, elevators, rasps, low speed and high torque drill and a fluoroscope.

Patient set up: The patient is supine, under regional or local anaesthesia, with the foot free over the end of the table to allow fluoroscopic control.

Portals: A small skin incision (1 or 2 mm) is made with the Beaver® blade next to the metatarsal head, parallel to the extensor tendon (Fig. 11.1). The portal can be more distal, at the level of the metatarso-phalangeal joint in case of dorsal release of this joint.

T. Bauer
Ambroise Paré Hospital, West Paris University, Department of Orthopaedic Surgery,
9a vC harlesde G aulle, 92100B oulogne, France
e-mail:thoma s.bauer@apr.aphp.fr

N. Maffulli and M. Easley (eds.), *Minimally Invasive Surgery of the Foot and Ankle*,
DOI: 10.1007/978-1-84996-417-3_11, © Springer-Verlag London Limited 2011

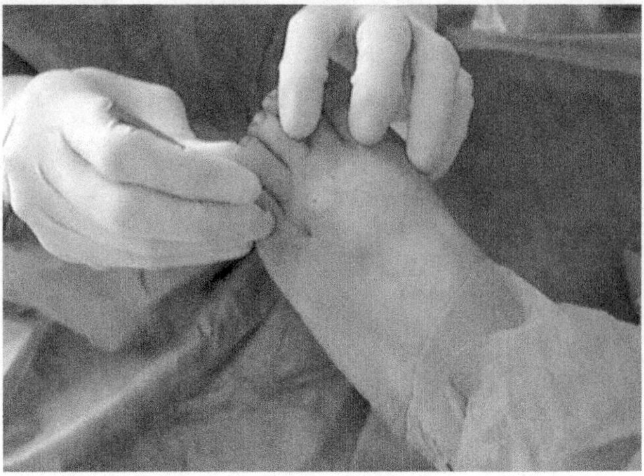

Fig. 11.1 Portals for DMMO of the second, third and fourth metatarsals

Distal Metatarsal Mini-invasive Osteotomy (DMMO): After subcutaneous dissection, an elevator is introduced with a 45° direction from dorsal distal to plantar proximal and is sliding down the lateral cortex of the metatarsal shaft just proximal to the head. This produce a working area avoiding soft tissue damages with the burr. The straight burr is then introduced in the same direction in contact with the bone (Fig. 11.2). The osteotomy is more proximal than the Weil osteotomy and is extra-articular. The osteotomy is in a 45° direction from dorsal distal to plantar proximal (Fig. 11.3). During the osteotomy, a circular movement of the burr is made around a fixed axis at the level of the skin incision. The osteotomy is begun on the lateral cortex 2–3 mm proximal from the articular surface with the burr parallel to the shaft and then the plantar and medial cortexes are cut (Fig. 11.4). The osteotomy ends on the dorsal cut with the burr perpendicular with the metatarsal shaft (Fig. 11.5). The toe is then pulled and pushed to check the osteotomy is complete and to release periosteal attachments that would prevent the shortening and rising up of the distal metatarsal fragment (Fig. 11.6). The same procedure is performed for each ray needing an osteotomy.

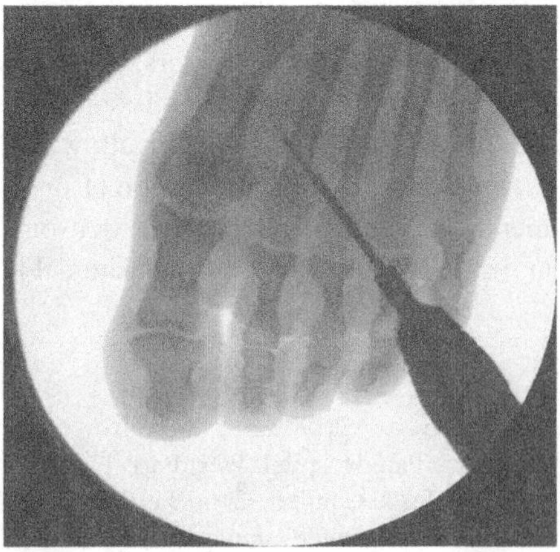

Fig. 11.2 Positioning of the burr

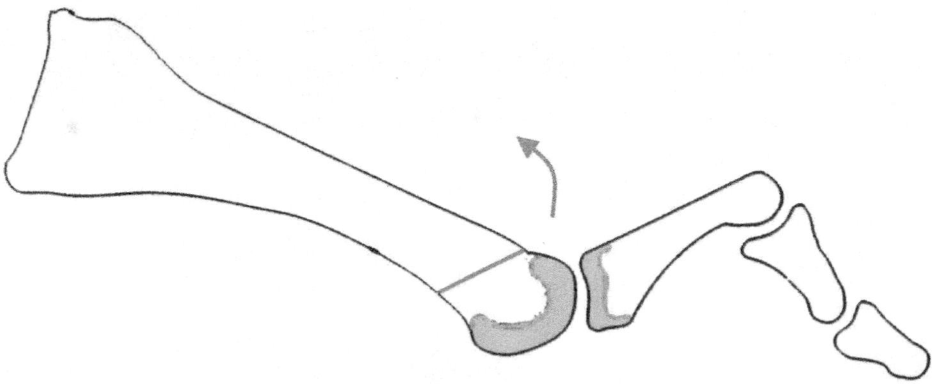

Fig. 11. 3 Principlesofth eD MMO

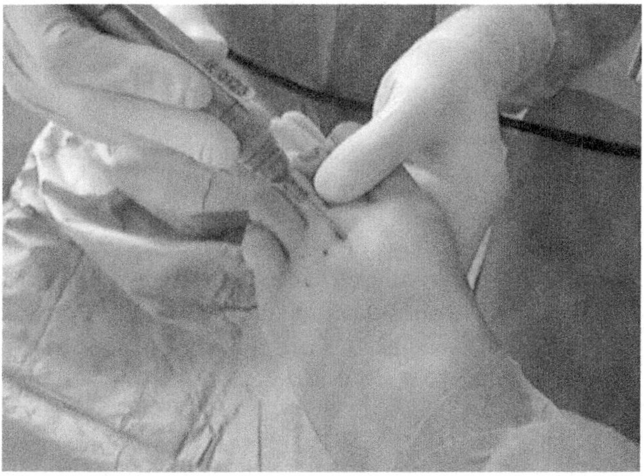

Fig. 11. 4 DMMO:be ginning of the osteotomy (the burr is paralleltothe me tatarsal)

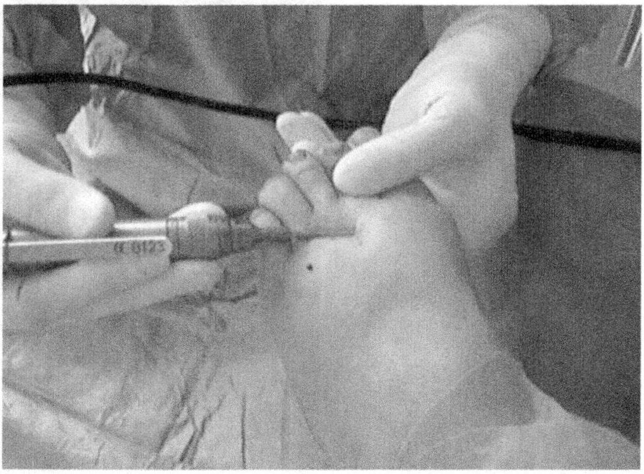

Fig. 11. 5 DMMO: end of the osteotomy (the burr is perpendicular to the metatarsal)

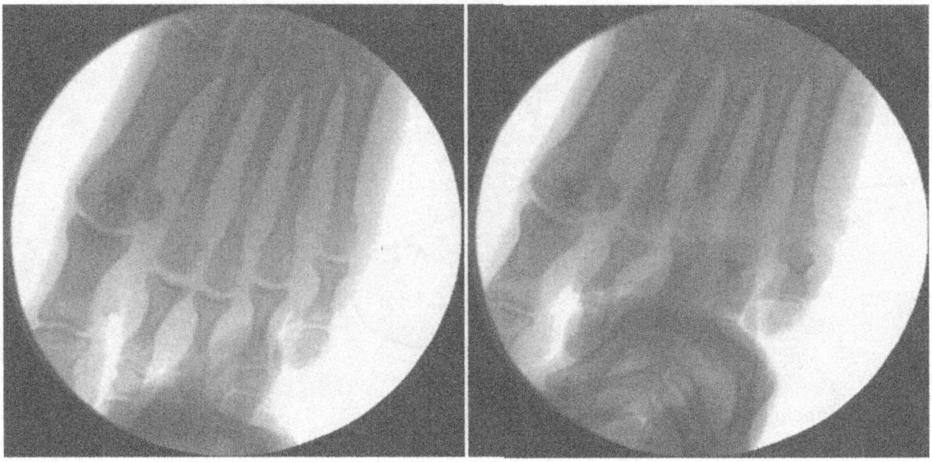

Fig. 11.6 Mobilizationof t het oesa fterD MMO

11.3 Post-OperativeC are

The portals are not closed. A post-operative dressing with specific bandage is made to keep the good alignment of the different toes. The dressing is changed after 10 days and a cohesive bandage is applied for 1 month (Fig. 11.7). Immediate full weight bearing is allowed in a shoe with a complete flat and rigid insole. Radiographs are taken after 10 days and 1 month from the operation. Normal shoe wearing is begun after 1 month according to the clinical and radiographic control.

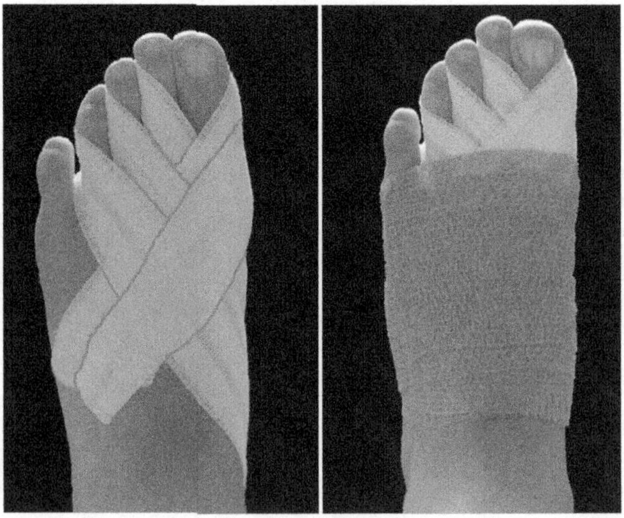

Fig. 11.7 Post-operative dressing with cohesive bandage

11.4 Indications:R esults

The indications for DMMO are basically all static metatarsalgias of the lateral rays with plantar hyperkeratosis after failure of conservative treatment for 6 months. These are very frequent with or without first ray deformity, after failed previous surgery or in chronic inflammatory diseases.

One hundred and eighteen cases of metatarsalgias in whom a DMMO had been performed were studied prospectively with a mean follow up of 26 months. Plantar hyperkeratosis and metatarsalgias disappeared in all the cases within 2.5 months. The overall functional AOFAS forefoot score significantly improved from a mean 60/100 pre-operatively to a mean 94/100 post-operatively ($p < 0.001$). Two patients had marked stiffness (ROM < 30°) of the metatarso-phalangeal joint of one ray: in both patients, the osteotomy was intra-articular, and was revised. In four patients in whom DMMO were performed only on the second and third ray, a transfer metatarsalgia appeared under the fourth ray after the post-operative month. A prolonged swelling of 2 months was often seen. Bone healing was achieved in all but one case with a very variable delay (6 weeks to 18 months). The only patient with one metatarsal non-union was still asymptomatic after 4 years. Antero-posterior radiographs showed shortening of the metatarsal with a lining up of the metatarsal heads from the first to the fifthm etatarsal.

11.5 Discussion

Percutaneous surgery for metatarsalgia using the DMMO is simple, effective and reproducible. Complications are rare, and can be avoided if appropriate care is exerted:

- The risk of skin burn decreases with the experience and learning curve in percutaneous forefoots urgery.
- Metatarso-phalangeal joint stiffness is avoided by performing a more proximal extra-articular osteotomy at the level of the distal third of the metatarsal shaft.
- Transfer metatarsalgia is avoided by performing simultaneous DMMO on the second, third and fourth metatarsal to obtain an harmonic lining up of the central metatarsal headsw itha na utomatica djustmentw ithf ullw eightbe aring.

References

1. Feibel JB, Tisdel CL, Donley BD. Lesser metatarsal osteotomies. A biomechanical approach to metatarsalgia. *Foot Ankle Clin.* 2001 Sept;6:473–489.
2. Leventen EO, Pearson SW. Distal metatarsal osteotomy for intractable plantar keratosis. *Foot Ankle Int.* 1987;10:247–251.

3. Gauthier G. Maladie de Freiberg ou deuxième maladie de Koehler. Propositions dun traitement de reconstruction au stade évolué de laffection (34 cas traités). *Rev Chir Orthop.* 1974;60:337–341.
4. Kitaoka HB, Patzer GL. Chevron osteotomy of lesser metatarsals for intractable plantar callosities. *J Bone Joint Surg (Br).* 1998;80:516–518.
5. Leemrijse T. Ostéotomie de Weil. In: Valtin B, Leemrijse T, ed. *Chirurgie de lavant-pied.* 2ème éd. Paris: Elsevier; 2005:126–141. Cahiers denseignement de la SOFCOT.
6. Wolf MD. Metatarsal osteotomy for the relief of painful metatarsal callosities. *J Bone Joint Surg (Am).* 1973;55:1760–1762.
7. Helal B. Metatarsal osteotomy for metatarsalgia. *J Bone Joint Surg (Br).* 1975;57:187–192.
8. Giannestras NJ. Plantar keratosis treatment by metatarsal shortening. *J Bone Joint Surg (Am).* 1966;48:72–76.
9. Giannestras NJ. Shortening of the metatarsal shaft in the treatment of plantar keratosis. An end-result study. *Foot Ankle Int.* 1995;16:529–534.
10. Delagoutte JP, Jarde O. Ostéotomies métatarsiennes à lexception de la technique de Weil. In: Valtin B, Leemrijse T, ed. *Chirurgie de lavant-pied.* 2ème éd. Paris: Elsevier; 2005:149–152. Cahiers denseignement de la SOFCOT.
11. Denis A, Huber-Levernieux C, Goutallier D. Notre expérience de lostéotomie métatarsienne dans le traitement des métatarsalgies statiques. *Méd Chir Pied.* 1984;1:85–88.
12. Toullec E, Barouk LS, Rippstein P. Ostéotomie de relèvement basal métatarsienne BRT. In: Valtin B, Leemrijse T, ed. *Chirurgie de lavant-pied.* 2ème éd. Paris: Elsevier; 2005:142–148. Cahiers denseignement de la SOFCOT.
13. De Prado M, Ripoll PL, Golano P. Metatarsalgias. In: De Prado M, Ripoll PL, Golano P, ed. *Cirurgia percutanea del pie.* Barcelona, Spain: Masson SA; 2003:167–182.
14. Coillard JY, Laffenetre O, Cermolacce C et al. Traitement chirurgical des métatarsalgies statiques par technique percutanée. In: Valtin B, Leemrijse T, ed. *Chirurgie de lavant-pied.* 2ème éd. Paris: Elsevier; 2005:153–157. Cahiers denseignement de la SOFCOT.

Percutaneous Treatment of Static Metatarsalgia with Distal Metatarsal Mini-InvasiveO steotomy

12

J. Y. Coillard, Olivier Laffenetre, Christope Cermolacce, Patrice Determe, Stéphane Guillo, Christopede L avigne,a ndP .G olano
GRECMIP (Groupe de Recherche et d'Etude en Chirurgie Mini-Invasive du Pied)

12.1 Introduction

Metatarsalgia is frequent. Most patients respond to 6 to 12 months of conservative management. At times,, usually from structural abnormalities of the foot, especially first-ray shortening, surgery provides considerable benefit. Historically, the first osteotomies described to manage metatarsalgia were diaphyseal,[5,6,7] then proximal metaphyseal,[8,9] and finally distal[10]. In 1991, Weil[1] described a technique, still widely used in Europe, which enables perfect control of the planned proximal migration of the metatarsal head. Consolidation is ensured by appropriate internal fixation. The technique, however, involves penetrating the metatarso-phalangeal joint, and frequently causes stiffening of the metatarso-phalangeal joint.

A minimally invasive distal metatarsal osteotomy[2,3,4] avoids these disadvantages, and is recommended in these patients.

12.2 Aimsand P rinciples

As in open surgery, the minimally invasive procedure which we describe aims to shorten the operated metatarsal and raise the metatarsal heads via a minimally invasive approach to limit dorsal fibrosis, avoiding to penetrate the joint to prevent stiffening, and without internal fixation to ensure appropriate bony callus in optimal weight-bearing position.

The aim is to shorten and dorsiflex the relevant metatarsal (Figs. 12.1–12.3). The indications for surgery are basically clinical, although antero-posterior weight-bearing forefoot radiographs also provides precious information about the metatarsal formula,

J.Y. Coillard(✉)
CliniqueduPa rcL yon, 155bdSt alingrad, 69006, Lyon, France
e-mail:jy .coillard@cliniqueduparclyon.com

N. Maffulli and M. Easley (eds.), *Minimally Invasive Surgery of the Foot and Ankle*,
DOI: 10.1007/978-1-84996-417-3_12, © Springer-Verlag London Limited 2011

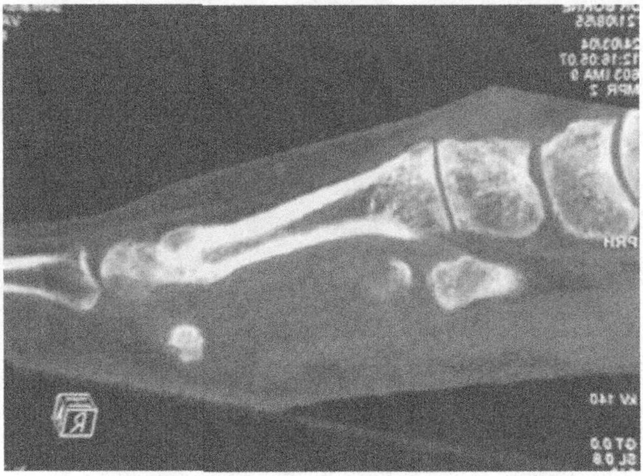

Fig.12. 1 (ProfileV iew)C T aspects of DMMO which produces a real vicious callus with elevation and shortening

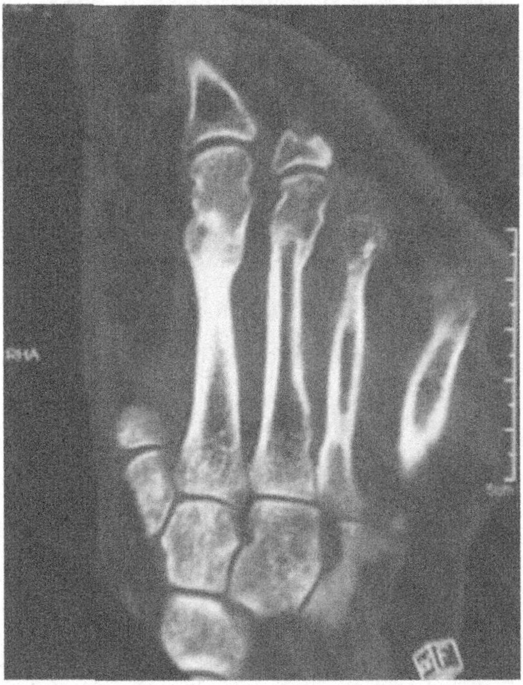

Fig.12. 2 (Front Side View) CT aspects of DMMO which produces a real vicious callus with elevation and shortening

acknowledging that it does not take into account sagittal metatarsal mobility. There is no pre-operative planning of the sort required, for example, when undertaking a Weil osteotomy. The osteotomized metatarsal heads find their own positions when weight-bearing postoperatively.

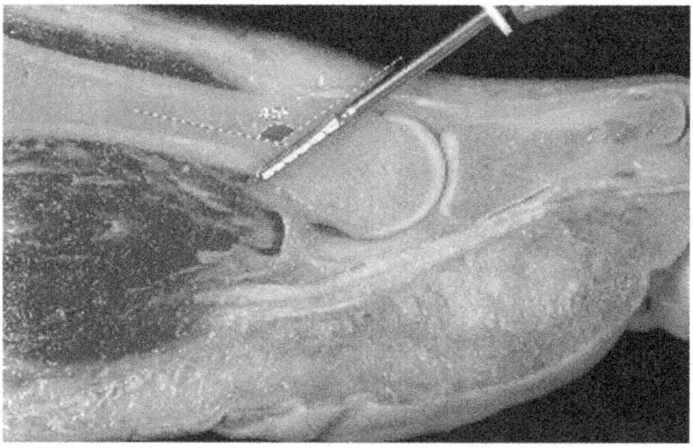

Fig. 12.3 Place of the burr in contact with the metatarsal cortexa t45°

12.3 Materials

To undertake minimally invasive surgery, a dedicated instrumentation, an image intensifier and a dedicated mini-motor are necessary.

The following are recommended:

(a) Beaver®t ypes calpel
(b) As mallpe riosteale levator
(c) Rasp(littleus edi nt hisi ndication)
(d) Slowr otation(<15,000r pm)m ini-motor
(e) Longor w ideS hannon44bur r
(f) Lowr adiation ani magei ntensifier

12.4 Surgical Technique

12.4.1 Anaesthesia

We normally use a popliteal or posterior tibial block supplemented by extensor brevis and anterior coronal midfoot block.

12.4.2 PatientP ositioning

Appropriate positioning of the patient depends on how the first ray is to be realigned. Peroperative control radiographs should, however, be planned.

12.4.3 Osteotomy

A small incision using the beaver knife is performed in the inter-metatarsal space just next to the head (to the right, for a right-handed surgeon) parallel to the extensor tendons. The scalpel is pointed at 45° to the metatarsal neck. The elevator is then introduced, to prepare the subcapital edge of the metatarsal neck and avoid soft tissue damage. Radiographs allow to check the most appropriate position for the osteotomy. The wide or long Shannon 44 burr is then introduced through the incision, in direct contact with the metatarsal cortex. During the osteotomy, the burr is maintained at 45°, milling a clear cortical groove to prevent any error in angulation or displacement of the burr. With a rotational movement, the medial, then planar, then lateral and finally dorsal cortex are osteotomised, with the burr at 45° throughout.

It is also possible to proceed by a simple lateral movement of the burr, without rotation around the metatarsal axis, but there is a greater risk of soft tissue injury. At this point, a further radiographic check can be made, together with clinical assessment that the metatarsal head is freely mobile.

The number of osteotomies depends on the pattern of plantar hyperkeratosis: when this lies exclusively under the second metatarsal head, the second and third metatarsals are osteotomised. If the plantar hyperkeratosis is located under the second and third metatarsal heads, the second, third and fourth metatarsals are osteotomised. The fifth ray is very mobile, and it seldom requires an osteotomy.

Finally, the wound is closed, with one suture per incision, it is also possible not to closed it to avoid hematoma and dressed with gauze compresses orienting the operated heads towards the hallux; this is especially important in patients in whom hallux valgus correction is associated with the distal metatarsal osteotomy of the lesser metatarsals, so that the deviation of the lesser toes caused by the hallux valgus deformity is corrected as theos teotomiesc onsolidate.

12.5 Post-OperativeF ollow-Up

Surgery may be performed on an out-patient basis or with overnight admission. Patient are allowed to weight bear immediately in a stiff-soled shoe, but should walk as little as possible during the first 3 weeks, to avoid pain and post-surgical oedema. The patients are recommended to spend as much time as possible with the foot raised during the day. When surgery to the first ray is associated, the dressing can be left unchanged for a week if the procedure was entirely minimally invasive; after that, the dressing is renewed, taking care that the bandage is fashioned so that the toes are pushed towards the hallux for 3 weeks to preventm al-union(Fig. 12.4).

A second postoperative check is made at 4 weeks to counsel about shoe wear, then at 3 or 4 months for consolidation. The fibrous callus forms as of week 3, limiting pain and mobility in the metatarsal heads, and a hypertrophic bony callus can be seen from the secondpos t-operativem onth(Fig. 12.5–12.7).

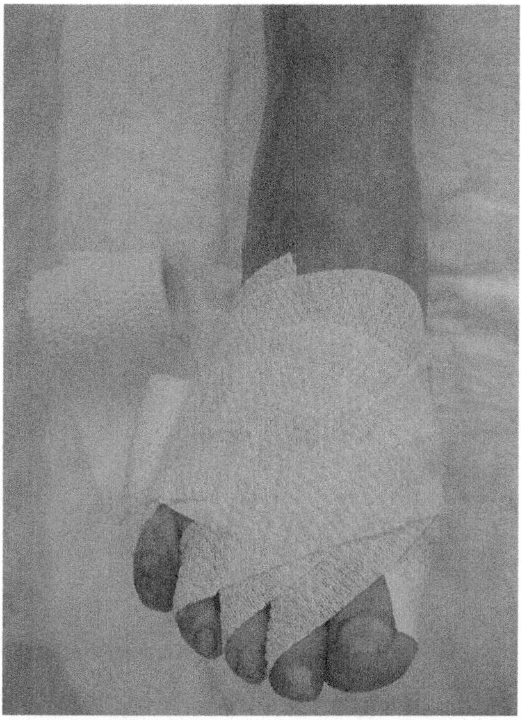

Fig. 12.4 Specific cohesive bandaging of the toes towards the hallux to prevent mal-uniona noe dema

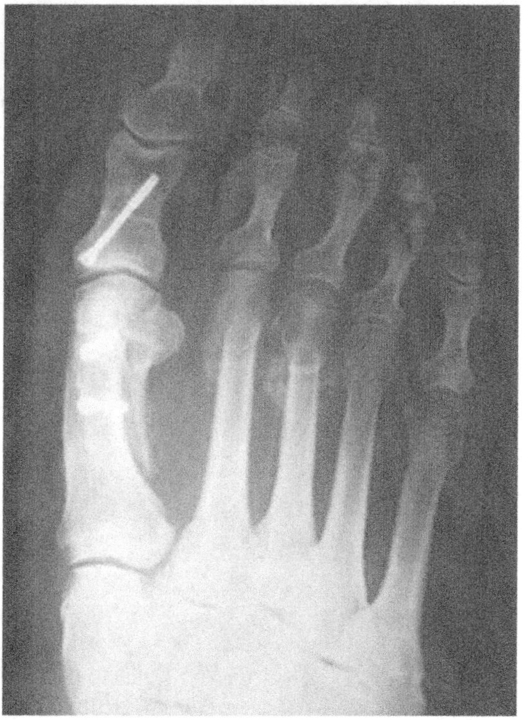

Fig. 12.5 Normal aspect of callus after 2 monthsfors econda ndt hirds hafts

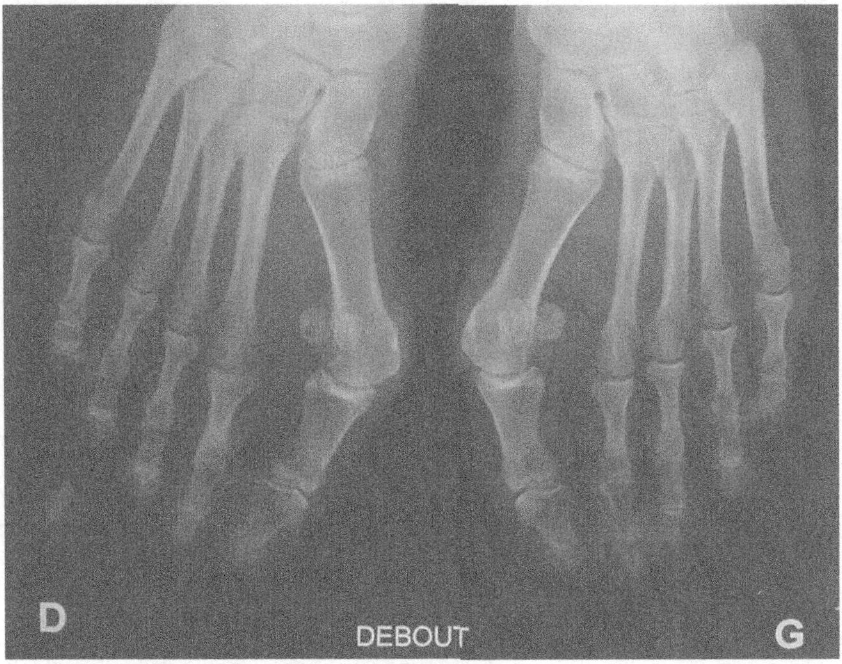

Fig.12.6 Preoperativer adiographpr iort ohyb ridm inii nvasives urgery

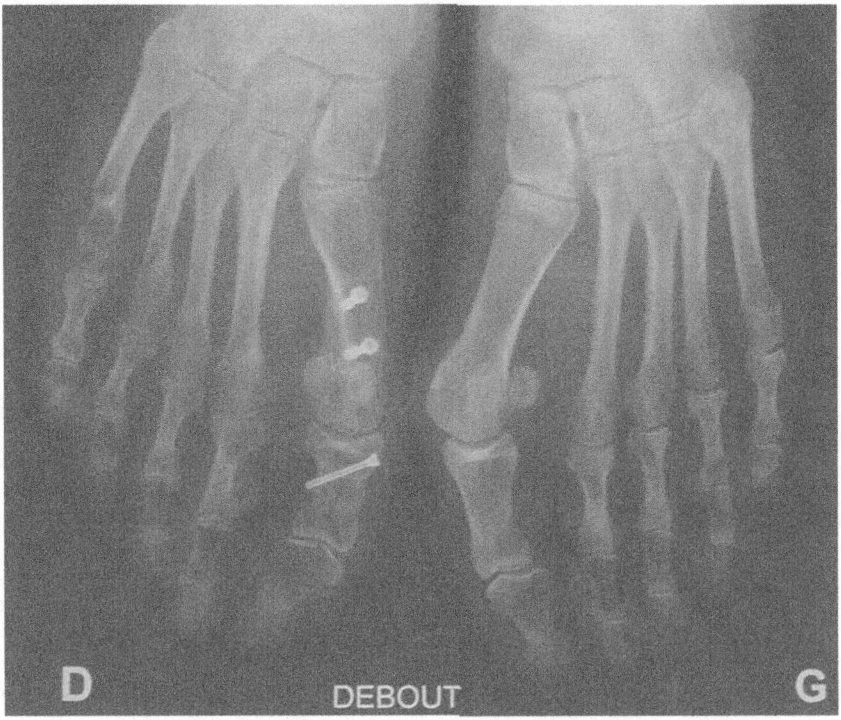

Fig. 12.7 Hybrid mini invasive surgery which has combined DMMO 2 to 5, percutaneous Akin osteotomy and classical scarf osteotomy. Post-operative (18 months follow-up) aspect

12.6 Conclusion

Minimally invasive distal osteotomy for static metatarsalgia provides satisfactory clinical and anatomical results avoiding the medium-term stiffness and pain typical of open surgery.

References

1. Barouk LS. Weil's metatarsal osteotomy in the treatment of metatarsalgia. *Orthopade*. Aug 1996;25:338–344(German).
2. De Prado M, Ripoll PL, Golano P. In: *Cirugia percutanea del pie*. Barcelona, Spain: Masson; 2003:165–174. Part 4 Capitulo 10, métatarsalgias.
3. Coillard JY, Laffenetre O, Cermolacce C, Determe P, Guillo S, Jambou S, de Lavigne C. *Traitement chirurgical des métatarsalgies statiques par technique mini-invasive*. 2e éd. Paris: Elsevier Ed; 2005:89,153–157. Conférences d'Enseignement de la Sofcot.
4. Darcel V, Villet L, Chauveaux D, Grecmip group, Laffenetre O. Treatment of static metatarsalgia using distal percutaneous metatarsal osteotomy: a prospective study of 222 feet *Rev Chir Orthop*.2009 ;5:229–242.
5. Meisenbach RO. Painful anterior arch of the foot, an operation for its relief by means of raising the arch. American Journal of Orthopaedic Surgery, 1916;14, 206–211.
6. Helal B. Metatarsal osteotomy for metatarsalgia. J Bone Joint Surg (Br) 1975; 57: 187–192.
7. Giannestras NJ. Shortening of the metatarsal shaft for the correction of plantar keratosis. Clinical Orthopaedics, 1954;4, 225–231.
8. Mau C. Eine Operation des kontrakten Spreizfuf3es. Z. Chit. 67. 1940; 667–670.
9. Delagoutte JP. Mainard D La double oste´otomie dans le traitement de l'hallux valgus. Rev Chir Orthop 76suppl 1990;1: 121–122.
10. Borggreve J. Zur operativen Behandlung des kontrakten Spreizfuf3es. Z. Orthop. 78. 1949; 581–582.

Isham Hammertoe Procedures for the Correction ofL esserD igitalD eformities

13

Stephen A. Ishama nd Orlando E. Nunez

These Minimal Invasive surgical (MIS) procedures are utilized for the treatment of a variety of hammertoe deformities. Performing transverse, combination, or wedge osteotomies in the proximal or middle phalanxes of the deformed digits preserve the functional articular surfaces of the metatarsal phalangeal and interphalangeal joint resulting in the correction of the structural deformity of lesser digits. Performing percutaneous tenotomies and capsulotomies will result in correction of the soft tissue deformities of this pathology. MIS permits the surgeon to utilize different surgical procedures to address the different components of a given deformity.

These surgical procedures are reserved for surgeons with experience, not only in minimal invasive, but also traditional surgery. These surgical procedures are performed through a very small incision. If the surgeon is not precise, important structures can be damaged and lead to predicted complications.

13.1 Definition

Hammertoe, including claw toe and mallet toe, deformities are a combination of one or more deformities of the digits at the metatarsal phalangeal joints (MPJ) and interphalangeal joint (IPJ). These deformities can be in sagittal, transverse, and frontal planes. Most commonly, the deformed digit is dorsal flexed at the metatarsal phalangeal joint and plantarflexed at the middle interphalangeal joints or distal phalangeal joints. These deformities contain both soft tissue and osseous components called positional and structural deformities.

S.A.Is ham(✉)
SanFra nciscoH ospital,Sa natorioS anF rancisco, MexicoD F, Mexico
ema il:dris ham@frontier.com

N. Maffulli and M. Easley (eds.), *Minimally Invasive Surgery of the Foot and Ankle*,
DOI: 10.1007/978-1-84996-417-3_13,

13.2 Etiology

One of the most common manifestations of biomechanical functional abnormalities of the foot is expressed in painful deformities of the lesser digits. This manifestation can be expressed by soft tissue and structural components caused by normal adaptive changes on soft tissue and osseous structures. Digital deformity can occur at the MPJ joint, the proximal IPJ joint, and the distal IPJ joint of the involved digit.

The primary cause of hammertoe deformities is the abnormal foot structure which, as dictated by genetic code, is exposed to abnormal pronatory forces. This results in hypermobility of the osseous structures and over dependence on soft tissue structure for stability during weight bearing and in particular during the last phase of the propulsive stage of gait. The severity of the hammertoes is proportionate to the severity of the abnormal pronatory forces present and how long the deformity has existed. Other causes of hammertoe deformities are systemic diseases such as gout, rheumatoid arthritis, neurological disorders, or trauma causing permanent osseous or soft tissue damage to the digit. Footwear, though not a primary cause, can definitely aggravate the symptoms of the deformity. When more than one cause is present the surgeon can expect the progression and the severity of the deformity to increase.

13.3 Classification

The classification of deformities is a tool that enables the surgeon to select or modify procedures to achieve the best results for each patient. To classify the severity of hammertoe deformities, the following observations are commonly used by the author. Most deformed digits that we are called upon to correct have been long term enough to have both structural and soft tissue components. The component of the deformity is the result of adaptive changes taking place at the involved joint or joints of the digits. The longer period of time the contracture exists, the more adaptive changes will occur. The classifications are *flexible and rigid.*

The aim of the Isham Hammertoe Procedures is directed at correcting the soft tissue structures by doing soft tissue releases of the extensor and flexor tendons and a capsulotomy at the metatarsal phalangeal joint, if indicated for rigid classification, and correcting the structural deformities while conserving the articulation and utilizing the adaptive changes that are occurring at these joint structures. By using conservative osteotomy and soft tissue procedures, we can redirect the biomechanical function and improve the appearance and symptoms of the deformed digit.

13.4 PhalangealO steotomyP rocedures

Development of surgical procedures is an evolution based on the work of previous surgeons. Diaphyseal osteotomy procedures of the phalanx have been utilized for years for the correction of hammertoe deformities. The author has modified these procedures by using a transverse, combination, and wedge osteotomies at the base of the proximal phalanx, in conjunction when indicated with a combination osteotomy of the middle phalanx and a wedge osteotomy when indicated along with exostectomies and soft tissue corrections.

Transverse osteotomy is an osteotomy performed in the diaphysis or metaphysis completely severing the phalanx thereby shortening the osseous structure.

Wedge osteotomy is an osteotomy procedure where a wedge is performed in the diaphysis or metaphysis whereby a cortical or periosteal hinge is conserved redirecting or realigning the osseous structures on an anatomical guideline.

Combination osteotomy is an osteotomy procedure in the diaphysis or metaphysis of the bone where a transverse bone shortening osteotomy is performed through the cortex and periosteum but also wedged to realign the osseous structures and improve function.

13.5 IshamH ammertoeP rocedures

I-1 procedure. This procedure is a combination osteotomy at the base of the proximal phalanx with soft tissue releases of the two extensor and flexor tendons and, if necessary, a capsulotomy on the dorsal aspect of the metatarsal phalangeal joint. This procedure is indicated in a hammertoe deformity where a majority of the deformity takes place at the metatarsal phalangeal joint (MPJ) (Fig. 13.1).

I-2 procedure. This procedure is a combination osteotomy performed on the base of the proximal phalanx and an exostectomy performed on the dorsal aspect of the head of the proximal phalanx along with extensor and flexor soft tissue releases. This is indicated in a deformity at the metatarsal phalangeal joint (MPJ) with an exostosis on the head of the proximalpha lanx(Fig. 13.2).

I-3 procedure. This procedure is a combination osteotomy at the base of the proximal phalanx, an exostectomy on the dorsal aspect of the head of the proximal phalanx, and a dorsal wedge osteotomy through the head of the proximal phalanx with extensor and flexor soft tissue releases resulting in a realignment and straightening of the articular surface of the proximal interphalangeal joint (PIPJ). This is indicated at the metatarsal phalangeal joint (MPJ) and proximal interphalangeal joint (PIPJ) (Fig. 13.3).

I-4 procedure. This procedure is a combination osteotomy at the base of the proximal phalanx and a combination osteotomy procedure in the diaphysis of the middle phalanx

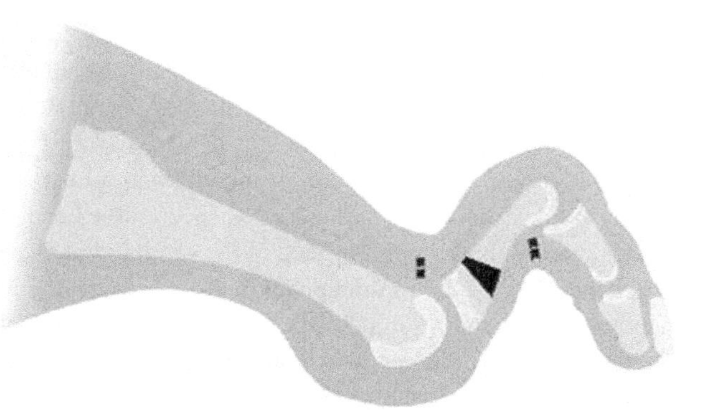

Fig.13.1 IshamH ammertoe procedure I-1. This procedure is a combination osteotomy at the base of the proximal phalanx with soft tissue releases of the two extensor and flexor tendons and, if necessary, a capsulotomy on the dorsal aspect of the metatarsal phalangeal jointaspect of the metatarsalpha langealjoi nt

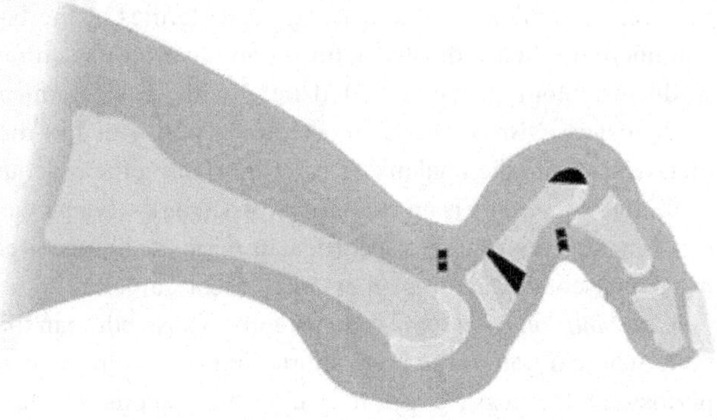

Fig. 13.2 IshamH ammertoe procedure I-2 procedure. This procedure is a combination osteotomy performed at the base of the proximal phalanx and an exostectomy performed on the dorsal aspect of the head of the proximal phalanx along with extensor and flexors oftt issuer eleases

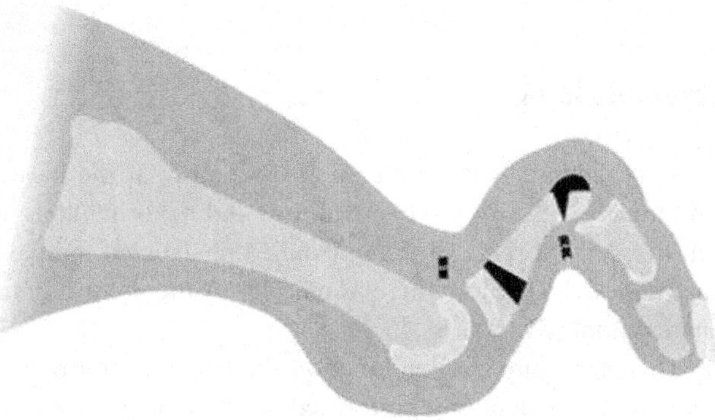

Fig. 13.3 Isham Hammertoe procedure I-3 procedure. This procedure is a combination osteotomy at the base of the proximal phalanx, an exostectomy on the dorsal aspect of the head of the proximal phalanx, and a dorsal wedge osteotomy through the head of the proximal phalanx with extensor and flexor soft tissue releases resulting in a realignment and straightening of the articular surfaceof t hepr oximali nterphalangealj oint(PIPJ)

with associated extensor and flexor releases. This is indicated for deformities where the deformity is not only at the metatarsal phalangeal joint (MPJ), but also at the proximal and distal interphalangeal joints (IPJ). This hammertoe procedure is most commonly utilized by the author (Fig. 13.4).

I-5 procedure. This procedure is a combination osteotomy at the base of the proximal phalanx and an exostectomy at the hypertrophied exostosis on the dorsal aspect of the proximal phalanx and a combination osteotomy of the middle phalanx. This is indicated where the deformity is not only at the metatarsal phalangeal joint (MPJ), but also at the proximal and distal interphalangeal joints (IPJ) with an exostosis on the dorsal aspect of the proximal phalanx (Fig. 13.5).

I-6 procedure. This procedure is a combination osteotomy at the base of the proximal phalanx, an exostectomy on the dorsal aspect of the head of the proximal phalanx, a dorsal wedge osteotomy through the head of the proximal phalanx, and a combination osteotomy at the diaphysis of the middle phalanx. This is indicated when the deformities exist at the metatarsal phalangeal joint (MPJ) and both interphalangeal joints (IPJ's) with exostosis of the dorsal aspect of the proximal phalanx. This procedure is mostly seen to be needed in a seconddi gitde formity(Fig. 13.6).

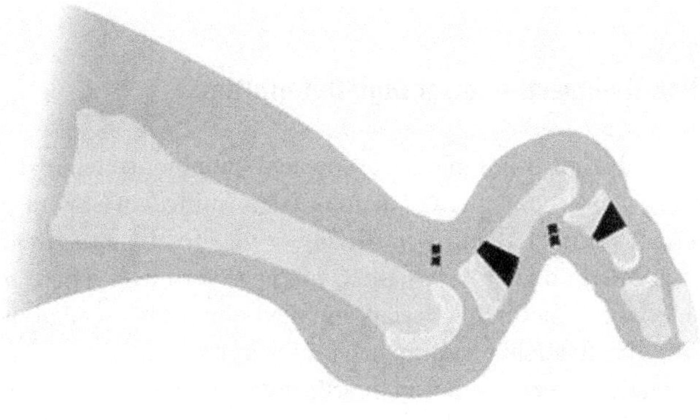

Fig.13. 4 IshamH ammertoe procedure I-4 procedure. This procedure is a combination osteotomy at the base of the proximal phalanx and a combination osteotomy procedure in the diaphysis of the middle phalanx with associated extensor and flexorre leases

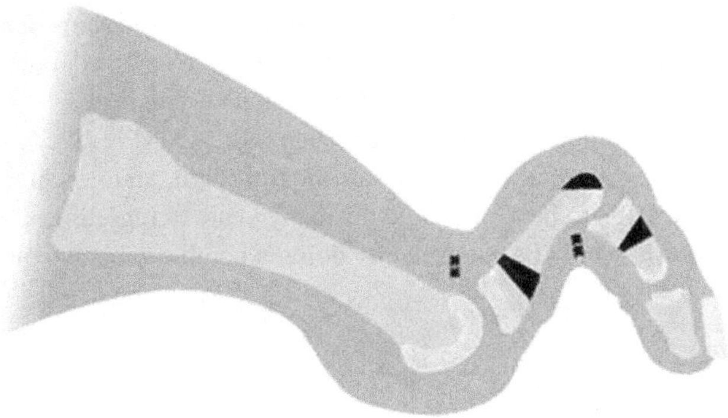

Fig.13. 5 IshamH ammertoe procedure I-5 procedure. This procedure is a combination osteotomy at the base of the proximal phalanx and an exostectomy at the hypertrophied exostosis on the dorsal aspect of the proximal phalanx and a combination osteotomy of the middle phalanx

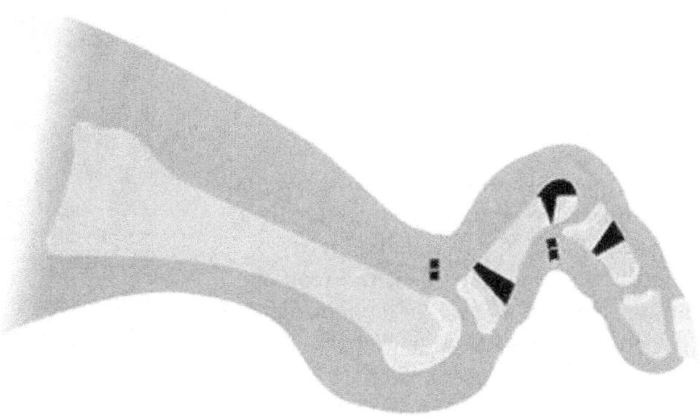

Fig. 13.6 Isham Hammertoe procedure I-6 procedure. This procedure is a combination osteotomy at the base of the proximal phalanx, an exostectomy on the dorsal aspect of the head of the proximal phalanx, a dorsal wedge osteotomy through the head of the proximal phalanx, and a combination osteotomy at the diaphysis of the middle phalanx

13.6 Non-Hammertoe Lesser Digit Deformities

Digital deformities may be associated with biomechanical or non-biomechanical deformities, such as congenital or acquired deformities. In a laterally or medially deviated digit the PASA is affected either positively or negatively at the metatarsal phalangeal joint (MPJ). It is often noticed with hallux valgus deformities where the lesser digit is deviated also laterally or medially overlapping the hallux. This medial deviation is caused by a plantarflexed metatarsal resulting in over stress of the metatarsal phalangeal joint (MPJ). A lateral deviation is very common in arthritic conditions such as rheumatoid arthritis.

If the digital deformity is associated strictly with a deformity at the metatarsal phalangeal joint (MPJ) and there is no metatarsal deformity, keratosis or symptomatology on the metatarsal, then a wedge phalangeal osteotomy may be performed to straighten the digit. This procedure is performed without or in conjunction with soft tissue releases, as needed.

A wedge osteotomy procedure may be performed to straighten out a laterally deviated or medially deviated digit conjunction with a Modified Isham Osteotomy through the head or neck of the metatarsal correcting the PASA as well as elevating the metatarsal head for a painful lesion underneath the metatarsal head area. Again, soft tissue procedures are infrequent and only performed when indicated (Fig. 13.7a and b).

On congenital deformities of the fifth digit, an overlapping fifth digit to the fourth digit has proven to be a challenge for many years to regarding correction of this deformity. This deformity may be corrected by doing a combination osteotomy at the base of the proximal

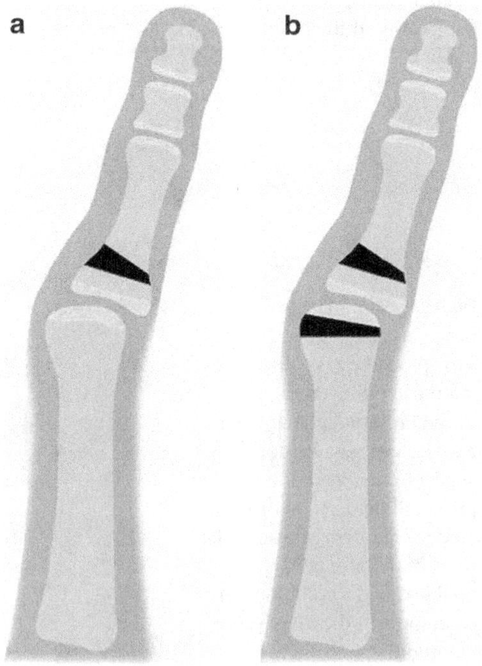

Fig.13.7 A wedge osteotomy procedure may be performed to straighten out a laterally deviated or medially deviated digit (**a**) together with a modified Isham osteotomy through the head or neck of the metatarsal (**b**) correcting the PASA as well as elevating the metatarsal head for a painful lesionunde rneatht hem etatarsalhe ada rea

phalanx in conjunction with an extensor tenotomy and capsulotomy releases. On occasion, should the adaptive cartilage of the fifth digit be significantly dorsal at the metatarsal phalangeal joint (MPJ) on the metatarsal head, a combination osteotomy is needed on the metatarsal plantarly in order to re-position the adaptive cartilage more towards normal function position directly in front of the metatarsal head (Fig. 13.8).

Exostosis excisions may be performed using percutaneous incisions on any hyperostosis on the phalanx such as on the distal aspect of the digit, at the distal interphalangeal joint (IPJ), the proximal interphalangeal joint (IPJ) either dorsal, medial, or lateral (Figs. 13.9 and 13.10).

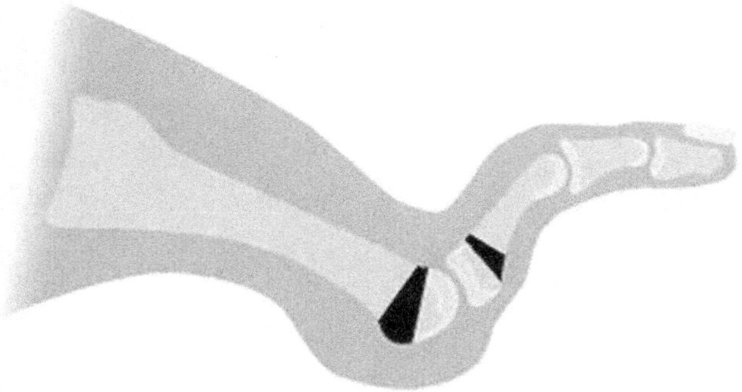

Fig. 13.8 A fifth digit overlapping on the fourth digit may be corrected by a combination osteotomy at the base of the proximal phalanx together with an extensor tenotomy and capsulotomy releases

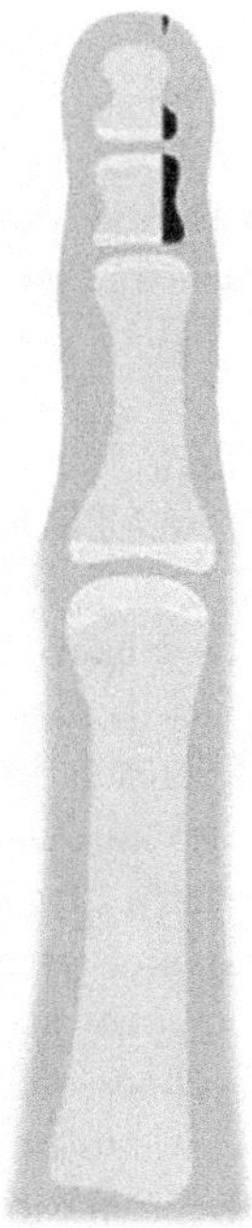

Fig. 13.9 Exostosis excisions can be performed using percutaneous incisions on any hyperostosis on the phalanx such as on the distal aspect of the digit, at the distal interphalangeal joint (IPJ), the proximal interphalangeal joint (IPJ) either dorsal, medial, or lateral

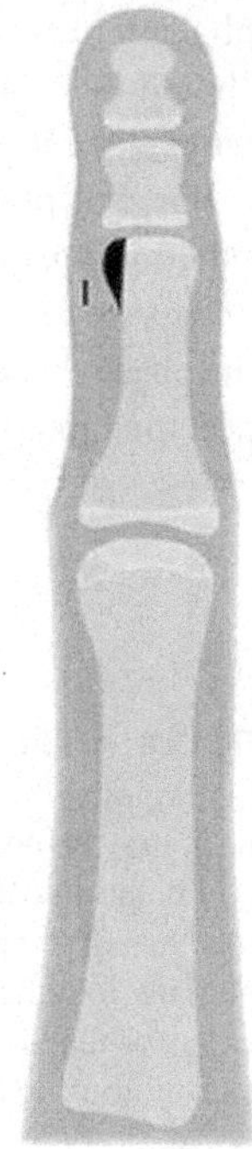

Fig. 13.10 Exostosis excisions can be performed using percutaneous incisions on any hyperostosis on the phalanx such as the proximal interphalangeal joint (IPJ)e itherdor sal,m edial,or l ateral

For a congenitally long digit that has no deformity factors at either the interphalangeal joint (IPJ) or metatarsal phalangeal joint (MPJ), a shortening osteotomy procedure may be performed in both the base of the proximal phalanx and in the middle phalanx without soft tissue releases in order to render the digit a more normal length (Fig. 13.11).

13.6.1 Operative Technique

The Isham Hammertoe Procedures are performed using 2 mm percutaneous incisions. These portals are performed using an MIS 64 or MIS 67 blade (BD Beaver Blades, Becton Dickinson, 1 Becton Drive, Franklin Lakes, NJ 07417). The first procedure is to release the soft tissue structures if indicated. A 2 mm incisions is made over the dorsal aspect of the metatarsal phalangeal joint (MPJ) over the extensor tendon apparatus. Tenotomy of the extensor longus is performed, and if necessary, the extensor brevis and a deeper capsulotomy may also be performed if indicated. On the plantar aspect of the involved digit 2 mm incisions are also performed using the same instrumentation. These incisions are performed to allow passage of a bone cutting instrument, a rotary burr (Isham Short by Vilex). These incisions are centered on the phalanx plantarly, extended deep allowing a channel

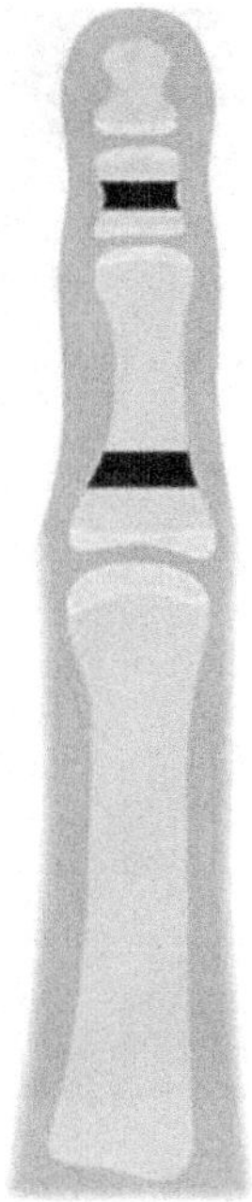

Fig. 13.11 A shortening osteotomy procedure may be performed in a congenitally long digit that has no deformity factors at either the interphalangeal joint (IPJ) or metatarsal phalangeal joint (MPJ)

for the cutting instrument. Through the same or separate incisions a percutaneous tenotomy of both the flexor brevis and longus is performed.

The author utilizes a combination osteotomy on the proximal and middle phalanxes when indicated to correct the majority of hammertoe deformities. The combination osteotomy permits the surgeon to correct the angle of a deformity and reposition the digit in its correct position, following the laws of Wolff (Figs. 13.12a–c Preoperative and Postoperative).

13.6.2 PostO perativeB andaging

Minimal invasive procedures by design are very atraumatic with minimal amount of soft tissue disruption. Although internal fixation is not required, external splinting is required to maintain the correction and enable the patient to bare weight.

Post operative dressings in minimal invasive foot surgery should stabilize the surgical site in its correct position, be comfortable to the patient and easy to apply and while maintaining a sterile barrier.

My post operative dressings present in phases. The first phase represents the type of dressing used during the first post operative 3 days. These dressings are applied by the

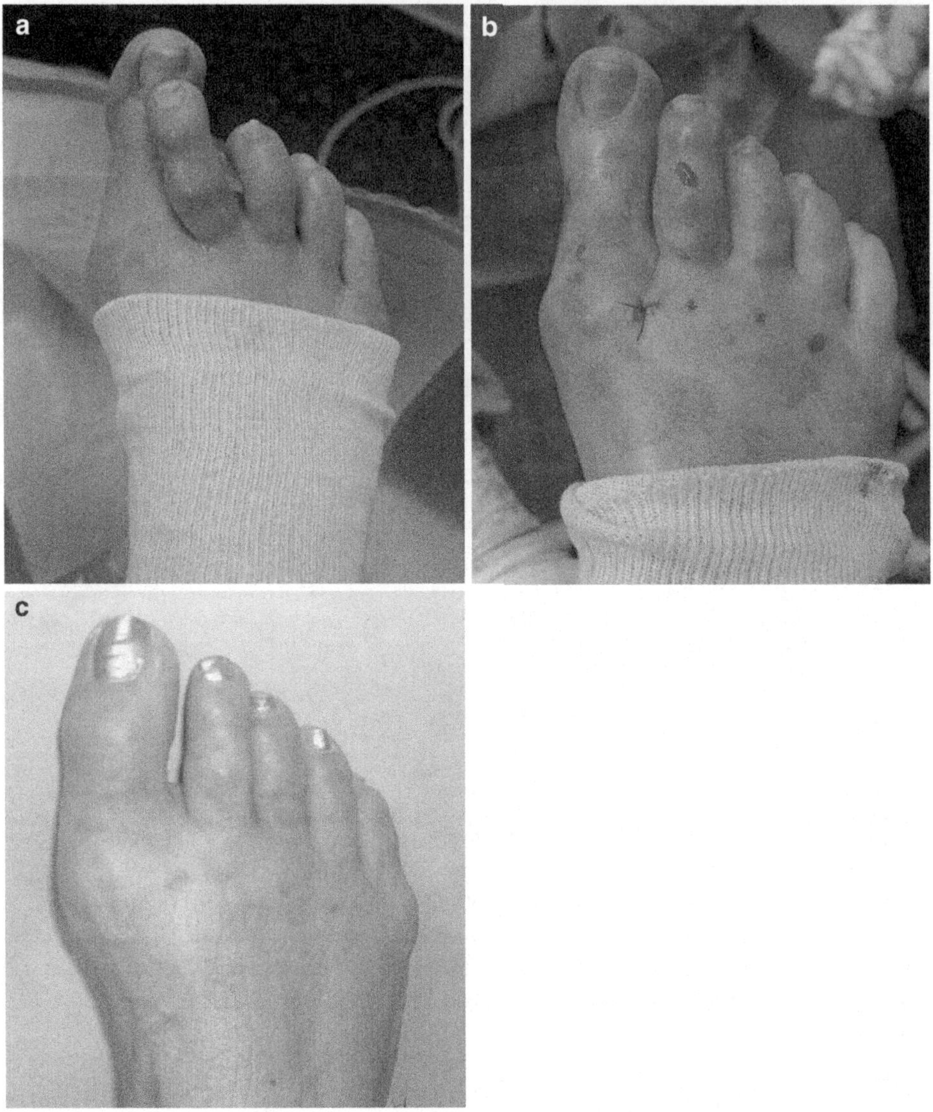

Fig. 13.12 Combination osteotomy on the proximal and middle phalanxes can be performed to correct most hammertoe deformities. The combination osteotomy allows to correct the deformity and reposition the digit in its correct position: pre-operative, post-operative and 19 weeks post-operative

surgeon. The second phase of the dressings are splint dressings that are used for the following 2 weeks. Figure 13.13a–c represents phase one dressing and Fig. 13.14a,b represents phase two dressing. The phase two dressings are initially applied by the surgeon and changed daily by the patients after they have been instructed in their application. Bathing is permitted on a daily basis after the first post operative week if the incisions are healed.

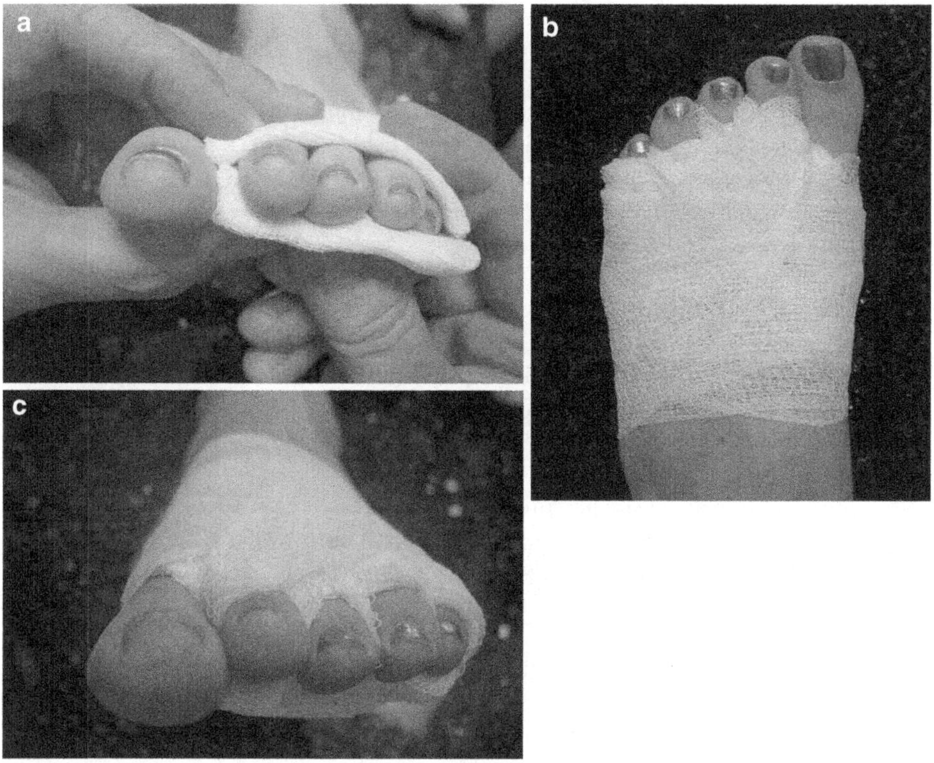

Fig. 13.13 Post-operative dressings present in phases: the first phase represents the type of dressing used during the firstpo st-operative3da ys

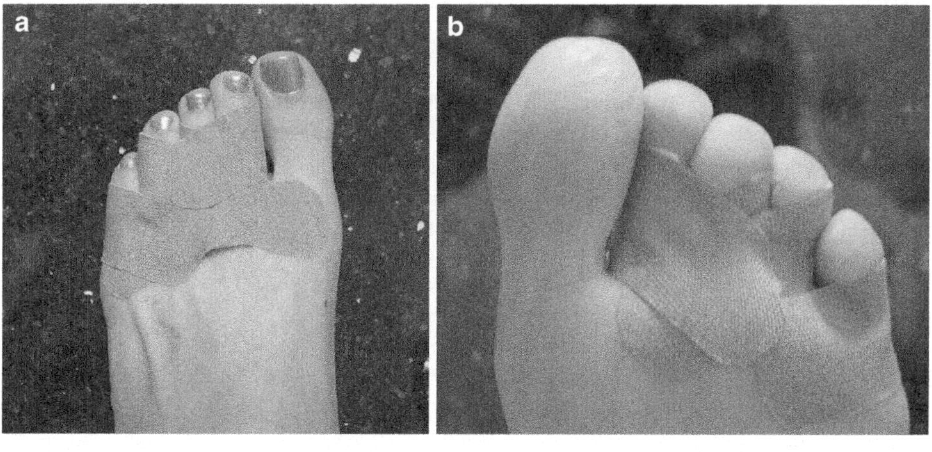

Fig. 13.14 Post-operative dressings present in phases: the second phase of the dressings are splint dressings that are used for the following 2 weeks

Advantages of the Isham Hammertoe Procedures

- Good healing due to minimal soft tissue trauma.
- Minimal fixation required because the procedure is minimally traumatic and neurovascular structures are intact resulting in shortened healing time.
- Tri-plane correction of the structural deformity is provided.
- Minimal amount of post-operative complication and disability. The patient remains ambulatorya ndpr oductive.

Disadvantages of the Isham Hammertoe Procedures

- Limitation of flexion at the proximal interphalangeal joint (IPJ) occurs in approximately 20% of the procedures performed; this is associated with fibrous adhesions around the joint structures. These are almost always asymptomatic and do not interfere with normal function during gait.
- Failure to adequately release the soft tissue structures in semi-rigid and rigid deformities may result in telescoping of the osseous segments at the osteotomy site. This will result in slower healing times and possibly malposition or malunion at the osteotomy site.
- Fibrous clinical union occurs quite rapidly in less than 3 weeks at the osteotomy sites. However, due to lack of highly vascularized soft tissue structures bony ossification is approximately twice as long as with metatarsal osteotomies. This is an asymptomatic finding.
- The goal of the procedure is to functionally realign the osseous segment and not realign the osseous segment anatomically. Should symptomatic failure of the procedure occur, then a traditional or Minimal Invasive Arthroplasty or partial head resection may be performedus ingp ercutaneouspr ocedures.

13.7 Summary

Correction of lesser digital deformities using percutaneous procedures using exostectomy but primarily combination osteotomies with soft tissue releases correct the vast majority of digital pathology. These procedures are very conservative however, and should we have a rare failure, the use of traditional hammertoe procedures would be a viable option. In most cases, however, a repetition or modification of the original Isham Hammertoe Procedure is effective.

References

1. Akin OF. The treatment of hallux valgus: a new operative and its results. *Med Sentinel.* 1925;33:678–679.
2. Collof B, Weitz EN. Proximal phalangeal osteotomy and hallux valgus. *Clin Orthop.* 1967;54:105.

3. De Prado M, Ripoll P, Golano P. *Cirugia percutanea del pie*. Barcelona, Spain: Masson; 2003.
4. Funk JF, Wells R. Bunionectomy with distal osteotomy. *Clin Orthop Rel Res*. June 1972;85:71–74.
5. Garcia NE. *Techniques of Minimal Incision*. Madrid, Spain: Mileto Ediciones; 2004.
6. Garcia NE. *Estructuras Anatomicas Implicadas en la Practica de la Cirugia de Minima Incision del Pie*. Barcelona, Spain: Editorial Glosa, S.L.; 2009.
7. Gerbert J. *Textbook of Bunion Surgery*. Mount Kisco, New York: Futura Publishing; 1981.
8. Gerbert J, Mercado OA, Sokoloff TH. The surgical treatment of hallux abducto-valgus and allied deformities. In: Fielding MD, ed. *Podiatric Medicine and Surgery: Monograph Series*. Mount Kisco, New York: Futura Publishing; 1973.
9. Gorman J, Plon M. *Minimal Incision Surgery and Laser Surgery in Podiatry*. Jack B. Gorman; 1983.
10. Isham SA. The Reverdin-Isham procedure for the correction of hallux abducto-valgus. *Curr Podiatric Med*. June 1985:11–13.
11. Kelikian H. *Hallux Valgus, Allied Deformities of the Forefoot and Metatarsalgia*. Philadelphia, PA: W.B. Saunders Co.; 1965.
12. Peabody CW. Surgical cure of hallux valgus. *J Bone Joint Surg*. 1931;13a:273.
13. Podiatrics Sino-American Conference on Foot Disorders. October 1987, Beijing, China.
14. Sanchez Pulgar JA. El Tratamiento Percutaneo Del Hallux Valgus Con La Tecnica De Reverdin-Isham, Tesis Doctoral, 2007.
15. Teatino JA. Cirugia por minima incision en los dedos medios-I. *Podoscopio 2 Epoca*. Marzo-Abril 1995;I(20).
16. Teatino JA. Cirugia por minima incision en los dedos medios-(II). *Podoscopio 2 Epoca*. Mayo-Junio 1995;I(21).
17. Teatino JA. Cirugia por minima incision en los dedos medios-(III). *Podoscopio 2 Epoca*. Julio-Agosto 1995;I(22).
18. Viladot A. Deformaciones de los dedos. Patologia del antepie. Capitulo X, 1984:181–189.
19. Watson A, Anderson R, Hodges W. Deformaciones de los dedos menores. In: Kelikian AS, ed. *Tratamiento quirurgico de pie y tobillo*. Cap 8. Madrid, Spain: McGraw-Hill Interamericana; 1999:97–113.

14 Minimally Invasive Management of Dorsiflexion Contracture at the Metatarsophalangeal Joint and Plantarflexion Contracture at the Proximal Interphalangeal Joint of the Fifth Toe

Mariano de Prado, Pedro-Luis Ripoll, Pau Golanó, Javier Vaquero, Filippo Spiezia,a nd Nicola Maffulli

14.1 Introduction

Surgical management of persistent dorsiflexion contracture at the metatarsophalangeal joint and plantarflexion contracture at the proximal interphalangeal joint of the fifth toe is indicated in patients with marked rigidity and pain, following failure of conservative management with appropriate orthoses and shoes with a wide toe box.

In this chapter we describe procedure of Augustine and Jacobs[1] to correct this deformity of the fifth toe using a minimally invasive approach. This technique consists of a plantar closing wedge osteotomy of the fifth toe at the base of its proximal phalanx associated with an exostosectomy of the head of the proximal phalanx and at the base of the middle phalanx. Lastly, a complete tenotomy of the deep and superficial flexor tendons and of the tendon of the extensor digitorum longus is undertaken (Fig. 14.1a and b).

14.2 Surgical Technique

The procedure can be performed under regional nerve bloc either at the level of the ankle or of the fifth metatarsal. The patient is supine with the foot to be operated overhanging the end of the operating table. It is not necessary to use a tourniquet.

M. de Prado (✉)
DepartmentofO rthopaedics, HospitalU SPS anC arlos, Murcia, España
e-mail:de prado@hospitalsancarlos.net

N. Maffulli and M. Easley (eds.), *Minimally Invasive Surgery of the Foot and Ankle*,
DOI: 10.1007/978-1-84996-417-3_14, © Springer-Verlag London Limited 2011

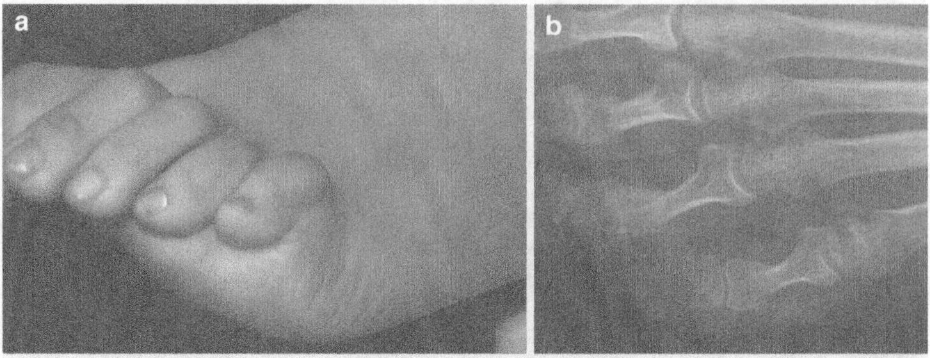

Fig. 14.1 (**a**) Clinical and (**b**) radiographical appearance 12 months after the procedure, showing stablec orrectionof t hede formity

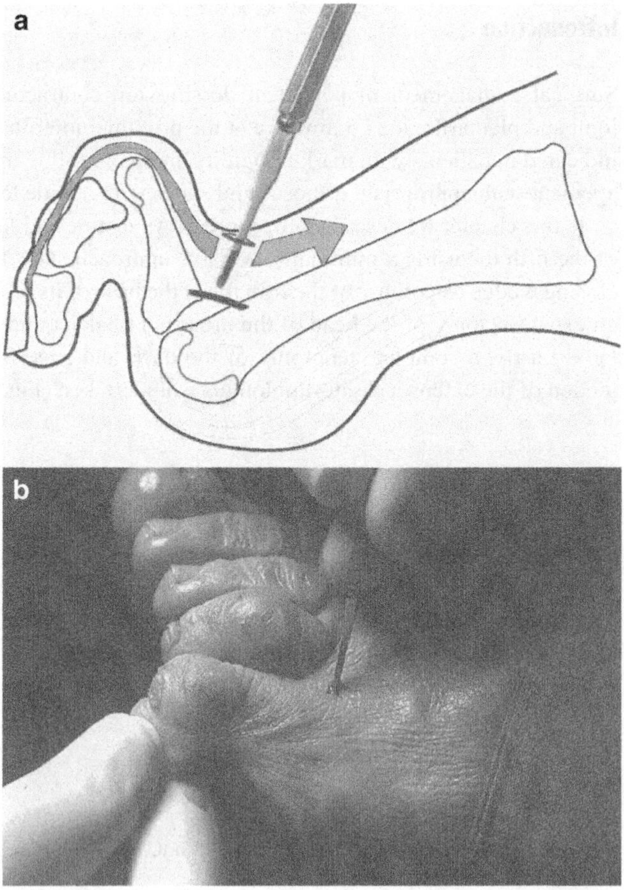

Fig.14. 2 (**a**)Sc hematic representation, and (**b**) clinical picture of the tenotomy of the tendon of extensor digitorum longus througha 2m mi ncision

1. Tenotomy of the tendon of extensor digitorum longus to the fifth toe
   A 2 mm incision is performed just above the extensor tendon and parallel to it at the level of the metatarsophalangeal joint. The patient is then asked to extend the fifth toe, allowing to better locate the tendon, which is fully tenotomised (Fig. 14.2a and b).
2. Dorsalm etatarsophalangealc apsulotomy
   In patients with severe rigidity, capsulotomy of the metatarsophalangeal joint is performed, releasing only the superior portion of the capsule and the extensor sling. Correctionof t hehype rextensioni sr emarkable.
3. Lateralc ondylectomy
   If the hyper-flexion of the interphalangeal joints is difficult to correct, there often is an exostosis at the lateral condyle of the proximal phalanx of the fifth toes and at the base of the middle phalanx. If this is the case, a lateral condylectomy is indicated. A 2 mm incision is made over the dorso-lateral aspect of the fifth toe. The blade is introduced until it touches the underlying bone. The periosteum is detached from the bone with a rasp, and the exostosis is removed with the short Shannon 44 burr (Fig. 14.3a, b) at slow speedw ithge ntleos cillatingm ovements.

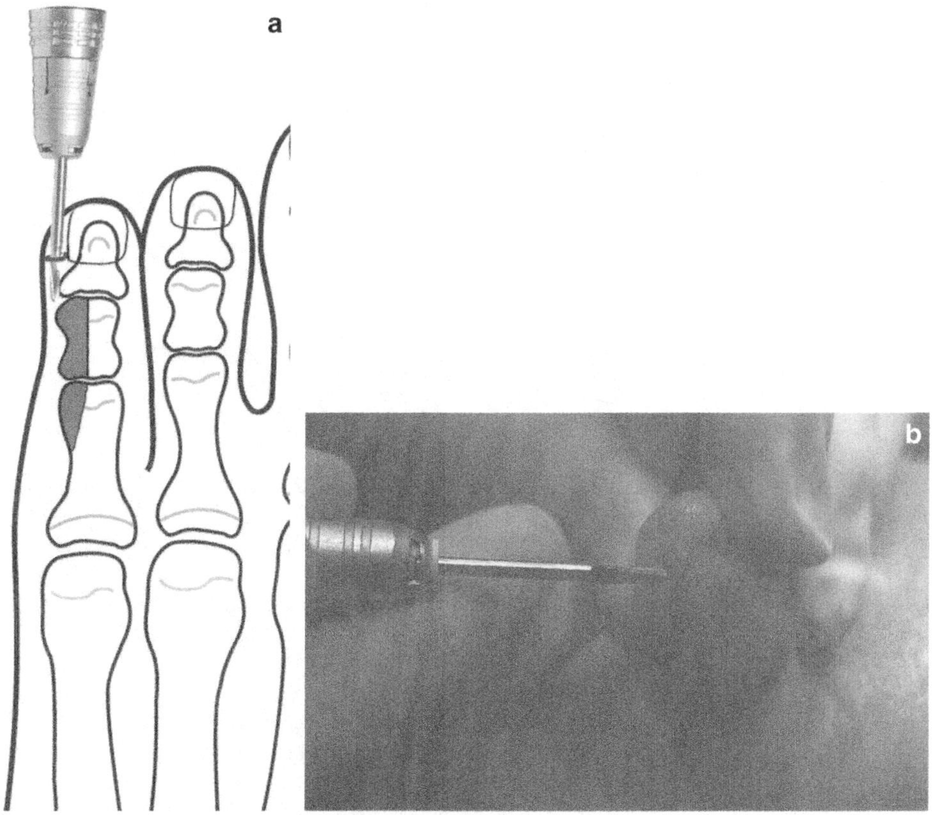

Fig. 14.3 (**a**) Schematic representation, and (**b**) clinical picture of the condilectomy performed with a short Shannon 44 drill using a 2 mm lateral approach

4. Tenotomyof t hefl exor tendons
   A 2 mm incision is performed just proximal to the plantar fold of the toe, just medial to the toe itself. The surgeon extends the fifth toe to tense the flexor tendon, which is severed with the tip of the scalpel. It should then be possible to appreciate the loss of resistance to extension in the proximal and distal interphalangeal joints.
5. Osteotomyof thepr oximalpha lanx
   A rasp is introduced through the same incision used for the tenotomy of the flexor tendons, and the periosteum is detached from the lateral aspect of the phalanx. A plantar based closing wedge osteotomy is performed (Fig. 14.4a, b) using the short Shannon 44 burr. Complete correction of deformity is thereby achieved (Fig. 14.5a and b).

The skin is sutured using a 4.0 monofilament suture. A bandage is put in place placing a strip of gauze to keep the proximal phalanx of the fifth toe in flexion. Another strip of gauze is applied to keep the interphalangeal joint in extension. Both dressings are joined by a bandage placed behind the interdigital pleats acting as a metatarsal spacer.

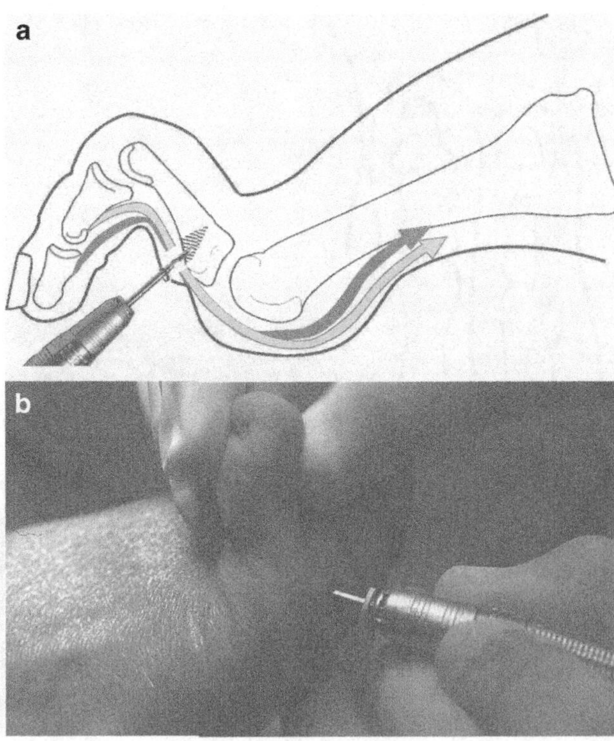

Fig.14. 4 (**a**)Sc hematic representation, and (**b**) clinical picture of the plantar based closing wedge osteotomy at the base of the proximal phalanx to correct the hyperextension deformity

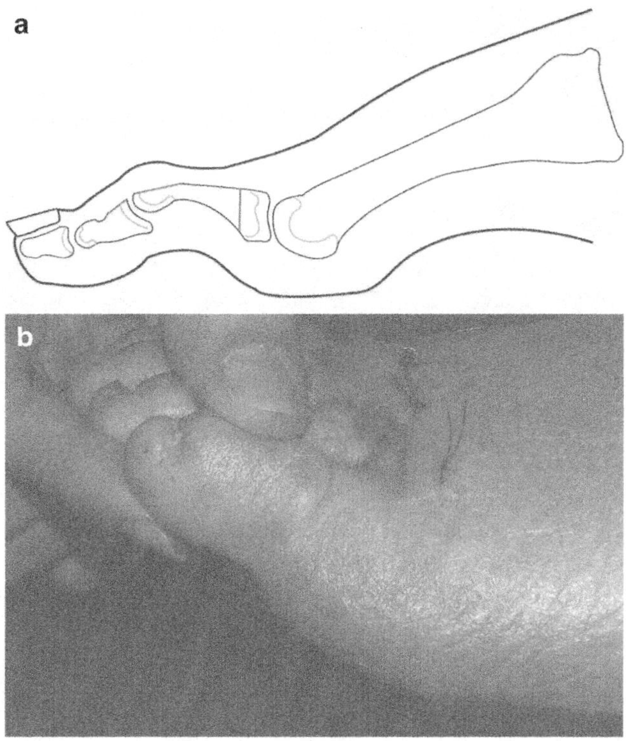

Fig. 14.5 (**a**)Sc hematic representation, and (**b**) clinical picture of the correctionobta ined

14.3 PostoperativeM anagement

Immediate mobilisation is encouraged, wearing an orthopaedic shoe for 7 days, when the stitches are removed and an adhesive bandage put in place, taking care to keep the deformity reduced. Patients are taught how to change the bandage, and told to change it every day after washing the foot for the following 6 weeks.

Around that time, complete consolidation of the osteotomies is achieved and the use of comfortable footwear is recommended.

14.4 Discussion

Several surgical options have been described to manage persistent dorsiflexion contracture at the metatarsophalangeal joint and plantarflexion contracture at the proximal interphalangeal joint of the fiftht oe.

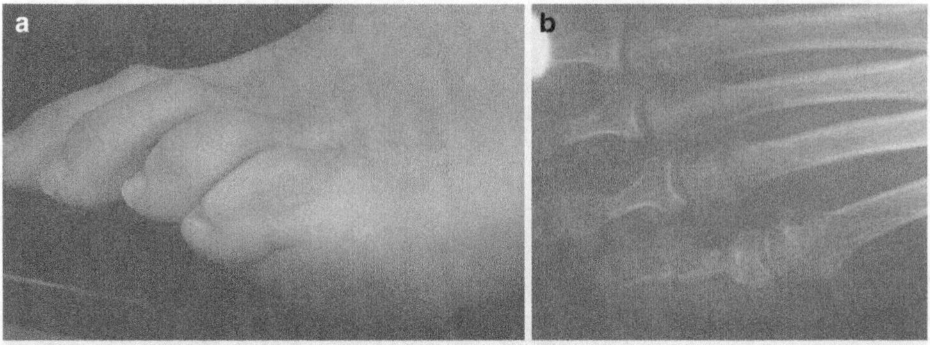

Fig. 14.6 (**a**) Clinical and (**b**) radiographical appearance of cock-up deformity of the fifth toe. Note the dorsiflexion of the metatarsophalangeal joint and the flexionof t hei nterphalangealj oint

This technique consists in a plantar closing wedge osteotomy of the fifth toe at the base of its proximal phalanx associated with a lateral condylectomy of the head of the proximal phalanx and at the base of the middle phalanx. Lastly, a complete tenotomy of the deep and superficial flexor tendons and of the tendon of the extensor digitorum longus is undertaken.

Possible complications of this procedure are iatrogenic bunionette, a floppy toe, extensive shortening of the fifth toe and subsequent hammertoe deformity of the fourth toe. In addition, some techniques involve the excision of an elliptical portion of the plantar skin is excised, a possible cause of vascular impairment of the fifth toe and hypertrophic scarring.[23]

This technique permits correction of the deformity using a minimally invasive approach without interfering with the joint surface and producing only minimal shortening of the fifth toe, and no vascular or skin compromise (Fig. 14.6a and b).

References

1. Augustine DF, Jacobs JF. Restoration of toe function with minimal traumatic procedures including advanced diaphysectomy. *Clin Podiatry.* 1985; 2:457–470.
2. Dyal CM, Davis WH, Thompson FM, et al. Clinical evaluation of the Ruiz-Mora procedure: long-term follow-up. *Foot Ankle Int.* 1997; 18:94–97.
3. Janecki CJ Jr. Triggering of the finger caused by flexor-tendon laceration. *J Bone Joint Surg Am.* 1976;58:1 174–1175.

Arthroscopic Assisted Correction of Lesser ToeDe formity

15

Tun Hing Lui

15.1 Introduction

Claw toe deformity is common. Hyperextension of the metatarsophalangeal joint is the key component of this deformity. The proximal and distal interpahalangeal joints remain flexed. The plantar plate is one of the structures responsible for the stability of the metatarsophalangeal joint.[1–4] The plantar plate experiences extension forces imposed by toe-off. The weak attachment of the plantar plate at the metatarsal neck attenuates or ruptures, allowing the plate to subluxate distally and dorsally, until rupture of the thin proximal synovial attachment occurs and the metatarsophalangeal joint dislocates. The intrinsic axis alters and the intrinsic muscles fail to act as efficient flexors of the metatarsophalangeal joint.[5–7] Painful callosity of the overlying the proximal interphalangeal joint and beneath the metatarsal head are thus presentation. Conservative management consists of taping, padding, shoewear modification or insoles. All may help to relieve the symptoms, but do not correct the deformity. Surgical options can be divided into soft tissue[8–12] and bony[13–17] procedures. Flexor tendon transfer has been reported as the most consistently successful treatment in stabilizing the metatarsophalangeal joint and correcting the flexible claw toe deformity. It works as a static tenodesis. However, the function of the tendon of flexor digitorum longus is lost and patient satisfaction has been limited due to stiffness and residual discomfort at the metatarsophalangeal joint. A shortening osteotomy, such as Weil's osteotomy, can be another option. It is indicated if the joint cannot be adequately decompressed by soft tissue release. However, a stiff toe commonly results. Resection arthroplasty or arthrodesis will result in loss of the joint integrity. Plantar plate tenodesis tackles the primary pathology of plantar plate attenuation. Postoperative stiffness and discomfort should be less of a factor if the stabilization is addressed at the level of the plantar plate rather than performing a tendon transfer.[18] Moreover, early toe mobilization is allowed and this can minimize the risk of toe stiffness.

T.H.Lui
Department of Orthopaedics and Traumatology, North District Hospital, 9 Po Kin Road, Sheung Shui, NT, Hong Kong SAR, China
e-mail:luithde rek@yahoo.co.uk

N. Maffulli and M. Easley (eds.), *Minimally Invasive Surgery of the Foot and Ankle*,
DOI: 10.1007/978-1-84996-417-3_15,

In claw toe deformity, the attenuation or rupture of the plantar plate is usually at the proximal end or the middle grooved area, while the phalangeal insertion is usually intact. We anchor the distal central part of the plantar plate and suture to the extensor digitorum longus tendon in figure of eight pattern. By this configuration, the middle central grooved area is closed up and the plantar plate is shifted proximally to its proximal insertion. Moreover, the tension produced by the extensor digitorum longus is redirected plantarward to move the plantar plate and the proximal phalanx proximally. The tension of the extensor digitorum longus distal to the suture is relieved. This, together with the arthroscopic dorsal capsular release, will release the hyperextension deforming force of the metatarsophalangeal joint. The joint is kept in neutral and the interosseous tendons become plantar to the axis of rotation of the metatarsal head. The intrinsic minus toe will then be corrected.[19,20]

In overriding toe deformity, there is medial deviation deformity of the toe in addition to the sagittal plane deformity of claw toe. Both the plantar plate and the collateral ligaments are involved. The plantar plate is deformed and displaced dorsomedially and the flexor tendons are medially displaced.[21] Under direct arthroscopic guidance, the contracted medial capsule and collateral ligament are released, and the lateral capsule is plicated. With the flexor tendon sheath attachment to the plantar plate, release of the collateral ligament will not recenter the subluxed plate and pull the flexor tendons back into alignment.[21] The figure of eight configuration of the "plantar plate tenodesis" suture will realign and centralize the plantar plate to the longitudinal axis of the metatarsal. Hopefully, this will reduce the risk of recurrence of the overriding toe deformity.

This procedure is indicated in case of claw toe or overriding toe deformity without complete dislocation of the metatarsophalangeal joint. It is contraindicated in patients in whom the plantar plate is attenuated at the phalangeal insertion, in rigid deformity, in the presence of arthrosis of the involved metatarsophalangeal joint, or deformity resulting from a neuromuscular condition or polyarthritis. It is relatively contraindicated in lateral deviation deformity of the second toe and overriding toe with predominant medial deviation deformity. In case of lateral deviation deformity, we use the extensor digitorum brevis tendon graft to reconstruct the medial collateral ligament of the second metatarsophalangeal joint. Modified extensor digitorum brevis transfer[22] is the treatment of choice to correct the transverse plane deformity in patients with overriding toe predominant medial deviation deformity and mild clawed toe component.

Potential problems include digital nerve injury, tethering of the flexor tendon by the suture or the weakening of the suture by the haemostat. The haemostat should stay subperiosteally and deep to the flexor tendon and the segment of the suture that was crushed by the haemostat should not be left in the figure of eight construct.

15.1.1 Technique of Plantar Plate Tenodesis

The patient is positioned supine, with a pneumatic tourniquet applied to the thigh. Metatarsophalangeal arthroscopy is performed through the dorsomedial and dorsolateral portals at the medial and lateral sides of the extensor tendons. The metatarsophalangeal joint is then examined with a 1.9 mm 30° arthroscope. Intra-articular pathology can be addressed. The distal part of the plantar plate can be examined. Plantar plate tenodesis can be performed if the phalangeal insertion of the plantar plate is intact. The dorsal capsule is stripped from the metatarsal neck with a small soft tissue stripper (Kokubun dissector) under arthroscopic guidance (Fig. 15.1).

In case of overriding toe deformity, the medial capsule and the medial collateral ligament are stripped from the medial side of the metatarsal head under arthroscopic guidance.

With the arthroscope in the dorsolateral portal, a PDS 1 suture is passed through the medial part of the plantar plate with a straight eyed needle. The needle should be pointed slightly towards the midline of the joint just after the penetration of plantar plate to ensure the suture is kept within the boundary of the fibrous flexor tendon sheath. Finally, the needle is passed through the skin of the plantar aspect of the toe (Fig. 15.2).

The suture is then retrieved from the plantar surface of plantar plate through the lateral side of the metatarsal to a proximal dorsal wound with a curved haemostat at the level of mid shaft of the second metatarsal (Fig. 15.3).

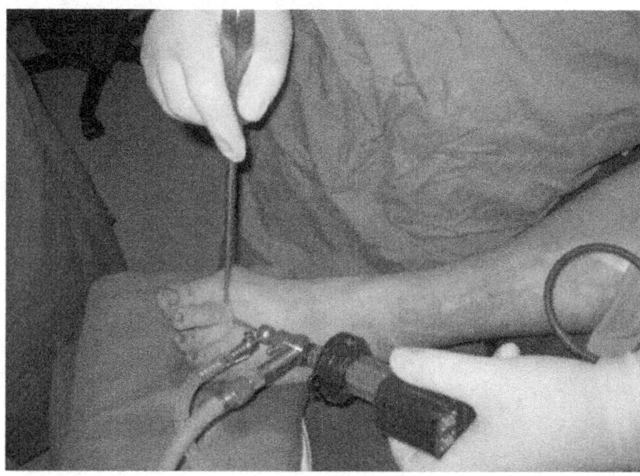

Fig. 15. 1 Thedors alc apsule is stripped from the metatarsal neck with a small soft tissue stripper (Kokubun dissector) under arthroscopic guidance

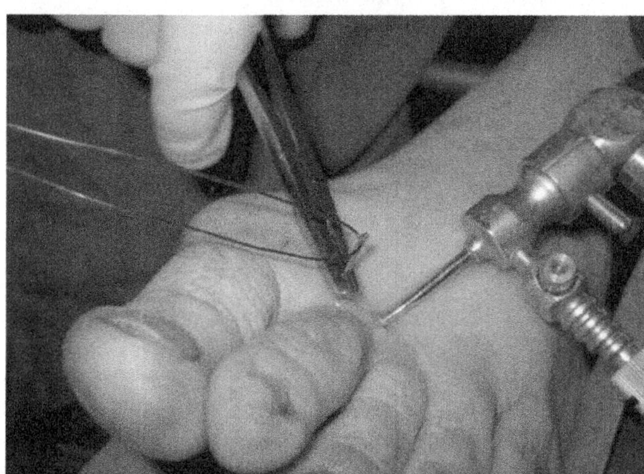

Fig. 15. 2 Witht he arthroscope in the dorsolateral portal, a PDS 1 suture is passed through the medial part of the plantar platew itha s traightne edle

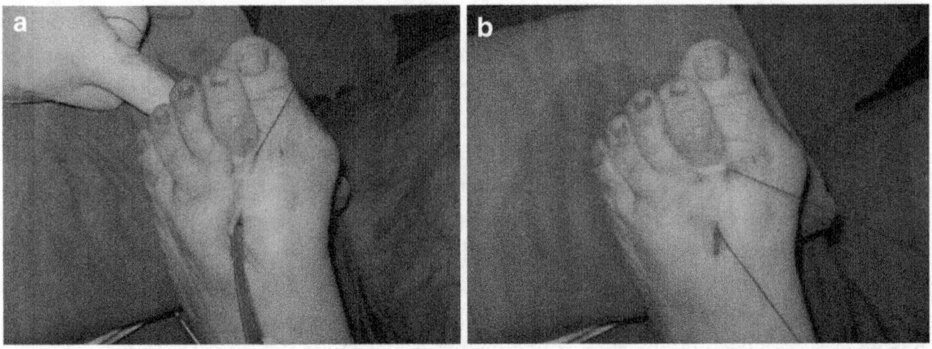

Fig.15.3 (**a**,**b**) The retrieval of suture to the proximal wound

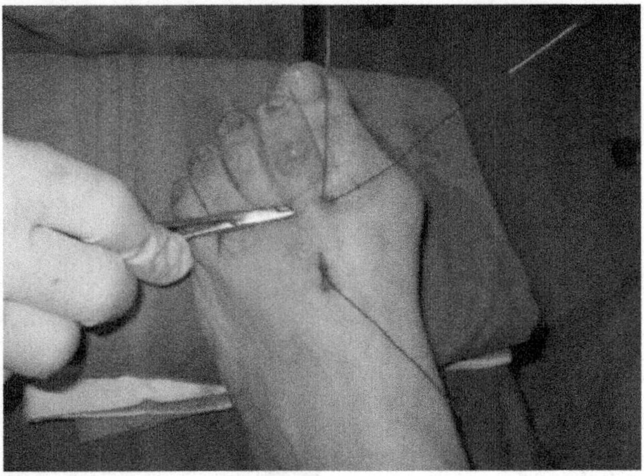

Fig.15.4 Thes utureis retrieved to the dorsolateral portal

The other limb of the suture is passed from the dorsomedial portal to the dorsolateral portal deep inside the joint (Fig. 15.4).

The suture is then passed through the lateral part of the plantar plate via the dorsolateral portal with the arthroscope in the dorsomedial portal. The suture is then retrieved through the medial side of the metatarsal to the proximal wound. It is important to maintain a loop of suture so that tension can be applied to the suture to aid the retrieval of the suture to the proximalw ound(Fig. 15.5).

The suture is anchored to the extensor digitorum longus tendon to the affected toe. Then a figure of eight configuration of suture connecting plantar plate to extensor digitorum longus is constructed. The suture is then tensioned with the ankle in neutral, so that the affected metatarsophalangeal joint is reduced spontaneously, and suture is tied over the long extensor tendon.

In case of overriding toe correction, the lateral capsule of the metatarsophalangeal joint is plicated with a PDS 1 suture in a figure of eight pattern. The distal limb of the figure of eight suture is inserted close to the base of proximal phalanx through the dorsolateral portal with the arthroscope in the dorsomedial portal. The proximal limb of the figure of eight is inserted close to the metatarsal head origin of the medial collateral ligament and exit

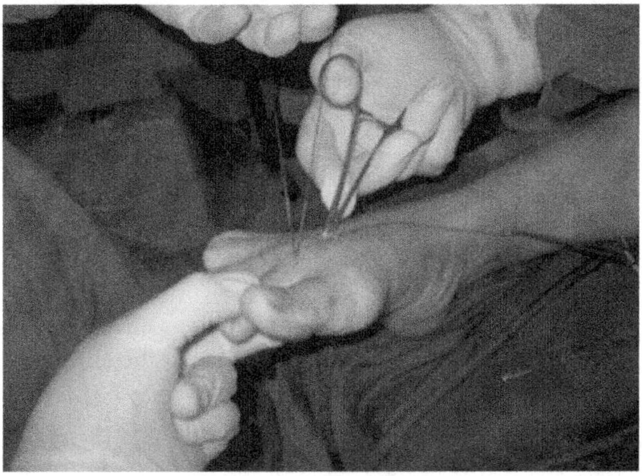

Fig. 15.5 The suture is then retrieved through the medial side of the metatarsal to the proximal wound. It is important to maintain a loop of suture so that tension can be applied to the suture to aid the retrieval of the suture tothe proxima lw ound

through the proximal wound. The suture is then retrieved back to the dorsolateral portal. It is important to tension the "plantar plate tenodesis" suture before the lateral capsule suture is tied. This can prevent the correction of medial deviation deformity with the toe in hyper-extension position. Finally, fine adjustment of tension of the "plantar plate tenodesis" suture and tired over the long extensor tendon to achieve full correction of the overriding toe deformity(Fig. 15.6).

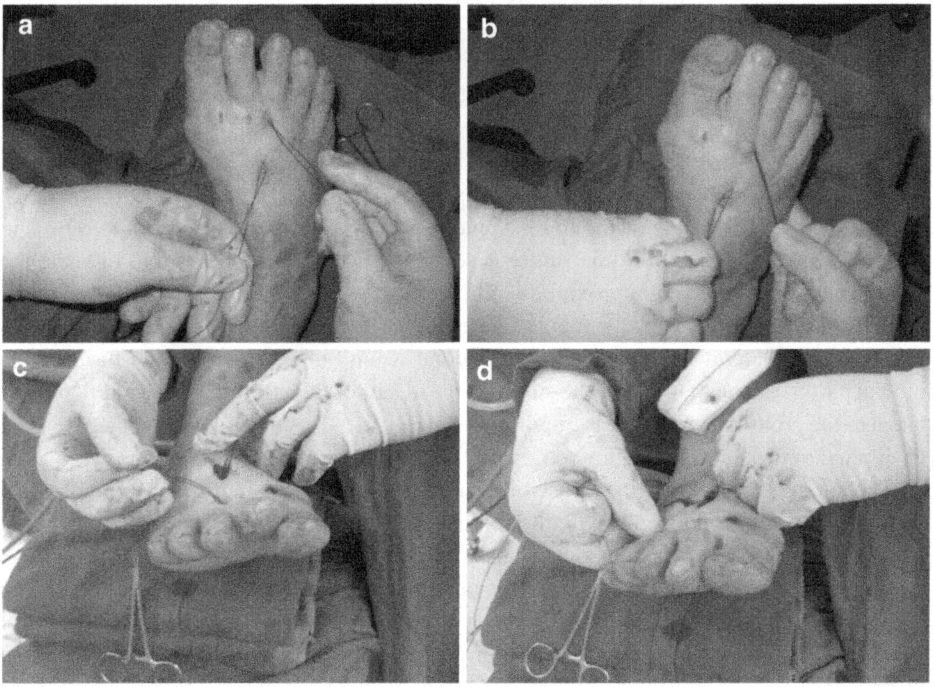

Fig. 15.6 (**a**, **b**, **c**, **d**) the overriding toe deformity can be corrected by tensioning of the lateral plication suture and the plantar plate tenodesis suture

The day after the operation, patients are advised on active toe mobilization and passive plantar mobilization of the affected metatarsophalangeal joint. Weight bearing walking with post-operative sandal is allowed.

15.2 ModifiedP lantarP late Tenodesis

Because of the confined space of the fibrous flexor tendon sheath and the presence of the flexor tendons within the sheath, it can be difficult to retrieve the suture at the surface of the plantar plate. Extensive blunt dissection may be needed to retrieve the suture. This may disrupt the extra-osseous arterial blood supply to the metatarsal head.[23,24]

15.2.1 Technique

Dorsomedial and dorsolateral stab wounds are produced at the sides of the extensor tendon at the level of the joint line of the second metatarsophalangeal joint. The dorsal capsule is stripped from the metatarsal neck with a small periosteal elevator. A PDS 1 suture is passed through the lateral part of the plantar plate with a straight needle through the dorsolateral wound. The needle should point slightly away from the midline of the joint to avoid the pass the suture through the flexor tendon. Finally, the needle pieces through the fibrous flexor tendon sheath and the plantar skin. The second toe is dorsiflexed passively with the suture kept in tension to make sure that the suture has not tethered the flexor tendon. Another dorsal longitudinal incision is made at the level of mid shaft of the metatarsal. A curved hemostat is introduced on the medial side of the metatarsal to the plantar aspect of the distal portion of the metatarsal deep to the interosseous muscles and the flexor tendons, and then to the lateral side of the fibrous tendon sheath. The suture is kept in tension and the plantar skin together with the suture is squeezed from distal to proximal to bring the plantar segment of the suture proximally. This will allow easy retrieval of the suture to the dorsal wound without extensive plantar dissection. The other limb of the suture is passed from the dorsolateral wound to the dorsomedial wound and is then passed through the medial part of the plantar plate. The suture is retrieved through the lateral side of the metatarsal to the proximal wound. It is important to maintain a loop of suture so that tension can be applied to the suture to aid the retrieval of the suture from the proximal wound.

The suture is sutured to the extensor digitorum longus tendon at the proximal dorsal wound. The suture is tensioned with the ankle in neutral, so that the affected metatarsophalangeal joint is reduced spontaneously, and suture is tied over the long extensor tendon. A figure of eight configuration of suture connecting the plantar plate-flexor tendon sheath complex to extensor digitorum longus is constructed.

The postoperative rehabilitation is along the same lines described for the original technique.

References

1. Deland JT, Lee KT, Sobei M, DiCarlo EF. Anatomy of the plantar plate and its attachments in the lesser metatarsal phalangeal joint. *Foot Ankle Int.* 19 95;16:480–486.
2. Green DR, Brekke M. Anatomy, biomechanics and pathomechanics of lesser digital deformities. *Clin Podiatr Med Surg.* 1996; 13:179–200.
3. Johnston RB, Smith J, Daniels T. The plantar plate of the lesser toes: an anatomical study in human cadavers. *Foot Ankle Int.* 1994; 15:276–282.
4. Stainsby GD. Pathological anatomy and dynamic effect of the displaced plantar plate and the importance of the integrity of the plantar plateÐdeep transverse metatarsal ligament tie-bar. *Ann R Coll Surg Engl.* 1997; 79:58–68.
5. Coughlin MJ. Subluxation and dislocation of the second metatarsophalangeal joint. *Orthop Clin North Am.* 1989; 20:539–551.
6. Coughlin MJ. Crossover second toe deformity. *Foot Ankle.* 1987; 8:29–39.
7. CoughlinM J.Le ssert oede formities. *Orthopedics.* 1987 ;10:63–75.
8. Barbari SG, Brevig K. Correction of clawtoes by the Girdlestone-Taylor flexor-extensor transfer procedure. *Foot and Ankle.* 1984; 5:67–73.
9. Feeney MS, Williams RL, Stephens MM. Selected lengthening of the proximal flexor tendon in the management of acquired claw toes. *J Bone Joint Surg.* 2001; 83B:335–338.
10. Frank GR, Johnson WM. The extensor shift procedure in the correction of clawtoe deformities in children. *South Med J.* 1966; 59:889–896.
11. Kuwuda GT, Dockery GL. Modification of the flexor tendon transfer procedure for the correction of flexible hammertoes. *J Foot Surg.* 1980; 19:38–40.
12. Thompson FM, Deland JT. Flexion tendon transfer for metatarsophalangeal instability of the second toe. *Foot Ankle.* 1993; 14:385–388.
13. Berens TA. Laterally closing metatarsal head osteotomy in the correction of a medially overlapping digit. *Clin Podiatr Med Surg.* 1996; 13:293–307.
14. Caterini R, Farsetti P, Tatantino U, Potenza V, Ippolito E. Arthrodesis of the toe joints with an intramedullary cannulated screw for correction of hammertoe deformity. *Foot Ankle Int.* 2004; 25:256–261.
15. Karlock LG. Second metatarsophalangeal joint fusion: a new technique for crossover hammertoe deformity. A preliminary report. *J Foot Ankle Surg.* 2003; 42:178–182.
16. O'Kane C, Kilmartin T. Review of proximal interphalangeal joint excisional arthroplasty for the correction of second hammer toe deformity in 100 cases. *Foot Ankle Int.* 2005;26:320–325.
17. Miller SJ. Hammer toe correction by arthrodesis of the proximal interphalangeal joint using a cortical bone allograft pin. *J Am Podiatr Med Assoc.* 200 2;92:563–569.
18. Ford LA, Collins KB, Christensen JC. Stabilization of the subluxed second metatarsophalangeal joint: flexor tendon transfer versus primary repair of the plantar plate. *J Foot Ankle Surg.* 1998;37:217–222.
19. Lui TH. Arthroscopic-assisted correction of claw toe or overriding toe deformity: plantar plate tenodesis. *Arch Orthop Trauma Surg.* 2007; 127:855–857.
20. Lui TH. Current concept: arthroscopy and endoscopy of the foot and ankle: indications for new techniques. *Arthroscopy.* 2007; 23:889–902.
21. Deland JT, Sung I-H. The medial crossover toe: a cadaveric dissection. *Foot Ankle Int.* 2000;21:375–378.
22. Lui TH, Chan KB. Modified extensor digitorum brevis tendon transfer for crossover second toe correction. *Foot Ankle Int.* 2007; 28:521–523.
23. Bayliss NC, Klenerman L. Avascular necrosis of lesser metatarsal heads following forefoot surgery. *Foot Ankle Int.* 1989; 10:124–128.
24. Peterson WJ, Lankes JM, Paulsen F, Hassenpflug J. The arterial supply of the lesser metatarsal heads: a vascular injection study in human cadavers. *Foot Ankle Int.* 2002; 23:491–495.

Percutaneous Fixation of Proximal Fifth MetatarsalF ractures

16

AaronT . Scotta nd JamesA . Nunley

16.1 Introduction

Fractures of the fifth metatarsal base have garnered a significant amount of attention since Sir Robert Jones' classic description of his own such fracture suffered while dancing.[10] Despite numerous publications on the topic, controversy continues to exist regarding nomenclature, classification, indications for surgery, and optimal surgical technique.

Stewart is credited with publishing the first anatomic classification scheme,[30] but the three zone classification system devised by Lawrence and Botte[16] is currently the most commonly cited anatomic classification system for proximal fifth metatarsal fractures (Fig. 16.1). In this system, Zone I injuries are tuberosity avulsion fractures. Zone II injuries are

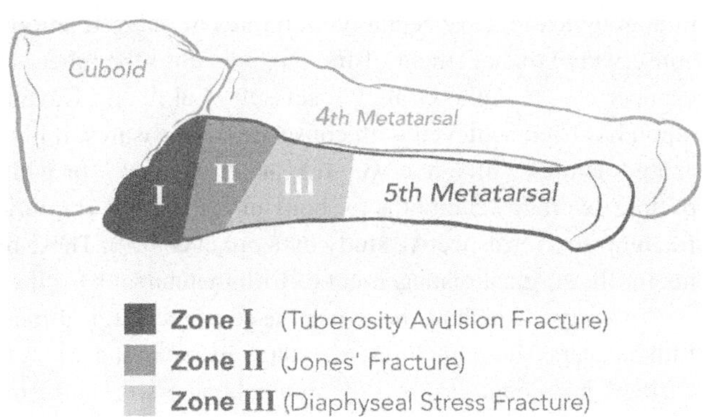

Fig.16.1 Lawrencea ndB otte classification of proximal fifthme tatarsalfra ctures

A.T.Sc ott(✉)
Department of Orthopaedic Surgery, Wake Forest University Baptist Medical Center, NorthC arolina, USA
e-mail:a ascott@wfubmc.edu

N. Maffulli and M. Easley (eds.), *Minimally Invasive Surgery of the Foot and Ankle*, DOI: 10.1007/978-1-84996-417-3_16, © Springer-Verlag London Limited 2011

considered "true Jones fractures," and have previously been defined by Stewart[30] as transverse fractures occurring at the level of the metaphyseal-diaphyseal junction with medial extension of the fracture line into the fourth-fifth intermetatarsal joint. The third zone in this classification is represented by the proximal diaphyseal stress fracture. In yet another classification system, Torg et al.[31] used radiographic criteria to divide fractures distal to the tuberosity into acute fractures, delayed unions, and non-unions. Acute fractures displayed a narrow fracture line and no intramedullary sclerosis, delayed unions a widened fracture line and a variable degree of intramedullary sclerosis, while the nonunions were characterized by a complete obliteration of the medullary canal. This radiographic classification has prognostic implications, and when combined with the anatomic classification of Lawrence and Botte, provides a basis for treatment recommendations.[24]

Lewis Carp in 1927 was the first to describe the fifth metatarsal's propensity for problematic healing when he reported four nonunions in his subset of 12 fifth metatarsal base fractures that returned for follow-up, a finding that he attributed to this bone's tenuous blood supply.[2] Although Stewart[30] was the first to suggest a differing prognosis for tuberosity avulsion fractures and true Jones fractures, Dameron[5] is credited with presenting the first large series of fifth metatarsal fractures that showed a clear-cut difference in healing rates based on anatomic location (in fractures treated non-operatively). Of the 100 tuberosity fractures in this series, all but one demonstrated a radiographic union at final follow-up and even this nonunion was asymptomatic. In contrast to the overwhelmingly successful non-operative treatment of tuberosity fractures, Dameron observed five nonunions in the 20 patients who were treated conservatively for fractures occurring within the proximal 1.5 cm of the shaft. In addition to these five nonunions which were later treated surgically, three other patients in this group required greater than 12 months to achieve osseous union radiographically. Unacceptably high rates of delayed unions and nonunions following the conservative management of fractures distal to the tuberosity have also been reported by Clapper et al.,[4] Zelko et al.,[36] Josefsson et al.,[11] and Kavanaugh et al.[12] When successful union has been achieved with conservative measures, it has been done so in the setting of acute fractures with a non-weightbearing regimen,[31] or with weightbearing at the expense of time (average 3.5 months for bony union in Zone II injuries and 4.8 months for Zone III fractures in a retrospective study by Konkel et al.[14]). These results have provided the impetus for the surgical management of fifth metatarsal base fractures in select circumstances.

A variety of methods have been used in the surgical management of acute and chronic fifth metatarsal base fractures, including open pinning,[30] percutaneous pinning,[1] tension band wiring,[27] inlay bone grafting,[17 31] sliding bone grafts,[5] and intramedullary screw fixation.[7, 8, 11, 12, 15, 18–20, 22–26, 32, 35] Kavanaugh et al.[12] were the first to advocate intramedullary screw fixation in competitive athletes and in non-athletes with delayed unions or re-fracture following non-operative management. In their 13 patients who underwent this procedure, there was a 100% union rate and no re-fractures at a mean follow-up of 3.5 years. Lending further support to this method of treatment, DeLee et al.[7] used a percutaneous intramedullary screw in the treatment of ten athletes with fifth metatarsal stress fractures. In these patients, they were able to achieve clinical union, radiographic union, and return to sports at 4.5, 7.5, and 8.5 weeks, respectively. There were no refractures or nonunions, and pain at the screw head or metatarsal head in seven of the ten patients was successfully managed with local shoe modifications. Other authors[18, 21–23] have reported similar rates of success with clinical and radiographic union rates approaching 100%, early return to sports, and no re-fractures.

Despite the success of intramedullary screw fixation, re-fractures, delayed unions, and nonunions[8, 15, 35] have been reported and have prompted a closer look at screw diameter, screw type, and post-operative protocols. Wright et al.[35] presented six re-fractures following intramedullary screw fixation and found that all of their re-fractures occurred in patients who were fixed with screws with diameters of 4.5 mm or less. In a retrospective review, Larson et al.[15] noted four re-fractures and two symptomatic nonunions following intramedullary screw fixation. In their failure group, the authors found a higher proportion of elite athletes, and found that patients in the failure group returned to full activity at 6.8 weeks following surgery versus 9 weeks in the non-failure group, prompting them to recommend postponing return to sports until radiographic union is confirmed. A myriad of biomechanical studies have been conducted to evaluate the various screws available.[9, 13, 21, 25, 28, 29, 33] In the biomechanical arm of a combined clinical and biomechanical study by Reese et al.,[25] it was shown that screws greater than 6.5 mm in diameter were superior to those under 4.0 mm, that stainless steel screws were superior to titanium screws, and that solid screws were superior to cannulated screws in terms of resistance to fatigue failure with a cyclic three-point bending protocol. In other studies, the 6.5 partially threaded lag screw was shown to have greater pull-out strength than the 5.0 mm partially threaded lag screw[13] and 4 mm leading thread-5 mm trailing thread tapered, variable pitch screw,[29] despite the lack of a significant difference in terms of bending stiffness. In yet another study, Horst et al.[9] showed that 5.0 and 6.5 mm screws provided equal torsional rigidity. However, to achieve stability equal to that of the 6.5 mm screw, the 5.0 mm screw required a length sufficient enough to gain purchase in the distal fragment which subsequently had a tendency to straighten out the normally curved fifth metatarsal, thus creating a gap at the lateral aspect of the fracture site. These findings have led to the current recommendations for selecting the ideal screw.

16.2 Surgicall ndications

Percutaneous intramedullary screw fixation is indicated in the competitive athlete with a Zone II or Zone III fracture of the proximal fifth metatarsal. Other indications include the non-athlete with a delayed union or a non-union, or any patient with a recurrent fracture. When attempting to decide between operative and non-operative intervention, there is no need to distinguish between the "true Jones" (Zone II) and proximal diaphyseal (Zone III) fractures.[3] Contra-indications for operative fixation include: active sepsis, skin infection or other cutaneous lesions in the vicinity of the skin incision, medical comorbidities that would prohibit a surgical procedure, and Charcot arthropathy.[19, 20, 32]

If surgery is not indicated or if the patient elects for non-operative management, we prefer to manage Zone II and Zone III fractures non-weightbearing in a short leg cast, bearing in mind that the time to union may be prolonged. In patients unwilling to comply with casting and a non-weightbearing status, we have used an in-shoe orthotic device that elevates and unloads the base of the fifth metatarsal as described by Dameron[6] (Figs. 16.2a, b). Despite anecdotal success, we are unaware of any published results regarding the use of this type of orthosis. We continue to manage Zone I fractures with weightbearing as tolerated in a hard-soled shoe.

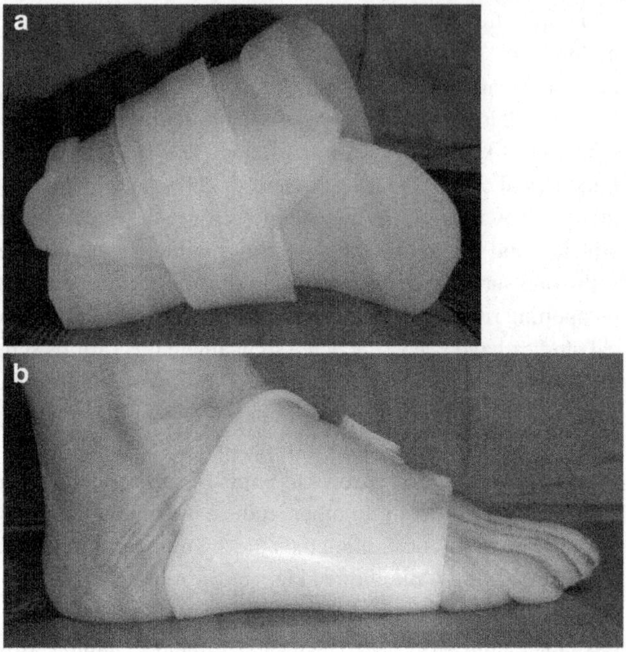

Fig.16.2 ((**a**) and (**b**)) Dameron-typeor thosis

16.3 Pre-operative Work-Up

Thorough physical examination of the injured foot with an emphasis on hindfoot alignment is essential. The presence of hindfoot varus, whether congenital or acquired, must be identified pre-operatively and corrected at the same time as the fifth metatarsal base fracture to prevent lateral column overload and subsequent non-union or refracture. Following physical examination, high quality radiographs of the foot are obtained in the anterior-posterior (AP), lateral, and oblique planes (Figs. 16.3a–c). Although pre-operative templating has been described,[32] we do not routinely do this, nor do we feel that it is necessary. In general, screw length and diameter are chosen intra-operatively based on fluoroscopic imaging and torque resistence of the cannulated tap.

Female athletes deserve special consideration. The combination of disordered eating, amenorrhea, and osteoporosis has been termed the "female athlete triad,"[34] and is a serious syndrome which has been associated with an increased risk of stress fractures. Following fixation of the fracture in a patient with the signs and symptoms of this condition, a multi-disciplinary approach to this complex, multi-faceted condition is warranted.

16.4 Surgical Technique

The procedure is performed under regional anesthesia, and we use either an ankle or a calf tourniquet. Perioperative antibiotics are optional.

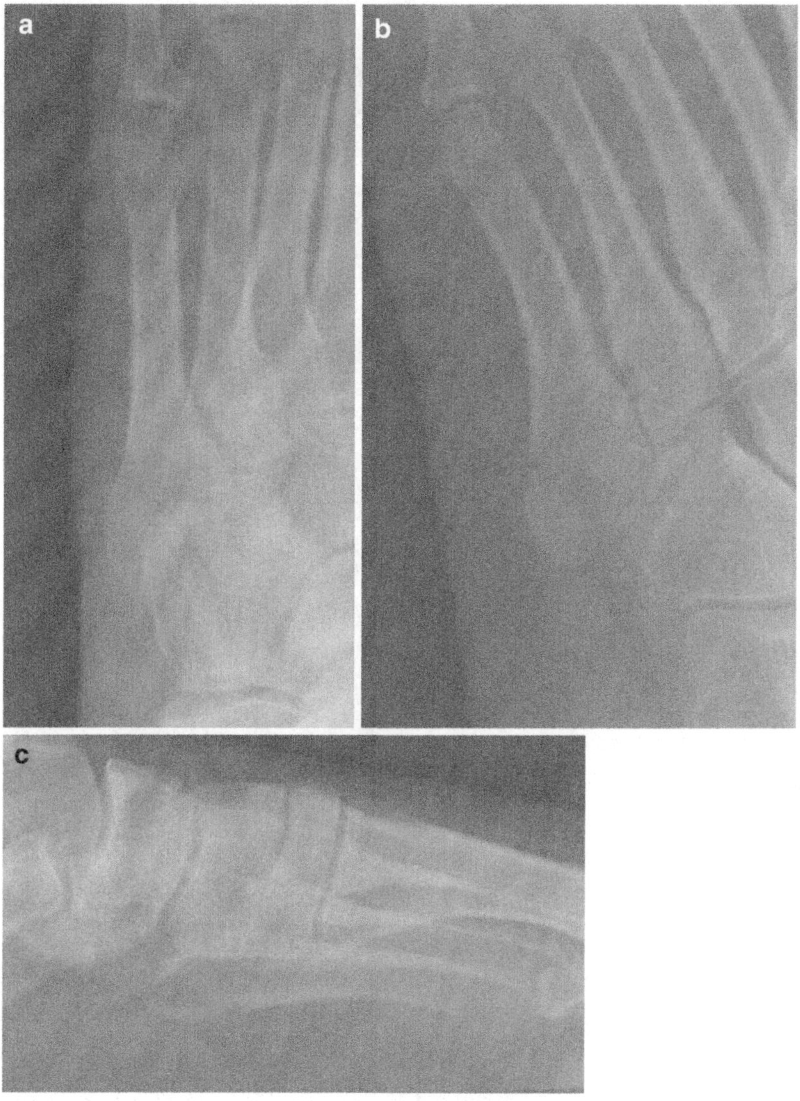

Fig. 16.3 (**a**, **b**, **c**) Pre-operative plain radiographs demonstrating a Zone II fracture of the proximal fifthme tatarsal

The patient is positioned supine with a bump under the ipsilateral greater trochanter to internally rotate the operative extremity, thereby permitting the foot to be placed plantigrade on the image intensifier platform of a standard fluoroscopy unit when the knee is flexed. The foot and ankle are prepped and draped in a standard, sterile fashion and the tourniquet is inflated after Esmarch exsanguination. With the knee flexed, the foot is positioned flat on the fluoroscopy platform and a free guide pin is placed on the dorsolateral skin overlying the intramedullary canal of the fifth metatarsal shaft (Fig. 16.4). Proper alignment is confirmed with fluoroscopy and a line is drawn along the path of the guide pin (Fig. 16.5a, b). This procedure is repeated in the lateral plane giving two lines that

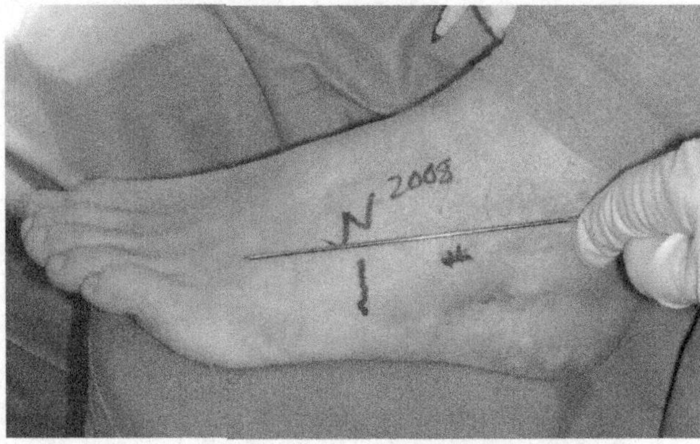

Fig.16.4 Footfl at on the image intensifier and free guide pin placed along dorsal aspect of fifth metatarsals haft

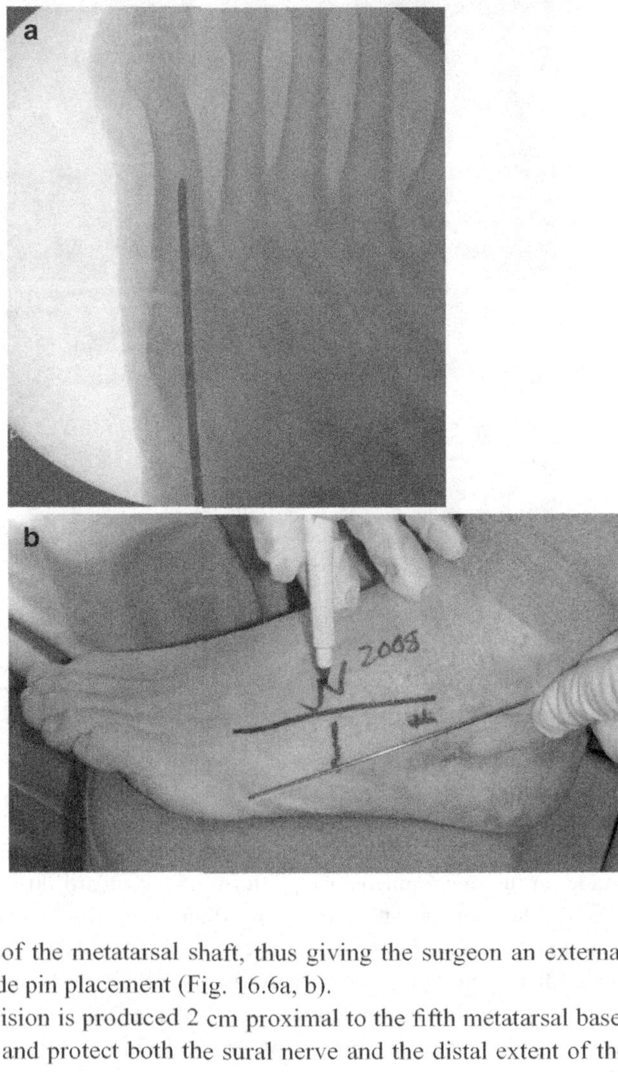

Fig.16.5 (**a**)Fluoros copic image demonstrating alignment of guide pin along metatarsal shaft. (**b**)L ine drawn on the skin corresponding to the alignment obtained in Fig. 16.5a

correspond to the trajectory of the metatarsal shaft, thus giving the surgeon an external reference for subsequent guide pin placement (Fig. 16.6a, b).

A 1.5 cm longitudinal incision is produced 2 cm proximal to the fifth metatarsal base, taking great care to identify and protect both the sural nerve and the distal extent of the

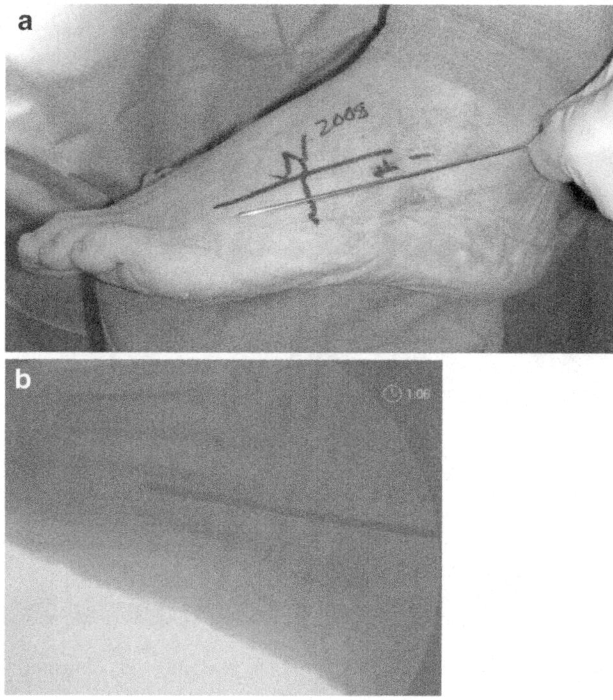

Fig. 16.6 ((**a**) and (**b**)) Intra-operative photograph and corresponding fluoroscopic image demonstrating correct alignment in the sagittal plane

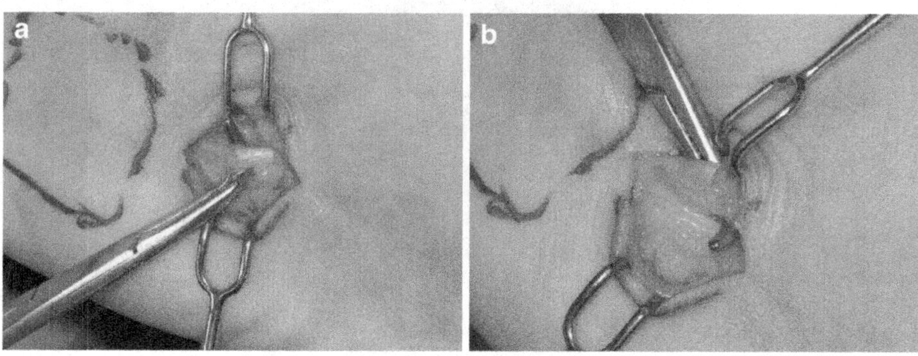

Fig. 16.7 (**a**) Sural nerve identified within the surgical wound. (**b**) Peroneus brevis tendon identified withint hes urgicalw ound

peroneus brevis tendon (Fig. 16.7a, b). Utilizing a tissue protector (sleeve), a guide pin is placed in the dorsomedial quadrant ("high and inside" position) of the fifth metatarsal base. Under fluoroscopic guidance, this guide pin is then advanced within the center of the medullary canal confirming proper position in the AP, lateral, and oblique planes (Fig. 16.8a, b). Throughout its advancement, the pin must lie against the lateral skin overlying the calcaneus to avoid penetration of the medial cortex of the shaft. The guide pin is advanced until its tip is approximately 2 cm beyond the fracture line, and then is over-drilled using a 3.2 mm drill bit under fluoroscopic guidance (Fig. 16.9). The drill is

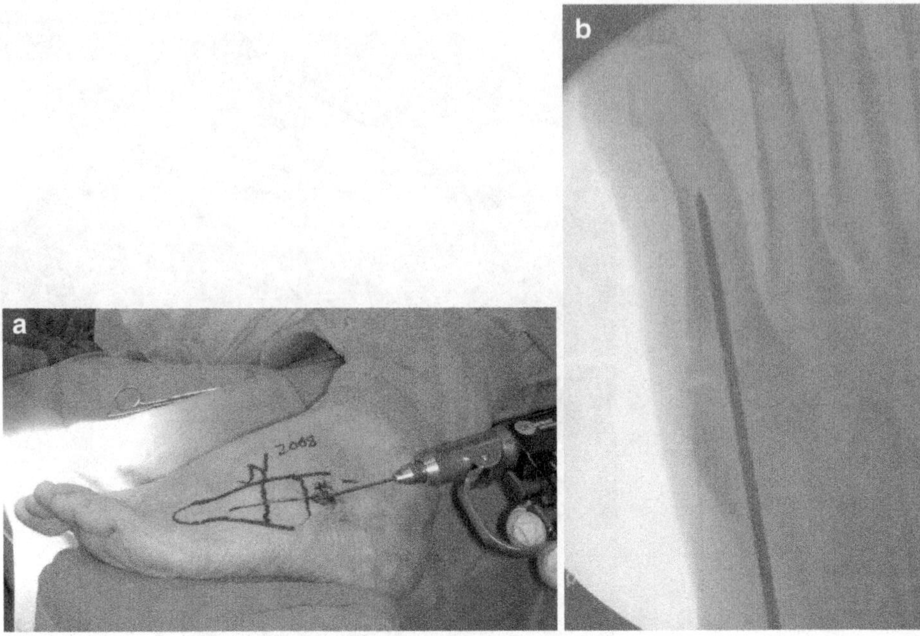

Fig.16.8 ((**a**) and (**b**)) Correct guide pin placement is confirmed fluoroscopically

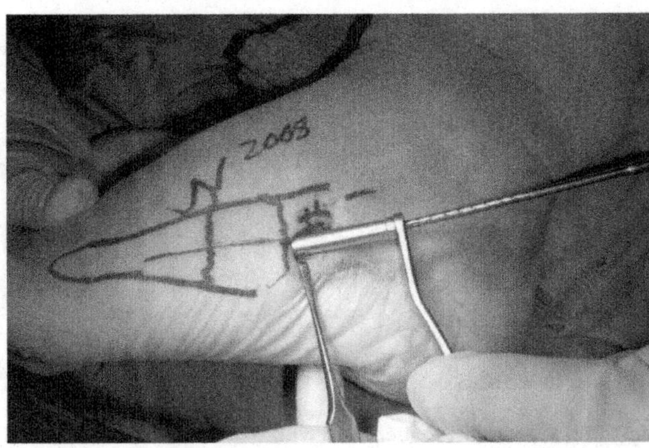

Fig.16.9 Overdrilling oft he proximal fifth metatarsal with the 3.2 mm drill bit using a tissue protector sleeve

withdrawn, and a 4.5 mm cannulated tap is advanced over the guide pin (Fig. 16.10). Tapping proceeds under fluoroscopic guidance across the fracture site to the curved portion of the fifth metatarsal shaft, but not beyond this region (Fig. 16.11). Sequential tapping with the 4.5, 5.5, and 6.5 mm taps is performed until a substantial amount of resistence is encountered within the medullary canal. When the surgeon observes external rotation of the right fifth metatarsal or internal rotation of the left fifth metatarsal with the final half-turn of the tap, the tap diameter corresponds to the desired screw diameter. It is essential

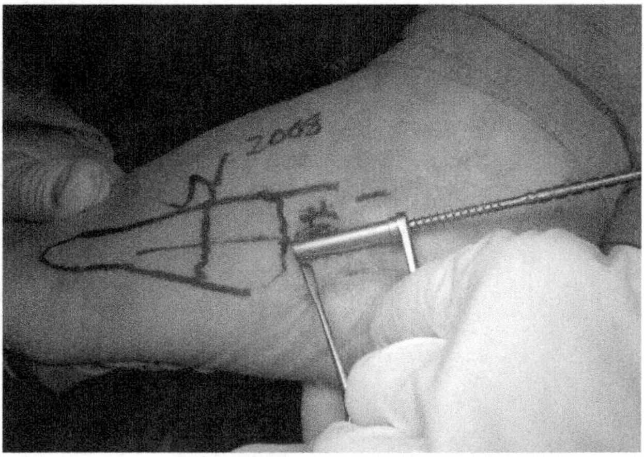

Fig. 16.10 Sequential tapping of the fifth metatarsal through the protective sleeve

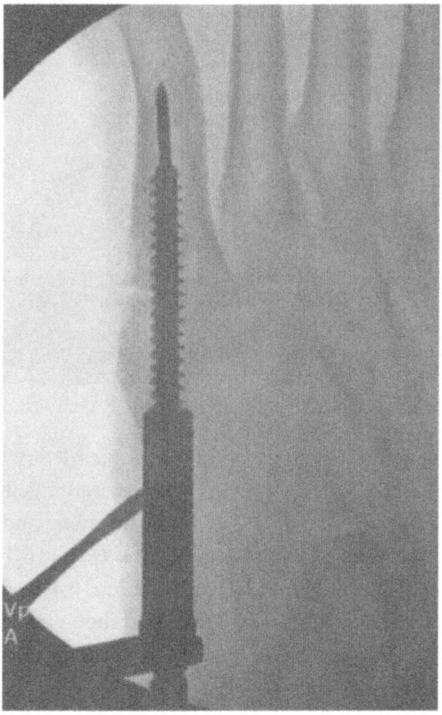

Fig. 16.11 Verification of the correct depth of the cannulated tap. Tapping proceeds across the fracture site and stops just proximal to the curved portion of the shaft

throughout the process of drilling and tapping that a soft tissue protector is used to prevent inadvertent damage to the sural nerve, peroneus brevis tendon, or the surrounding skin. Once the canal has been tapped to the desired diameter, screw length is measured using a cannulated depth gauge (Fig. 16.12) and double-checked by placing a screw of the measured length on the lateral aspect of the foot and taking an oblique fluoroscopic image (Fig. 16.13). The ideal screw should be long enough that all of the threads lie beyond the fracture line, yet not so long that its tip enters the curved portion of the medullary canal. If the

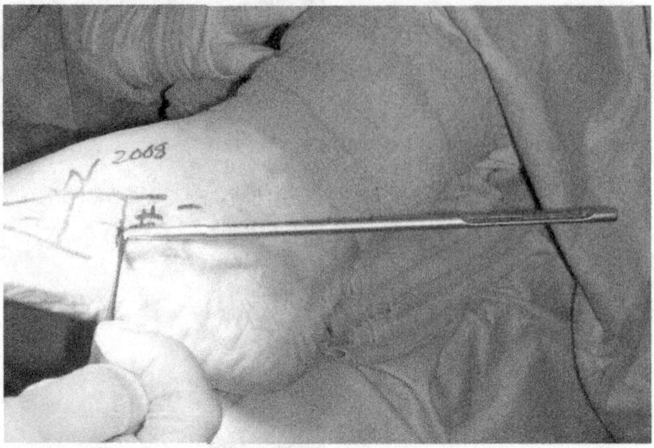

Fig.16. 12 Lengthofth e proper screw is measured using a cannulated depth gauge

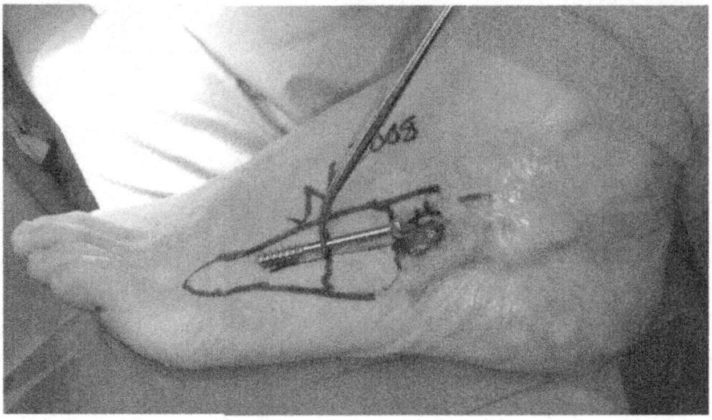

Fig.16. 13 Thea ppropriate length of the screw may alternatively be checked by placing a screw of the projected length on the skin, and verifying its selection fluoroscopically. The appropriate length screw should have all of its threads distal to the fracture line, and its tip should not enter the curved portion of the medullaryc anal

screw is too long, it will have a tendency to straighten out this normally curved bone, thus distracting the fracture site laterally. After determining the correct screw diameter and length, the guide pin is withdrawn, and immediately replaced with a solid, partially-threaded, stainless steel screw (Fig. 16.14). The screw is fully seated, and final fluoroscopici magesa reobt ained(Fig. 16.15).

The wound is irrigated and then closed using 4–0 nylon horizontal mattress sutures. A sterile dressing is applied, and the extremity is placed in a well padded short leg plaster splint or cast boot (Fig. 16.16).

16.5 Post-operativeP rotocol

Following rigid fixation, patients are kept non-weightbearing in their post-operative splint. At 2 weeks, sutures are removed and the patient is fashioned with an in-shoe clamshell orthosis as described by Dameron.[6] At the 4-week mark, three plain radiographic views of

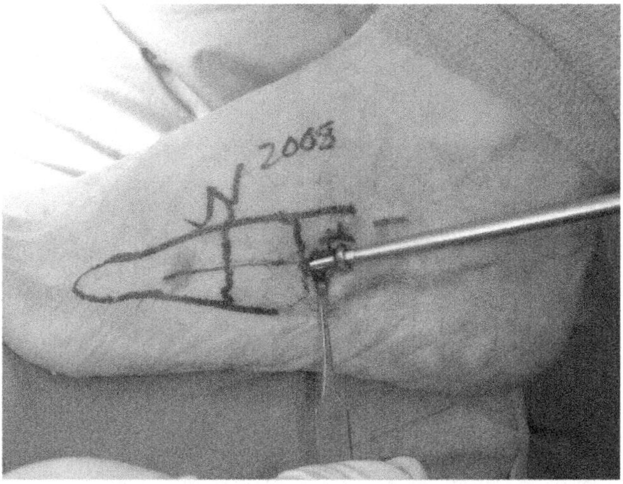

Fig. 16.14 Afterre movalof the guide pin, the solid, partially threaded, stainless steels crewis ins erted

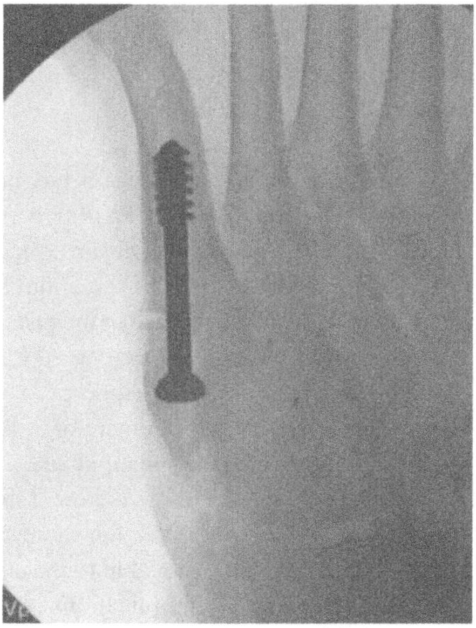

Fig. 16.15 Finalfl uoroscopic images are obtained

the operative foot are obtained and, if early bony healing is noted, the patient is allowed to commence weightbearing as tolerated in a CAM Walker with their orthotic device. At 6 weeks, the CAM Walker is exchanged for a regular tennis shoe (with the orthosis), and, if full radiographic healing is noted at the 12-week visit, the orthosis may be discontinued.

In the competitive athlete, the post-operative protocol parallels that of the non-athlete with a few exceptions. In these patients, we routinely employ a bone stimulator and begin upper body conditioning at the 2-week mark. At 3 weeks, partial weightbearing in the CAM Walker with clamshell orthosis is commenced, as well as a daily regimen of 30 min on the stationary bike. If radiographs taken at the 6 week follow-up appointment show

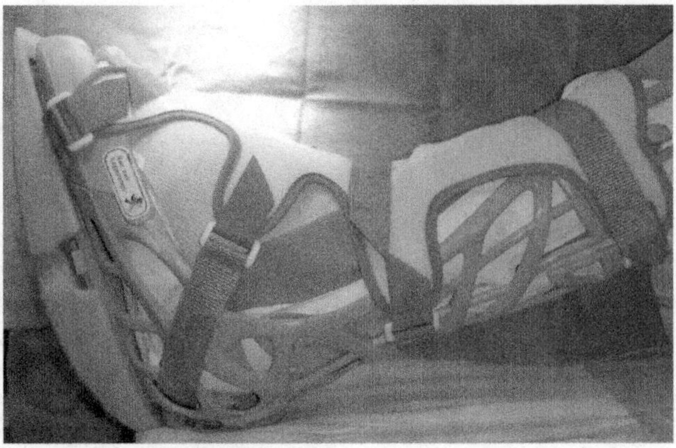

Fig. 16.16 Atthe c ompletion of the procedure, the patient is placed in a cast boot or shortl egs plint

adequate fracture healing, the patient starts progressive on-field work-out. Full, unrestricted return to sports is allowed at 8-weeks postoperatively, barring any set-backs.

16.6 Complications

Delayed union, nonunion, and refracture have all been reported following an otherwise successful percutaneous fixation of a fifth metatarsal base fracture,[8, 11, 15, 25, 35, 36] and are generally the result of a technical or diagnostic error. Common technical errors include: failure to fully cross the fracture site with the screw threads, placement of a screw that lacks an adequate diameter to gain solid purchase in the distal fragment, or insertion of a screw that is too long and subsequently straightens the curved fifth metatarsal thereby distracting the lateral aspect of the fracture site.[20] From a diagnostic standpoint, failure to identify an associated hindfoot varus may lead to the development of a delayed union, nonunion, or refracture, and should therefore be addressed with a simultaneous Dwyer calcaneal osteotomy or other corrective procedure.[20] In thin athletes, irritation of the peroneus brevis tendon by the screw head may be observed.[20] However, given the significant risk of refracture following screw removal,[11] we do not recommend removal until the athlete has completed their competitive careers.

Two other potential complications include injury to the sural nerve or peroneus brevis tendon.[20] These important structures must be identified during this limited percutaneous approach and protected throughout the entire procedure. The importance of gentle retraction with the use of the soft tissue protector sleeve cannot be overstated.

References

1. Arangio G. Transverse proximal diaphyseal fracture of the fifth metatarsal: a review of 12 cases. *Foot Ankle.*1992; 13:547–549.
2. Carp L. Fracture of the fifth metatarsal bone with special reference to delayed union. *Ann Surg.*1927;86:30 8–320.

3. Chuckpaiwong B, Queen RM, Easley ME, Nunley JA. Distinguishing Jones and proximal diaphyseal fractures of the fifth metatarsal. *Clin Orthop Rel Res*.2008; 466:1966–1970.
4. Clapper MF, O'Brien TJ, Lyons PM. Fractures of the fifth metatarsal: analysis of a fracture registry. *Clin Orthop Rel Res*.1995; 315:238–241.
5. Dameron TB. Fractures and anatomical variations of the proximal portion of the fifth metatarsal. *J Bone Joint Surg*.1975; 57-A:788–792.
6. Dameron TB. Fractures of the proximal fifth metatarsal: selecting the best treatment option. *J Am Acad Orthop Surg*.1995; 3:110–114.
7. DeLee JC, Evans JP, Julian J. Stress fracture of the fifth metatarsal. *Am J Sports Med*. 1983;11:349–353.
8. Glasgow MT, Naranja RJ, Glasgow SG, Torg JS. Analysis of failed surgical management of fractures of the base of the fifth metatarsal distal to the tuberosity: the Jones fracture. *Foot Ankle Int*.1996;17 :449–457.
9. Horst F, Gilbert BJ, Glisson RR, Nunley JA. Torque resistance after fixation of Jones fractures with intramedullary screws. *Foot Ankle Int*.2004; 25:914–919.
10. Jones R. Fracture of the base of the fifth metatarsal bone by indirect violence. *Ann Surg*. 1902;35:697–700.
11. Josefsson PO, Karlsson M, Redlund-Johnell I, Wendeberg B. Jones fracture: surgical versus nonsurgical treatment. *Clin Orthop Rel Res*.1994; 299:252–255.
12. Kavanaugh JH, Brower TD, Mann RV. The Jones fracture revisited. J Bone Joint Surg. 1978;60-A:776–782.
13. Kelly IP, Glisson RR, Fink C, Easley ME, Nunley JA. Intramedullary screw fixation of Jones fractures. *Foot Ankle Int*.2001; 22:585–589.
14. Konkel KF, Menger AG, Retzlaff SA. Nonoperative treatment of fifth metatarsal fractures in an orthopaedic suburban private multispecialty practice. Foot Ankle Int. 2005;26:704–707.
15. Larson CM, Almekinders LC, Taft TN, Garrett WE. Intramedullary screw fixation of Jones fractures: analysis of failure. *Am J Sports Med*.2002; 30:55–60.
16. Lawrence SJ, Botte MJ. Foot Fellow's review: Jones' fractures and related fractures of the proximal fifth metatarsal. *Foot Ankle*.1993; 14:358–365.
17. Lehman RC, Torg JS, Pavlov H, DeLee JC. Fractures of the base of the fifth metatarsal distal to the tuberosity: a review. *Foot Ankle*.1987; 7:245–252.
18. Mindrebo N, Shelbourne D, Van Meter CD, Rettig AC. Outpatient percutaneous screw fixation of the acute Jones fracture. *Am J Sports Med*.1993; 21:720–723.
19. Nunley JA. Fractures of the base of the fifth metatarsal: the Jones fracture. *Orthop Clin North Am*.2001;32:171– 180.
20. NunleyJ A.J onesf racturet echnique. *Techn Foot Ankle Surg*.2002; 1:131–137.
21. Pietropaoli MP, Wnorowski DC, Werner FW, Fortino MD. Intramedullary screw fixation of Jones fractures: a biomechanical study. *Foot Ankle Int*.1999; 20:560–563.
22. Porter DA, Duncan M, Meyer SJF. Fifth metatarsal Jones fracture fixation with a 4.5-mm cannulated stainless steel screw in the competitive and recreational athlete: a clinical and radiographic evaluation. *Am J Sports Med*.2005; 33:726–733.
23. Portland G, Kelikian A, Kodros S. Acute surgical management of Jones' fractures. *Foot Ankle Int*.2003;24:829–833.
24. Quill GE. Fractures of the proximal fifth metatarsal. *Orthop Clin North Am*. 1995;26:353–361.
25. Reese K, Litsky A, Kaeding C, Pedroza A, Shah N. Cannulated screw fixation of Jones fractures: a clinical and biomechanical study. *Am J Sports Med*.2004; 32:1736–1742.
26. Rosenberg GA, Sferra JJ. Treatment strategies for acute fractures and nonunions of the proximal fifth metatarsal. *J Am Acad Orthop Surg*.2000; 8:332–338.
27. Sarimo J, Rantanen J, Orava S, Alanen J. Tension-band wiring for fractures of the fifth metatarsal located in the junction of the proximal metaphysis and diaphysis. *Am J Sports Med*. 2006;34:476–480.

28. Shah SN, Knoblich GO, Lindsey DP, Kreshak J, Yerby SA, Chou LB. Intramedullary screw fixation of proximal fifth metatarsal fractures: a biomechanical study. *Foot Ankle Int.* 2001;22:581–584.
29. Sides SD, Fetter NL, Glisson R, Nunley JA. Bending stiffness and pull-out strength of tapered, variable pitch screws, and 6.5-mm cancellous screws in acute Jones fractures. *Foot Ankle Int.* 2006;27:821–825.
30. Stewart IM. Jones's fracture: fracture of the base of the fifth metatarsal. *Clin Orthop.* 1960;16:190–198.
31. Torg JS, Balduini FC, Zelko RR, Pavlov H, Peff TC, Das M. Fractures of the base of the fifth metatarsal distal to the tuberosity: classification and guidelines for non-surgical and surgical management. *J Bone Joint Surg.*1984; 66-A:209–214.
32. Tsaknis R, Leumann A, Valderrabano V, Pagenstert G, Hintermann B. Fixation of proximal fifth metatarsal fractures. *Techn Foot Ankle Surg.*2008; 7:115–119.
33. Vertullo CJ, Glisson RR, Nunley JA. Torsional strains in the proximal fifth metatarsal: implications for Jones and stress fracture management. *Foot Ankle Int.*2004; 25:650–656.
34. West RV. The female athlete: the triad of disordered eating, amenorrhea, and osteoporosis. *Sports Med.*1998; 26:63–71.
35. Wright RW, Fischer DA, Shively RA, Heidt RS, Nuber GW. Refracture of proximal fifth metatarsal (Jones) fracture after intramedullary screw fixation in athletes. *Am J Sports Med.* 2000;28:732–736.
36. Zelko RR, Torg JS, Rachun A. Proximal diaphyseal fractures of the fifth metatarsal – treatment of the fractures and their complications in athletes. *Am J Sports Med.*1979; 7:95–101.

Part IV

Hindfoot

Minimally Invasive Realignment Surgery oft heC harcotF oot

17

Bradley M. Lamm

17.1 Introduction

Charcot neuroarthropathy may produce joint subluxation or dislocation, loss of the bone quality, and osseous malalignment, which produces abnormal osseous prominences that become potential areas for ulceration. The deformed Charcot foot position causes aberrant weight bearing forces and altered muscle-tendon balance that also increase the risk for infection and amputation. When treating the Charcot neuroarthropathic foot, the best results are achieved when intervention is initiated early and the treatment is performed accurately and efficiently.[1,2]

The main goal in treating acute Charcot neuroarthropathy (i.e., Eichenholtz stage I) is to stabilize the bony anatomy and to avoid joint subluxation/dislocation.[3–5] In the acute stage of Charcot neuroarthropathy, the foot becomes extremely unstable at the level of the Charcot event. The traditional treatment is total contact casting for immobilization and to attempt to maintain the foot position. However, total contact casting has disadvantages due to the patient's inability to weight bear while in the cast, producing osteopenia of the ipsilateral foot and an increase in the weight bearing forces on the contralateral foot. Osteopenia makes subsequent surgery difficult, and contralateral foot ulceration can occur. In addition, patients with neuroarthropathy can have significant difficulty maintaining non-weight-bearing status for multiple reasons (e.g., obesity, muscle atrophy, diminished proprioception).[1,2]

The chronic Charcot foot (i.e., Eichenholtz stage II or III) can be stable or unstable. The unstable Charcot foot is difficult to shoe or brace, and typically results in ulceration. The stable Charcot foot is easier to shoe or brace but is still prone to ulceration. The main goal of surgical treatment in cases of chronic Charcot neuroarthropathy (i.e., Eichenholtz stage II or III) is to establish a stable plantigrade foot. Achilles tendon lengthening, ostectomy, débridement, osteotomy, arthrodesis, and open reduction with internal fixation aim to re-establish the normal foot position. Acute correction via open

B.M.La mm
International Center for Limb Lengthening, Rubin Institute for Advanced Orthopedics, Sinai HospitalofB altimore, 2401W estB elvedereA venue, Baltimore, MD, 21215, USA
e-mail:bla mm@lifebridgehealth.org

N. Maffulli and M. Easley (eds.), *Minimally Invasive Surgery of the Foot and Ankle*,
DOI: 10.1007/978-1-84996-417-3_17,

reduction with rigid internal fixation or plantar plating is frequently used for reconstruction.[6] Also, acute correction via open reduction with application of static external fixation has been reported.[3]

17.2 PreoperativeE valuation

Foot and ankle Charcot deformities are observed at isolated or multiple anatomic locations at various stages (i.e., Eichenholtz stages I, II, and III) with varying degrees of severity.[1,5–8] Plantar ulcers correlate to the anatomic location of the Charcot neuroarthropathy and are associated with the degree of stability of the foot. Plantar central or plantar lateral ulcers are associated with midfoot Charcot neuroarthropathy and are typically unstable. Instability of the lateral column leads to recurrent ulcers, whereby complex surgical reconstruction often becomes necessary.[8,9] Ulcers along the medial column are generally associated with Lisfranc Charcot deformities and medial column collapse. Lisfranc Charcot deformities are typically stable because of the interlocking anatomy and are successfully treated conservatively or with a limited surgical approach.[7,10]

The Charcot foot and ankle have subluxed/dislocated joints which causes the bones to become superimposed and makes the radiographs difficult to interpret. In addition, the Charcot process of bone fragmentation and proliferation adds to the complexity of radiographic readings. Weight bearing radiographs should be obtained in all planes to identify the level of Charcot deformity. Axial view radiographs are very helpful to evaluate hindfoot and ankle deformity.[11,12]

17.3 SurgicalP lanning

An unstable Charcot foot, whether in the chronic or acute phase of Charcot neuroarthropathy, is at risk for collapse and subsequent ulceration. The treatment of these Charcot neuroarthropathic feet and ankles depends on multiple factors including the stage, the location, stability, and ulcer osteomyelitis. The first goal of surgical intervention is to accurately diagnose the stage and location of the Charcot event. The second goal of surgical intervention is to convert an unstable Charcot foot into a stable, realigned (plantigrade) foot.

Recently, a method was described for treating acute Charcot neuroarthropathy by applying a static external fixator, which acts like a cast by stabilizing the affected joints and bones.[13] However, a static frame maintains the current foot position. In most instances, the foot is already deformed, collapsed, or malpositioned, and realignment of the subluxed/dislocated Charcot joint is therefore necessary. I have previously published a new, minimally invasive method of gradual distraction with external fixation that provides both realignment and stabilization.[14]

17.4
Minimally Invasive Charcot Foot Reconstruction

The goals of surgical intervention for the Charcot foot are to restore anatomic alignment, impart stability, prevent amputation, prevent foot shortening, and allow the patient to be ambulatory. Traditionally, open reduction with internal fixation was the mainstay for the management of Charcot foot deformities. Large open incisions were made to remove the excess bone, reduce the dislocated bone, and stabilize with internal fixation (screw fixation or plantar plating). These invasive surgical procedures typically resulted in a nonanatomic correction (e.g., shortening of the foot or incomplete deformity correction), and occasionally resulted in neurovascular compromise, incision healing problems, infection, and the use of casts or boots for patients who were non-weight-bearing.

Even though open reduction has disadvantages, in patients with tarsometatarsal Charcot deformity, it is advantageous. Typically, Charcot neuroarthropathy of the tarsometatarsal joints is associated with mild to moderate deformities because these joints are structurally interlocked. Acute realignment is achieved by performing a wedge resection or open reduction with fusion and internal fixation to produce a stable foot.

In patients with acute Charcot neuroarthropathy, static external fixation is placed to stabilize the Charcot process. The smooth wire fixation for the external fixation is applied so as to avoid the "hot" or Charcot joint region of the foot. In addition, the static fixator is applied strategically so gradual realignment can begin after the acute phase of Charcot has passed. Thus, the external fixator serves a dual purpose: it stabilizes the acute Charcot joint and provides subsequent realignment of the dislocated osseous anatomy. Once the bony anatomy is realigned, the external fixation is removed and a formal minimally invasive fusion of the Charcot joint is performed. Rigid intramedullary metatarsal screws are used to maintain the fusion.

Chronic stable or coalesced Charcot foot deformities require an osteotomy for correction of the deformity. I prefer a percutaneous Gigli saw osteotomy technique. Midfoot osteotomies can be performed across three levels (i.e., talar neck and calcaneal neck, cubonavicular osseous level, and cuneocuboid osseous level). Performing Gigli saw osteotomy across multiple metatarsals should be avoided because of the risk of neurovascular injury.[11]

For an unstable or an incompletely coalesced Charcot foot, correction can be obtained through gradual distraction. Despite the radiographic appearance of coalescence (superimposition of the dislocated/fragmented pedal bone because of the Charcot process), most Charcot deformities can undergo distraction without osteotomy to realign the pedal anatomy. An Achilles tendon lengthening is performed and held in a neutral position with the external fixation. This restores the normal calcaneal pitch and hindfoot position. Then, under fluoroscopy, the surgeon attempts to reduce the forefoot acutely and, if possible, insert intramedullary metatarsal screws. Acute reduction of the forefoot is rarely successful, but if accomplished, fusion of the midtarsal joint through a small medial and lateral incision would be required. I prefer percutaneously inserted intramedullary metatarsal screws for fixation. The patient maintains a short leg cast (no weight bearing allowed) for 2 months and a boot (weight bearing allowed) for 1 to 2 additional months. If the forefoot cannot be acutely reduced, an external fixator is used to hold the hindfoot position while gradually lengthening and realigning the forefoot. After realignment, the correction is maintained by minimally invasive arthrodesis of the Charcot joint(s) and fixed with percutaneous intramedullary metatarsal screws.

17.5 Surgical Technique for Gradual Correction

The first step consists of soft tissue realignment that is achieved by performing a percutaneous Achilles tendon lengthening to correct the hindfoot position. The second step consists of gradual soft tissue distraction with the Taylor spatial frame (TSF) (Smith & Nephew, Memphis, TN). The adjustments that the patient makes to the TSF (forefoot 6 × 6 butt frame) provide gradual correction of the forefoot on the fixed hindfoot.

The external fixation is mounted as follows. The distal tibia, talus, and calcaneus are fixed with two U-plates joined and mounted orthogonal to the tibia in both the anteroposterior and lateral planes. The U-plate placed around the anterior aspect of the ankle is affixed to the tibia with one lateral-to-medial 1.8 mm wire and two to three additional points of fixation (combination of smooth wires or half-pins). For additional tibial stability, a second more proximal tibial ring can be added to construct a distal tibial fixation block. To achieve hindfoot fixation, the ankle is dorsiflexed and the hindfoot manually held in a neutral position. The vertical U-plate is fixed to the calcaneus with two crossing 1.8 mm wires in the frontal plane. A 1.8 mm medial-to-lateral talar neck wire also is inserted and fixed to the U-plate. It is essential to fix the hindfoot in a neutral position. Next, two 1.8 mm stirrup wires are inserted through the osseous segment just proximal and distal to the Charcot joint(s). Stirrup wires are bent 90° just outside the skin to extend and attach but are not tensioned to their respective external fixation rings. Stirrup wires capture osseous segments that are far from an external fixation ring, thereby providing accurate and precise Charcot joint distraction. A full external fixation ring is then mounted to the forefoot by two 1.8 mm crossing metatarsal wires and the aforementioned distal stirrup wire. Digital pinning often is required, whereby the digital wires (1.5 or 1.8 mm) are attached to the forefoot ring. Finally, the six TSF struts are placed. Final orthogonal postoperative anteroposterior and lateral view fluoroscopic images are obtained of the reference ring; these images provide the mounting parameters that are needed for the computer planning. The choice of which ring (distal or proximal) to use as the reference ring depends on the surgeon's preference; typically, a distal reference ring is chosen for foot deformity correction. Superimposition of the reference ring on the final films is essential for accurate postoperative computer deformity planning. Computer planning of the TSF is a critical part of this procedure. The surgeon enters the deformity and mounting parameters into an Internet-based software program (www.spatialframe.com) that produces a daily schedule for the patient to perform adjustments on each of the six struts. The rate of correction and duration of treatment is controlled by the surgeon's data entry. The patient is clinically and radiographically followed in the office weekly or biweekly.

External fixation construction is challenging because of the small size of the foot. When applying the forefoot 6 × 6 butt frame, it is important to mount the U-plate on the hindfoot as posterior as possible and the forefoot ring as anterior as possible. The greater the distance between the forefoot ring and hindfoot ring, the more space for the TSF struts. Bone segment fixation is important; otherwise, failure of Charcot joint separation or incomplete anatomic reduction occurs. Small wire fixation is preferred in the foot because of the size and consistency of the bones. When treating a patient with neuropathy, construction of extremely stable constructs is of great importance. External fixation for Charcot deformity correction should include a full distal tibial ring with a closed foot ring.

Gradual distraction for realignment of the dislocated Charcot joint(s) is obtained in approximately 1–2 months. After gradual distraction with the TSF has realigned the anatomy of the foot, a second stage surgery is performed. The external fixator is removed along with simultaneously performing minimally invasive arthrodesis of the affected joints through small incisions (2–3 cm in length) overlying the appropriate joint(s). Minimally invasive arthrodesis is easily preformed because the Charcot joint(s) are already distracted. Under fluoroscopic guidance, guidewires for the large-diameter cannulated screws are inserted percutaneously through the plantar aspect of the metatarsal head by dorsiflexing the metatarsophalangeal joint. After the lateral and medial column guidewires (fourth, first, and second metatarsals) are inserted to maintain the corrected foot position, the frame is removed, and the foot is prepped again. Typically, three large-diameter cannulated intramedullary metatarsal screws are inserted: medial and lateral column partially threaded screws for compression of the arthrodesis site and one central (second metatarsal) fully threaded screw for additional stabilization. These screws span the entire length of the metatarsals to the calcaneus and talus, provide compression across the minimally invasive arthrodesis site, and stabilize adjacent joints. The intramedullary metatarsal screws cross an unaffected joint, the Lisfranc joint, thereby protecting the Lisfranc joint from experiencing a future Charcot event. The minimally invasive incisions are then closed, and a well-padded L and U splint is applied. At the time of hospital discharge, the patient is placed in a non-weight-bearing short leg cast applied for 2–3 months, and then gradual progression to weight bearing is achieved. Thus, the entire treatment is completed in 4–5 months(Fig. 17.1).

17.6 Results

Gradual deformity correction with external fixation is preferred for large deformity reductions of the dislocated Charcot joint(s) of the foot. Correction with external fixation allows for gradual, accurate realignment of the dislocated/subluxated Charcot joints.

I have performed this gradual distraction technique during the past 5 years and have achieved good to excellent success. Feet were treated at various stages of Charcot deformity: Eichenholtz stage I, Eichenholtz stage II, and Eichenholtz stage III. No deep infection, no screw failure, and no recurrent ulcerations were observed during follow-up. No amputations were necessary. Gradual Charcot foot correction with the Taylor spatial frame followed by minimally invasive arthrodesis has constituted a safe and effective treatment.

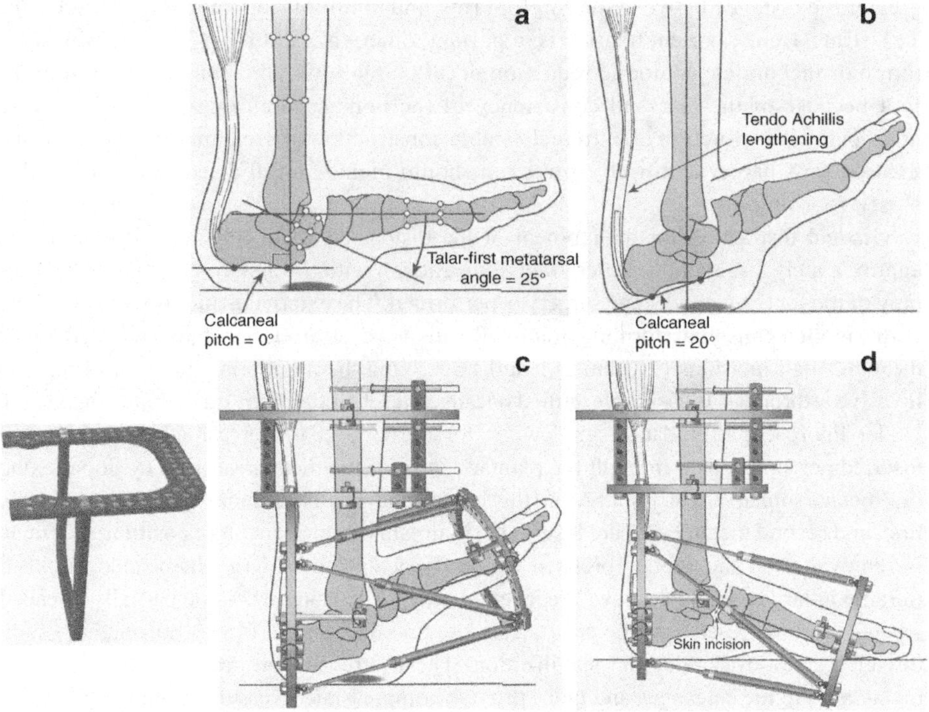

Fig. 17.1 (**a**) Illustration shows midfoot Charcot neuroarthropathy with equinus deformity (Eichenholtz stage II or III, with ulceration). Equinus (calcaneal pitch, 0°) and rockerbottom (talar-first metatarsal angle, 25°) is shown in the lateral view. (**b**) Equinus deformity is acutely corrected by performing a percutaneous Achilles tendon Z-lengthening. (**c**) Taylor spatial frame (forefoot 6 × 6 butt) is used to fix the hindfoot and ankle in the corrected position. Then the forefoot is fixed to the distal foot ring. Note the initial forefoot position. (**d**) Fixator is used to gradually distract (5–15 mm) and realign the forefoot to the hindfoot. A minimally invasive fusion of the midtarsal joint is performed immediately before fixator removal. (**e**) Fixator is removed after inserting the percutaneous guidewires for the large-diameter cannulated screws. The medial and lateral columns of the foot are compressed by inserting partially threaded intramedullary metatarsal cannulated screws beneath the metatarsal head. (**f**) Anteroposterior view shows a third fully threaded screw inserted to increase midfoot stability. Note the accurate anatomic reduction, restoration of foot length, healed ulceration, and preservation of the subtalar and ankle joints (Copyright 2009, Rubin Institutef orA dvancedO rthopedics,Si naiH ospitalof B altimore)

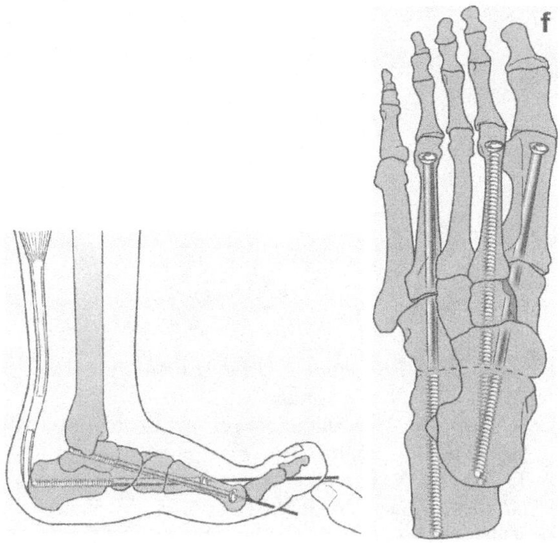

Fig. 17.1 (Continued)

17.7 Conclusion

Our short-term results are promising. The advantages of our method when compared with the resection and plating method reported by Schon et al.[6] or the resection and external fixation method reported by Cooper[15] are preservation of foot length (no bone resection), accurate anatomic realignment of soft tissues and bone, and a stable foot. Furthermore this method is much less invasive and allows for partial weight bearing.

17.8 Acknowledgements

The authors thank Joy Marlowe, MA, for her excellent illustrative artwork. Special thanks to Amanda Chase, MA, for her exceptional editing.

References

1. Frykberg RG, ed. *The High Risk Foot in Diabetes Mellitus*. New York, NY: Churchill Livingstone; 1991.
2. Trepman E, Nihal A, Pinzur MS. Current topics review: Charcot neuroarthropathy of the foot and ankle. *Foot Ankle Int*. 2005;26:46–63.
3. Jolly GP, Zgonis T, Polyzois V. External fixation in the management of Charcot neuroarthropathy. *Clin Podiatr Med Surg*. 2003;20:741–756.
4. Shibata T, Tada K, Hashizume C. The results of arthrodesis of the ankle for leprotic neuroarthropathy. *J Bone Joint Surg Am*. 1990;72:749–756.
5. Eichenholtz SN. *Charcot Joints*. Springfield, IL: C. C. Thomas; 1966.
6. Schon LC, Easley ME, Weinfeld SB. Charcot neuroarthropathy of the foot and ankle. *Clin Orthop Relat Res*. 1998;349:116–131.
7. Brodsky JW, Rouse AM. Exostectomy for symptomatic bony prominences in diabetic Charcot feet. *Clin Orthop Relat Res*. 1993;296:21–26.
8. Catanzariti AR, Mendicino R, Haverstock B. Ostectomy for diabetic neuroarthropathy involving the midfoot. *J Foot Ankle Surg*. 2000;39:291–300.
9. Paley D. *Principles of Deformity Correction*. 1st ed., Corr. 3rd printing. Rev ed. Berlin, Germany: Springer; 2005.
10. Simon SR, Tejwani SG, Wilson DL, Santner TJ, Denniston NL. Arthrodesis as an early alternative to nonoperative management of Charcot arthropathy of the diabetic foot. *J Bone Joint Surg Am*. 2000;82:939–950.
11. Lamm BM, Paley D. Charcot neuroarthropathy of the foot and ankle. In: Rozbruch RS, Ilizarov S, eds. *Limb Lengthening and Reconstruction Surgery*. New York, NY: Informa Healthcare; 2006:221–232.
12. Lamm BM, Paley D. Deformity correction planning for hindfoot, ankle, and lower limb. *Clin Podiatr Med Surg*. 2004;21:305–326.
13. Wang JC, Le AW, Tsukuda RK. A new technique for Charcot's foot reconstruction. *J Am Podiatr Med Assoc*. 2002;92:429–436.
14. Lamm BM. Surgical reconstruction and stepwise approach to acute Charcot neuroarthropathy. In: Zgonis T, ed. *Surgical Reconstruction of the Diabetic Foot and Ankle*. Philadelphia, PA: Lippincott Williams & Wilkins; 2009:223–229.
15. Cooper PS. Application of external fixators for management of Charcot deformities of the foot and ankle. *Foot Ankle Clin*. 2002;7:207–254.

Arthroscopic Triple Arthrodesis

18

Tun Hing Lui

18.1 Introduction

Triple arthrodesis play a significant role in the management of hindfoot osteoarthrosis and deformity. Traditionally, this is performed as an open procedure with extensive soft-tissue dissection and bone resection especially at the talonavicular joint. Arthroscopy can provide better intra-articular visualization, minimal bone removal, and better fusion surface preparation, especially of the talonavicular joint. This may reduce the nonunion rate of the talonavicular joint. Furthermore, "4-corner arthrodesis" at the junction site among the four hindfoot bones will aid stabilization of the position and fusion of the subtalar, talonavicular, and calcaneocuboid joints.[1–3]

18.2 Description of Technique

Arthroscopic triple arthrodesis comprises arthroscopic subtalar arthrodesis and arthroscopic midtarsal arthrodesis.[1–3]

Under general or regional anesthesia with the patient supine with a support over the buttock. We use a thigh tourniquet to maintain bloodless field. No traction is required. To avoid painful neuroma formation, portals are produced using the nick and spread technique.

Subtalar arthroscopy is performed through the anterolateral and middle portals. The anterolateral portal is just above the angle of Gissane. The middle portal is just anterior and distal to the tip of the lateral malleolus. The articular cartilage of subtalar joint is denuded with small periosteal elevator, arthroscopic curette and arthroscopic osteotome. The subchondral bone is then micro-fractured with the arthroscopic awl (Fig. 18.1).

We then proceed to mid-tarsal joint arthroscopy through lateral, dorsolateral, dorsomedial and medial portals.[1,4] The lateral and dorsolateral portals are established for

T.H. Lui
Department of Orthopaedics and Traumatology, North District Hospital, 9 Po Kin Road, Sheung Shui, NT, Hong Kong SAR, China
e-mail: luithderek@yahoo.co.uk

N. Maffulli and M. Easley (eds.), *Minimally Invasive Surgery of the Foot and Ankle*,
DOI: 10.1007/978-1-84996-417-3_18,

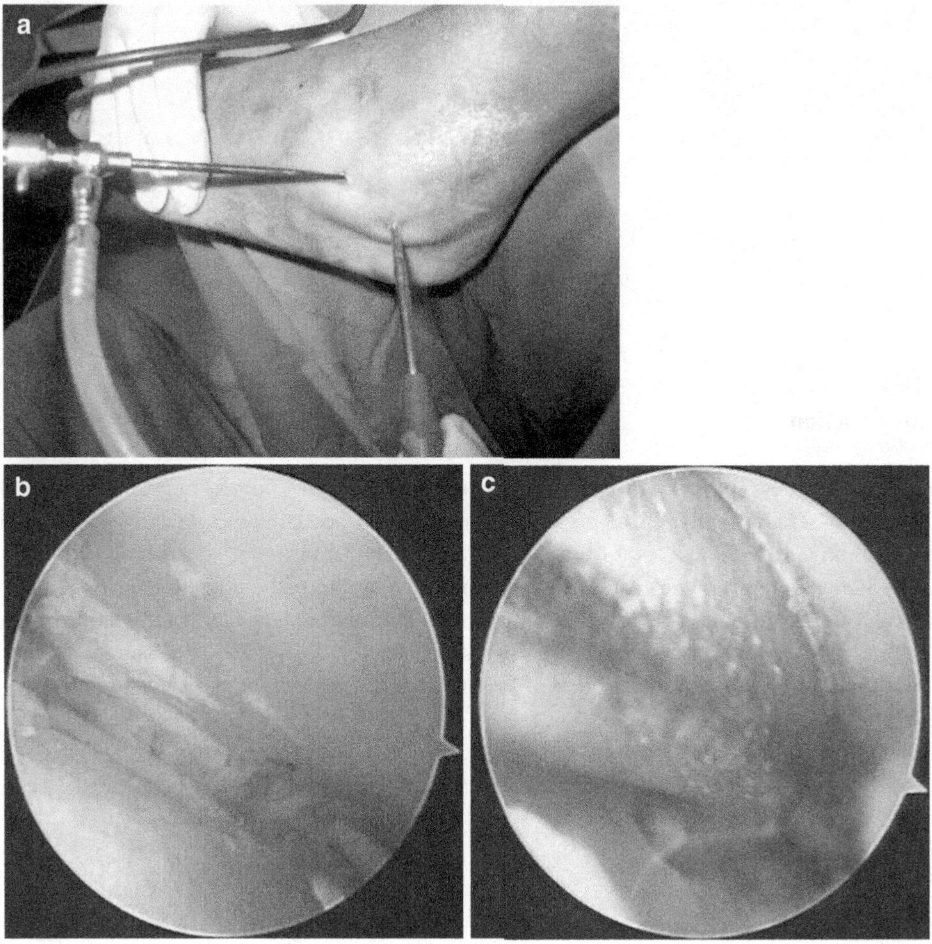

Fig. 18.1 (**a**) Subtalar arthroscopy through the anterolateral and middle portals. (**b**) The articular cartilage is denuded, leaving the subchondral bone intact. (**c**) Micro-fracture of the subchondral bonew itha rthroscopica wl

calcaneocuboid arthroscopy. The lateral portal is established at plantar-lateral corner of the calcaneocuboid joint. The structures at risk include the peroneal tendons and the sural nerve. The dorsolateral portal is directly over the space between the talonavicular and calcaneocuboid joints. It is the most important portal of this procedure, since through it we can approach the medial aspect of the calcaneocuboid joint, the lateral and plantar aspects of talonavicular joint, the junction between talus, calcaneum, navicular and cuboid, and the anterior subtalar joint. The long extensor tendons and intermediate dorsal cutaneous branch of superficial peroneal nerve are close to this portal. The medial portal is established at the medial aspect of the talonavicular joint, just dorsal to the insertion of the posterior tibial tendon. The dorsomedial portal is at the mid-point between the medial and dorsolateral portals. The extensor hallucis longus tendon and the deep peroneal nerve are at risk when producing the dorsomedial portal. The portals are located with a needle and checked by fluoroscopy.

During calcaneocuboid arthroscopy, the dorsolateral and lateral portals are interchangeable as visualization and instrumentation portals. The articular cartilage is denuded with a small periosteal elevator, and the subchondral bone is micro-fractured with arthroscopic awl.

The talonavicular joint is approached through the medial, dorsomedial and dorsolateral portals. These three portals are interchangeable as visualization and instrumentation portals, and through them most of the articular surface of talonavicular can be reached. Sometimes, the anterolateral subtalar portal and the lateral midtarsal portal can be used as visualization portals. The articular cartilage is denuded and the subchondral bone prepared for fusion as described above. Because of the tight talonavicular and calcaneocuboid joints, the arthroscope is introduced along the side of the joint and the joint line is located before the insertion of instruments to remove the articular cartilage. In case of degenerated midtarsal joint, the dorsal osteophytes may need to be removed before the joint line can be identified arthroscopically.[5] It is useful to locate the joint under fluoroscopy and mark with a needle in patients with severe joint degeneration. The needle can serve as the landmark of the joint line during arthroscopy (Fig. 18.2).

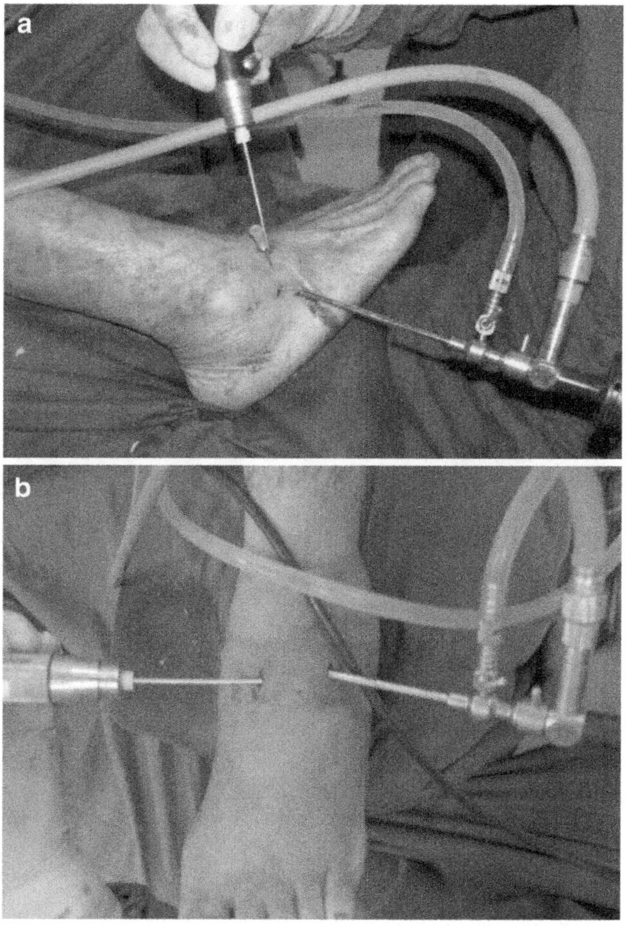

Fig. 18.2 (**a**) Calcaneocuboid arthroscopy with dorsolateral and lateral midtarsal portals. A needle is inserted in the joint in patients with severe osteoarthritis as a landmark of the joint during arthroscopy. (**b**) Talonavicular arthroscopy using the dorsomedial and dorsolateral portals. Finally, the dorsomedial portal, dorsolateral and lateral portals can be used to prepare the space between calcaneum, talus, navicular and cuboid for fusion. Usually, dorsomedial and lateral portals are the visualization portals and dorsolateral portal are the working ones. The cortical bone of the boundary of this space is prepared for fusion using arthroscopic burr

After the fusion sites are prepared, subtalar joint and mid-tarsal joints are reduced into the desirable positions, and the subtalar joint is transfixed with a 7.3 mm cannulated screw and talonavicular and calcaneocuboid joints are transfixed with a 4.0 mm cannulated screw using percutaneous techniques. The junction space between the four bones and the three joint spaces can be grafted with autologous bone graft or hydroxyapatite granules using a drill guard as the delivery channel.

Post-operatively, patients are put on short leg cast and non-weight-bearing walking for 8 weeks, and then protected weight bearing walking with rocker boot for another 4 weeks wasa llowed.

18.3 DeformityC orrection

18.3.1 Arthroscopic Lateral Subtalar Release

In patients with valgus hindfoot deformity from intra-articular pathology, e.g., rheumatoid arthritis, the lateral capsuloligamentous structures can be released arthroscopically (Fig. 18.3).[6]

18.3.1.1 Technique

Subtalar arthroscopy is performed via the anterolateral subtalar portal, middle subtalar portal and the posterolateral subtalar portal at the lateral side of the Achilles tendon just above the posterosuperior tubercle of the calcaneus. Arthroscopic subtalar release is performed in stages. The lateral subtalar capsule and lateral subtalar ligamentous structures are stripped from the lateral calcaneal cortical surface through the portals with a small

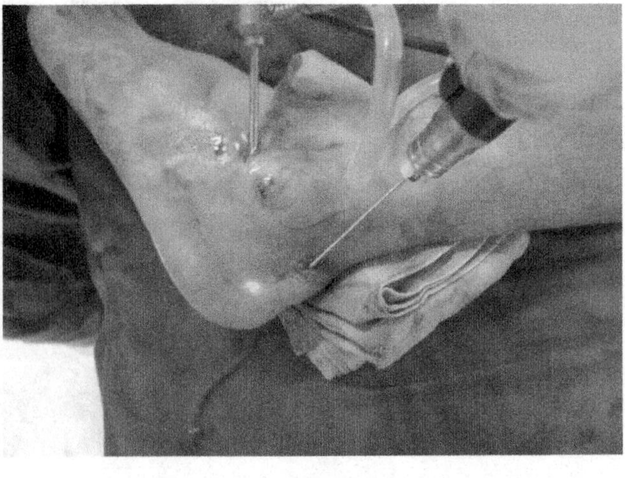

Fig.18.3 Arthroscopicl ateral releaseof t hes ubtalarj oint

periosteal elevator. If the correction is still not sufficient, the ligamentous structures of the sinus tarsi, especially the interosseous ligament, are released through the anterolateral and middle portals. The posterior subtalar capsule can be released through the anterolateral, middle and posterolateral portals. The lateral gap resulting after the correction of the valgus deformity can be packed with bone graft through the subtalar portals.

18.3.2 "Closing Wedge"P rocedure

In case of varus hindfoot deformity, the articular cartilage can be removed as described above. After the fusion surfaces are prepared, a "closing wedge" procedure[7] of the subtalar joint is performed with the Isham straight flute burr (Vilex Inc.). The burr is inserted through the subtalar portals. A lateral wedge of bone, especially the lateral talar process, is burred while applying valgus force to the heel and the varus heel will be corrected (Fig. 18.4). If the correction is hindered by midtarsal joint deformity e.g., in neglected clubfoot deformity,

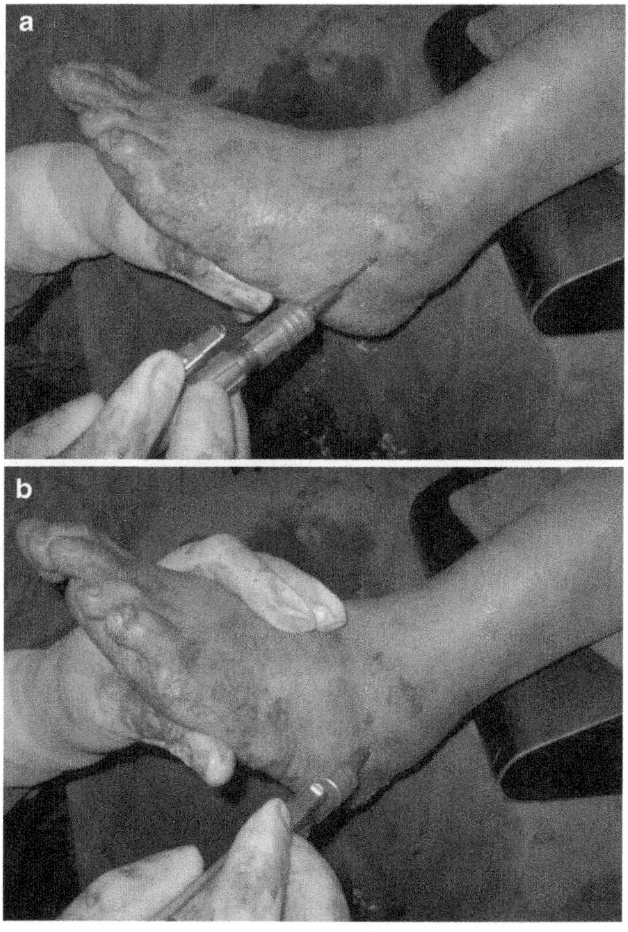

Fig.18.4 (**a**) A "closing wedge" procedure of the subtalar joint is performed with the Isham straight flute burr (Vilex Inc.). The burr was inserted through the subtalar portals. (**b**) A lateral wedge of bone especially the lateral talar process is burred while applying valgus force to the heel and the varus heel willbe c orrected

a 2.0 mm Kirschner wire is inserted into the navicular to de-rotate the midfoot. If this fails to de-rotate the midfoot, the medial capsuloligamentous structure can be released from the navicular through the medial and dorsomedial midtarsal portals. The Spring ligament can be released by anterior subtalar arthroscopy as described below. The derotation is repeated and the Isham straight flute burr is inserted into the talonavicular portals to remove the impinging bone encountered.

18.3.3 AnteriorS ubtalarA rthroscopy

The anterior subtalar joint and the spring ligament can be approached by the anterior subtalar arthroscopy.[8] Arthroscopic resection of the talocalcaneal coalition and release of the spring ligament are feasible with this arthroscopic approach.

18.3.3.1 Technique

The anterolateral subtalar portal is the primary visualization portal. The dorsolateral midtarsal portal is the primary working portal (Fig. 18.5). These two portals can be switched. With the 2.7 mm, 30° arthroscope in the anterolateral subtalar portal, the soft tissue at the junction between the talonavicular and calcaneocuboid joint is removed with an arthroscopic shaver through the dorsolateral midtarsal portal. The inferior corner of the medial side of the talar head will be exposed. The contour of the talar head is then traced proximally to expose the Spring ligament and the articulation between the talar head and the anterior and middlec alcaneal facets.

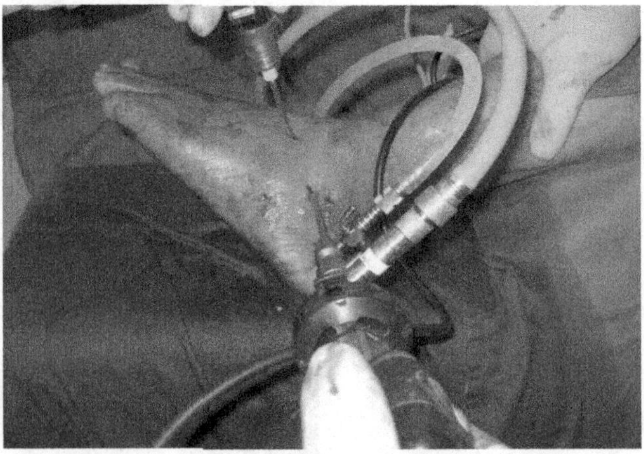

Fig.18. 5 Anteriors ubtalar arthroscopy. The anterolateral subtalar portal is the primary visualization portal. The dorsolateral midtarsal portal is the primaryw orkingpor tal

18.3.4 Extra-Articular Procedure: Percutaneous Tendon Release or Transfer or Percutaneous Osteotomy

Frequently, both soft tissue and osteo-articular pathology should be dealt with to correct the foot deformity. Various soft tissue balancing procedures e.g., percutaneous tendon release or transfer and percutaenous osteotomy may be needed together with an arthroscopic triple arthrodesis to achieve adequate correction of the deformity and prevent recurrence.

References

1. Lui TH. New technique: arthroscopic triple arthrodesis. *Arthroscopy.*2006; 22:464.e1–464.e5.
2. Lui TH. Current concepts: foot and ankle arthroscopy and endoscopy: indications of new technique. *Arthroscopy.*2007; 23:889–902.
3. Lui TH. Arthroscopic triple arthrodesis in patients with Müller Weiss disease. *Foot Ankle Surg.* Inpre ss.
4. Oloff L, Schulhofer SD, Fanton G, Dillingham M. Arthroscopy of the calcaneocuboid and Talonavicular Joints. *J Foot Ankle Surg.*1996; 35:101–108.
5. Lui TH, Chan LK. Cadaveric study on the safety and efficacy of talonavicular arthroscopy in arthroscopic triple arthrodesis. *Arthroscopy.*I npr ess.
6. Lui TH. Arthroscopic subtalar release of post-traumatic subtalar stiffness. *Arthroscopy* 2006;22:1364e 1–e4.
7. Lui TH. Case report: correction of neglected club foot deformity by Arthroscopic Triple Arthrodesis. *Arch Orthop Trauma Surg.*2010; 130:1007–1011.
8. Lui TH. Anterior subtalar (talocalcaneonavicular) arthroscopy. *Foot Ankle Int.* 2008;29: 94–96.

Percutaneus Calcaneal Displacement Osteotomy

19

Lawrence A. DiDomenico, Joseph M. Anain Jr..a nd Michael D. LaCivita

19.1 Introduction

Calcaneal osteotomies are commonly performed procedures in the correction of compound deformities in the foot and ankle.[1] They have been utilized for over 100 years in foot surgery with their first introduction by Gleich in 1893.[1–11] Complications in the performance of the calcaneal osteotomy are rare.[3,6,11] Among the complications seen through the standard lateral approach of a calcaneal osteotomy are: wound dehiscence, sural nerve damage, sural neuritis, delayed union, non–union, infection, and invasion of the medial neurovascular structures.[3,6,9–11]

The Percutaneous Calcaneal Displacement Osteotmy approach has been developed to help avoid the complications commonly seen with the traditional standard open calcaneal osteotomy.[3,6,9–11] Wound dehiscence is a problem encountered when performing these osteotomies open. Large incisions on the lateral aspect of the foot can also cause fibrosis in the area that leads to painful nerve symptoms. When performing these osteotomies open, the surgeon must be cautious about exiting the medial aspect too aggressively due to the neurovascular structures that lie in this area.[10,12]

In an effort to avoid these complications, the percutaneous technique of performing the posterior calcaneal displacement osteotomy has been employed. This technique is performed through four small stab incisions to avoid the open osteotomy incision, which can be prone to dehiscence.[6,9] The technique is also unique in that it avoids major neurovascular structures if performed properly.

In the past 5 years, over 100 percutaneous calcaneal displacement osteotomies have been performed. There has been success in performing an effective calcaneal displacement osteotomy, avoiding wound problems, and avoiding invasion of neurovascular structures.

L.A.D iDomenico(✉)
Reconstructive Rearfoot and Ankle Surgical Fellowship, Ankle and Foot Care Centers/Ohio CollegeofPodia tricM edicine, Cleveland, OH, USA
e-mail:ld5353@ aol.com

N. Maffulli and M. Easley (eds.), *Minimally Invasive Surgery of the Foot and Ankle*,
DOI: 10.1007/978-1-84996-417-3_19, © Springer-Verlag London Limited 2011

19.2 Indications

Calcaneal valgus: The medial displacement osteotomy is presently described throughout foot and ankle literature for the treatment of the flexible flatfoot with good results reported in adults and children.[1,3–8,11,13–19,20,21] Flexible flatfoot is one of the most common orthopedic problems found in children.[18,19] Torosian et al. found that the medial slide calcaneal osteotomy is a simple and effective treatment for hindfoot valgus.[20] When valgus malalignment is detected, medializing the calcaneus provides satisfactory outcomes.[22] In advanced stages of the deformity the medial column may be affected and the need for tendon transfers or joint fusions are effective treatments when combined with the medial calcaneal displacement osteotomy.[22]

Posterior tibial tendon dysfunction: Posterior tibial tendon dysfunction is when the adult aquired flatfoot becomes evident with the heel in valgus position, the flattening of the medial longitudinal arch, and forefoot abduction.[15,17,23] Presently in the literature surgeons are using calcaneal osteotomies in the treatment of posterior tibial tendon dysfunction combined with various ancillary procedures.[3–6,13–18,22,24–33]

Without surgical intervention, the deformity is likely to progress to a fixed malformation.[33] Mann, and Myerson both describe a posterior calcaneal osteotomy in which the posterior aspect of the calcaneus is moved medially. This osteotomy is performed in conjunction with a flexor digitorum longus transfer in the treatment of patients with stage II posterior tibial tendon dysfunction. Both authors are reporting satisfactory results.[5,6,28–30]

Mann describes the foot as a tripod.[5,6] The three legs being – the first metatarsal head, the fifth metatarsal head, and the calcaneus. If too much heel valgus is present, as in the above mentioned indications, the tripod does not function properly and the medial aspect of the foot decreases in height. Performing the posterior medial calcaneal displacement osteotomy places the calcaneus back into its correct position.[5,6]

Loss of calcaneal height status post calcaneal fracture: Loss of hindfoot height or leg length is often times seen status post calcaneal fracture.[22] A posterior calcaneal osteotomy is an effective way of restoring the height of the hindfoot or leg.[22] The osteotomy is performed and the posterior aspect of the calcaneus is shifted plantarly to restore this height.[22]

Calcaneal Varus, and lateral ankle instability: The posterior calcaneal slide osteotomy is also reported in literature for correction of abnormal heel alignment that is rectus or varus.[22,34] The objective of the osteotomy is to reposition the Achilles tendon, plantar fascia and the bone which will reduce stress on the lateral ligaments. The tripod theory is once again applicable here.[34,35] The calcaneal displacement osteotomy can be manipulated and reduce abnormal stresses on the lateral aspect of the foot.[22]

The above mentioned deformities are the indications in which the open posterior calcaneal displacement osteotomy is used. These remain the same indications for the use of the percutaneous calcaneal displacement osteotomy. The percutaneous calcaneal displacement osteotomy can be performed on any patient that would benefit from the traditional open calcaneal displacement osteotomy. There are no contraindications to a percutaneous calcaneal displacement osteotomy versus an open calcaneal displacement osteotomy. The advantages are as follows: better cosmesis, low postoperative morbidity, absence of significant wound problems, less blood loss, minimize the risk for postoperative infection, faster rehabilitation and mobilization (if performed as an isolated procedure), decrease time of union, less stress to the local tissues, less trauma to the tissues and bone, and fewer neurovascular complications. This is probably because periosteal stripping is not necessary and the local circulation remains intact.

19.3 Considerations for Preoperative Planning

A thorough history and physical examination should be performed. This is necessary to evaluate the patients overall health and decide if the patient is the appropriate candidate to undergo reconstructive foot surgery. The examination should focus on vascular, neurological, dermatological and biomechanical function. If deficits are found they should be fully investigated.

Radiologic evaluation of the foot and ankle is very important in assessing the entire deformity. Routine views of the foot should include an anteriorposterior view, a medial oblique view and lateral view.[16,22,36,37] The anteriorposterior view allows one to evaluate loss of normal alignment of Kite's angle, the talus and first metatarsal, and the degree of subluxation of the talus and navicular.[38] The lateral radiograph demonstrates the calcaneal pitch.[38,39] A study was performed by Smith, Sima, and Reischl which deemed this a very reliable radiographic angle in the evaluation of flatfoot and cavus deformities.[38,39] Twenty to twenty–five degrees would be considered normal, less then 15° would been seen in a flatfoot, and greater then 30° in a cavus deformity.[38,39] One may also evaluate subluxation of the talonavicular and navicular cuneiform joints through lateral radiographs.[38] Ankle radiographs should be obtained as well, and should include anteriorposterior, lateral, and mortise views.[16,22] These views will allow for proper assessment of the ankle joint for degenerative processes and malalignment.[38] A long axial view should also be performed to quantify the amount of valgus or varus present.[38,40] Paley describes a method (modified from Salzman and El–Khoury's method, in which the alignment between the body of the calcaneus and the tibia are measured to assess the degree of varus or valgus deformity.[41]

Unless there is trauma all foot and ankle radiographs should be obtained weight bearing, with the knee straight, and comparative contralateral views should be taken.[16,22,36,38] The knee should be straight because deformities of the hind foot, and mid foot are frequently associated with a tight gastrocnemius.[22]

19.4 Surgical Technique

The equipment needed to perform the percutaneous calcaneal displacement osteotomy is minimal and includes: #15 blade, curved Kelly hemostat, straight hemostat, 12 in. flexible gigli saw, large cannulated cancellous screw set, and appropriate suture for closure. A fluoroscopy unit will be necessary to perform this osteotomy. We recommend a small fluoroscopy unit for its ease of use in the operating room.

This procedure is partly designed to limit, if not eliminate, neurovascular compromise when performing a calcaneal osteotomy. Greene et al. performed a study evaluating the medial neurovascular structures that crossed the site of the traditional open calcaneal displacement osteotomy.[10] In this study they found that an average of four neurovascular structures crossed each osteotomy site, most were branches of the Lateral Plantar Nerve and branches of the Posterior Tibial Artery.[10] The sensory branch of the Lateral plantar nerve crossed the osteotomy in 86% of the subjects studied.[10] Baxter's nerve (a distal branch of the Lateral Plantar Nerve) crossed in 95% of the specimens.[10] The Posterior tibial artery distributed from zero to three branches that crossed the osteotomy at variable intervals.[10] It is evident that there are a number of structures to be concerned with on the medial aspect of the foot when performing a calcaneal osteotomy. On the lateral aspect, the Sural nerve and its branches are in the vicinity of the calcaneal displacement osteotomy. The approach of this procedure is through four small stab incisions placed away from neurovascular structures, and the tunnels that are made when performing this procedure are deep to the neurovascular structures that come into play when performing the osteotomy.

The plantar aspect of the foot is also of concern. The origin of musculature, ligaments, and nerves all are in very close proximity to the exit site of the saw when performing this osteotomy. It is of the utmost importance to not violate these structures when exiting the plantar cortex whether performing the procedure open or percutaneously.

19.5 Procedure

The patient should be placed on the operating table in the supine position. Using a marking pen, mark out the four stab incision sites. Two on the lateral aspect of the heel, and two on the medial aspect of the heel. Palpate the plantar medial calcaneal tubercle, make a small mark along the lines of the proposed ostetomy approximately 5 mm distal to the tubercle. Palpate the posterior, superior aspect of the calcaneus medially. Make a skin mark following the skin lines posterior to the Posterior tibial nerve and anterior to the Achilles tendon. Direct your attention to the lateral aspect of the foot. Make the inferior mark along the lines of the proposed osteotomy and parallel with the medial inferior incision approximately 5 mm distal to the plantar lateral tubercle. Palpate the posterior superior aspect of the calcaneus laterally. Make a skin mark here following the skin lines. This mark is posterior to the course of the sural nerve and peroneal tendons, and anterior to the Achilles tendon (Fig. 19.1).

The first stab incision is made at the inferior medial calcaneal mark. Make a stab incision along the lines of the proposed osteotomy full thickness. Using a curved hemostat, bluntly deepen the incision down to the calcaneus. Next, with the curved end pointing toward the skin, create a tunnel toward the superior incision making sure that the tip of the hemostat is directly over the calcaneus as this blunt dissection is performed. The tunnel is made deep to the neurovascular structures. It is important to keep the tip of the hemostats against the calcaneus while tunneling superiorly. Once the superior medial landmark is reached, tent the skin and make a stab incision with in the resting skin line. The tip of the curved hemostat is then exited out the incision site. This is the site that the gigli saw will be introduced. Open the tip of the hemostat and clamp a 12 in. flexible gigli saw. Pull the hemostats inferiorly through the tunnel, and through the inferior incision. One loop of the gigli saw is now exiting the medial inferior incision. Unclamp the hemostat from the end of the gigli saw (Fig. 19.2).

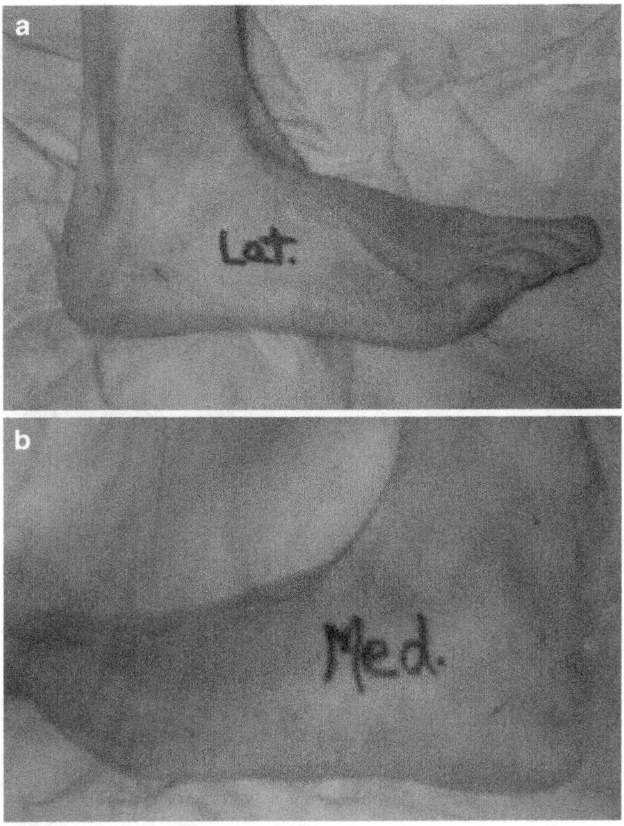

Fig.19. 1 (**a**) A lateral view of the foot with stab incisions for a percutaneous calcaneal displacement osteotomy marked. (**b**) A medial view of the foot with the stab incisions for the percutaneous calcaneal displacement osteotomy marked

Redirect your attention back to the superior medial incision. Using the straight hemostat bluntly tunnel across the superior aspect of the calcaneus. This tunnel is made anterior to the Achilles tendon and posterior to the posterior facet of the calcaneus in Kagers's triangle. Be sure to keep the hemostat on the superior aspect of the calcaneus while tunneling across. Tent the skin at the lateral superior skin mark and make a stab incision within the resting skin line. Remove the hemostat from the foot. Enter the straight hemostat through the superior lateral incision, follow the tunnel just made and exit the superior medial incision. Open the tips of the hemostat and place the free end of the gigli saw into the tip. Clamp down and pull the hemostat back through the tunnel. Exit the superior lateral incision pulling the end of the gigli saw through the incision (Fig. 19.3). Unclamp the hemostat.

Make the fourth stab incision at the lateral inferior incision mark along the lines of the proposed osteotomy. Bluntly deepen this incision down to the calcaneal body. Once again make a tunnel superiorly toward the superior incision being sure to keep the tip of the hemostat against the body of the calcaneus. This tunnel is deep to the neurovascular structures. Exit the superior incision on the lateral aspect and open the tip of the hemostat. Insert the loop of the gigli saw into the tip of the curved hemostat. Pull the hemostat back through the tunnel out the lateral inferior incision. Release the hemostat. Hook the gigli saw handles to the loops of the gigli saw on the medial and lateral aspects of the foot. Pull the gigli saw taught being sure not to kink the saw and to have equal amounts of the gigli saw

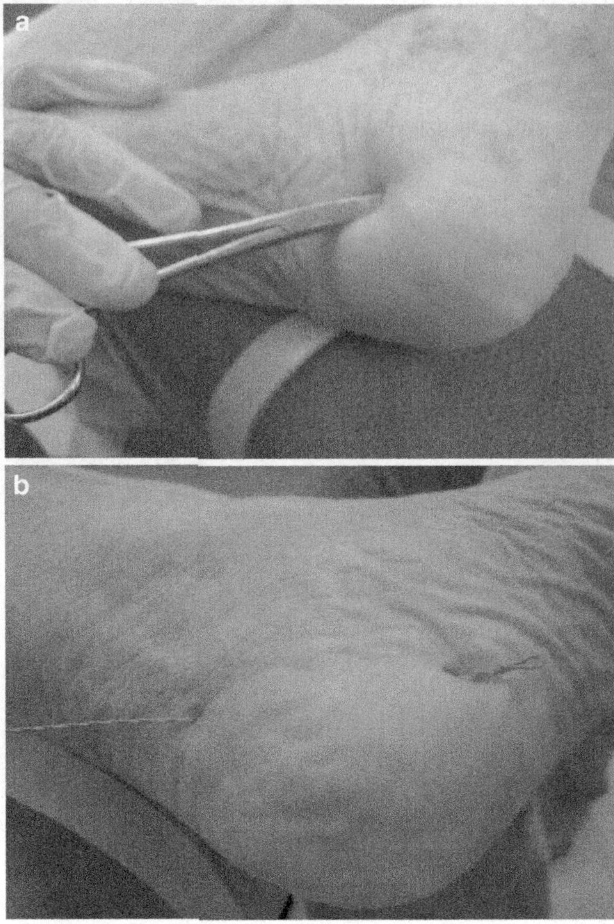

Fig.19. 2 (**a**) The first stab incision is made and deepened on the medial side down to the calcaneus to perform the medial tunnel for the gigli saw. (**b**) The gigli saw in place in the medialt unnel

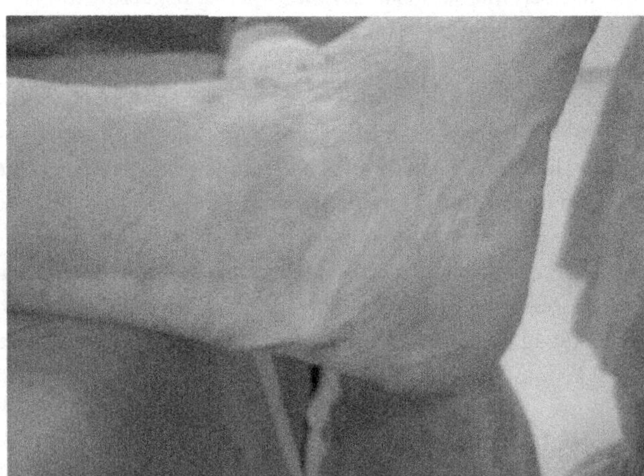

Fig.19. 3 Thes traight hemostat creates a tunnel in Kager's triangle and tents the skin before the superior laterals tabi ncisioni sm ade

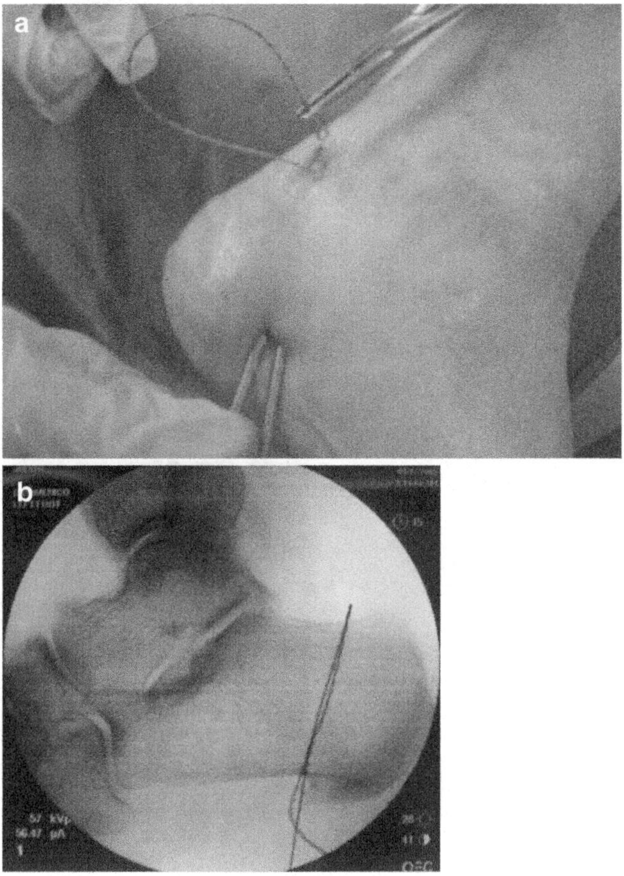

Fig. 19.4 (**a**) Lateral aspect of the foot, using the curved hemostat to grip the gigli saw and pull through the lateral tunnel. (**b**)La teral view of the foot with fluoroscopy to view the placement of the gigli saw before performing the osteotomy

exiting each inferior incision. The gigli saw should now be taut to the calcaneus, deep to all neurovascular structures, across the superior aspect and along the medial and lateral body of the calcaneus (Fig. 19.4).

Using a mini fluoroscopy unit, take a lateral view of the foot. This will ensure proper placement of the saw. Check to be sure there are no kinks in the saw and that the saw is in the desired placement. It is now time to perform the osteotomy. The placement of the incisions ensures that the osteotomy is performed in the proper plane, which should be inclined posteriorly at 45° to the plantar surface of the rear foot.[4] Grip the gigli saw handles and perform the osteotomy. Your assistant needs stabilize the lower leg, dorsiflex the foot, to tighten the plantar fascia, and Achilles tendon to lock the osteotomy in place.via dynamic stabilization. As the saw advances through the calcaneus the surgeon should widen his/ her arms to avoid harming the skin as the cut is made. As the surgeon advances toward the plantar aspect of the calcaneus extreme care should be taken to not exit the calcaneus forcefully and violate the vital plantar structures. If necessary another lateral view can be taken as the plantar cortex is approached. Once the osteotomy is completed cut one end of the gigli saw to the incision line. Pull the opposite end of the saw out of the foot (Fig. 19.5).

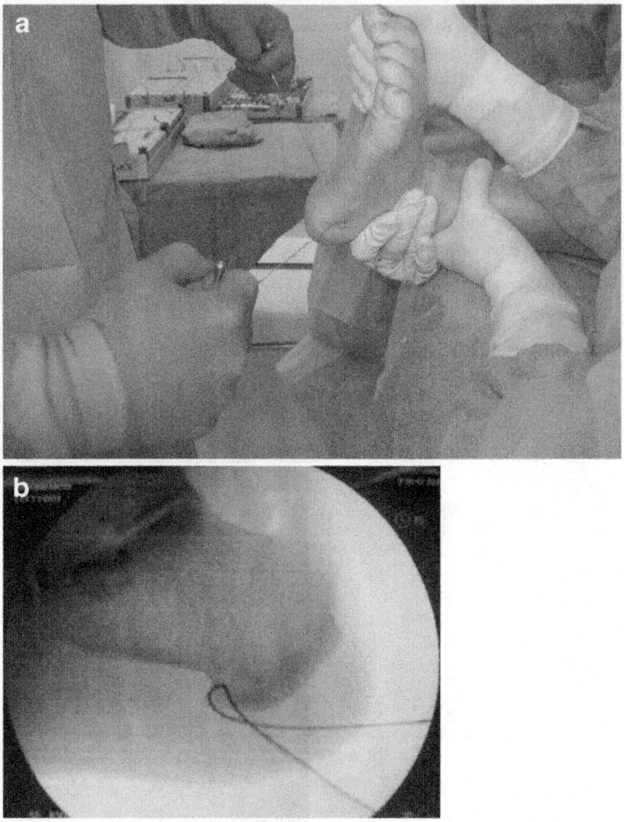

Fig.19.5 (**a**) Performing the percutaneous calcaneal displacement osteotomy, note the surgeons arms are spread to not harm the skin of the inferior incisions with the gigli saw. (**b**)A fluoroscopic view of the foot aftert heos teotomyi sm ade

Now displace the free posterior calcaneus to the desired plane of correction. As you displace the osteotomy your assistant should plantarflex the foot. This will loosen the plantar fascia, and Achilles tendon to allow one to manipulate the posterior aspect of the calcaneus into the desired position with very little resistance. Once in desired position dorsiflex the foot to tighten the plantar fascia, and Achilles tendon to lock the osteotomy in place via dynamic stabilization. Next drive two guide wires perpendicular to the osteotomy site, from the large cannulated cancellous screw set, through the plantar posterior aspect of the foot. Using fluoroscopy check the wire placement with a lateral, calcaneal axial and anteriorposterior view. The surgeon should try to purchase the sub cortical bone just inferior to the posterior calcaneal facet. This bone allows for strong screw purchase. Once the desired placement is achieved make two stab incisions at the entrance site of the wires. Deepen the incisions down to the calcaneus. Measure and drive two cannulated cancellous screws. Once again check the screw position with fluoroscopy using lateral, calcaneal axial and anteriorposterior views (Fig. 19.6). It is very important not to violate the posterior facet of the calcaneus. Close all incisions.

Postoperative management is 2 weeks in a below the knee posterior splint non–weight bearing. Ancillary procedures will dictate the course of postoperative management. If the osteotomy was performed as an isolated procedure, the first postoperative visit the patient can be placed in a cast boot, partial weight–bearing, for 4 more weeks. Physical therapy is recommended after 6 weeks to strengthen the musculature.

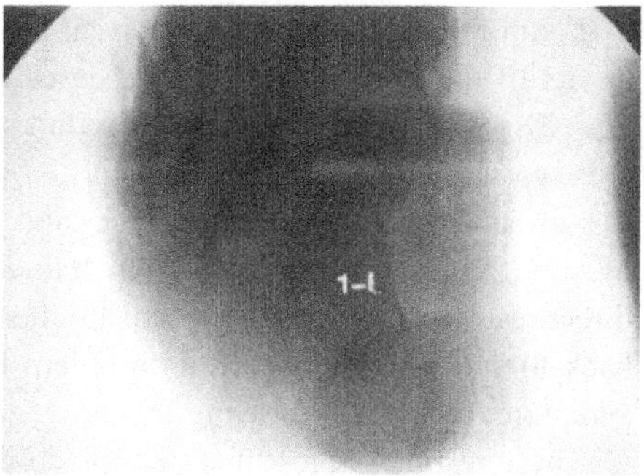

Fig.19.6 Aninte roperativefl uoroscopic view of the foot with the posterior aspect of the calcaneus in the desired position after the osteotomyis pe rformed

19.6 Pitfallsand B ailouts

Intraoperative complications while performing this procedure are few. If the gigli saw used is not flexible enough the surgeon may encounter kinks in the saw. We recommend the use of the Depuy 12 in. gigli saw due to it's flexibility. It is also recommended to have a ¼ inch straight osteotome present. This can be used to pry the osteotomy apart and/or complete the osteotomy if any difficulties are encountered when trying to manipulate the posterior aspect of the osteotomy.

For the surgeon who is not experienced in this particular procedure two guide wires can be placed in the calcaneus as an osteotomy guide. This is not necessary but can be helpful in guiding the surgeon through the osteotomy. The guide wires are placed along the lines of the desired osteotomy.

If the assistant is not holding the leg and foot very stable, it is possible the gigli saw can get stuck in the bone partially through the osteotomy. If this occurs, cut one end of the gigli saw close to the skin and pull out the other end. At this time use the same incisions and insert a new gigi saw within the tunnels. Be sure to have the assistant dorsiflex the toes/foot and stabilize the leg very well.

To date the percutaneous calcaneal displacement osteotomy has not encountered much difficulty in which an open procedure was needed. If any problem should occur, this can easily be converted to an open procedure by connecting the lateral incisions to produce the traditional incision for the open calcaneal displacement osteotomy.

19.7 Outcomes

In the evaluation of over 100 percutaneous calcaneal displacement osteotomies one of the most prevalent complication encountered with the technique was painful fixation. In the patients who encountered this complication all of them had the fixation removed and all of the patients' pain associated with the fixation were relieved.

Four of the patients that underwent the procedure had neuritis complaints on the lateral aspect of the foot. In all of these cases these were transient symptoms that resolved in 10–12 weeks time. Ancillary procedures were performed with the osteotomy on all of these patients. Our theory is that neuritis symptoms may be due to the ancillary procedures, in particular the gastrocnemius recession, or post–operative swelling. There was one case of skin irritation in a patient in which there was a prominent lateral shelf of calcaneus as a direct result of the osteotomy causing the skin irritation. This patient was revised by taken back to surgery to correct this problem by resecting the prominent bone. The patient's symptoms resolved following this procedure.

These results suggest that the low complication rate indicates that this procedure is an effective alternative to the traditional open calcaneal displacement osteotomy.

A cadaver lab was performed by the authors in which the osteotomy was performed on five specimens (Fig. 19.7). The neurovascular structures were dissected out on all of the specimens after performance of the osteotomy. There was no evidence of neurovascular injury to any of the specimens.

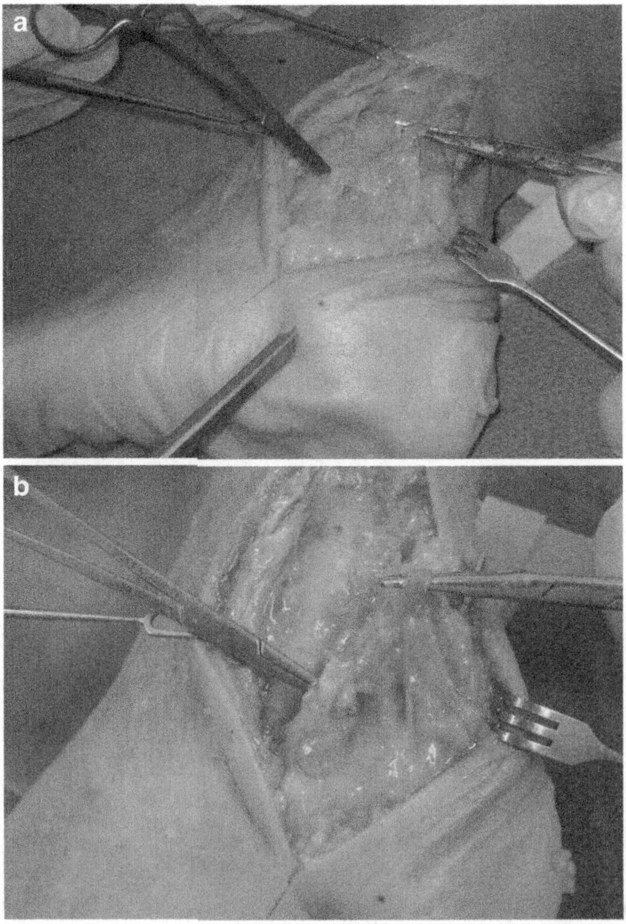

Fig.19.7 Ac adaveric study was performed to view the medial and lateral neurovascular structures following the percutaneous calcaneal displacement osteotomy. Note the intact neuro–vasculars tructures

To date no study has been performed on biomechanical outcome or pain relief after the performance of the percutaneous calcaneal displacement osteotomy. The literature is full of good results of posterior displacement osteotomies. This osteotomy parallels the correction of the open posterior displacement osteotomy and yields the same outcomes as far as biomechanical correction and pain relief (Figs. 19.8 and 19.9).

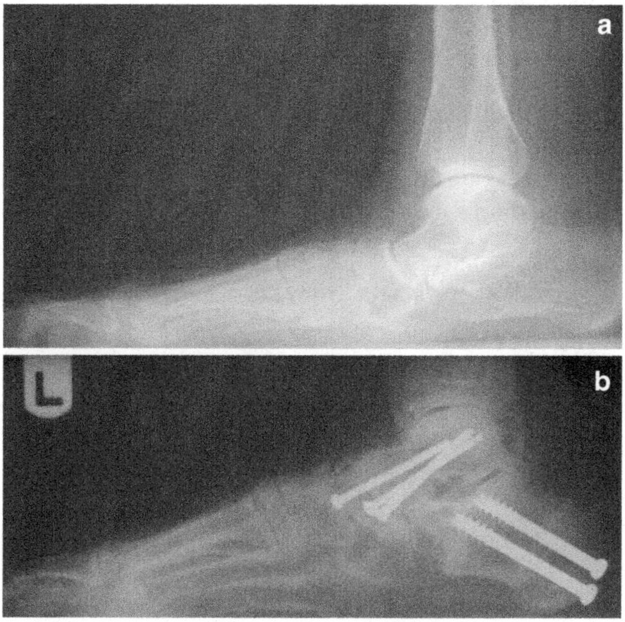

Fig.19.8 (**a**) Pre operative percutaneous calcaneal displacement osteotomy. (**b**) Post operative percutaneous calcanealos teotomy

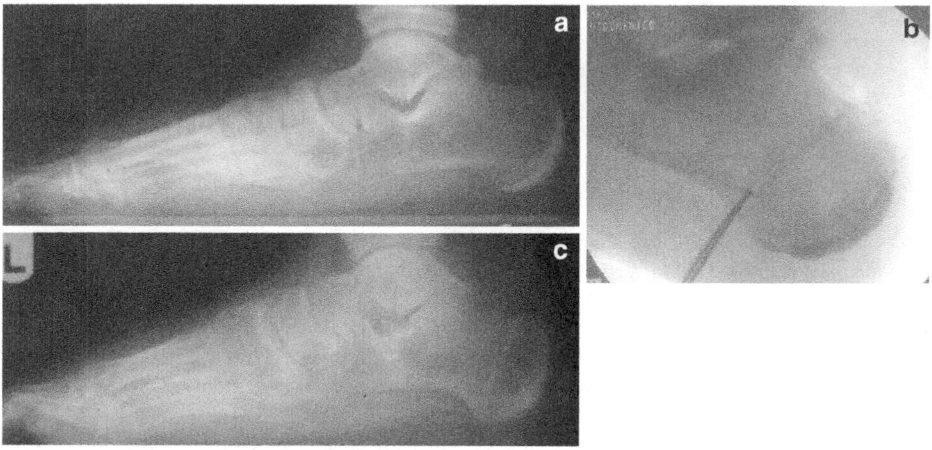

Fig. 19.9 (**a**) Pre operative lateral radiograph of a pediatric flatfoot deformity (**b**) Intraoperative lateral view demonstrating a Percutaneous Calcaneal Displacement Osteotomy utilizing a gigli saw (**c**) Post operative lateral view Percutaneous Displacement Calcaneal Osteotomy

19.8 Summary

Calcaneal osteotomies have and will remain a vital part in the surgical treatment of compound hind foot deformities. The percutaneous calcaneal displacement osteotomy is a very effective way of reducing hind foot deformities and avoiding post–operative complications.

Indications:

- Hind foot valgus
- Posterior Tibial Tendon Dysfunction
- Hind foot Varus
- Lateral ankle instability
- Status post calcaneal fracture

Complications:

- Infection
- Painful fixation
- Neuritis
- Prominent bone on side that posterior calcaneus is displaced

References

1. Mahan KT, Flanigan PK. Pathologic pes valgus disorders. In: Banks AS, Downey MS, Martin DE, Miller SJ, eds. *McGlamry's Comprehensive Textbook of Foot and Ankle Surgery*. Philadelphia, PA: Lippincott Williams and Wilkins; 2001:799–899
2. Koutsogiannis E. Treatment of mobile flat foot by displacement osteotomy of the calcaneus. *J Bone Joint Surg*.1971; 53B:96–100.
3. Steven WB. Medial slide calcaneal osteotomy technique, patient selection, and results. *Foot Ankle Clin*.2001 ;6:89–94.
4. Trnka H–J, Easley ME, Myerson MS. The role of calcaneal osteotomies for correction of adult flatfoot. *Clin Orthop Relat Res*.1999; 1:50–64.
5. Mann RA. Flatfoot in adults. In: Coughlin MJ, Mann RA, eds. *Surgery of the Foot and Ankle*. St Louis, MO: Mosby; 1999:733–767.
6. Mann RA, Guyton GP. Medial displacement osteotomy of the calcaneus and flexor digitorum longus transfer. In: Kitaoka HB, ed. *The Foot and Ankle*. Philadelphia, PA: Lippincott Williams and Wilkins; 2002:369–385.
7. Mendicino RW, Catanzariti AR, Reeves CL. Posterior calcaneal displacement osteotomy: a new percutaneous technique. *J Foot Ankle Surg*.2004; 43:332–335.
8. Dull JM, DiDomenico L. Percutaneous displacement calcaneal osteotomy. *J Foot Ankle Surg*. 2004;43:336–337.
9. Frankel J, Turf RM, Nichols D. Complications of calcaneal osteotomies. *Clin Podiatric Med Surg*.1991;8:409–423.
10. David GL, Michael TC, Dirk GS, Stanley GC. Anatomic study of the medial neurovascular structures in relation to calcaneal osteotomy. *Foot Ankle Int*.2001; 22:569–571.

11. David PM, Roya M. Posterior calcaneal displacement osteotomy with lateral wall reduction. *J Foot Ankle Surg.*2002; 41:135–137.
12. Andermahr J, Helling H, Rehm KE, Koebke Z. The vascularization of the os calcaneum and the clinical consequences. *Clin Orthop Relat Res.*1999; 363:212–218.
13. D'Souza NA, Kinchelow T, Lin S. Posterior tibial tendon dysfunction: tendon transfers, osteotomies, and lateral column lengthening. *Curr Opin Orthop.*2002; 13:81–88.
14. Guyton GP, Jeng C, Kreiger LE, Mann RA. Flexor digitorum longus transfer and medial displacement calcaneal osteotomy for posterior tibial tendon dysfunction: a middle term clinical follow–up. *Foot and Ankle Int.*2001; 22:627–636.
15. Lawrence SJ, Wright RD. Posterior tibial tendon dysfunction: current concepts including operative and nonoperative approaches. *Curr Opin Orthop.*2004; 15:62–68.
16. Pomeroy GC, Pike HR, Beals TC, Manoli A. Acquired flatfoot in adults due to posterior tibial tendon. *J Bone Joint Surg.*1999; 81–A:1173–1182.
17. Kohls–Galzoulis J, Angel JC, Singh D, Haddad F, Livingstone J, Berry G. Tibialis posterior dysfunction: a common and treatable cause of adult acquired flatfoot. *Brit Med J.* 2004;329: 1328–1333.
18. Murphy AG. Pes planus. In: Canale ST, ed. *Campbell's Operative Orthopedics.* St Louis, MO: Mosby;2003:4017–4045.
19. Giannini S, Ceccarelli F, Benedetti MG, Catani F, Faldini C. Surgical treatment of flexible flatfoot in children: a four year follow–up study. *J Bone Joint Surg.*2001; 83–A:73–79.
20. Torosian CM, Dias LS. Surgical treatment of severe hindfoot valgus by medial displacement osteotomy of the os calcis in children with myelomeningocele. *J Pediatr Orthop.* 2000;20: 226–229.
21. Buerk AA, Albert MC. Advances in pediatric foot and ankle treatment. *Curr Opin Orthop.* 2001;12:437–442.
22. Hansen ST. Atlas of standard operative techniques. In: Hurley R, ed. *Functional Reconstruction of the Foot and Ankle.* Philadelphia, PA: Lippincott Williams and Wilkins; 2000:283–512.
23. Johnson KA, Strom DE. Tibialis posterior tendon dysfunction. *Clin Orthop.* 1989;39: 196–206.
24. Marks R. Medial displacement calcaneal osteotomy with flexor digitorum longus tendon substitution for Stage II posterior tibial tendon insufficiency. *Techn Foot Ankle Surg.* 2003;2:222–231.
25. Johnson KA. Tibialis posterior tendon rupture. *Clin Orthop.*1983; 177:140.
26. Fayazi AH, Nguyen H–V, Juliano PJ. Intermediate term follow–up of calcaneal osteotomy and flexor digitorum longus transfer for treatment of posterior tibial tendon dysfunction. *Foot Ankle Int.*2002;23: 1107–1111.
27. Wacker JT, Hennessey MS, Saxby TS. Calcaneal osteotomy and transfer of the tendon of flexor digitorum longus for Stage–II dysfunction of the tibialis posterior. Three to five year results. *J Bone Joint Surg Br.*2002; 84:54–58.
28. Myerson MS, Corrigan J. Treatment of posterior tibial tendon dysfunction with flexor digitorum longus tendon transfer and calcaneal osteotomy. *Orthopaedics.*1996; 19:383.
29. Myerson MS, Corrigan J, Thompson F. Tendon transfer with calcaneal osteotomy for treatment of posterior tibial tendon insufficiency: a radiological investigation. *Foot Ankle Int.* 1996;16:383.
30. MyersonM S.A dulta cquiredfl atfoot deformity. *J Bone Joint Surg.*1996; 78A:780.
31. Sammarco GJ, Hockenbury T. Treatment of Stage II posterior tibial tendon dysfunction with flexor hallucis longus transfer and medial displacement calcaneal osteotomy. *Foot Ankle Int.* 2001;22:305.
32. Mizel MS, Hecht PJ, Marymont JV, Temple TH. Evaluation and treatment of chronic ankle pain. *J Bone Joint Surg.*2004; 622–632.
33. Mosier SM, Pomeroy G, Monoli A. Pathoanatomy and etiology of posterior tibial tendon dysfunction. *Clin Orthop Relat Res.*1999; 365:12–22.

34. MoscaV S.Th ec avusf oot. *J Pediatr Orthop.*2001; 21:423–424.
35. Paulos L, Coleman S, Samuelson K. Pes cavovarus: review of a surgical approach using selective soft–tissue procedures. *J Bone Joint Surg (Am).*1980; 62:942–953.
36. Watkins L. Radiology and imaging. In: *Pocket Podiatrics*,pp227–242.
37. Felton G, Yale I. Congenital pes planus. In: *Clinical Foot Roentgenology*. Baltimore, MD: The Williams & Wilkins Company; 1966:209–214.
38. Anderson R, Davis W. Management of the adult flatfoot deformity. In: Myerson MS, ed. *Foot and Ankle Disorders.* Philadelphia, PA: W.B. Saunders Company; 2000:1017–1039.
39. Smith R, Sima WF, Reischl S. Can we meaningfully measure the flatfoot? A multi–examiner comparison of radiographic arch structure measurements. Presented at: The American Foot and Ankle Society Meeting; July 22–25, 1993; Asheville, NC.
40. Saltzman CL, El–Khoury GY. The hindfoot alignment view. *Foot Ankle Int.* 1995;6:572–575.
41. PaleyD . *Principles of Deformity Correction.*N ewY ork,N Y:S pringer;2002: 46

Tendoscopy of the Flexor Hallucis Longus Tendon

20

Tun Hing Lui

20.1 Introduction

The tendon of flexor hallucis longus (FHL) can present several pathologies along its course, including rupture, laceration, longitudinal tears, stenosing tenosynovitis and pigmented villonodular synovitis. The flexor hallucis longus is a bipennate muscle which extends to the posterior part of the ankle. The tendon of FHL courses from the fibro-osseous tunnel posterior to the talus and passes into the fibrocartilaginous tunnel under the sustentaculum tali. The tendon is connected to the flexor digitorum longus tendon at the master knot of Henry. Distal to the master knot of Henry, the FHL tendon passes into the fibro-osseous tunnel between the sesamoid bones and insert into the base of distal phalanx of the hallux. Most of the course of the FHL tendon is deep and difficult to approach surgically. Surgical exploration of the tendon requires extensive soft tissue dissection. The course of the flexor hallucis longus tendon is divided into three zones. Zone 1 is located behind the ankle joint, from the musculotendinous junction to the orifice of the tunnel underneath the sustentaculum tali. Zone 2 is located from the tunnel underneath the sustentaculum tali to the knot of Henry. Zone 3 is located from the knot of Henry to the tendon insertion to the base of the distal phalanx of the hallux.[1] Zone 2 tendon sheath can be subdivided into proximal fibrous sheath (Zone 2A) and distal fascial sheath (Zone 2B)[2] (Fig. 20.1). Using a different endoscopic approach to the each zone of the FHL tendon, the course of the tendon can be examined arthroscopically from the musculotendinous junction to its insertion.

T.H.Lui
Department of Orthopaedics and Traumatology, North District Hospital,
9 Po Kin Road, Sheung Shui, NT Hong Kong SAR, China
e-mail:luithde rek@yahoo.co.uk

N. Maffulli and M. Easley (eds.), *Minimally Invasive Surgery of the Foot and Ankle*,
DOI: 10.1007/978-1-84996-417-3_20,

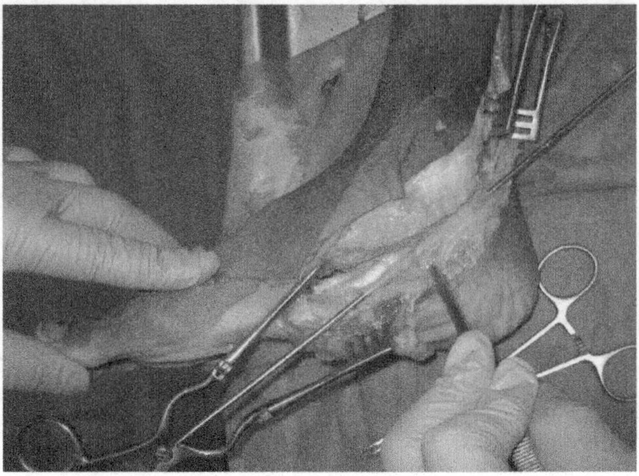

Fig. 20.1 Therodre present the portal tract of zone 2 FHL tendoscopy with proximal fibrous (**a**)t endon sheath and distal fascial (**b**)te ndons heath

20.2 Descriptionof Technique

The patient is prone with a pneumatic thigh tourniquet applied to the operated side. We use a 4.0 mm 30° arthroscope, a switching stick, an arthroscopic shaver and arthroscopic scissors.

van Dijk CN described an endoscopic approach to deal with posterior ankle pathology.[3] The FHL tendon pathology that is posterior to the ankle (Zone 1) e.g., stenosing tenosynovitis at the fibro-osseous tunnel of the talus, can be managed by posterior ankle endoscopy. The posteromedial portal is established at the intersection between the medial margin of the Achilles tendon and a line joining the sustentaculum tali and the inferior border of the medial cuneiform and first metatarsal (Fig. 20.2).

The posterolateral portal is lateral to the Achilles tendon and just above the posterosuperior calcaneal tubercle. A 4.0 mm 30° arthroscope is introduced into the posterolateral

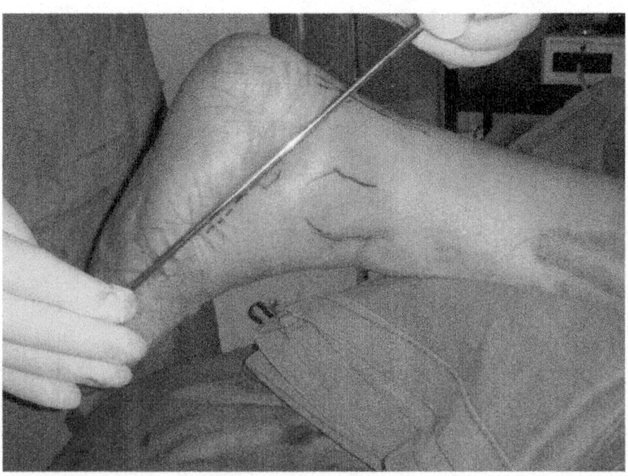

Fig. 20.2 The rod marked the undersurfaces of first metatarsal, medial cuneiform and sustentaculum tali. It intersects the medial border of the Achilles tendon and passes through the posteromedialpor tal

portal. The fatty tissue overlying the FHL tendon is removed with an arthroscopic shaver through the posteromedial portal. The FHL tendon can then be examined from the musculotendinous junction down to the orifice of the fibrous tendon sheath underneath the sustentaculum tali.

Under arthroscopic visualization, a Wissenger rod is introduced to the tendon sheath underneath the sustentaculum tali and the plantar aponeurosis is penetrated distal to the level of the cuneiforms. The plantar portal is then made (Fig. 20.3).

The zone 2 FHL tendon can then be examined through the posteromedial and the plantar portals which can be interchanged between visualization and instrumentation portals.

The zone 3 FHL tendon is examined with the toe flexor tendoscopy.[4] A plantar toe portal is created with a transverse skin incision close to the insertion of the FHL tendon. The tendon sheath is opened and the arthroscopic cannula together with the trocar is introduced through the toe portal to the plantar portal. The FHL tendon can then be examined with a 2.7 mm 30° arthroscope from the knot of Henry to its insertion at the distal phalanx of the hallux.

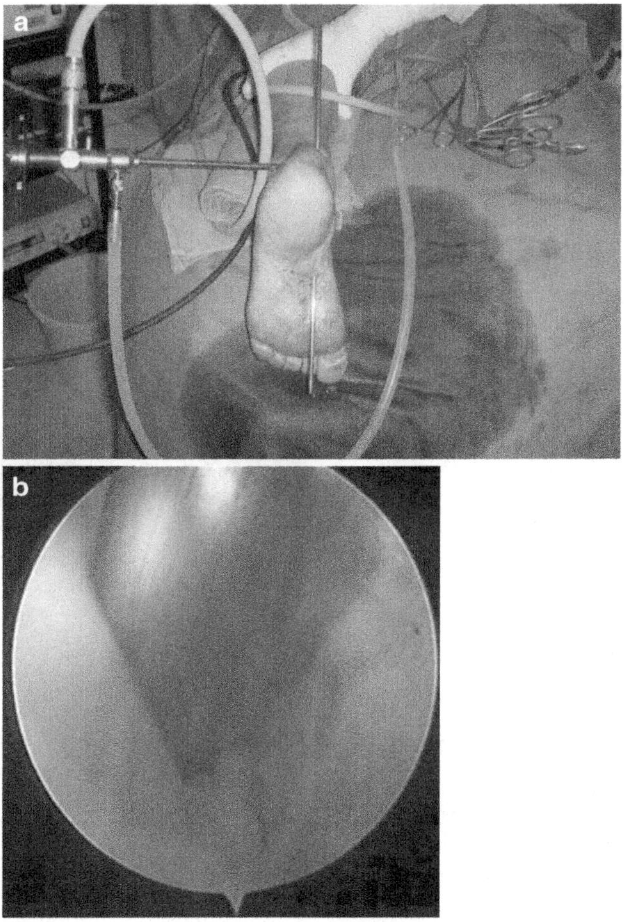

Fig. 20.3 The Wissenger rod is inserted into zone 2 FHL tendon sheath under arthroscopic guidance and exited at the plantar portal

20.3 Zone2 F HL Tendoscopy

Zone 2 FHL tendon sheath is a deep structure starting from the orifice of the zone 2A (fibrous) tendon sheath at the posterior ankle. The orifice is defined by the posterior talar tubercles and the ligament connecting the tubercles. Usually the posteromedial portal is the primary visualization portal and the plantar portal is the working portal. The Wissenger rod is inserted the zone 2 tendon sheath through the posteromedial portal. The cannula of the arthroscope is then introduced along the metal rod and exits through the plantar portal. The rod is exchanged with the arthroscope (Wissenger rod technique). The arthroscope is withdrawn from the plantar portal in a distal to proximal direction (Fig. 20.4).

As the arthroscope is withdrawn from the plantar portal, it will pass through the plantar aponeurosis, flexor digitorum brevis muscle, and then enter the Zone 2B (fascial) tendon sheath. The flexor digitorum longus tendon at the Knot of Henry is the first structure identifiable in the zone 2B tendon sheath. The flexor hallucis longus tendon at the proximal e nd of the Knot of Henry will be seen when the arthroscope is further withdrawn. Finally, the arthroscope will enter the Zone 2A (fibrous) tendon sheath which is underneath the sustentaculum tali.[2,5]

20.4 Application of Zone 2 Tendoscopy

1. *Endoscopic synovectomy*

Arthroscopic synovectomy (Fig. 20.5) in Zone 2A is a relatively safe procedure, since the tough fibrous tendon sheath is difficult to be perforated by the shaver and the medial plantar nerve is constantly at the plantar-medial side of the zone 2A tendon sheath.

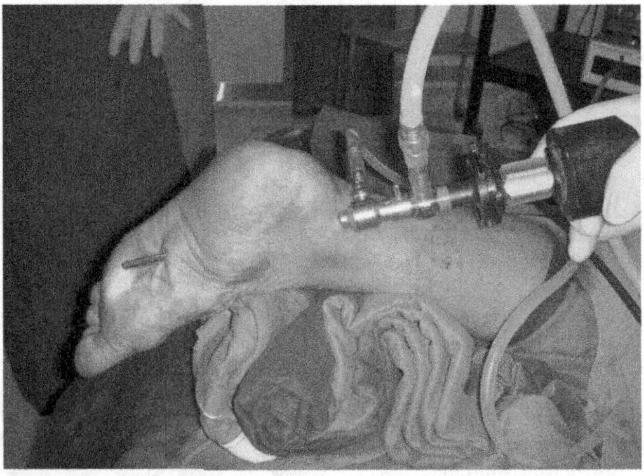

Fig.20. 4 TheFH L tendoscopy begins as the arthroscope is withdrawn fromt hepl antarpor tal

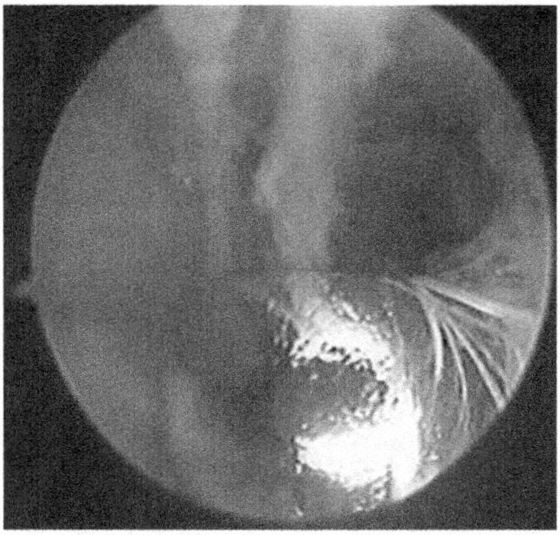

Fig.20.5 Synovitisofz one2F HLt endons heath

Arthroscopic synovectomy in the zone 2B can be risky because the zone 2B tendon sheath is a thin fibrous structure which can be easily perforated by the shaver. Also, the relationship of the medial plantar nerve to the zone 2B tendon sheath is variable and can be directly opposed to the sheath. Surgeons should pay particular attention during zone 2B synovectomy. The shaver opening should be kept towards the FHL tendon and suction should be kept to minimum in order to avoid damage of the medial plantar nerve.[2]

2. *Endoscopic FHL transfer*

It is indicated in patients with chronic Achilles tendon ruptures. The patient is prone with a pneumatic tourniquet applied to the thigh of the operated side. The posteromedial portal is established at the intersection point between the medial margin of the Achilles tendon and a line joining the sustentaculum tali and the inferior border of the medial cuneiform and first metatarsal. The posterolateral portal is located 1 cm anterior to the lateral margin of the Achilles tendon insertion. Posterior ankle endoscopy is then performed and the FHL tendon posterior to the ankle joint is identified. It is traced proximally towards the FHL muscle belly and the overlying fascia is released to facilitate the later tendon transfer. The opening of the zone 2A tendon sheath underneath the sustentaculum is identified, and a Wissenger rod introduced in the tendon sheath underneath the sustentaculum tali. The plantar fascia is penetrated distal to the cuneiform. The plantar portal is then made. The FHL tendon can then be examined through the posteromedial and the plantar portals. The tendon can be cut just proximal to the knot of Henry with the arthroscopic scissors (Fig. 20.6) and it is retrieved to the posteromedial portal. A stay stitch is applied to the free tendone nd(Fig. 20.7).

A 4.5 mm (6.0 mm if the FHL tendon graft is thick) bone tunnel is drilled at the posterior calcaneal tubercle through the posterolateral portal. The direction of drilling is from dorsolateral to plantar-medial (Fig. 20.8).

The medial exit point of the drill bit is then cut open. The free end of the FHL tendon is passed from the posteromedial portal wound to the distal wound and then through the bone tunnel to the posterolateral portal wound (Fig. 20.9).

It is then passed to the posteromedial portal wound again. The ankle is plantarflexed and the FHL tendon is tensioned and the stay stitches is sutured to the FHL tendon itself.

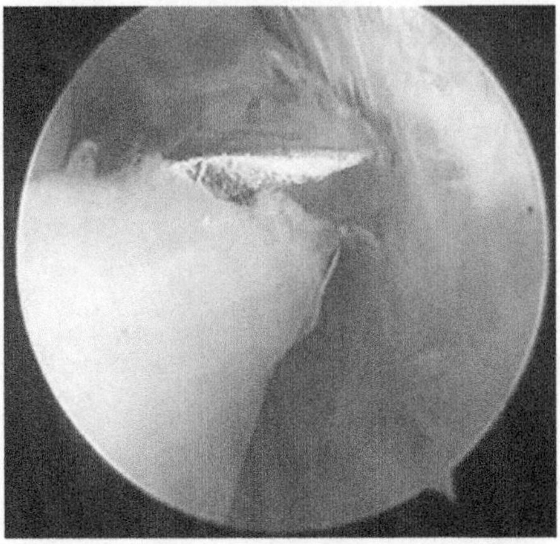

Fig. 20.6 The FHL tendon is cut with arthroscopics cissors

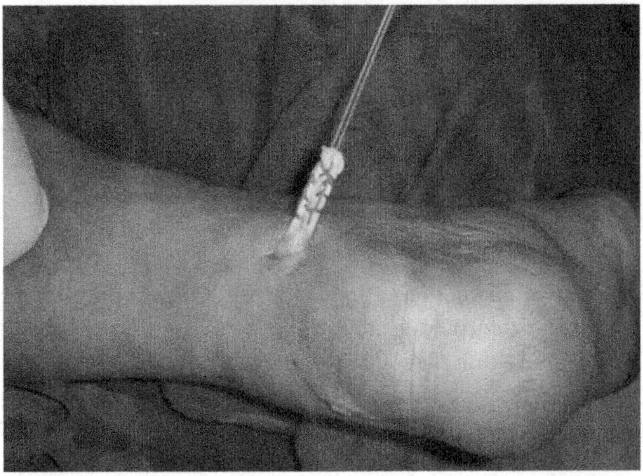

Fig. 20.7 The FHL tendon is retrieved from the posteromedial portal, and a stay stitch is applied to the freet endone nd

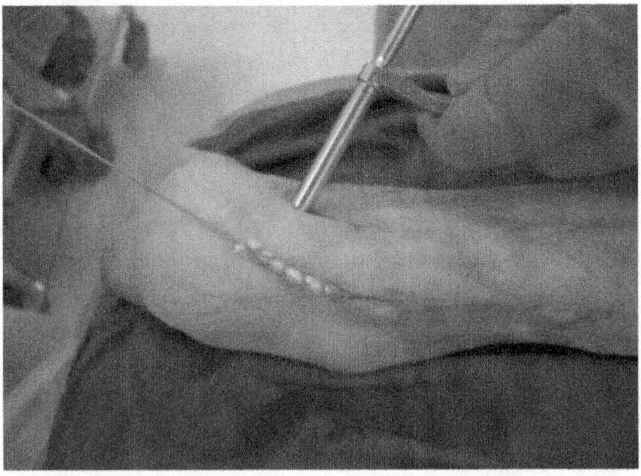

Fig. 20.8 A bone tunnel is drilled at the posterior calcanealt ubercle

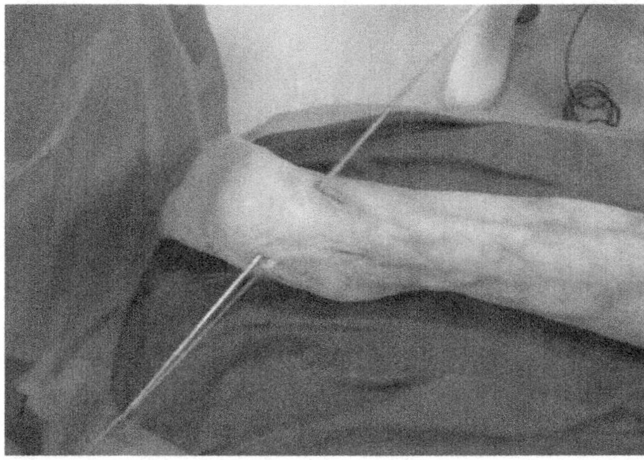

Fig.20.9 Thete ndonis passed from the distal medial wound to the posterolateral portal wound through the calcaneal bone tunnel

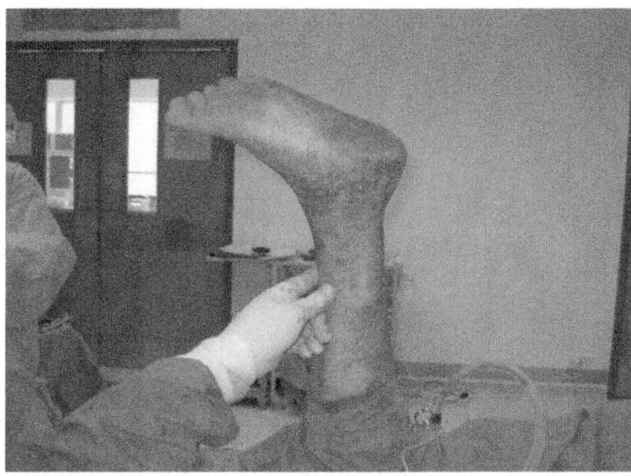

Fig.20.10 Thea nklere sumes the physiological plantarflexed position after thee ndoscopicFH Ltra nsfer

The distal stump of the Achilles tendon can be sutured to the FHL tendon at the posteromedial portal wound (Fig. 20.10).

The wounds are closed in a standard fashion, and a short leg cast in equinus is applied. The cast is kept for 6 weeks, and the patient is advised on non-weight-bearing walking during this period.[6]

3. *Excision of symptomatic talocalcaneal coalition*

The substentaculum tali and the plantar and posterior part of the talocalcaneal coalition can be removed with an arthroscopic burr during zone 2A FHL tendoscopy.[7] The anterior and dorsal part of the coalition can be removed with anterior subtalar arthroscopy.[8] Combination of both procedures will allow complete excision of symptomatic talocalcanealc oalition.

References

1. Lui TH. Flexor hallucis longus tendoscopy. *Knee Surgery, Sports Traumatology, Arthroscopy.* 2009;17:107–110.
2. Lui TH, Chan KB, Chan LK. Cadeveric study of Zone 2 flexor hallucis longus tendon sheath. *Arthroscopy.* Inpr ess.
3. van Dijk CN, Scholten PE, Krips R. A 2-portal endoscopic approach for diagnosis and treatment of posterior ankle pathology. *Arthroscopy.* 2000; 16:871–876.
4. Lui TH, Chow HT. Role of toe flexor tendoscopy in the management of an unusual cause of metatarsalgia. *Knee Surg Sports Traumatol Arthrosc.* 20 06;14:654–658.
5. Lui TH, Chan KB, Chan LK. Zone 2 flexor hallucis longus tendoscopy: an anatomic study. *Foot Ankle Int.* Inpr ess.
6. Lui TH. Endoscopic assisted flexor hallucis longus tendon transfer in management of chronic Achilles tendon rupture of Achilles tendon. *Knee Surg Sports Traumatol Arthrosc.* 2007;15:1163–1166.
7. Lui TH. Current concepts: foot and ankle arthroscopy and endoscopy: indications of new technique. *Arthroscopy.* 2007; 23:889–902.
8. Lui TH. Anterior subtalar (talocalcaneonavicular) arthroscopy. *Foot Ankle Int.* 2008;29:94–96.

Open Reduction and Internal Fixation of Calcaneal Fractures Through a Combined Medial and Lateral Approach Using a Small Incision Technique

21

Michael M. Romash

21.1 Introduction

Principles endure while technology advances. The evaluation and management of calcaneal fractures has evolved as new technology has been used to apply proven principles. Smaller incisions and the use of titanium locking plates designed for the limited incisions to accomplish ORIF of calcaneal fractures represent such an advance.

Ian McReynolds[13] described the principles which are now applied with newer technology.

21.2 TheF racture

Most fractures of the calcaneus occur as the heel is subjected to sudden axial loading.

The tuberosity, or point of plantar loading, is lateral to the axis of the tibia. This causes internal oblique stress across the posterior heel (Fig. 21.1). When failure of the bone occurs it does so along this line causing an oblique fracture. Burdeaux[5] was able to reproduce calcaneal fractures in this fashion (Fig. 21.2). When he inverted the foot and placed the tuberosity in line with the axis of the limb, he was unable to reproduce the fracture. The lack of oblique shear stress is implied by this more pure direct axial load.

The tuberosity translates laterally and proximally, and tilts into varus.

Simultaneously, the body of the talus impacts the posterior facet and drives the displacing portion of the articular surface downward into the body of the calcaneus. This sequence

M.M. Romash
Orthopedic Foot and Ankle Center of Hampton Roads, The Sports Medicine and Orthopedic Center, Chesapeake, VA, USA and
UnitedSe rvicesU niversityof H ealthSc iences, Bethesda, MD, USA

N. Maffulli and M. Easley (eds.), *Minimally Invasive Surgery of the Foot and Ankle*,
DOI: 10.1007/978-1-84996-417-3_21, © Springer-Verlag London Limited 2011

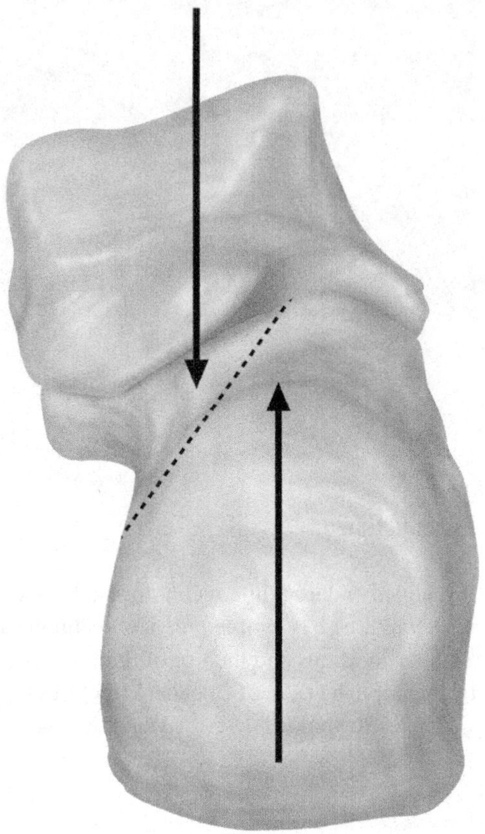

Fig. 21.1 Axial load causes internal oblique shear stress along plane of the primary fracturel ine

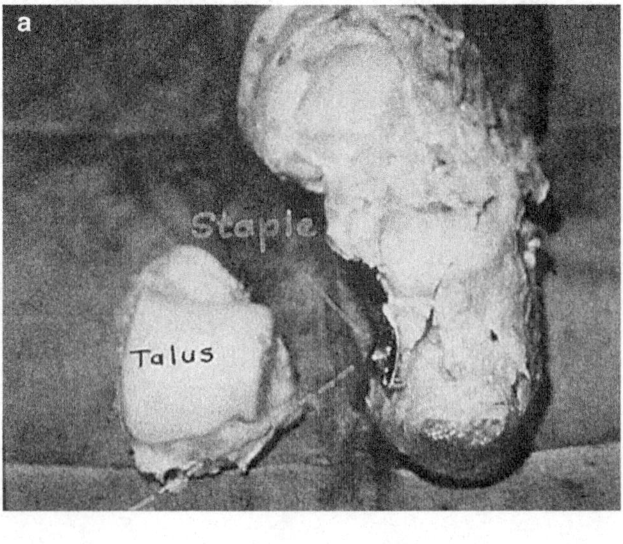

Fig. 21.2 Burdeaux'sc adaver fracture produced by axial load of the foot in neutral or slight eversion viewed from the posterior facet side (dorsal) and medial side of foot

Fig. 21.2 (continued)

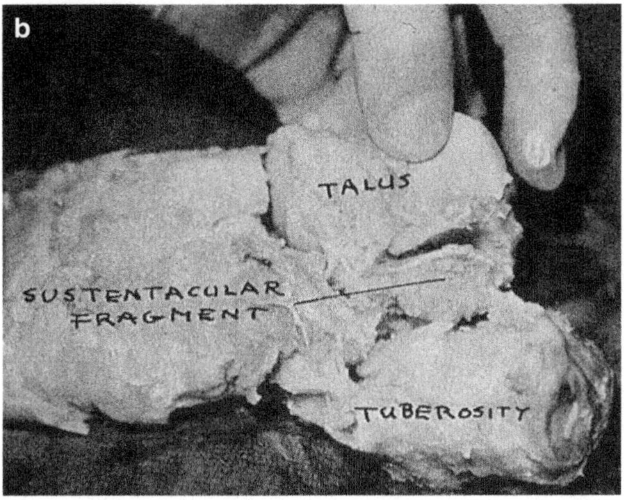

of events occurs in both a joint depression or tongue type pattern. The medial portion of the facet often remains in contact with the sustentaculum tali, and remains in anatomical position relative to the talus (Fig. 21.3). Palmer[15] described this in 1948, and his diagrams are as clear as present day CT studies (Fig. 21.41)

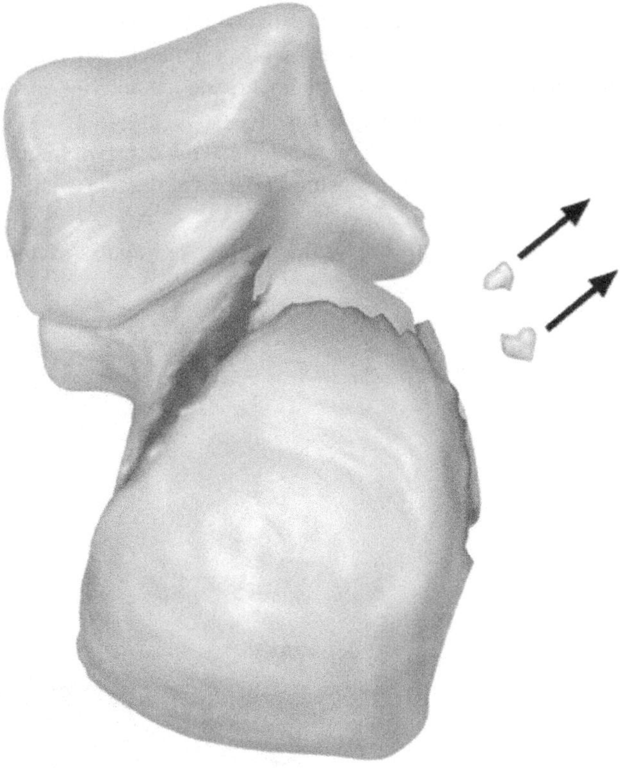

Fig.21. 3 Displacementof fracturefra gments

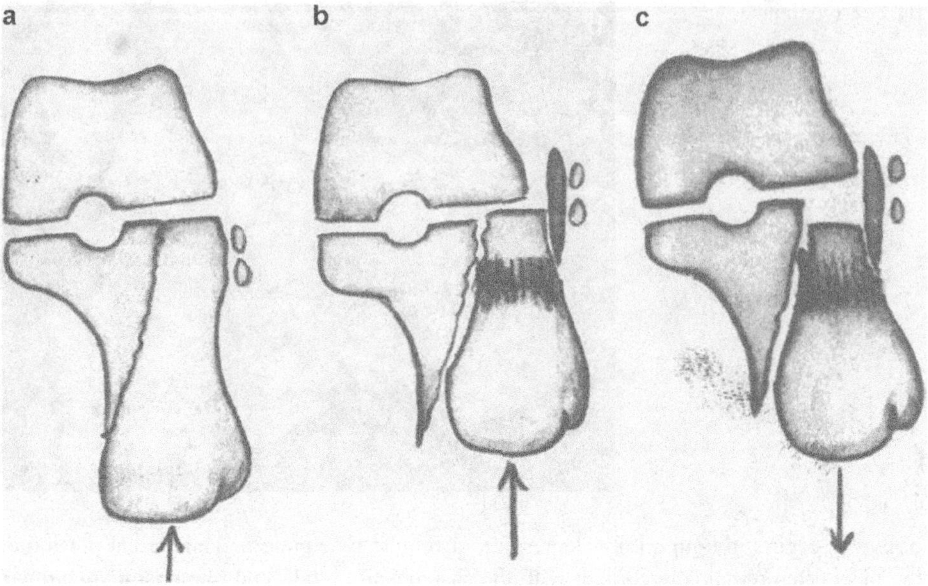

Fig.21.4 Palmersdia grams

The anterior aspect of the body of the talus impacts the calcaneus at the angle of Gissane causing a fracture that separates the anterior calcaneus from the body (Fig. 21.5).

This produces four major fracture fragments: the tuberosity, the posterior lateral facet fragment, the sustentacular fragment, and the anterior lateral fragment. Further comminution of the fragments may occur.

The sustentacular fragment is termed the constant fragment as it is usually the one fragment that is in anatomic position relative to the talus. The other fragments will be reduced to this fragment.

Sanders[18] classified these fractures according to the comminution of the posterior facet fragments.

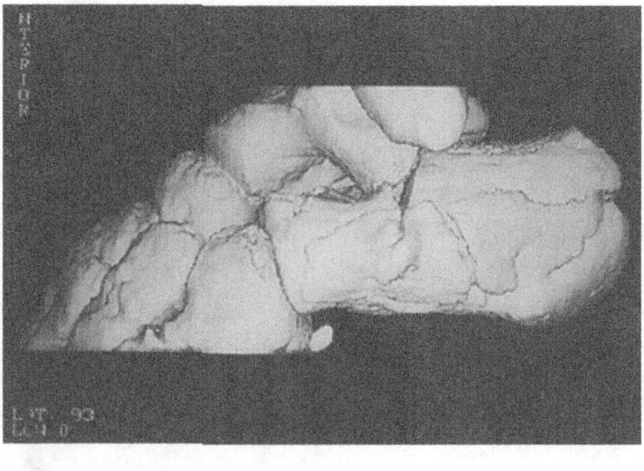

Fig.21.5 3DC T demonstrating antero lateral fragment

21.3 PastMe dicalHi story

Diabetes, smoking or a history of peripheral vascular disease increase the risk of surgical treatment and must be evaluated on a patient to patient basis.

21.4 PhysicalE xamination

The foot is swollen and often bruised. The heel may be widened and shortened. Fracture blisters may occur in the first 24–48 h (Fig. 21.6). Tenting of skin medially or posteriorly by a protruding spike of bone can produce skin necrosis. Neurapraxia of the medial or lateral plantar nerves can be present. Compartment syndrome may occur in the plantar spaces of the foot, producing painful limited motion of the toes.

21.5 RadiographicE valuation

Antero-posterior and lateral views of the foot, axial view of the heel, and Brodens views of the subtalar joint are taken. A lateral view of the uninjured foot for comparison can be helpful. An injury that masquerades as a "non" or "minimally" displaced fracture can be unmasked and identified as a significantly displaced fracture when Bohlers[2,3] angles can be compared.

The antero-posterior view of the foot shows the calcaneo-cuboid joint and the anterior aspect of the calcaneus (Fig. 21.7). The lateral foot view shows the loss of the height of the heel and loss of the congruity of the subtalar joint (Fig. 21.8). Measurement of Bohlers angle allows quantification of this change. It also demonstrates a joint depression or tongue type fracture pattern. The fracture at the angle of Gissane is discernible.

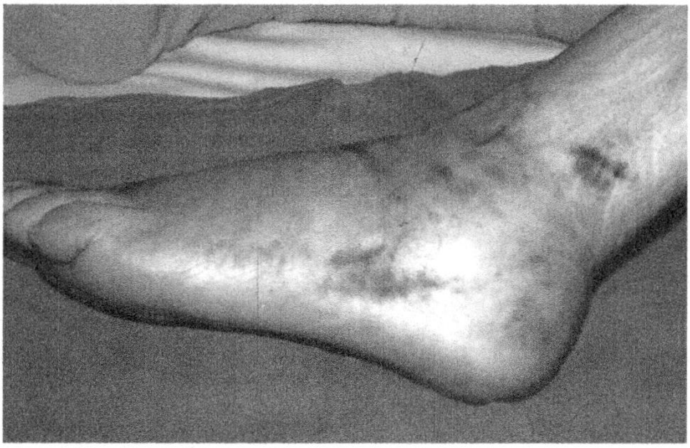

Fig.21.6 Blisterre mnants

Fig.21.7 Antero-posteriorvi ew demonstrating calcaneo cuboid involvement in primary fracture of anterol ateralf ragment

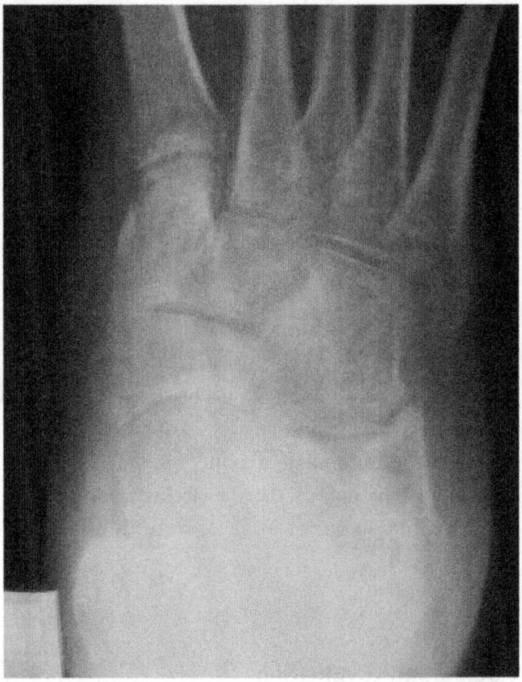

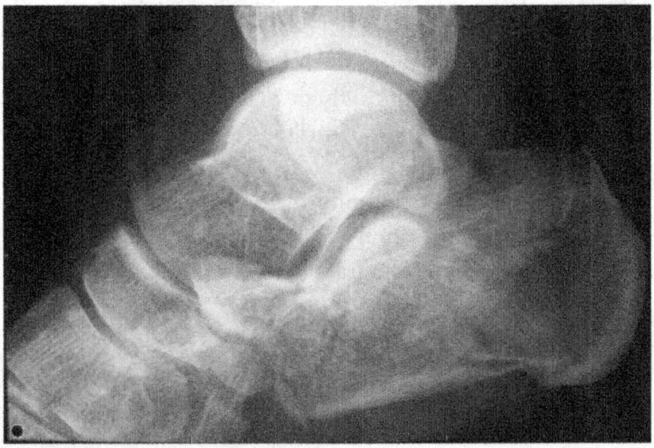

Fig.21.8 Lateralra diograph

The axial heel view demonstrates the oblique fracture line and displacement of the tuberosity(Fig. 21.9).

Brodens[1,4,5] view shows the disruption of the subtalar joint, the oblique fracture, and translation of the tuberosity (Fig. 21.10).

CT scans should be made, and high quality reconstructions in the axial, sagittal and semi-coronal views should be obtained to provide crucial information of the internal architecture of the fracture (Fig. 21.11a–c).

Three dimensional volumetric reconstructions of the heel provide a striking visual representation of the fracture, and prepare the surgeon to handle the surfaces that will be exposed(Fig. 21.12a–c).[7]

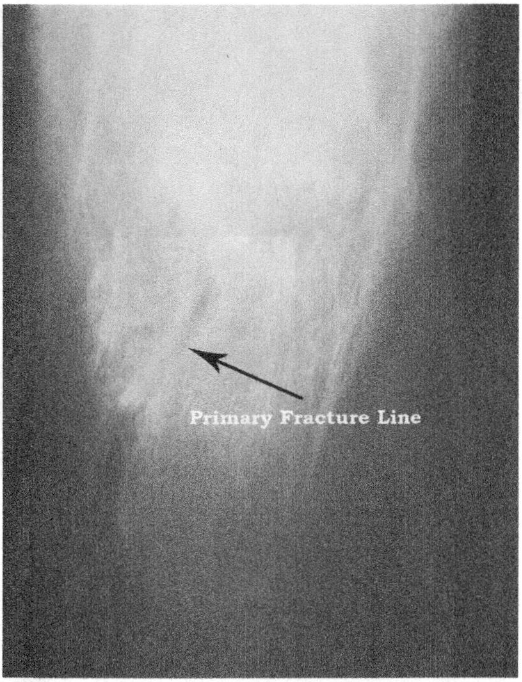

Fig.21. 9 Axialra diograph

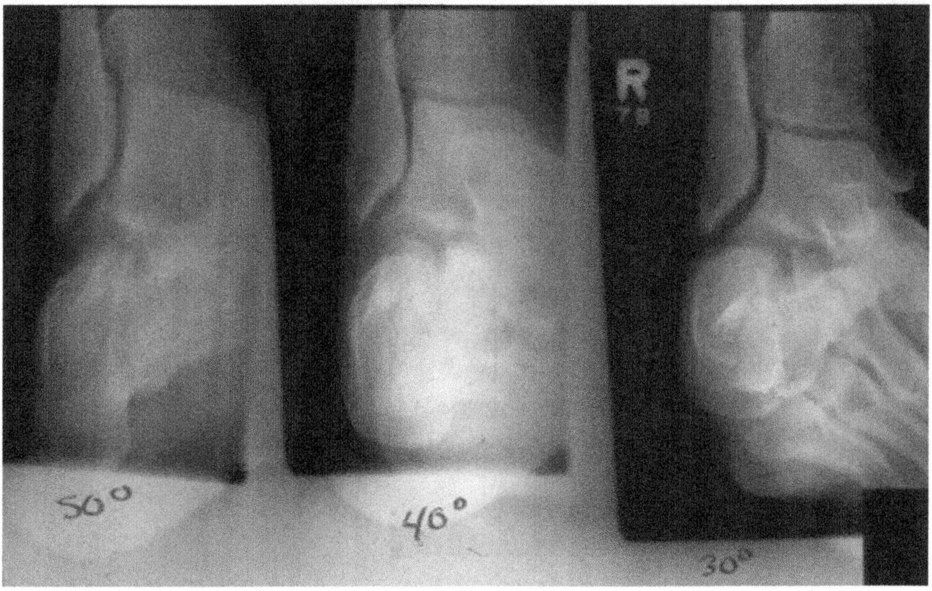

Fig.2 1.10 BrodensV iewpl ainr adiograph

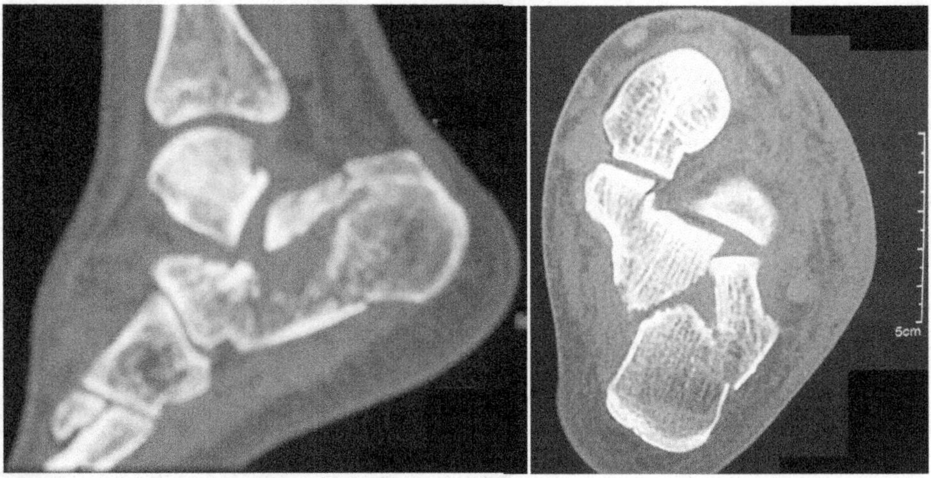

Fig.21.11 CTSc ans

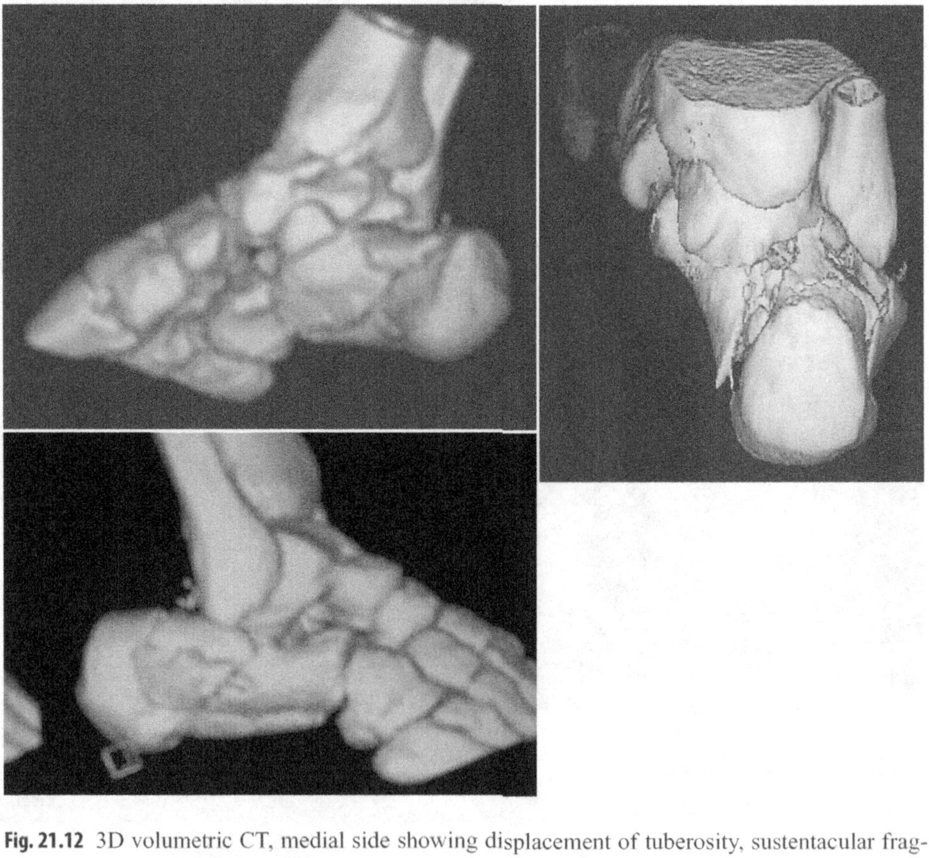

Fig. 21.12 3D volumetric CT, medial side showing displacement of tuberosity, sustentacular fragment and "shingle" effect medially, Axial and Lateral View

21.6 Timingt oS urgery

Some degree of tissue equilibrium must occur before surgery.

Tenting of the skin by bone should be treated as an emergent problem and reduction be effected immediately lest tissue necrosis occurs. The skin tenting may occur on the medial side where the skin is pulled against a spike of bone from the sustentacular fragment, or posteriorly when a tongue fracture occurs and the tuberosity fragment is pressed against the skin.

Blisters of the skin must be allowed to subside and be treated gently, as they reflect marked underlying soft tissue injury (Fig. 21.13).[8,9]

Surgery should generally be delayed until edema has subsided to the point that skin wrinkles are observed. This constitutes a "positive wrinkle sign."

Well padded compression dressings should be used from time of injury until surgery is performed.

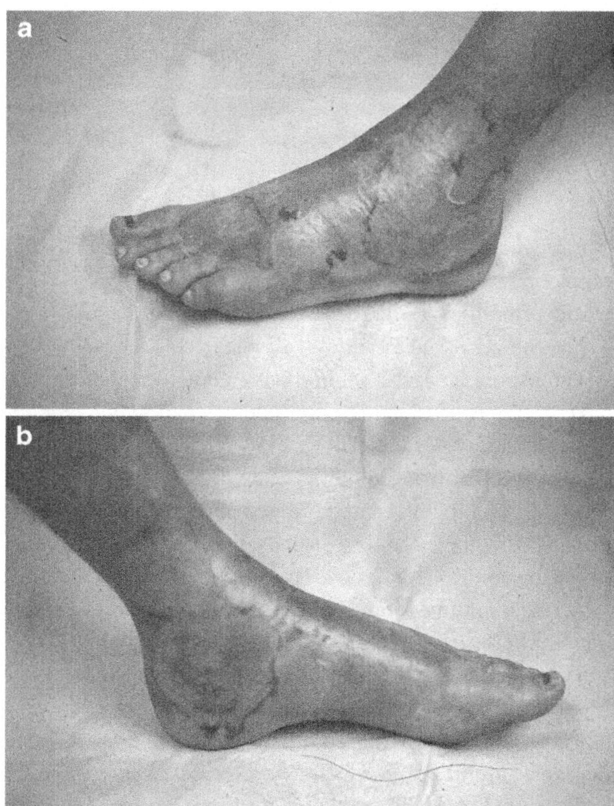

Fig.21.13 Footw ithfra cture blisters due to calcaneal fracture. Blisters have subsided. Blisteres area outlined

21.7 The Principles of Reduction

The displacements and angulations described above must be reversed.[12,19–22] Motion of the hind foot complex depends upon the smoothness of the articular surfaces of the calcaneus and the three dimensional spatial relationships that result between the talus, calcaneus, and cuboid due to the proper shape length and height of the calcaneus.

Carr[6] has described the concept of the medial and lateral columns of the calcaneus. It is necessary to reconstruct both columns.

Disimpaction of the fragments must be accomplished. Then reduction of the tuberosity to the sustentaculum re-establishes the medial wall of the calcaneus. This restores the height by reconstructing the medial column.

The posterior lateral facet fragment can then be elevated, de-rotated and fixed to the sustentacular fragment. After this is accomplished, the lateral wall can be molded into its anatomic position.

In the process of de-rotating the posterior facet fragment, its anterior margin provides the landmarks for the reduction of the anterior lateral fragment to the remainder of the construct, thus re-establishing the length of the lateral column. The articular surface of the anterior process may then be reduced.

21.8 Reduction and Internal Fixation

Reduction requires disimpaction of the fragments and reversal of the deformities. Internal fixation requires placement of appropriate implants to stabilize the reduced fracture fragments.

The principles of the reduction remain unchanged.[10,16,17]

The tuberosity and medial wall of the calcaneus are the starting points.

The patient is placed supine, with a bolster under the buttock the injured side. This will make access to the lateral side easier. A pad is placed under the affected leg to elevate it above the uninjured leg. This will also help position the limb for the lateral exposure and make intra-operative radiographic evaluation easier.

After the limb is prepared, draped and exsanguinated, the leg is placed in the figure four position (hip flexed and externally rotated, knee flexed and the foot and ankle brought across the contra lateral leg). The surgeon faces the medial aspect of the foot.

A horizontal incision 5–6 cm long is made over the posterior tuberosity three fingers breadths below the medial malleolus (Fig. 21.14).

The fascia over the abductor hallucis is opened and the muscle split down to its deeper fascia. This deeper fascia lies over the neurovascular bundle in the anterior aspect of the incision. This is incised carefully, entering the tarsal tunnel, and the vital structures are identified, mobilized, protected and retracted anteriorly. The short flexors of the foot are then elevated from the medial wall of the calcaneus to visualize the fracture (Fig. 21.15).

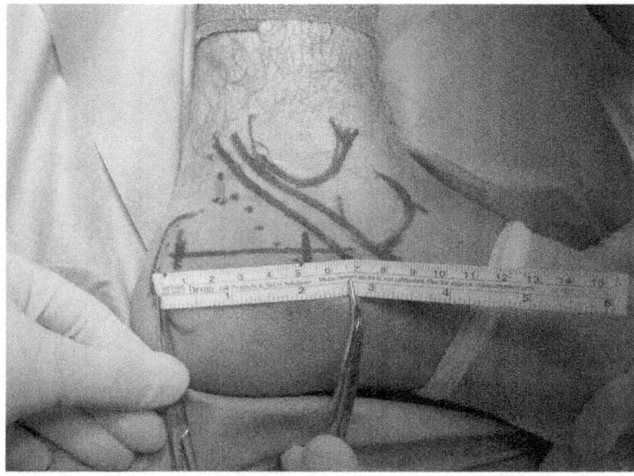

Fig.21.14 Medialinc ision

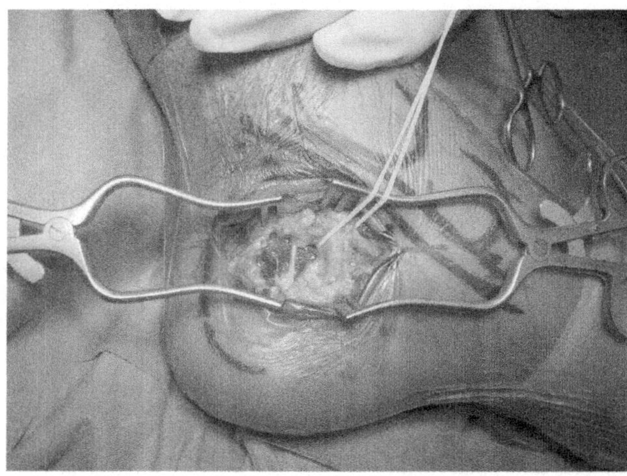

Fig.2 1.15 Mediala pproach, with the neuro-vascular bundlem obilized

The tuberosity has shifted laterally and proximally, therefore the medial wall of the sustentacular fragment overlaps and obscures the superior margin of the tuberosity fragment, much as a roofing shingle overlaps and obscures the superior margin of the shingle below. The medial wall of the sustentacular fragment may even fold in a Z collapse pattern. These nuances will be will visualized by CT scans of the fracture. Three dimensional volumetric reconstructions of the fracture give great insight to the fracture visualized in thise xposure(Figs. 21.16a nd 21.17).

The fracture is disimpacted using an instrument such as a "Joker" elevator placed though the medial fracture under the lateral facet to elevate the lateral facet as much a possible. This clears the space for the reduction of the tuberosity (Fig. 21.18).

A Steinman pin is placed through the tuberosity from medial to lateral. This should be posterior and inferior enough to avoid interfering with the later placement of the plate. The pin should protrude 2–3 in. laterally. The Steinman pin tip should be supported on surgical towels laterally. This will prevent puncturing the drapes and provide a firm surface for

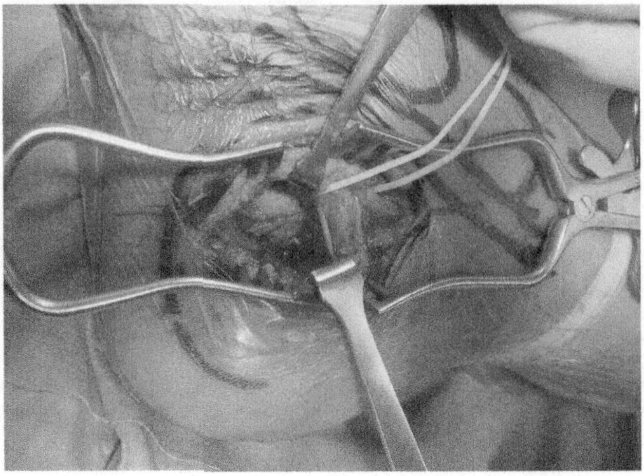

Fig.21. 16 Medialw all exposed

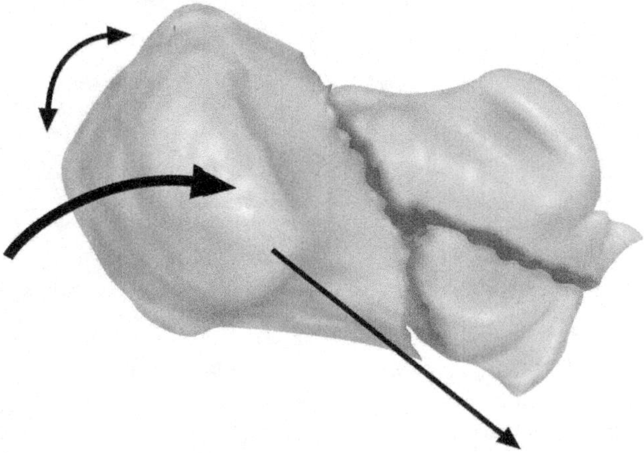

Fig.21. 17 Diagramof m edial shinglea nddi splacement

support. The Steinman pin is then used to reduce the tuberosity to its anatomical position (Figs. 21.19a nd 21.20).

The point of the pin acts as the fulcrum or hinge point for this maneuver. The longer end of the pin acts as a lever. The distance from the foot to the point of the pin produces a laterally offset hinge. When the lever is pulled distally and posteriorly, the tuberosity comes out of varus and translates back into position. The force of the pin from lateral to medial also contributes to the reversal of the displacement (Fig. 21.21).

If the fracture does not reduce, it may be blocked by the impacted posterior facet fragment. This problem is solved by going to the lateral side of the heel as described later.

Initial fixation is then placed. A locked titanium hindfoot plate (Ascension) is placed from the tuberosity to the sustentacular fragment. The curved contour of this plate, when placed with the convex side against the bone comes close to matching the contour of the medial wall. Small adjustments in the contour of the plate may be made. It may be necessary to mobilize the tendon of the flexor hallucis longus to access the solid portion of the medial wall of the sustentacular fragment. Short screws should be used

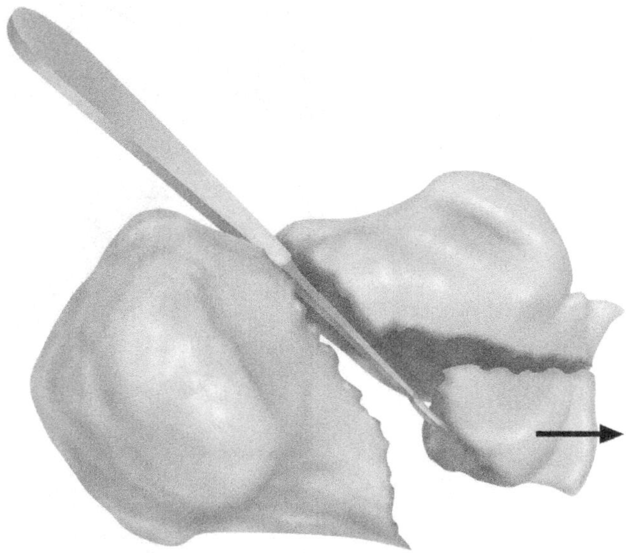

Fig.21.18 Diagramof disimpaction of fragments fromthe me dials ide

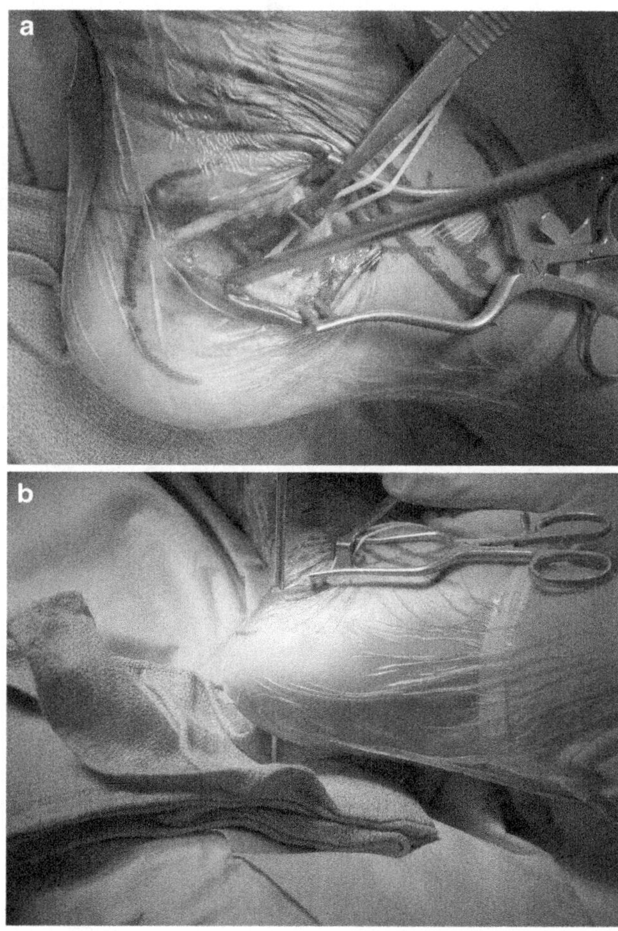

Fig.21.19 Steinmanpin placed through tuberosity fragment from medial to lateral, lateral side down. Pin tip exiting on lateral side becomes fulcrum or hinge point for reduction of tuberosity. Pin becomes lever to move tuberosity fragment

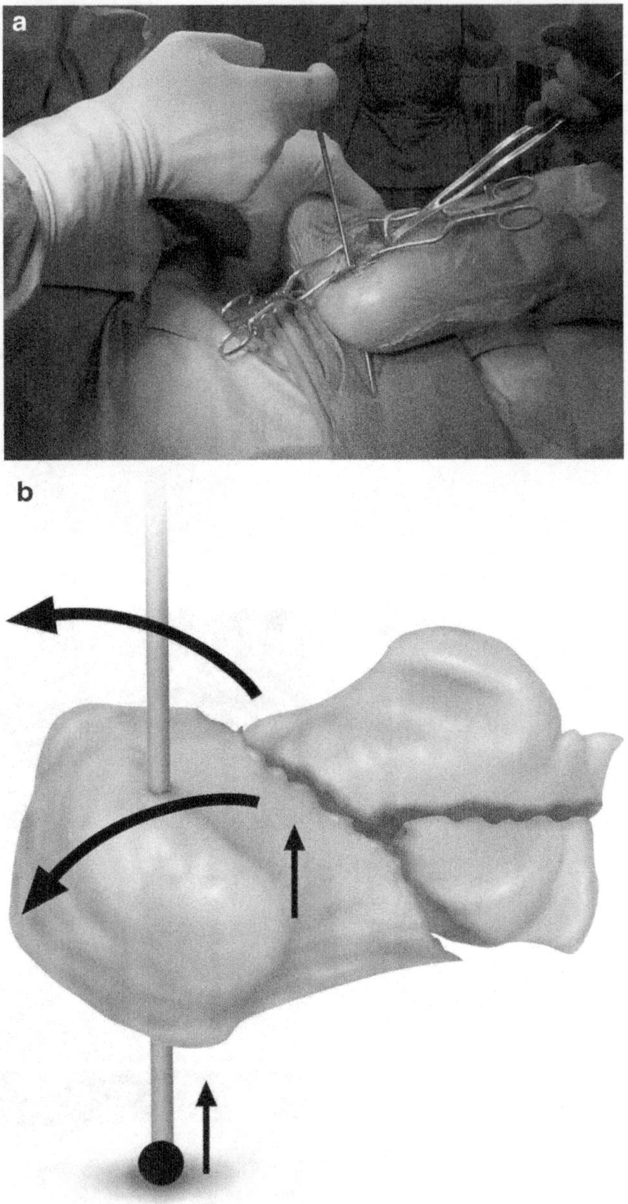

Fig. 21.20 Diagram of the reduction maneuver

at this point in the sustentacular fragment, as a long screws may impede the lateral reduction (Fig. 21.22).

The leg is then brought out of the figure four position and extended. The lateral incision is made. This goes from just behind the tip of the lateral malleolus for a distance of approximately 5 cm in the line of the fourth to fifth ray toward the cuboid, above the sural nerve (Fig. 21.23).

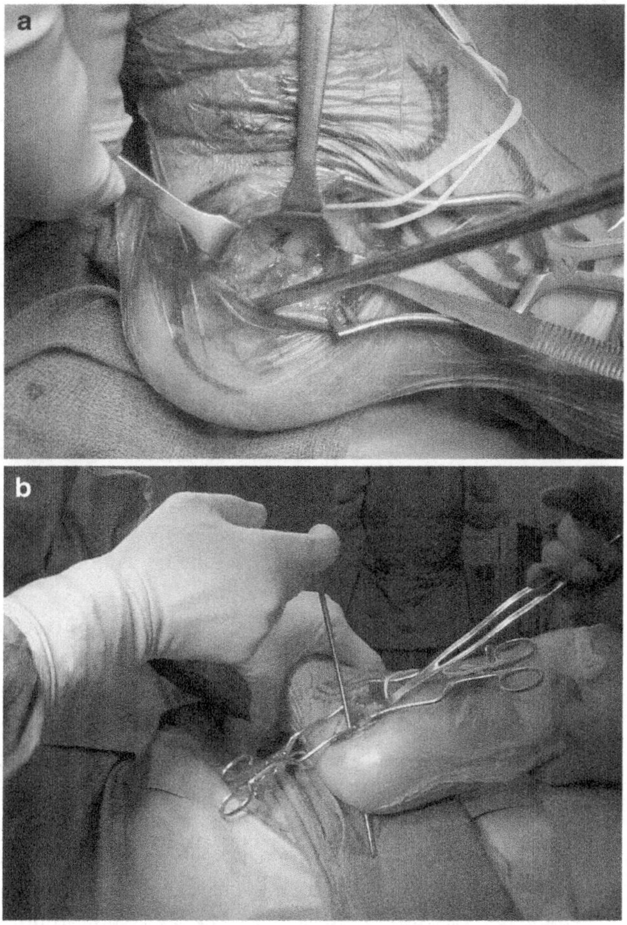

Fig.21.21 (**a**) Steinman pin used a lever has repositioned tuberosit fragment to permit reduction of medial wall. Toes to top of picture, ankle to right, neurovascular bundle in vessel loop. Medial wall reduction in depth of wound. (**b**) Steinman pin being used as lever with fulcrum at tip of pin lateral to foot (down side). Fulcrum point being lateral to foot guides translation of tuberosity in reduction

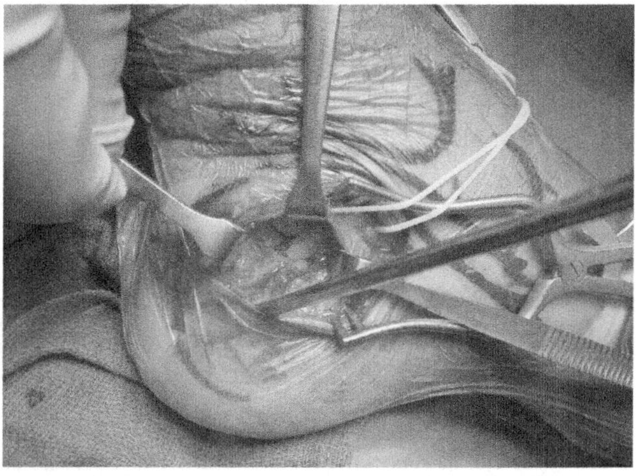

Fig.21.22 Medialw all reduction

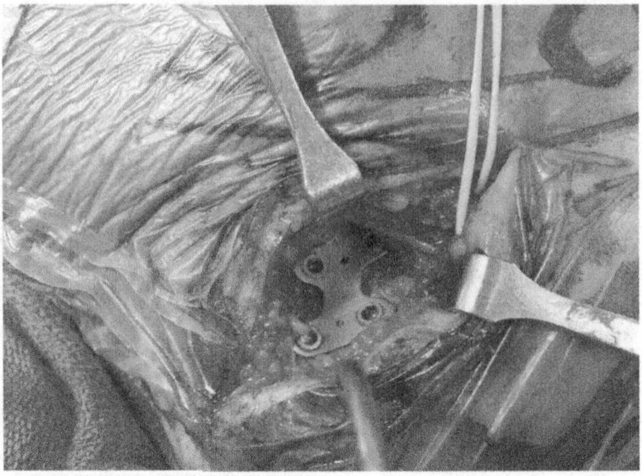

Fig. 21.23 Medialhind f oot platea pplied

The peroneal tendons are exposed and retracted. Placing an umbilical tape around the tendons is helpful. The umbilical tape may be wound around the Steinman pin which protrudes to provide a "self retaining retractor."

The extensor digitorum brevis proximally is mobilized and released and the sinus tarsi and the subtalar joint are exposed. The lateral wall of the calcaneus under the peroneal tendons is exposed. A baby Inge lamina spreader is placed in the sinus tarsi to help visualize the fracture of the posterior facet. The dorsal surface of the anterior calcaneus is exposed and visualized to assess the comminution (Fig. 21.24).

The lateral portion of the posterior facet is usually depressed and rotated forward, so that the anterior aspect of the posterior facet is further depressed. It may be buried under the anterior fragment. The disimpaction effort from the medial side does not produce anatomic reduction.

The underside of this fragment can be accessed through the lateral wall at the angle of Gissane where a fracture often exists. The fragment is elevated and derotated. Reduction

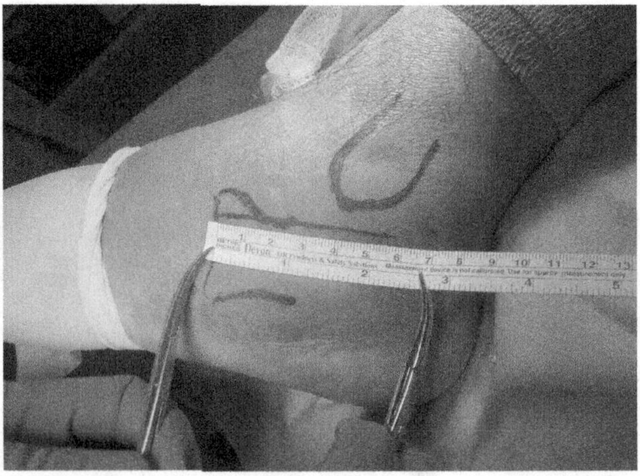

Fig. 21.24 Lateralinc ision

of a tongue fragment can be facilitated by placing a longitudinal Steinman pin from posterior into the fragment. This is used as a lever to reduce the fragment. Posterior "over reduction" can occur and should be looked for. Carr has advocated the use of arthroscopes to inspect the articular reduction. 0.45 or 0.62 in. Kirschner wires hold these fragments temporarily(Figs. 21.25a nd 21.26).

The anterior fragment and posterior fragments are then approximated. As the posterior lateral facet fragment is derotated into position, appropriate anterior reduction is often effected. Kirschner wire fixation is established.

At this point, image intensification via the C ARM is used to assess the reduction radiographically. The Brodens view, axial heel view, lateral view and AP foot view are made. If the reduction is satisfactory, the Mini Calcaneal Titanium locking plate (Ascension) is applied. This plate is designed to act as a washer allow compression from lateral to medial across the posterior facet and anterior calcaneus and to link the posterior construct to the anterior calcaneus. Screws go across the posterior fragment to the sustentacular fragment.

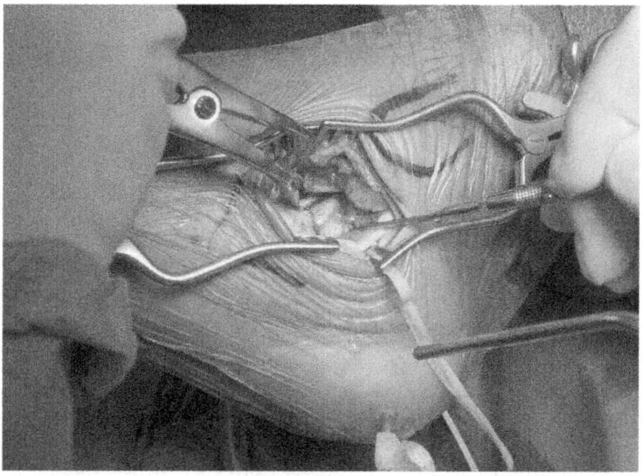

Fig.21.25 Laterale xposure

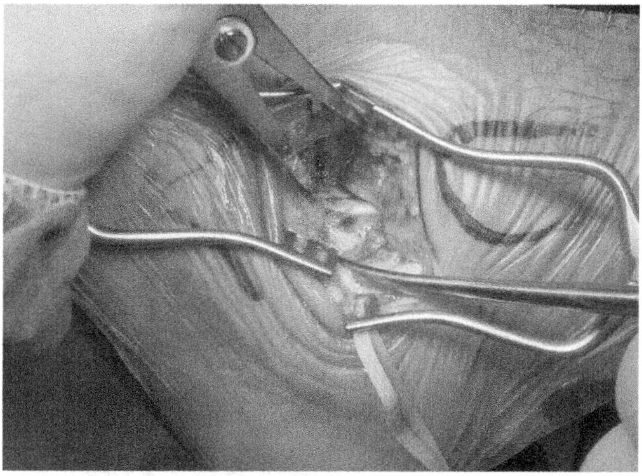

Fig.21.26 Lateralre duction

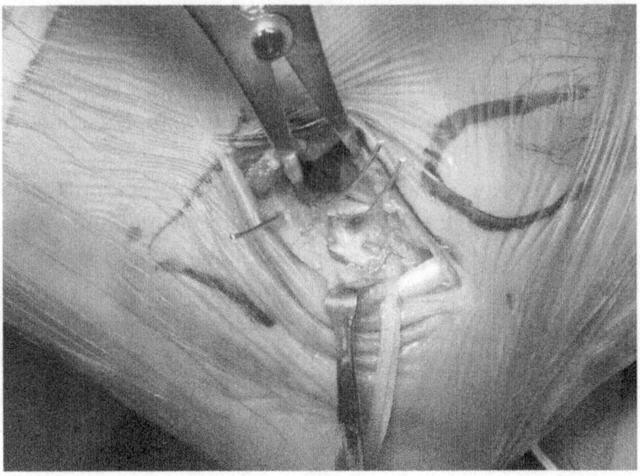

Fig. 21.27 Lateralre duction temporarily stabilized with Kirschnerw ires

3.5 mm fully threaded locking and non locking screws are used. A non locking screw may be used to provide compression across the facet fracture. The screws should aim slightly plantar as the subtalar surface drops medially (Fig. 21.27).

The locking and non locking screw heads are recessed into the plate, thus presenting a smooth surface. The peroneal tendons will move over this plate. Irritation of these tendons is minimized as there are no protruding screw heads.

The medial wound is again accessed. The short screws can now be changed to screws that span the width of the calcaneus.

The fixation pattern established is as follows. The tuberosity is reduced to and fixed to the sustentacular fragment. The posterior lateral fragment is reduced to and fixed to the tuberosity fragment. The anterior fragments are reduced to and fixed to the posterior construct. All four fragments are reduced and stabilized.

Note the construct on a saw bones model (Fig. 21.28a, b).

The principles of the procedure have been satisfied.

After taking and assessing final radiographs, the tourniquet is deflated. Small drains are used if needed, the wound in closed in layers, and a well padded short leg cast is applied

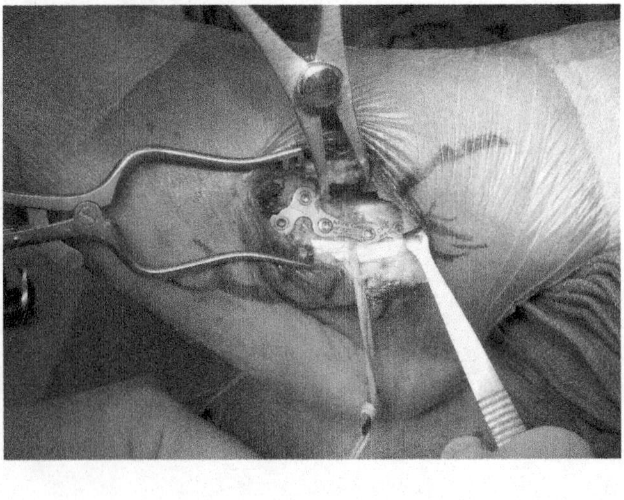

Fig. 21.28 Minic alcaneal platea ppliedt ol aterala spect

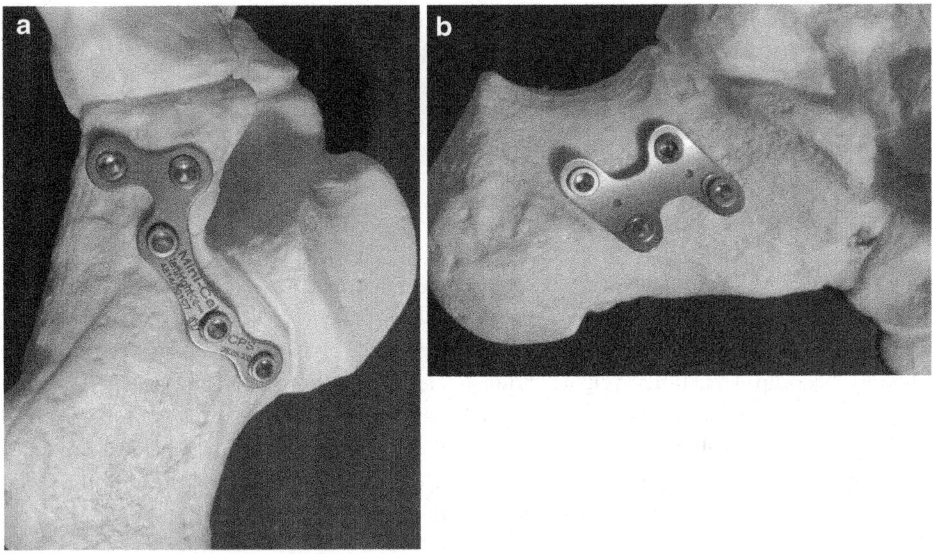

Fig.2 1.29 (**a**,**b**) Sawbo nesw ithpl atesa pplied

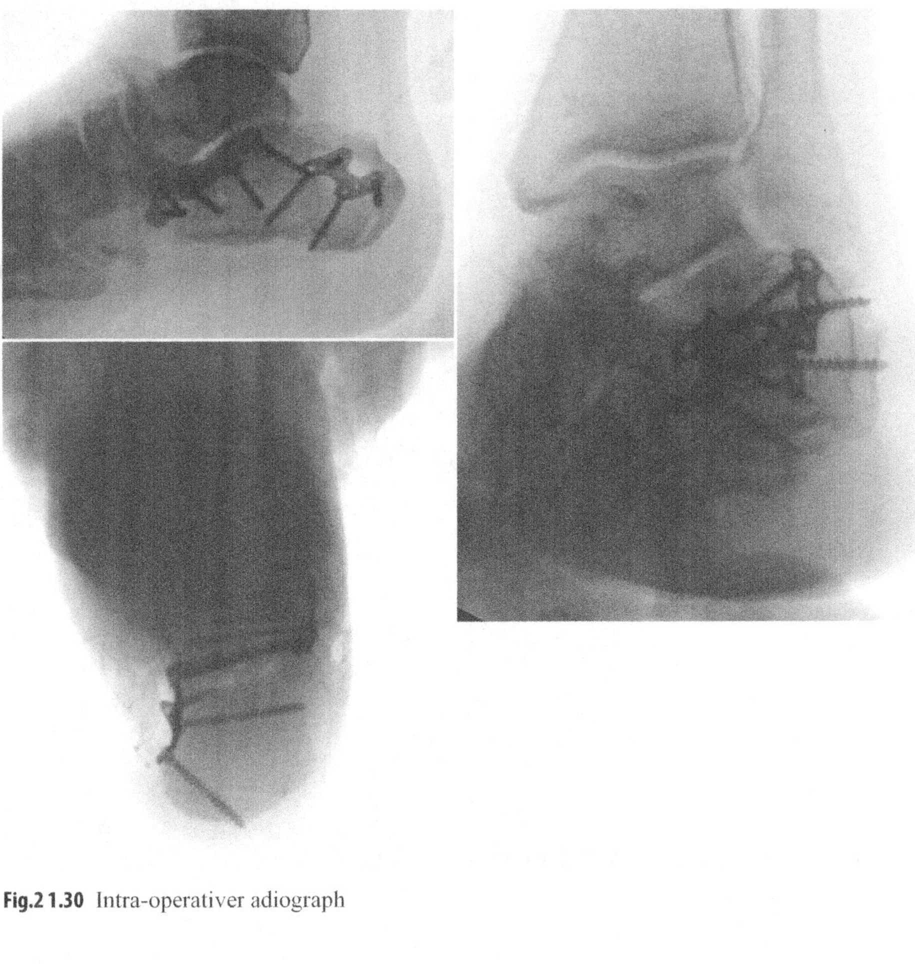

Fig.2 1.30 Intra-operativer adiograph

and bivalved within 12 h. AV Impulse foot compression pneumatic pumps can be used to decrease the inevitable post-operative swelling (Figs. 21.29 and 21.30).[14]

21.9 Post-operativeC are

The cast is changed during the first week and again at 2 weeks, when the sutures are removed. The patient is kept non weight bearing for 6 weeks, when patient are allowed 25% partial weight bearing at weeks 7 and 8. The cast is then removed (Fig. 21.31). Patients may wear a post op shoe and heel cup at that time. Weight bearing as tolerated is allowed, and physical therapy initiated. The efforts of the therapists are directed toward ankle and subtalar range of motion, and strengthening of the calf muscles. Gradual resolution of swelling occurs over the next 4 months. A very positive prognostic sign is the ability to perform a single foot toe raise and walking "tip toe." I advise patients that improvement may continue for up to a year from surgery.

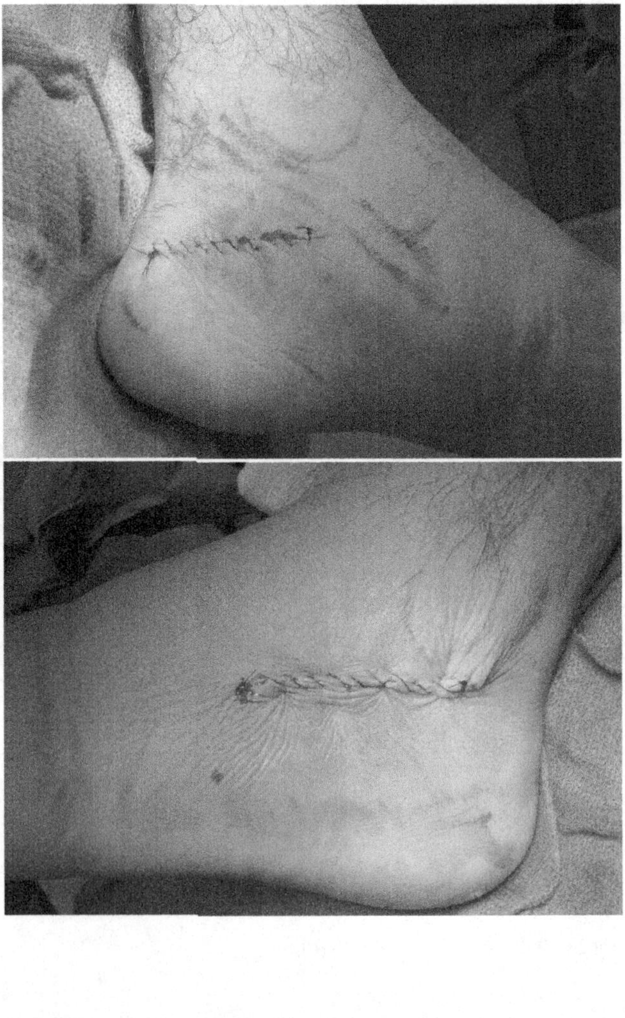

Fig.21. 31 Woundsa t closure

21.10 Experience

One hundred and thirty-six fractures have been treated with this technique over the past 13 years. There have been slight changes as the shape and thickness of the plate changed to its present form in 2008. The medial fixation changed from staples to the locking plate for the last 30 patients.

In general, the patients have regained 50% of their subtalar motion. Good to excellent results defined by the following parameters have been achieved in 80–90% of the injuries.

Patients have been able to wear standard shoes. Neurologic deficit beyond that noted on initial presentation has been negligible. Mobilization of the neurovascular bundle has not been a source of increased morbidity. Ankle motion has been unimpaired.

Smokers had more problems than the non smoking population. There were three incidents of delays in wound healing, all in smokers. Diabetes was not an absolute

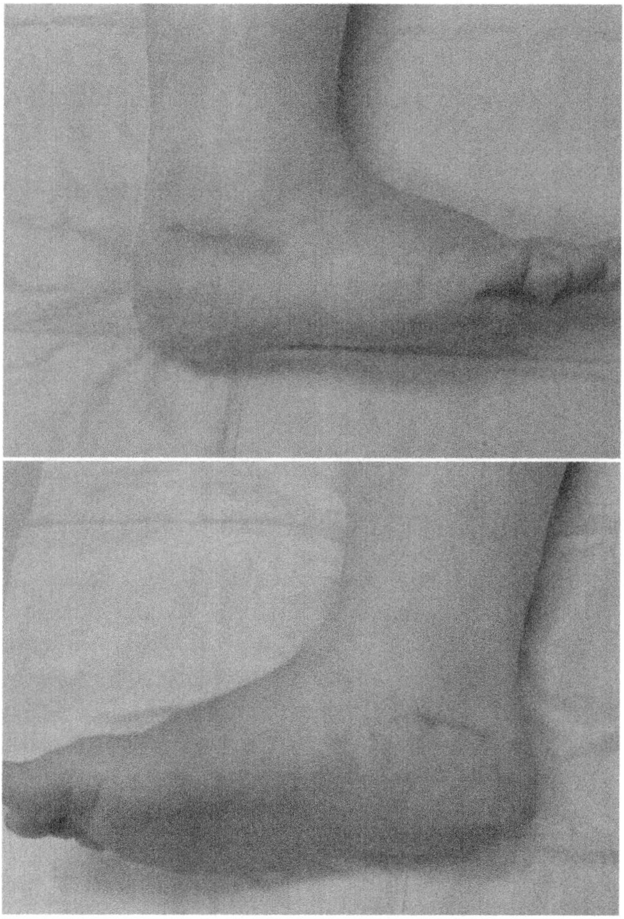

Fig.21.32 Woundsmore mature

contraindication to the procedure. One patient who had other previous Charcot changes in the forefoot had a primary subtalar arthrodesis performed with the ORIF.

Further surgery had to be performed rarely. One patient had screw threads penetrate the subtalar surface. Removal of the screws and plate was undertaken after union had occurred. Five patients required later subtalar arthrodesis. The initial lateral incision was well suited to this salvage procedure.

Associated simultaneous surgery: Ten patients had abductor hallucis flaps and skin grafts done with the index open reduction and internal fixation. The indication was medial blistering and "zone of injury" muscle damage on the medial side. There were no flap failures, and bone union progressed uneventfully (Fig. 21.32).[11]

One patient who was referred more than a week after injury developed skin necrosis directly posteriorly at the point of a "tongue" fragment severely displaced. He was a smoker and developed delayed healing of a fascial flap. This patient also bore weight early causing failure of his fixation.

An elderly man began immediate full weight bearing, and lost the reduction of the height of his heel but maintained the congruity of the subtalar joint surface. The patient needed no further surgery.

21.11 Discussion

Whether or not to perform an ORIF of a comminuted intra articular calcaneal fracture continues to remain slightly controversial. The decision of course lies in the hands of the surgeon managing this injury. This was once the territory of the Foot and Ankle Specialist. Residency training now prepares many young physicians to face this problem. Surgeons should not be didactic and prescriptive in managing these fractures. There are opportunities to apply any of many treatments to the fracture, from "benign neglect" to immediate reduction and subtalar arthrodesis. Each method of treatment has its own advantages and disadvantages.

The extensile lateral approach permits excellent visualization of the lateral wall of the calcaneus, anterior calcaneus and posterior facet, but no visualization of the medial wall. The medial side is reduced indirectly. Large plates are applied from the lateral side. Large skin flaps are raised. Salvage procedures often require reusing the initial incision and raising the large flap again.

The dual incision technique does not require the raising of large skin flaps. All portions of the fracture are reduced and fixed directly. The key is direct fixation of the displaced fragments to the "constant" fragment of the sustentaculum which is in anatomic relation with the talus. The neurovascular bundle is mobilized medially, but this is not a source of increased morbidity. Salvage procedures can be performed through the initial lateral incision which is the same incision that would be used for the primary approach to pathology in the subtalar complex.

The plates that are applied through the extensile lateral approach encompass the perimeter of the calcaneus and have an oblique strut from the tuberosity toward the subtalar joint. This plate was introduced as there were problems with failure of previous plates supporting the subtalar joint.

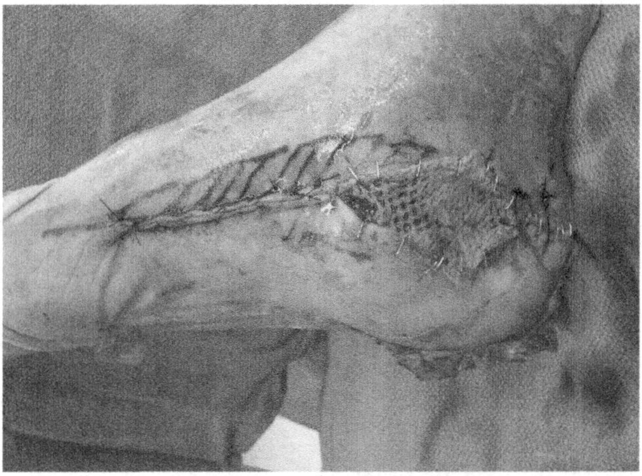

Fig.21. 33 Abductorfl ap and skingra ft

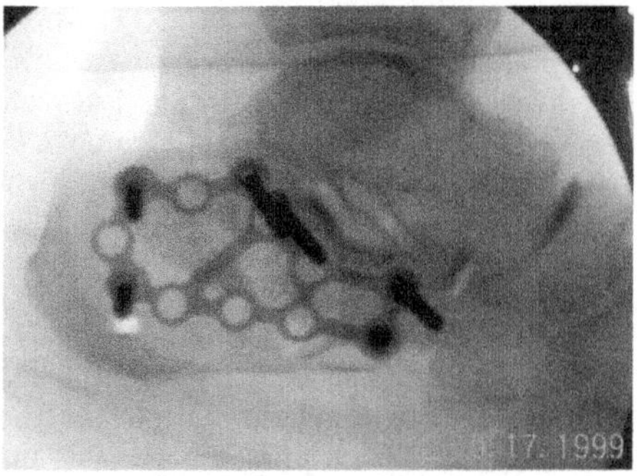

Fig. 21.34 Extensile lateral plate, lateral radiograph

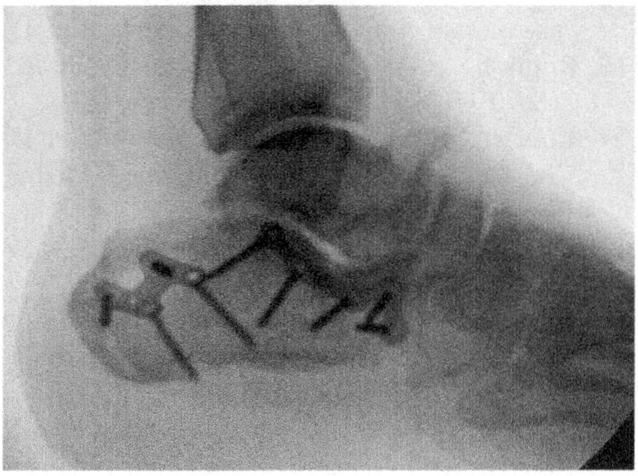

Fig.21. 35 Medial and lateral plate lateral radiographs

The fixation pattern achieved with the dual small incision technique attends to this by means of the medial staples. When lateral radiographs of the fracture fixed by both techniques are compared, the staples and now the locking plate and the reinforcing strut of the plate are similarly oriented and almost superimposable (Figs. 21.33–21.35).

The results of treatment are not compromised by use of the dual small incision technique.

References

1. Atones W. An oblique projection for roentgen examination of the talo-calcaneal joint, particularly regarding intra articular fractures of the calcaneus. *Acta Radiol.* 1943;24:306.
2. Bohler L. Diagnosis, pathology and treatment of fractures of the os calcis. *JBJS.* 1931;13:75.
3. Bohler L. *The Treatment of Fractures.* Vol. 3. New York, NY: Grune and Stratton; 1958:2045–2108.
4. Broden B. Roentgen examination of the subtaloid joint in fractures of the calcaneus. *Acta Radiol.* 1949;31:85.
5. Burdeaux BD. Reduction of calcaneal fractures by the McReynolds medial approach technique and its experimental basis. *Clin Orthop.* 1983;177:87–103.
6. Carr JB, Hamilton JJ, Bear LS. Experimental intra-articular calcaneal fractures: anatomic basis for a new classification. *Foot Ankle.* 1989;10:81–87.
7. Carr JB. Three dimensional CT scanning of calcaneal fractures. *Orthop Trans.* 1989;13.
8. Giordano CP, Koval KJ. Treatment of fracture blisters: a prospective study of 53 cases. *J Orthop Trauma.* 1995;9:171.
9. Giordano CP, Koval KJ, Zuckerman JD, Desai P. Fracture blisters. *Clin Orthop.* 1994;292:214.
10. Johnson EE, Gebhardt JS. Surgical management of calcaneal fractures using bilateral incisions and minimal internal fixation. *Clin Orthop.* 1993;290:117–124.
11. Levin LS, Nunley JA. The management of soft tissue problems associated with calcaneal fractures. *Clin Orthop.* 1993;290:151–156.
12. Le Tournel E. Open reduction and internal fixation of calcaneal fractures. In: Spiegel P, ed. *Topics in Orthopaedic Surgery.* Baltimore, MD: Aspen; 1984:173.
13. McReynolds IS. Trauma to the os calcis and heel cord. In: Jahss M ed. *Disorders of the Foot and Ankle.* Philadelphia, PA: WB Saunders; 1984:1497.
14. Myerson MS, Henderson MR. Clinical applications of a pneumatic intermittent impulse compression device after trauma and major surgery to the foot and ankle. *Foot Ankle.* 1993;14:198.
15. Palmer I. The mechanism and treatment of fracture of the calcaneus. Open reduction and the use of cancellous grafts. *JBJS.* 1948;30 A:2–8.
16. Romash MM. Calcaneal fractures; three dimensional treatment. *Foot Ankle.* 1988;8: 180–197.
17. Romash MM. Open reduction and internal fixation of comminuted intra articular fractures of the calcaneus using the combined medial and lateral approach. *Op Techn Ortho.* July 1994;4:157–164.
18. Sanders R, Dipasquale T. Intra – operative Brodens views in the operative treatment of calcaneus fractures. *Orthop Trans.* 1989;13.
19. Sanders R, Fortin P, Di Pasquale T, Walling A. Operative treatment in 120 displaced intra articular calcaneal fractures: results using a prognostic computed tomography scan classification. *Clin Orthop.* 1993;290:87.
20. Sangeorzan BJ. Open reduction and internal fixation of calcaneal fractures. In: Kitaoka H, ed. *Master Techniques in Orthopaedic Surgery, The Foot and Ankle.* Chapter 30. Philadelphia, PA: Lippincott Williams and Wilkins; 2002:425–447.
21. Soeur R, Remy R. Fractures of the calcaneus with displacement of the thalamic portion. *JBJS [Br].* 1975;57:413–421.
22. Stephenson JR. Treatment of displaced intra articular fractures of the calcaneus using medial and lateral approaches, internal fixation and early motion. *JBJS.* 1987;69A:115.

EndoscopicP lantarF asciotomy

22

Amol Saxena

22.1 Introduction

Plantar fasciopathy can be chronic and debilitating, with recent histopathological studies showing that the condition is actually a failed healing response.[1] Surgical solutions have evolved over the years from traditional open surgical release (with and without spur resection), percutaneous fasciotomy, and, most recently, to endoscopic release.[2–19] Endoscopic release has the benefit of direct v?sualization of the plantar fascia with minimal soft tissue trauma.[2,3,8–10,14–17]

Indications for endoscopic plantar fasciotomy ("EPF") are the same for open and percutaneous approaches. Patients should have recalcitrant symptoms of plantar fasciopathy for at least 6 months despite traditional non-surgical treatment, which should include rest, medication, ice, stretching, inserts, shoe modification, night splints and appropriate physical therapy measures, including extracorporeal shock wave therapy.[3,9–11,14,18] Stress fracture, nerve entrapment, compartment syndrome, tumor and inflammatory arthropathy should be excluded.[9–11,14]

EPF was first described by Barrett and Day in the early 1990s.[2] Since then, several studies of the technique have taken place. Most studies are favorable, though post-operative complications of lateral column pain, stress fracture and nerve entrapment have been described.[3,5,6,12–16,19,20] Lateral column symptoms occurred in the early case series, as surgeons allowed for immediate weightbearing post-operatively and transected the entire central fascia attachment.[3,5,6,12–16] Subsequently, authors recommended post-operative non-weightbearing and transection of only the medial half of the central fascial band, yielding better results.[6,12,14–16]

A.Sa xena
Department of Sports Medicine, PAFMG, Palo Alto, CA 94301, USA
e-mail:he ysax@aol.com

N. Maffulli and M. Easley (eds.), *Minimally Invasive Surgery of the Foot and Ankle*,
DOI: 10.1007/978-1-84996-417-3_22,

22.2 Technique

EPF is performed on an out-patient ("same-day") basis. General or regional anesthesia can be used. Care is taken not to infiltrate local anesthetic in the direct region of the surgical field, as the extra fluid could hamper visualization. The procedure begins with a medial incision at the level of the medial tubercle, approximately 1 cm distal to a perpendicular line from the medial malloleous. The incision is made obliquely within the skin creases in this region. Care is taken to place the incision above the plantar skin, which avoids a hypertrophic scar (Figs. 22.1 and 22.2). After the skin incision, blunt dissection is performed down to the level of the plantar fascia, avoiding neurovascular structures. A fascial elevator is used to produce a pathway for the obturator/cannula assembly inferior to the plantar fascia (Figs. 22.3 and 22.4). Next, a 4 mm 30° endoscope is placed in the medial portal to visualize the plantar fascia superiorly (Figs. 22.5 and 22.6). The endoscope is

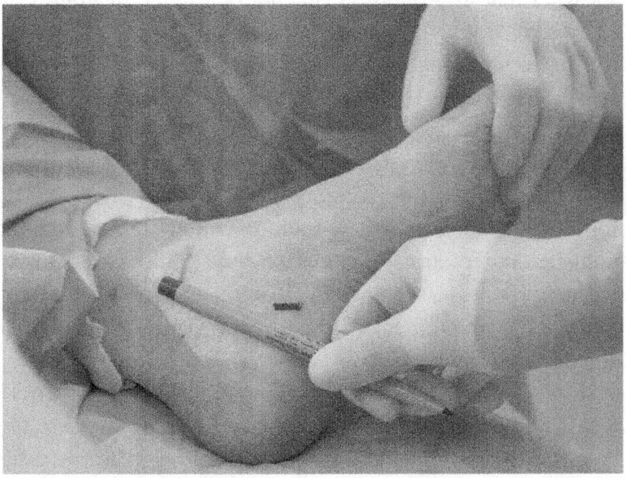

Fig.22.1 Placementofs kin incision 1 cm distal to the medial malleolus at the level of thepl antarf ascia

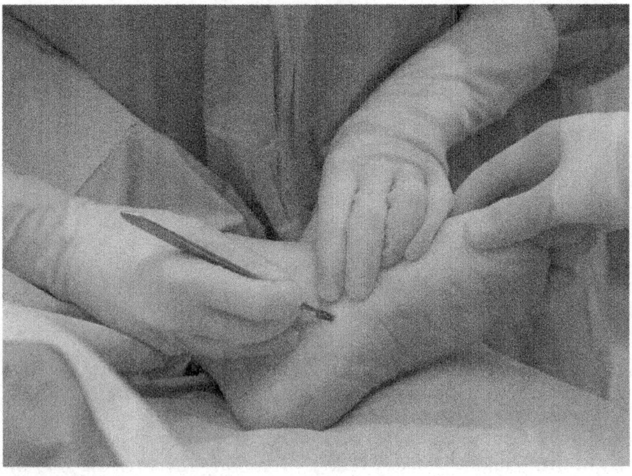

Fig.22.2 Skininc isionw ithin skinc reases

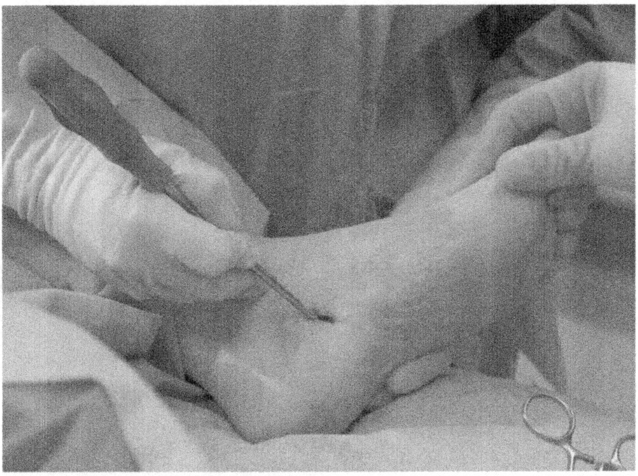

Fig. 22.3 Fasciale levatort o create a pathway superficial tothe pla ntarfa scia

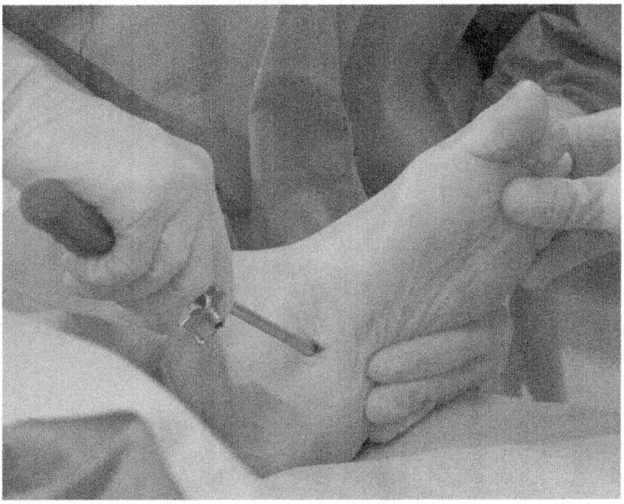

Fig. 22.4 Insertionofth e cannula

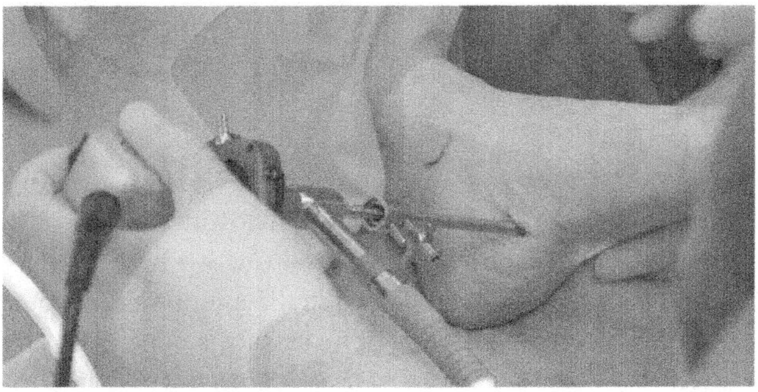

Fig. 22.5 Endoscopeins erted medially

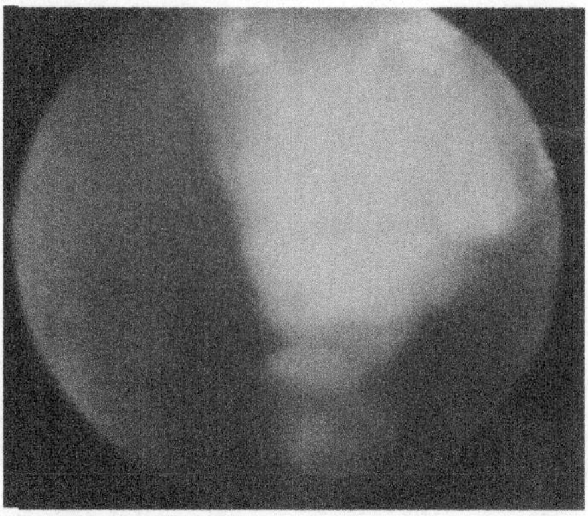

Fig. 22.6 Medial view of the plantar fascia superiorly (white)

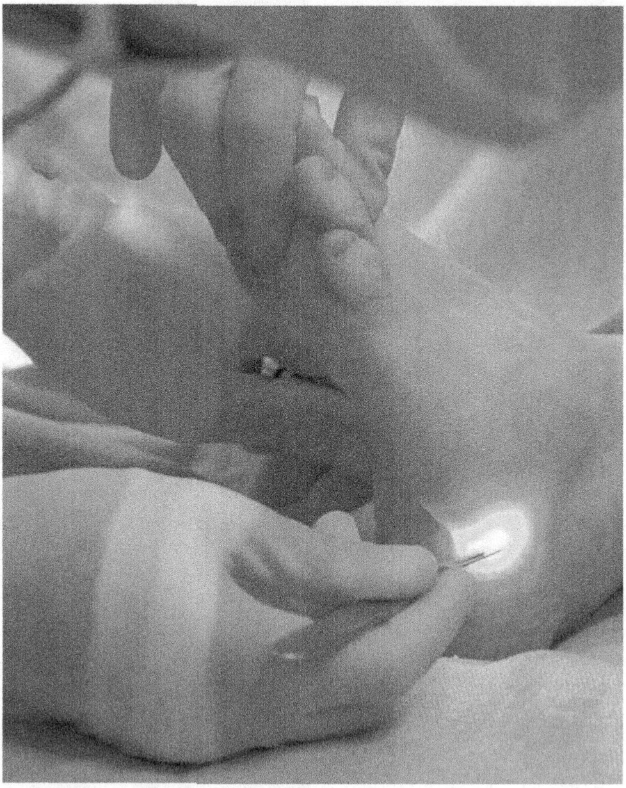

Fig. 22.7 Transillumination laterally for incision for lateral portal

advanced laterally to transilluminate the lateral aspect of the foot, and produce a lateral portal (Fig. 22.7). The cannula is then advanced through the lateral portal and then stabilized with a locking device (Mondeal, Inc.) (Figs. 22.8a nd 22.9).

The endoscope is then placed in the lateral portal, again viewing the plantar fascia. If necessary, suction or cotton-tipped swabs can help remove extraneous fluid (Figs. 22.10 and 22.11). The endoscope is then temporarily rotated to help identify the demarcation of the medial half of the plantar fascia via transillumination (Fig. 22.12). The endoscope

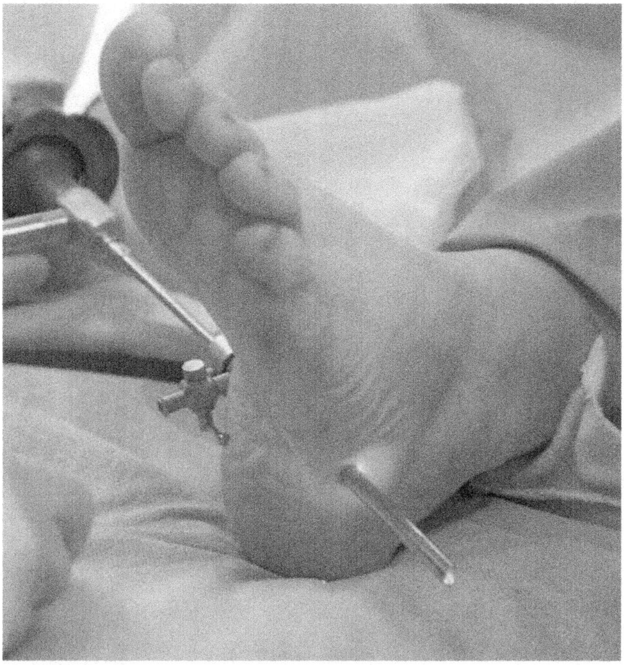

Fig. 22.8 Advancement of the cannula through the lateral incision

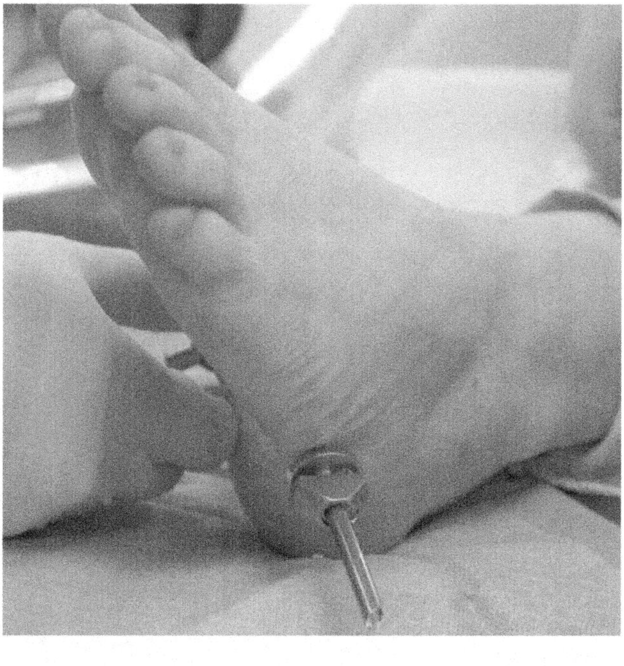

Fig. 22.9 Stabilization of cannula with "Cannlock" (Mondeal NA, Inc.)

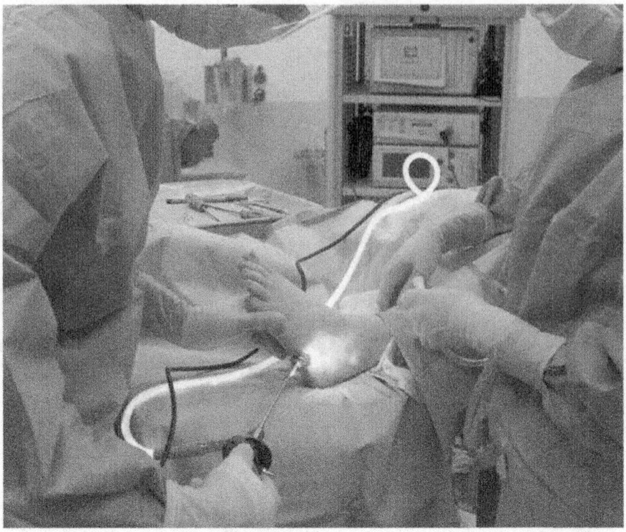

Fig.22. 10 Endoscopepl aced laterally

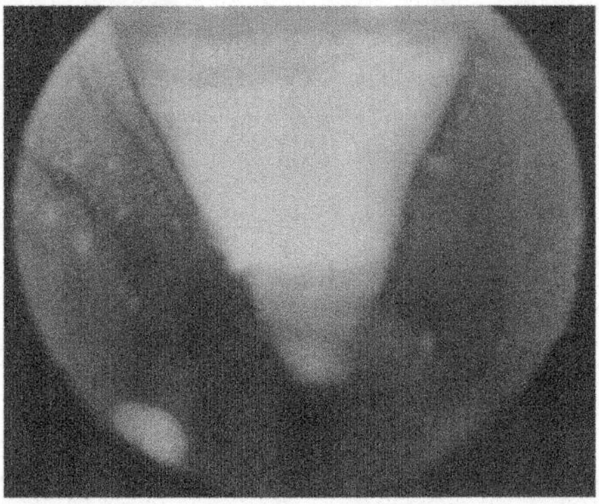

Fig.22. 11 Endoscopic view of plantar fascia froml ateralpor tal

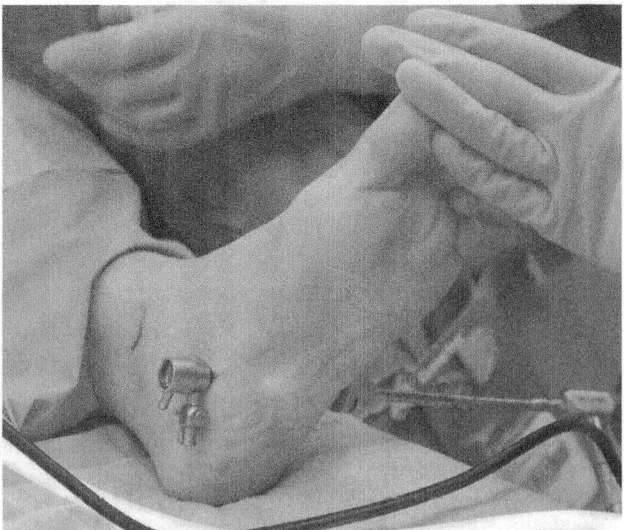

Fig.22. 12 Endoscoper otated inferiorly, transilluminating to show level for transection of medial50%

is rotated back so the fascia is visualized superiorly. A forward cutting knife is inserted through the cannula medially to transect the medial plantar fascia (Mondeal, Inc.) (Fig. 22.13). Care is taken to keep the endoscope stable to avoid inadvertent transection of the fascia laterally. Dorsiflexing the toes makes transaction easier (Fig. 22.14). From the lateral portal, one can view the knife advancing as it transects the fascia, (white), exposing muscle above (red) (Fig. 22.15). The endoscope can then be replaced into the medial portal to verify the transection, with the lateral portion intact. Most often there is a fat globule in this region demarcating the lateral portion (seen as yellow) (Figs. 22.16–22.18). The surgical field is irrigated through the cannula, which is then removed (Figs. 22.19 and 22.20).

An injection of 1 cc of dexamethasone phosphate (4 mg/mL) and 3 cc of 0.5% bupivicaine is administered at the surgeons discretion (Fig. 22.21). The skin is approximated with 3-0 nylon interrupted horizontal sutures (Figs. 22.22 and 22.23) Post-operatively, patients are placed in a below-knee cast boot, and kept non-weightbearing for 2 weeks. Suture removal is performed at that time, and then patients begin to weightbear in the cast boot for an additional 2–3 weeks until they are pain-free. If needed, they use an arch support or orthoses. They often receive physical therapy, including soft-tissue mobilization and strengthening for up to12 weeks. Return to daily activities and sports range from 4 to 12 weeks.[11,14,15]

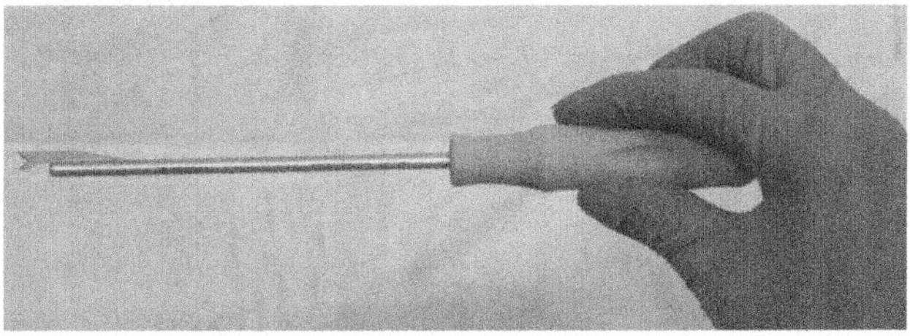

Fig.22. 13 Forwardc utting knife inserted through the medialporta l

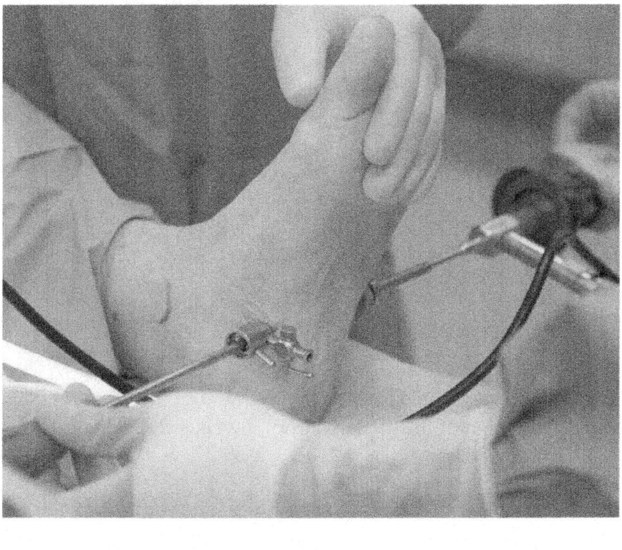

Fig.22. 14 Dorsiflexing the toesma kestra nsactione asier

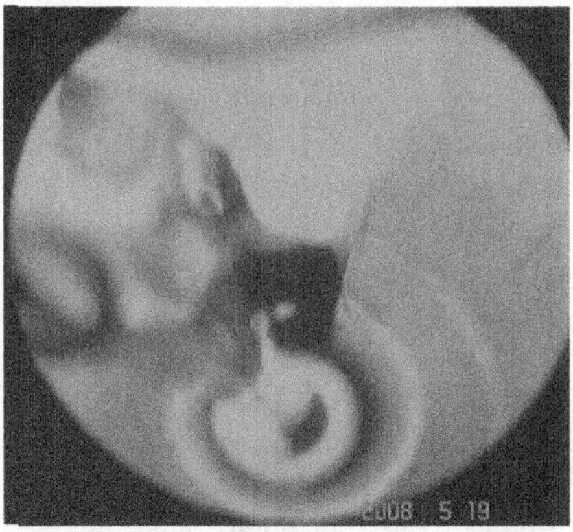

Fig.22. 15 Endoscopic view from the lateral side, cutting fascia medially (white) exposing musclea bove

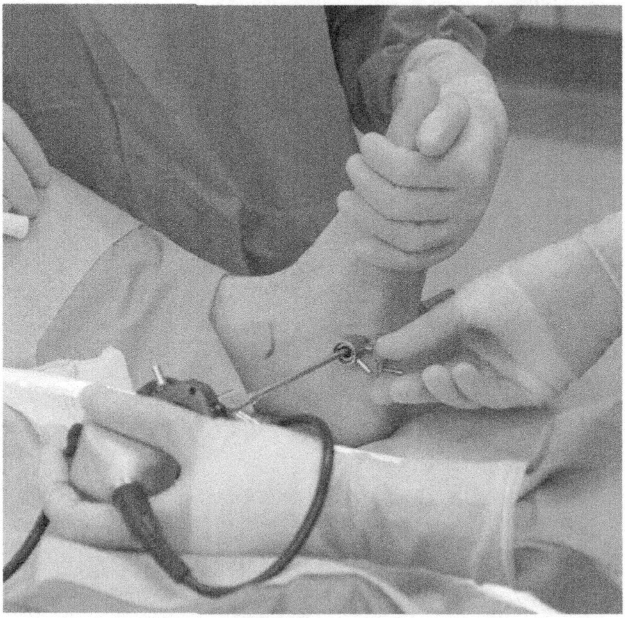

Fig.22. 16 Re-insertionof endoscopef romm edial

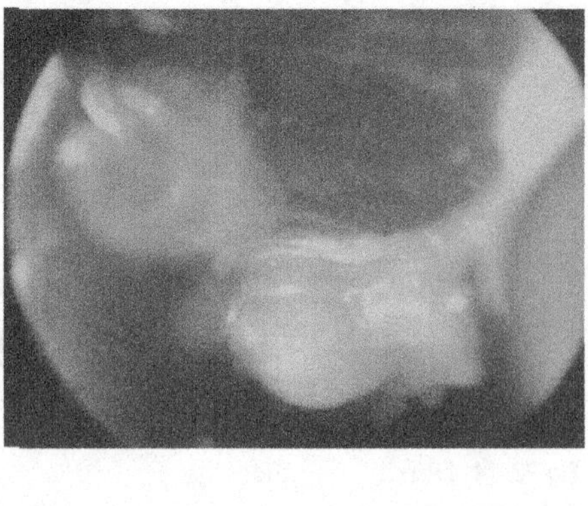

Fig.22. 17 A fat globule is often present at the demarcation of the medial half of the central plantarf asciaba nd

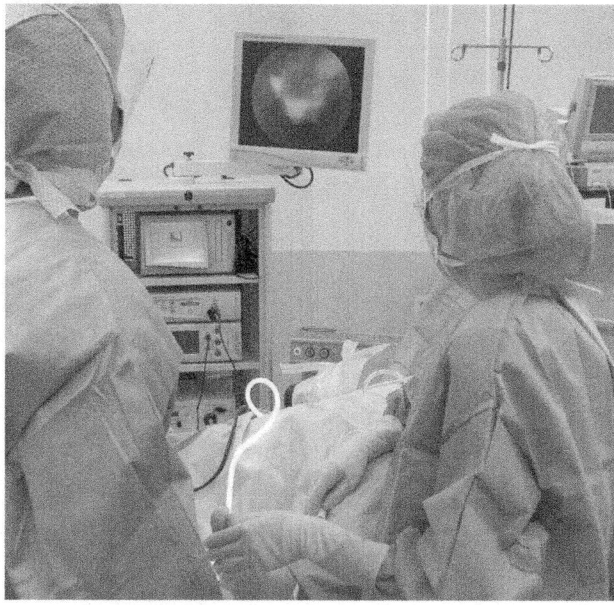

Fig.22. 18 Confirming appropriatetra nsection

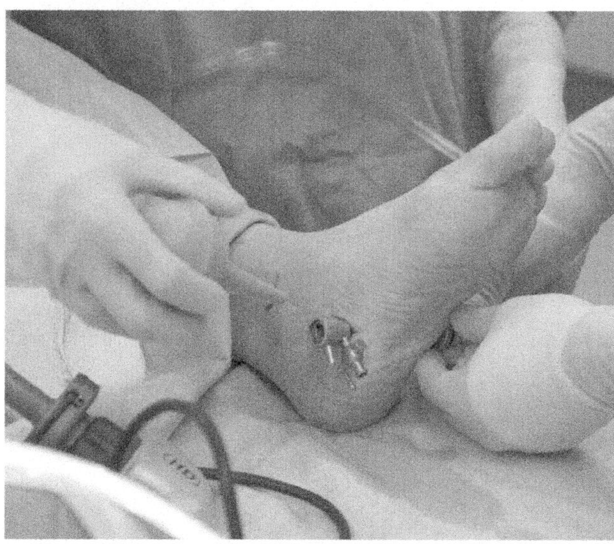

Fig.22. 19 Thes urgicalfi eld isirriga ted

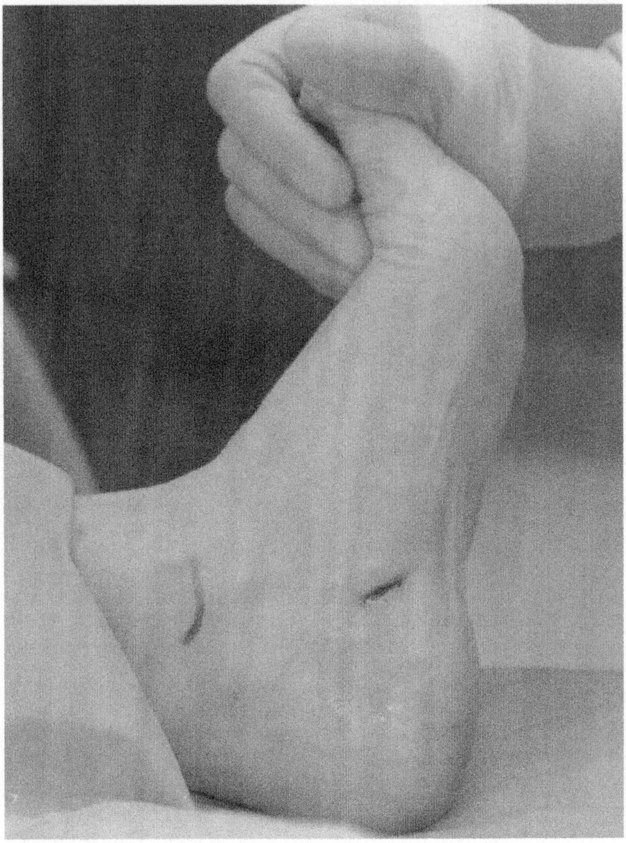

Fig.22.20 Thec annulai s removed

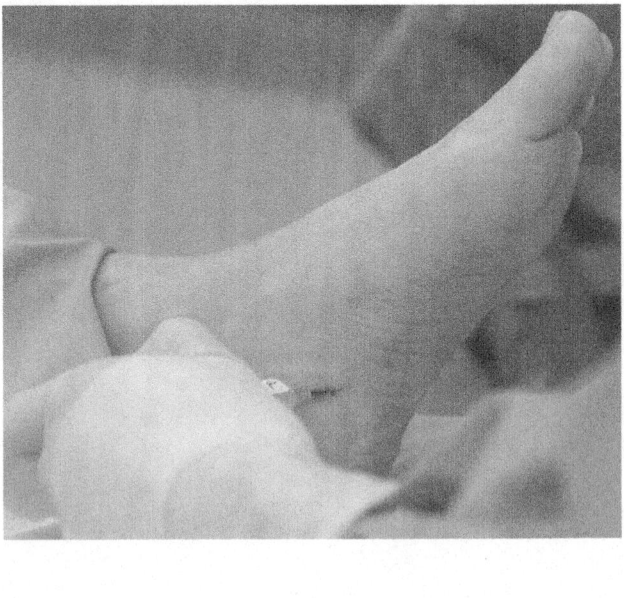

Fig.22.21 An injection of 1 cc of dexamethasone phosphate (4 mg/ml) and 3 cc of 0.5% bupivicaine is administered (at surgeons discretion)

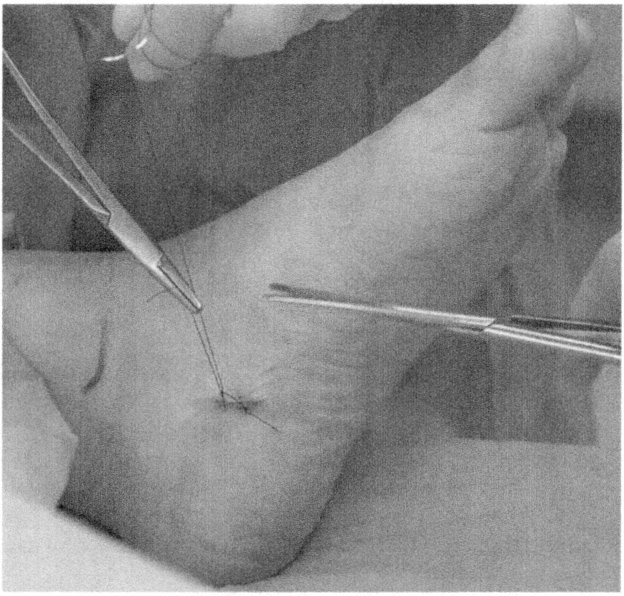

Fig.22. 22 Thes kinis approximated with 3-0 nylon interrupted horizontal sutures

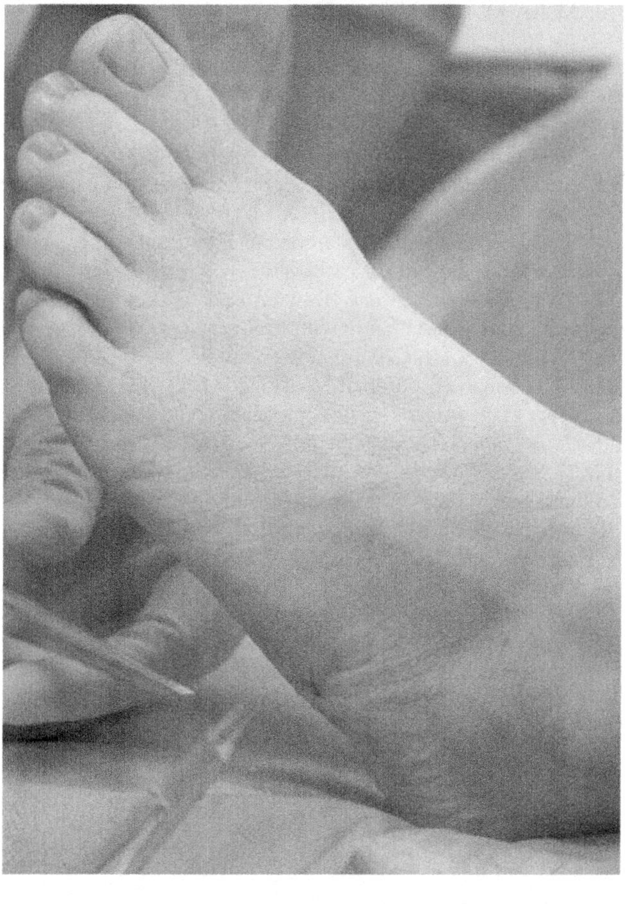

Fig.22. 23 Lateralporta la lso closedw ith3-0nylon

References

1. Lemont H, Ammirati K, Usen N. Plantar Fasciitis: a degenerative process (fasciosis) without acute inflammation. *J Am Podiatr Med Assoc.*2003; 93:234–237.
2. Barrett S, Day S. Endoscopic plantar fasciotomy: preliminary study with cadaveric specimens. *J Foot Ankle Surg.*1991; 30:568–570.
3. Barret S, Day S, Pignetti T, Robinson L. Endoscopic Plantar Fasciotomy: a multi-surgeon prospective analysis of 652 cases. *J Foot Ankle Surg.*1995; 34:400–406.
4. Boberg J, Dauphinee D. Plantar heel. In: Banks A, Downey M, Martin D, Miller S, eds. *McGlamrys Comprehensive Textbook of Foot and Ankle Surgery.* 3rd ed. Philadelphia, PA: Lippincott Williams & Wilkins; 2001:464–477.
5. Brekke M, Green D. Retrospective analysis of minimal incision, endoscopic, and open procedures for heel spur syndrome. *J Am Podiatr Med Assoc.*1998; 88:64–72.
6. Brugh A, Fallat L, Savoy-Moore R. Lateral column symptomatology following plantar fascia release: a prospective study. *J Foot Ankle Surg.*2002; 41:365–371.
7. Hawkins B, Langerman R, Gibbons T, Calhoun J. An anatomic analysis of endoscopic plantar fascia release. *Foot Ankle Int.*1995; 16:552–558.
8. Hofmeister E, Elliot M, Juliano P. Endoscopic plantar fascia release: an anatomical study. *Foot Ankle Int.*1995; 16:719–723.
9. Jeran D, McElgun T, Mirza A, King E. Single portal endoscopic plantar fascial release: operative technique with preliminary results. *Lower Extrem.*1997; 4:103–107.
10. Malley M, Page A, Cook R. Endoscopic plantar fasciotomy for chronic heel pain. *Foot Ankle Int.*2000;21:505 –510.
11. Schepsis A, Leach R, Gorzyca J. Planatr fasciitis: etiology, treatment, surgical results and review of the literature. *Clin Orthop Rel Res.*1991; 266:185–196.
12. Stone P, McClure L. Retrospective analysis of endoscopic plantar fasciotomy. 1994 through 1997. *J Am Podiatr Med Assoc.*1999; 90:89–93.
13. Stone P, Davies J. Retrospective review of endoscopic plantar fasciotomy- 1992 through 1994. *J Am Podiatr Med Assoc.*1996; 86:4141–4420.
14. Saxena A. Uni-portal endoscopic plantar fasciotomy: a prospective study on athletic patients. *Foot Ankle Int.*2004; 25:882–889.
15. Tomczak R, Haverstock B. A retrospective comparison of endoscopic plantar fasciotomy to open plantar fasciotomy with heel spur resection for chronic plantar fasciitis/heel spur syndrome. *J Foot Ankle Surg.*1995; 34:305–311.
16. Zimmerman B, Cardinal M, Cragel M, Goel A, Lane J, Schramm K. Comparison of three types of post-operative management for endoscopic plantar fasciotomy. A retrospective study. *J Am Podiatr Assoc.*2000; 90:247–251.
17. Kinely S, Frascone S, Calderone D, et al. Endoscopic plantar fasciotomy versus traditional heel spur surgery. A prospective study. *J Foot Ankle Surg.*1993; 32:595–603.
18. Rompe JD, Furia J, Weil L, Maffulli N. Shock wave therapy for chronic plantar fasciopathy. *Br Med Bull.*2007; 81–82:183–208.
19. Gentile A, Zizo C, Dahukey A, Berman S. Traumatic pseudoaneurysm of the Lateral plantar artery after endoscopic plantar fasciotomy. *Foot Ankle Int.*1997; 18:821–822.
20. Sammarco G, Idusuyl O. Stress fracture of the third metatarsal after endoscopic plantar fasciotomy: a case report. *Foot Ankle Int.*1998; 19:157–159.

Arthroscopic Os Trigonum Excision 23

Shuji Horibe and Keisuke Kita

23.1 Introduction

The os trigonum is a non-united lateral tubercle on the posterior aspect of the talus with an incidence of between 1.7% and 7.7%.[12] In general, this bone is asymptomatic and treatment is not necessary. However, in athletes with repeated full plantar flexion of the ankle, such as ballet dancers and kicking sports athletes, or even Zen monks, the os trigonum can impinge between the posterior edge of the tibial plafond and the calcaneus and become symptomatic.[3] For this lesion, conservative treatment such as anti-inflammatory medication, physical therapy, orthosis and steroid injection is indicated first. Hedrick and McBryde reported that 12 of 20 patients who had posterior bony impingement respond to nonoperative treatment.[4] Paulos et al. reported that ten of 20 patients respond to conservative treatment. Of these 20 patients, chronic injuries were observed in 17, and only seven of these 17 patients responded to nonoperative management.[11] After failure of conservative management, surgical removal should be considered. Many clinical series of open excision of the os trigonum through the medial or lateral approach are reported to be highly successful.[1,4,6,17] However, postoperative immobilization is usually necessary and it takes a relatively long time to return fully to the previous sports activity level.[1] Compared to the open approach, arthroscopic surgery is less invasive and gives patients a shorter recovery time. Marumoto and Ferkel have first reported the removal of the os trigonum in 11 patients under arthroscopic control in 1997. They used the anterolateral portal for the arthroscope and the posterolateral portal for instruments. [9] Van Dijk et al. advocated the two posterior portals approach for posterior ankle problems and successfully removed the os trigonum using the postero-lateral and postero-medial portals.[16] To avoid the technical difficulties in using the anterolateral portal, or higher risk of damaging posteromedial neurovascular structures during use of the posteromedial portal, we recommend the use of the accessory posterolateral portal for instruments instead.[5]

S. Horibe (✉)
Department of Orthopaedic Sports Medicine, Osaka Rosai Hospital, 1179-3, Nagasone-cho, Kita-ku, Sakai, Osaka, 591-8025, Japan
e-mail: horibe@orh.go.jp

N. Maffulli and M. Easley (eds.), *Minimally Invasive Surgery of the Foot and Ankle*, DOI: 10.1007/978-1-84996-417-3_23, © Springer-Verlag London Limited 2011

23.2 ClinicalExami nation

Patients complain of pain in the posterior part of the ankle. This pain is aggravated with activities involving repeated plantar flexion of the ankle, such as ballet and soccer. There is tenderness on palpation of the posterior aspect of the talus. Passive forced plantar flexion can be helpful to diagnose posterior impingement. If passive forced plantar flexion is negative following local anesthetic infiltration, the diagnosis is confirmed.

23.3 Imaging

Conventional radiographs should include routine antero-posterior and lateral films of the ankle. The os trigonum on the posterior aspect of the talus is best visualized on the lateral view (Fig. 23.1). Van Dijk recommends a lateral radiograph with the foot at 25° of external rotation because the posterolateral part is often superimposed in the medial talar tubercle on a standard lateral radiograph.[15] A stress film in the lateral plane is useful if there is a question of impingement. A Broden view will show any involvement of the posterior subtalar joint. As the radiography does not show the exact morphology of the os trigonum (Fig. 23.2a), a computed tomography (CT) scan, especially a multiple planar reconstruc-

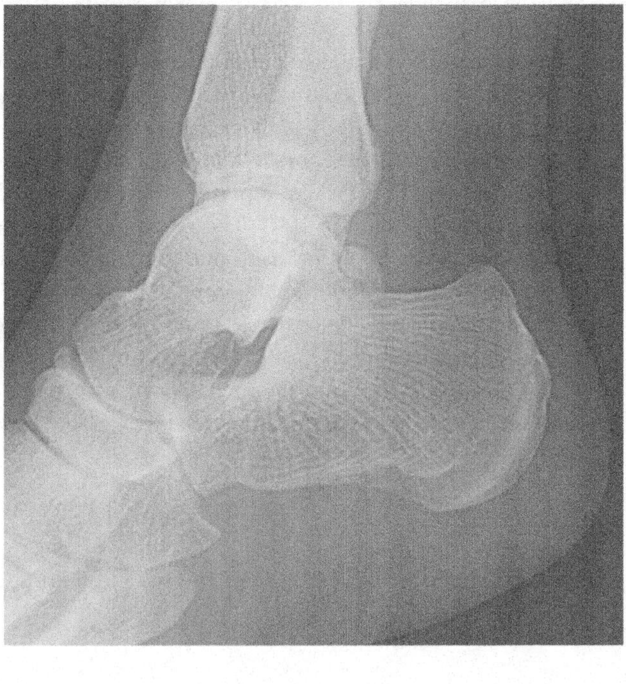

Fig.23.1 Lateralra diograph of the ankle. The os trigonum is shown on the posteriora spectof t het alus

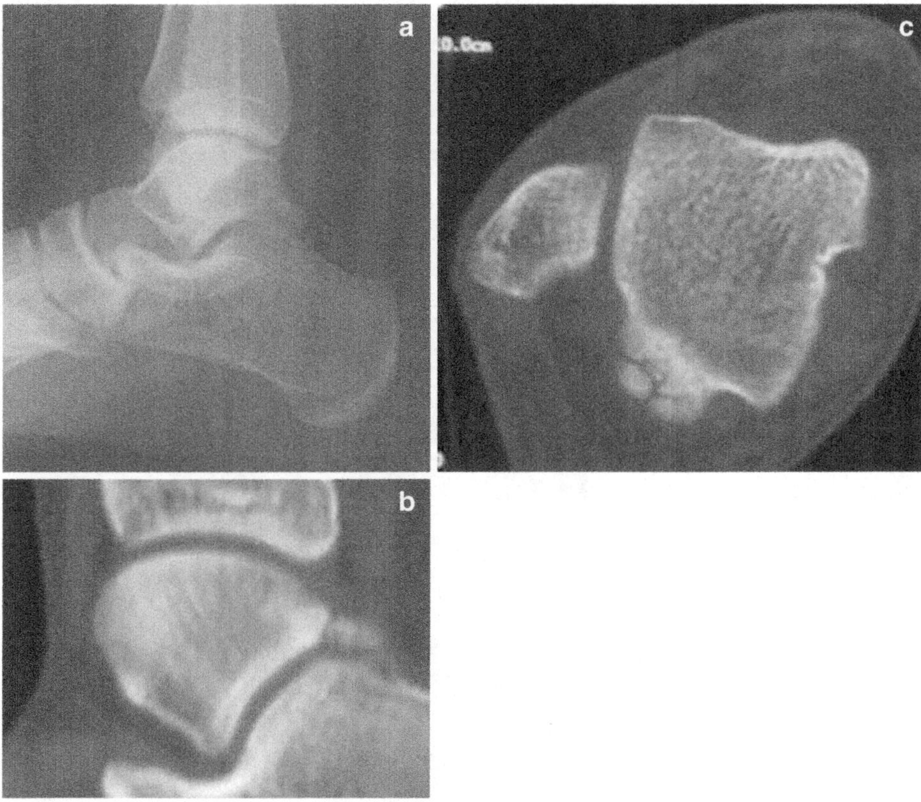

Fig. 23.2 Preoperative images (**a**) Lateral radiographs do not always show the exact morphology of the os trigonum. ((**b**) and (**c**))A C Tr econstructionc anhe lpp re-operative

tion, is helpful (Fig. 23.2b, c). As the morphology is varied, and multiple fragments of the os trigonum occasionally exist, reconstructed CT is necessary before operation (Fig. 23.3a, b). A bone scan can be used to determine whether the os trigonum is symptomatic, but care must be taken because the presence of increased uptake does not always correlate with symptoms(Fig. 23.4).[14]

23.4 Indication

The indication for surgical excision of the os trigonum is persistent pain in the posterior part of the ankle despite a minimum of 3 months of conservative treatment. Conservative treatment includes anti-inflammatory medication, physical therapy, orthosis, and local steroidi njection.

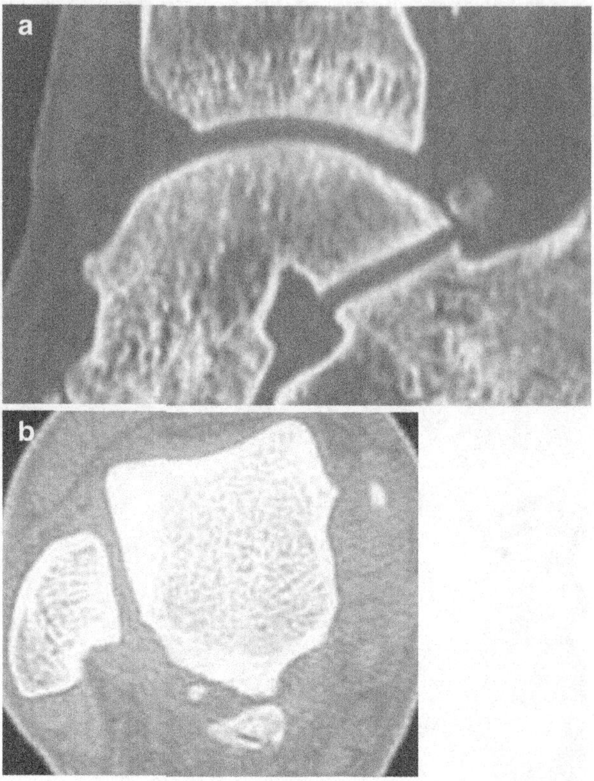

Fig.23.3 CTre construction. Multiple fragments of the os trigonum are occasionally present. Sagittal (**a**) and axial (**b**) CT scan images showed two fragmentsof t heos t rigonum

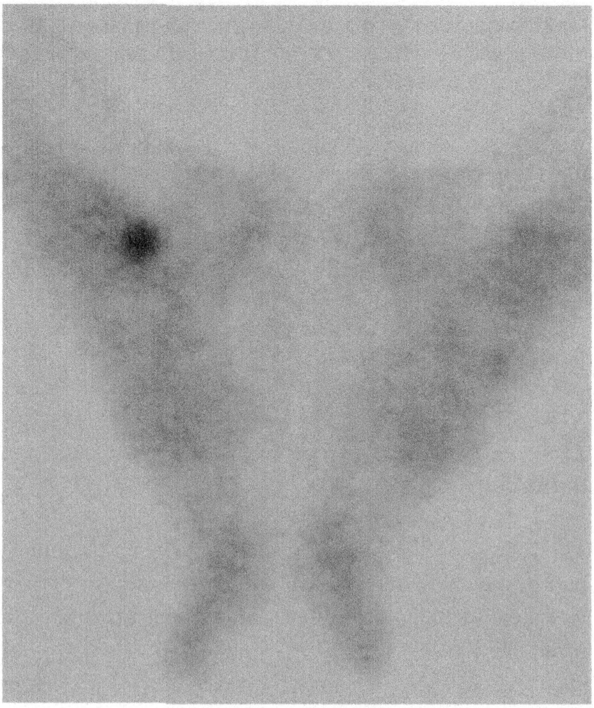

Fig.23.4 Bones can.Inc reased uptake on the posterior aspect of ther ighta nklej oint

23.5 Contraindication

All endoscopic or arthroscopic surgery requires technical proficiency. This technique can be performed easily and safely, but should be performed only by skilled arthroscopist.

23.6 Surgical Technique

The patient is placed in the prone position under general or spinal anesthesia. A small pillow is placed under the dorsal aspect of the ankle joint to leave the foot to drop under gravity. A thigh tourniquet or a distraction strap is necessary. A 23-gauge spinal needle is inserted into the posterior aspect of the subtalar joint 5 mm proximal to the tip of the fibula, just lateral to the border of the Achilles tendon (Fig. 23.5a). Ten milliliters saline are infused into the subtalar joint, and a 5 mm vertical skin incision is made using a # 11 scalpel in the same place where the needle stabs for a posterolateral portal. Only the skin is incised, and the subcutaneous tissue is bluntly split with a mosquito clamp not to damage the sural nerve (Fig. 23.5b). A blunt trocar with the attached cannula is introduced into the subtalar joint, followed by a 4 mm 30° arthroscope. The secondary accessory posterolateral portal for instruments is then established from the point just posterior to the peroneal tendon sheath at the same level as the posterolateral portal. A # 23 spinal needle is inserted for the orientation of the accessory posterolateral portal under arthroscopic control (Fig. 23.5c). As for the posterolateral portal, only the skin is incised for length of 5 mm and the subcutaneous tissue is bluntly split with a mosquito clamp under arthroscopic visualization. A power shaver is introduced through the accessory posterolateral portal, and the surrounding soft tissues are debrided (Fig. 23.5d). This makes it possible to visualize the os trigonum and expand the space to work, but the debridement of the soft tissues should be always performed under arthroscopic visualization not to damage other important tissues. An os trigonum usually has fibrous adhesions to the talus and a periosteal elevator is used to release bluntly the fibrous tissue between the os trigonum and the talus (Fig. 23.6a, b). Then the os trigonum is completely excised with a grasper to visualize the flexor hallucis longus tendon (Fig. 23.7a, b). The excision can be achieved piece by piece if en bloc excision is not successful. When a small piece of bone impinges the flexor hallucis longus tendon, it is carefully removed until the impingement is free (Fig. 23.8a, b). Radiographic control is helpful to check the position of the arthroscope, if it happens to be inserted into the ankle joint due to the reduced subtalar joint space (Fig. 23.9).

23.7 PostoperativeC are

No immobilization is necessary. Full weight bearing is allowed as tolerated, depending on the residual pain and the capability of the patient to walk normally. Rehabilitation of range

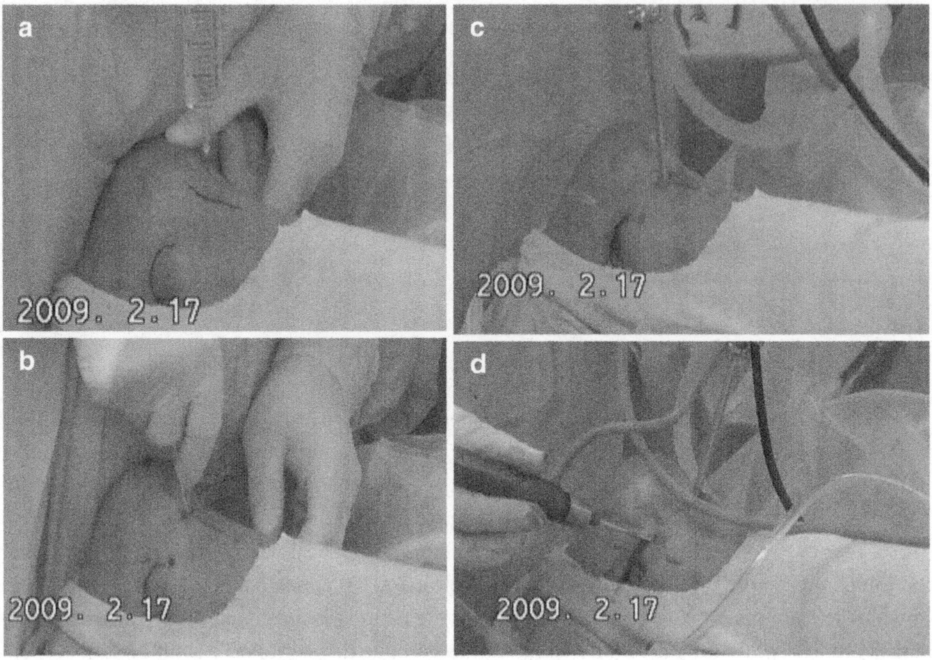

Fig. 23.5 Posterolateral and accessory posterolateral portals. (**a**) A 23-gauge spinal needle is inserted into the posterior aspect of the subtalar joint 5 mm proximal to the tip of the fibula, just lateral to the border of the Achilles tendon and 10 mL of saline are infused into the subtalar joint. (**b**) A 5 mm vertical skin incision is made using a #11 scalpel in the same location where the needle had been inserted to produce the postero-lateral portal. Only the skin is incised, and the subcutaneous tissues are bluntly split with a mosquito clamp. (**c**) A #23 spinal needle is inserted for the orientation of the accessory posterolateral portal under arthroscopic control. (**d**) As for the posterolateral portal, only the skin is incised for a length of 5 mm, and the subcutaneous tissues are bluntly split with a mosquito clamp under arthroscopic visualization. A power shaver is introduced through the accessory posterolateral portal, and the surrounding soft tissues are debrided

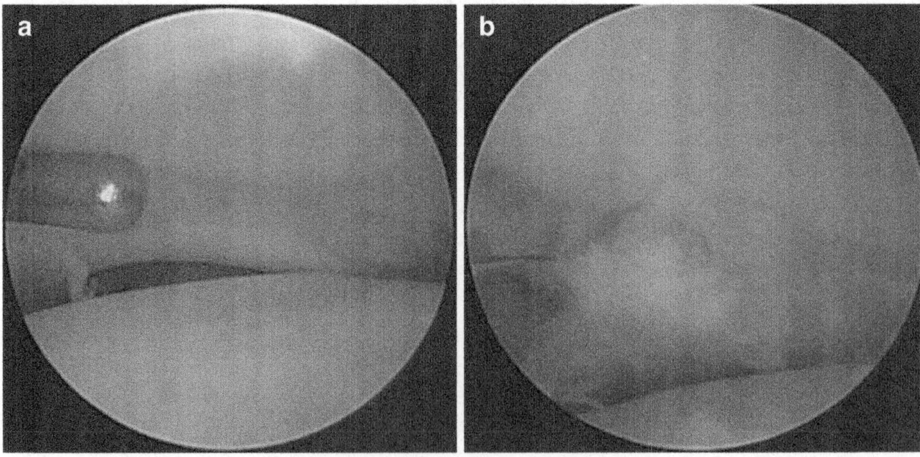

Fig. 23.6 Arthroscopic view (**a**) The os trigonum presents fibrous adhesions to the talus. (**b**) An elevator is used to release the fibrous tissue between the os trigonum and the talus

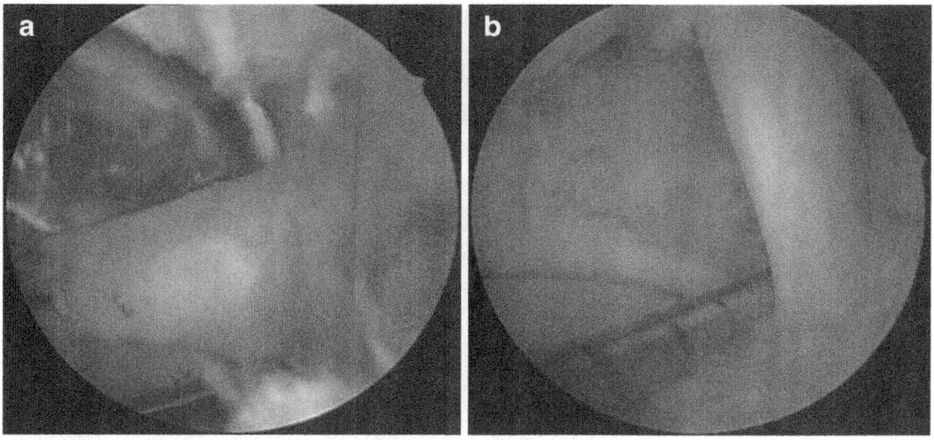

Fig. 23.7 Arthroscopic view (**a**) The os trigonum is removed with a grasper. (**b**) The bone is removed until the flexorha llucisl ongust endoni svi sualized

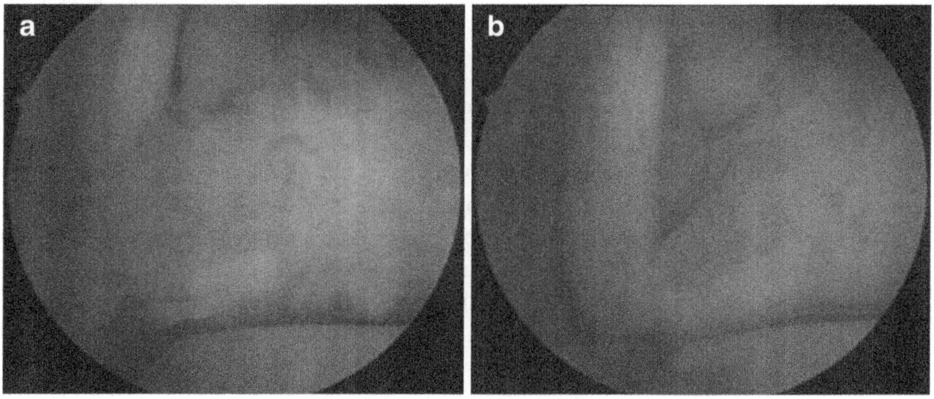

Fig. 23.8 Arthroscopic view (**a**) A small piece of bone still impinges on the tendon of the flexor hallucis longus. (**b**) The fragment is removed, and the impingement is freed

motion exercise and muscle strength training are not usually required. Previous sports activity is permitted once pain has subsided.

23.8 Resultsa ndC omplications

Fifteen feet in 12 patients have undergone arthroscopic os trigonum excision with sufficient follow-up time to determine the effectiveness of this procedure. There were nine

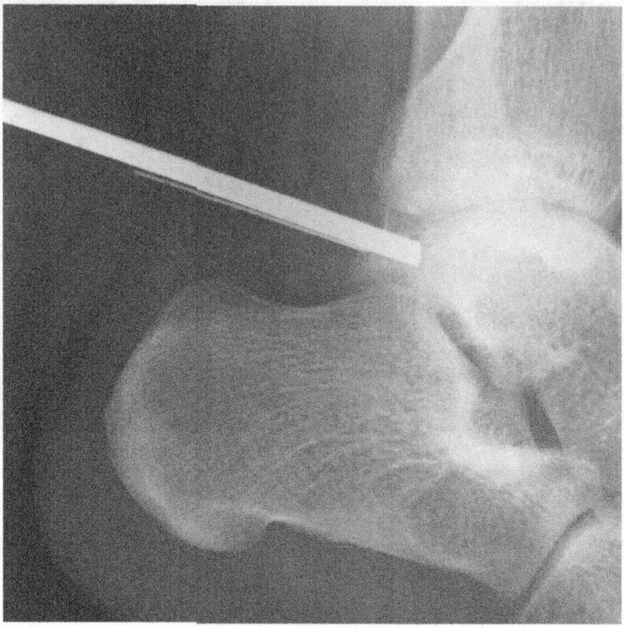

Fig. 23.9 Radiographic control. Radiographic control is helpful to check the position of the arthroscope

male and three female patients, with a mean age of 20, ranging from 14 to 30 years at the time of operation. All patients were engaged in sports. The mean time from the onset of symptoms to surgery was 17 months, with range of 5–50 months. The os trigonum was successfully removed under arthroscopic control in all patients. There were no complications such as neurovascular injuries. All patients returned to their previous sports activity within 3 months, and the mean American Orthopaedic Foot & Ankle Society score improved from 71 to 99. No patients had any symptoms except for one complaining of slight pain during strenuous sports activity at the 2-year follow-up.

23.9 Discussion

Arthroscopic surgery is less invasive, providing precise identification of the pathology and complete excision of the os trigonum, with an early return to the previous activity level while minimizing soft-tissue complication. Several reports on subtalar arthroscopy have been published since the first report by Parisien in 1985.[10] In 1997, Marumoto and Ferkel first described arthroscopic excision of an os trigonum. Their procedure involved using antero-lateral and postero-lateral portals, with the patients supine. They visualized the os trigonum through anterolateral portal using a 2.7 mm 70° arthroscope,[9] but the procedure is technically demanding. Lombardi et al. reported a single patient in whom the os trigonum was excised using two stacked posterolateral portals in the lateral decubitus position. The skin was incised horizontally, and two stacked portals were produced on the lateral border of the Achilles tendon.[8] Although the procedure was successful, sural nerve injury is a concern.

The two posterior portal arthroscopic approach with the patient prone was described in 2000.[16] The authors describe how to produce the postero-medial portal in a safe manner avoiding risk of injury to the posterior tibial neurovascular structures. In their study, the neurovascular structures are protected by using the arthroscope shaft from the posterolateral portal as a guide for the instrument to travel in the direction of the joint. To avoid possible injuries to the neurovascular bundle, a device from posteromedial portal should always be operated on the lateral side of the flexor hallucis longus tendon. Recent studies verified that this technique is relatively safe, and that it has the potential to increase the arthroscopic working area in the posterior subtalar joint.[7,13,18] Recently, Allegra et al.[2] has reported two postero-medial portals procedure in the supine position. This unique technique makes it possible to treat the patients with both the anterior and posterior pathologies of the ankle. However, this posteromedial approach still carries the risk of injury to the tibial nerve, which would be more serious as it could result in loss of the vital protective sensation on the sole of the foot. Unpublished data from the same group reported three cases with a temporary diminished sensibility of the heel out of the 140 cases of prone subtalar arthroscopy, probably due to the variable bifurcation of the calcaneal branch from the posterior tibial nerve.

There are two more posterior portals available: the trans–Achilles portal, and the accessory posterolateral portal. The trans-Achilles portal involves no risk to neurovascular structures, but nevertheless it is not advisable due to the risk of damage to the vulnerable Achilles tendon. On the other hand, no complication was found in our series in which the accessory portal close to the sural nerve and the small saphenous vein was utilized. To avoid injury to these neurovascular structures, the accessory posterolateral portal should be produced just posterior to the peroneal tendon sheath by blunt dissection of the soft tissues to the subtalar joint using a mosquito clamp at the same level as the posterolateral portal.

23.10 Conclusion

Compared to an open surgical resection requiring extensive exposure with the risk of infection or sural nerve injury, arthroscopic resection of the symptomatic os trigonum is a less invasive surgical technique with no risk of complications, a shorter recovery period and better clinical outcomes. Arthroscopic excision of a symptomatic os trigonum using the posterolateral portal for visualization and the accessory posterolateral portal for instrumentation is safe and effective.

Acknowledgments The authors report no conflictof i nterest.

References

1. Abramowitz Y, Wollstein R, Barzilay Y, London E, Matan Y, Shabat S, Nyska M. Outcome of resection of a symptomatic os trigonum. *J Bone Joint Surg Am.* 2003;85-A:1051–1057.
2. Allegra F, Maffulli N, Cerza F, Delianni E. Postero-medial approach procedure in the supine position for one-step anterior and posterior ankle arthroscopy. *Sports Med Arthrosc.* 2009;17:185–189.
3. Chao W. Os trigonum. *Foot Ankle Clin.* 2004;9:787–796, vii.
4. Hedrick MR, McBryde AM. Posterior ankle impingement. *Foot Ankle Int.* 1994;15:2–8.
5. Horibe S, Kita K, Natsu-ume T, Hamada M, Mae T, Shino K. A novel technique of arthroscopic excision of a symptomatic os trigonum. *Arthroscopy.* 2008;24:121 e1–4.
6. Howse AJ. Posterior block of the ankle joint in dancers. *Foot Ankle.* 1982;3:81–84.
7. Jerosch J, Fadel M. Endoscopic resection of a symptomatic os trigonum. *Knee Surg Sports Traumatol Arthrosc.* 2006;14:1188–1193.
8. Lombardi CM, Silhanek AD, Connolly FG. Modified arthroscopic excision of the symptomatic os trigonum and release of the flexor hallucis longus tendon: operative technique and case study. *J Foot Ankle Surg.* 1999;38:347–351.
9. Marumoto JM, Ferkel RD. Arthroscopic excision of the os trigonum: a new technique with preliminary clinical results. *Foot Ankle Int.* 1997;18:777–784.
10. Parisien JS, Vangsness T. Arthroscopy of the subtalar joint: an experimental approach. *Arthroscopy.* 1985;1:53–57.
11. Paulos LE, Johnson CL, Noyes FR. Posterior compartment fractures of the ankle. A commonly missed athletic injury. *Am J Sports Med.* 1983;11:439–443.
12. Sarrafian SK. Anatomy of the foot and ankle: descriptive, topographic, functional. *Lippincott.* 1983;18:52–53, 94.
13. Scholten PE, Sierevelt IN, van Dijk CN. Hindfoot endoscopy for posterior ankle impingement. *J Bone Joint Surg Am.* 2008;90:2665–2672.
14. Sopov V, Liberson A, Groshar D. Bone scintigraphic findings of os trigonum: a prospective study of 100 soldiers on active duty. *Foot Ankle Int.* 2000;21:822–824.
15. van Dijk CN. Anterior and posterior ankle impingement. *Foot Ankle Clin N AM.* 2006;11:663–683.
16. van Dijk CN, Scholten PE, Krips R. A 2-portal endoscopic approach for diagnosis and treatment of posterior ankle pathology. *Arthroscopy.* 2000;16:871–876.
17. Veazey BL, Heckman JD, Galindo MJ, McGanity PL. Excision of united fractures of the posterior process of the talus: a treatment for chronic posterior ankle pain. *Foot Ankle.* 1992;13:453–457.
18. Willits K, Sonneveld H, Amendola A, Giffin JR, Griffin S, Fowler PJ. Outcome of posterior ankle arthroscopy for hindfoot impingement. *Arthroscopy.* 2008;24:196–202.

Endoscopic Calcaneoplasty

24

Maayke Nadine van Sterkenburg, Peter Albert Johannes de Leeuw, and Cornelis Nicolaas van Dijk

24.1 Introduction

In 1928, the Swedish orthopedic surgeon Patrick Haglund described a patient with a painful hindfoot caused by a prominent posterosuperior aspect of the calcaneus in conjunction with a sharp rigid heel counter.[1] The term Haglund's disease, deformity and syndrome have been used interchangeably, but have also been described as different entities by others.

Nowadays, the term "Haglund's *deformity*" is used to describe tenderness and pain on the posterolateral aspect of the calcaneus. On physical examination, a bony prominence can be palpated at this location. This entity is described by a variety of different names such as "pump-bump,"[2] "cucumber heel,"[3] "high-prow heels"[4] and "winter heel."[3]

There is more uncertainty on the definition of Haglund's *disease*. It is described to be a synonym for deformity or syndrome, but has also been referred to as an osteochondrosis of the accessory navicular bone.[5–7] For this reason, it will not be considered in this chapter.

In Haglund's *syndrome*, the retrocalcaneal bursa is inflamed with concomitant swelling. The swelling is present on both sides of the Achilles tendon at the level of the posterosuperior calcaneal prominence, sometimes in combination with insertional tendinopathy of the Achilles tendon. The syndrome is caused by repetitive impingement of the retrocalcaneal bursa between the anterior aspect of the Achilles tendon and the enlarged posterosuperior aspect of the calcaneus. It occurs most often at the end of the second or the third decade, mainly in females, and is often bilateral. However, it may occur in both sexes and at any age.

In this chapter, the diagnosis and endoscopic treatment for patients with complaints of a retrocalcaneal bursitis as a part of Haglund's deformity and Haglund's syndrome are described.

M.N. van Sterkenburg (✉)
Department of Orthopaedic Surgery, Academic Medical Center, University of Amsterdam, 227001 100, DE Amsterdam, The Netherlands
e-mail: m.n.vansterkenburg@amc.uva.nl

N. Maffulli and M. Easley (eds.), *Minimally Invasive Surgery of the Foot and Ankle*,
DOI: 10.1007/978-1-84996-417-3_24, © Springer-Verlag London Limited 2011

24.2 Diagnosis

Patients typically describe the onset of pain when starting to walk after a period of rest.

The distinction between Haglund's deformity, Haglund's syndrome, and other pathologic conditions of the posterior aspect of the heel, most importantly Achilles tendinopathy, should be made.

Insertional tendinopathy is defined as a tendinopathy of the tendon at its insertion. The pain is most frequently located in the midline at the insertion into the calcaneus. Co-existence with retrocalcaneal bursitis is known.

In Haglund's deformity, a bony prominence can be seen at the posterosuperolateral aspect of the heel, which is painful on palpation. The superficial bursa may be swollen, and the overlying skin can be thickened and dyschromic. A retrocalcaneal bursitis occasionally develops as a result of this deformity.

In Haglund's syndrome, on physical examination swelling can be seen on both sides of the tendon at the level of the posterosuperior calcaneal prominence, and pain can be reproduced by palpation of the lateral and medial side of the Achilles tendon at this level (Fig. 24.1). With dorsiflexion of the ankle, the anterior part of the tendon impinges against the

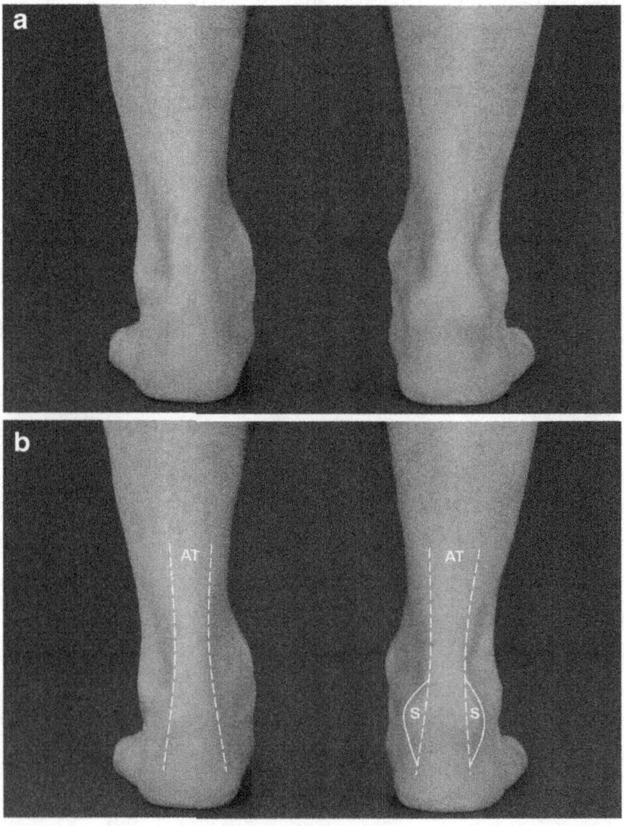

Fig.24. 1 (**a**) A patient with Haglund's syndrome in the right hindfoot. (**b**)The typical swelling (S) on both sides of the Achilles tendon (AT) at the level of the posterosuperior calcaneal prominencei si ndicated

posterosuperior rim of the calcaneus, leading to retrocalcaneal bursitis. A hindfoot varus and a pes cavus are both predisposing factors for heel pain. In the cavus foot, the calcaneus is not only in varus malalignment, but it is also more vertical, which results in a more prominent projection posteriorly.[8]

24.3 Management

Multiple options have been described to manage chronic retrocalcaneal bursitis, including avoidance of tight shoe heel counters, cast immobilization, NSAIDs, activity modification, padding, shock wave treatment, physical therapy and a single injection of corticosteroids into the retrocalcaneal space. If conservative management fails, there are essentially two distinct operative methods, and one endoscopic surgical technique. The open operative alternatives include resection of the posterosuperior part of the calcaneus or a calcaneal wedge osteotomy. Complications include skin breakdown, tenderness in the region of the operative scar, esthetically non-appealing operative scars and altered sensation around the heel.[9–13] More serious complications include Achilles tendon avulsions and calcaneal (stress) fractures.[11,12,14] Recurrent persistent pain secondary to an inadequate amount of bone resected, and stiffness of the Achilles tendon resulting in decreased dorsiflexion have also been reported.[15] Wound healing problems have been described in 30% of patients treated with open procedures.[16]

24.4 Endoscopic Treatment

Endoscopic treatment offers advantages that are related to any minimal invasive surgical procedure, such as a low morbidity, excellent scar healing, functional aftertreatment, short recovery time and a shorter time to sport resumption as compared to open surgical approaches. Here we describe the technique of endoscopic calcaneoplasty, and compare the results of this minimal invasive technique[17] with those reported for the open surgical techniques.

24.4.1 Indication

Patient complaints include pain at rest, when standing, walking (uphill), running and walking on hard surfaces. Conventional lateral radiographs show hypertrophy of the posterosuperior aspect of the calcaneus and deep retrocalcaneal bursitis, identified by diminished radiolucency of the retrocalcaneal recess and the lower portion of Kager's triangle (Fig. 24.2).

If conservative treatment fails, we undertake endoscopic surgery.

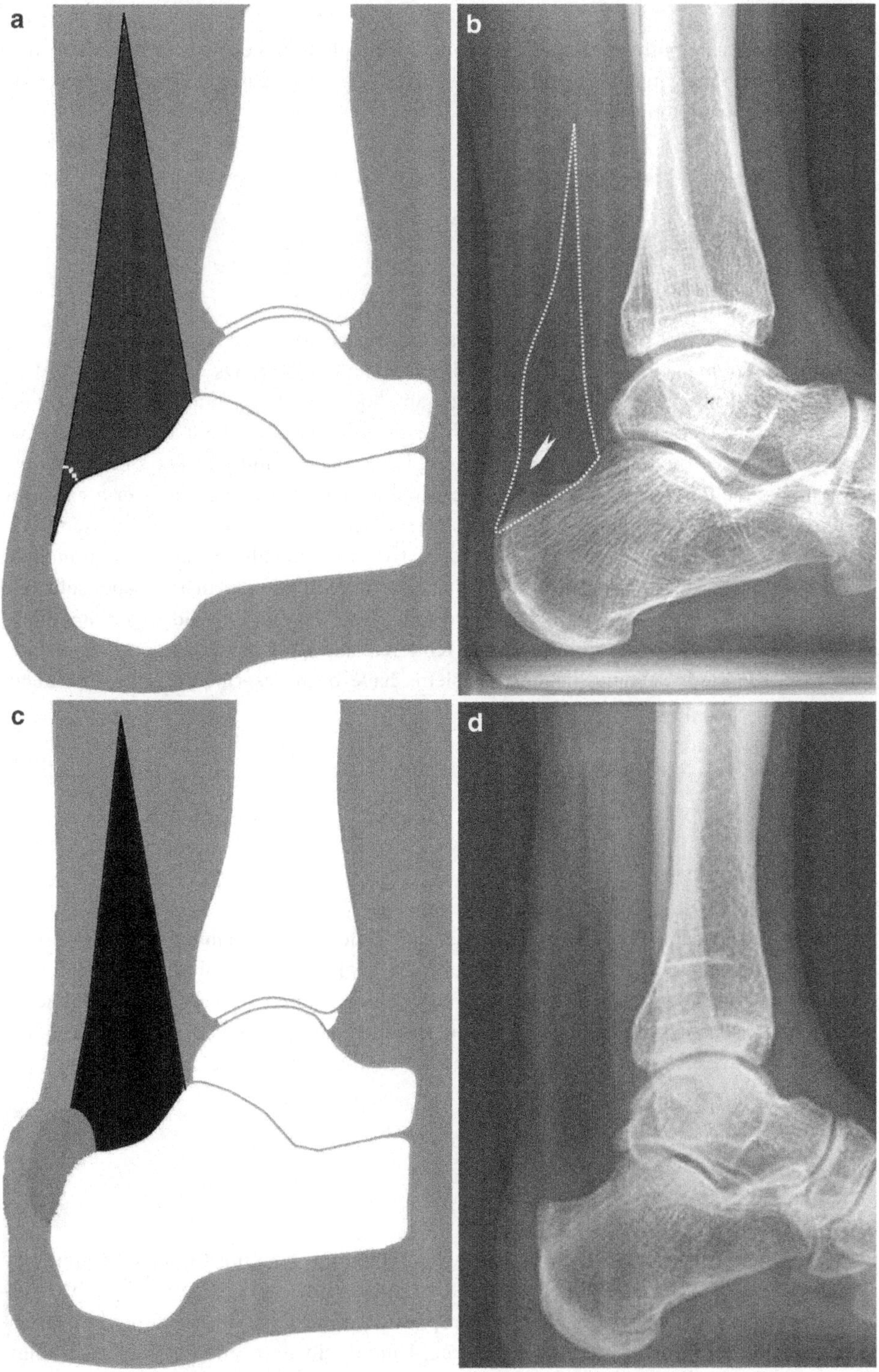
a
b
c
d

24.4.2 Surgical Technique

Surgery is performed with the patient in prone position under general or regional anesthesia. The involved leg is marked with an arrow by the patient, to avoid wrong side surgery. The feet are positioned just over the edge of the operation table. The involved leg is slightly elevated by placing a bolster under the lower leg (Fig. 24.3).

The position of the foot is in plantarflexion through gravity. Prior to surgery important anatomical structures are marked. These include the medial and lateral border of the Achilles tendon and the calcaneus (Fig. 24.4).

The lateral portal is made first, just lateral of the Achilles tendon at the level of the superior aspect of the calcaneus. This portal is produced as a small vertical incision through the skin only. The retrocalcaneal space is penetrated with a blunt trocar. A 4.5 mm arthroscopic shaft with an inclination angle of 30° is introduced (Fig. 24.5).

Irrigation is performed by gravity flow. A 70° arthroscope can also be used but is seldom necessary. Under direct vision, a spinal needle is introduced just medial to the Achilles tendon, again at the level of the superior aspect of the calcaneus, to locate the medial portal (Fig. 24.6).

After having prepared the medial portal by a vertical stab incision, a 5.5 mm bonecutter shaver (Dyonics Bonecutter, Smith & Nephew, Andover, USA) is introduced and visualized by the arthroscope. The inflamed retrocalcaneal bursa is removed first (Fig. 24.7) to provide a better view. Now the superior surface of the calcaneus is visualized and its fibrous layer and periosteum are stripped off. During resection of the bursa and the fibrous layer and periosteum of the superior aspect of the calcaneus, the full radius resector is facing the bone to avoid damage to the Achilles tendon.

When the foot is brought into full dorsiflexion, impingement between the posterosuperior calcaneal edge and the Achilles tendon can be perceived. The foot is subsequently brought into plantarflexion and now the posterosuperior calcaneal rim is removed. This bone is quite soft and can be removed by the aggressive synovial full radius resector or bone cutter. A burr is not needed at this point. The portals are used interchangeably for both the arthroscope and the resector, so as to remove the entire bony prominence. It is important to remove a sufficient amount of bone at the posteromedial and lateral corner (Fig. 24.8). These edges have to be rounded off by moving the synovial resector beyond the posterior edge onto the lateral respectively medial wall of the calcaneus.

Fig. 24.2 (**a**) Schematic lateral view of a hindfoot showing Kager's triangle (black). (**b**) Plain conventional lateral standing radiograph of an ankle with a normal aspect of the bony and soft tissues in the hindfoot. Kager's triangle is indicated (dotted line). The arrow points at the retrocalcaneal recess. (**c**) Kager's triangle is schematically drawn (black). Indicated in red is the fluid-filled retrocalcaneal bursa. (**d**) Lateral standing radiograph of a patient's right ankle showing hypertrophy of the posterosuperior aspect of the calcaneus with infiltration of the retrocalcaneal recess of Kager's triangle by the fluid-filledr etrocalcanealbur sa

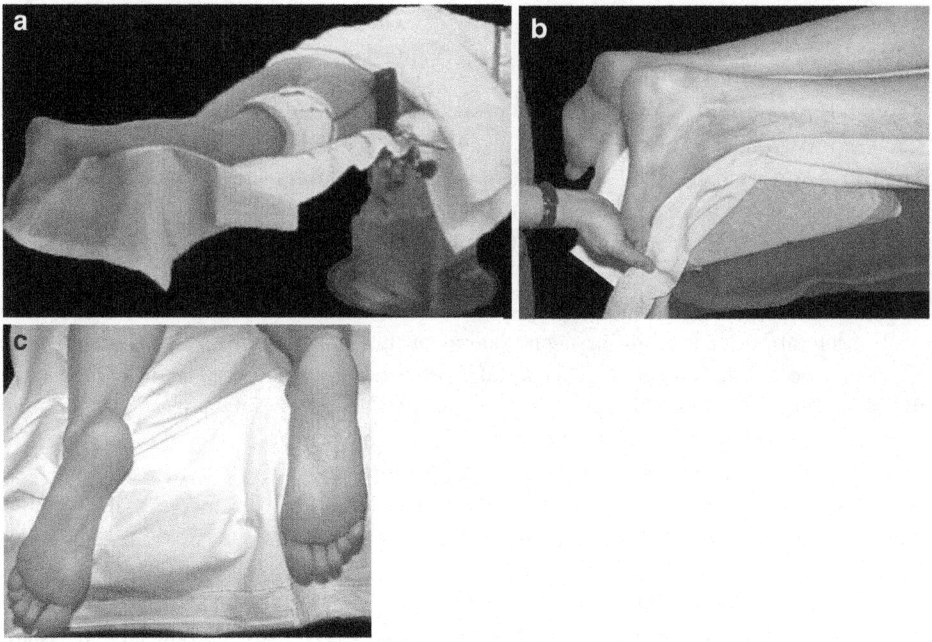

Fig. 24.3 The patient is placed in prone position (**a**). The affected right leg is placed on a bolster and right over the end of the table (**b**). The other foot is positioned in a way that the surgeon has sufficient working area (**c**)

The Achilles tendon is protected throughout the entire procedure by keeping the closed end of the resector against the tendon. With the foot in full plantarflexion, the insertion of the Achilles tendon can be visualized.

The bonecutter is placed on the insertion against the calcaneus to smoothen this part of the calcaneus. Finally, the resector is introduced to clean up loose debris and to smooth possible rough edges. In the first several patients, fluoroscopic control can be used to ascertain whether sufficient bone has been resected. With some experience, this will no longer be necessary. Figure 24.9 shows an endoscopic view of the end result.

To prevent sinus formation, at the end of the procedure the skin incisions are closed with 3.0 Ethilon sutures. The incisions and surrounding skin are injected with 10 mL of a 0.5% bupivacain/morphine solution. A sterile compressive dressing is applied (Klinigrip, Medeco BV, Oud Bijerland, The Netherlands).

24.4.3 Post-operativeM anagement

Postoperatively, the patient is allowed weight-bearing as tolerated and is instructed to elevate the foot when not walking. The dressing is removed 3 days postoperatively, after which the patient is allowed to shower. Patients are encouraged to perform active range

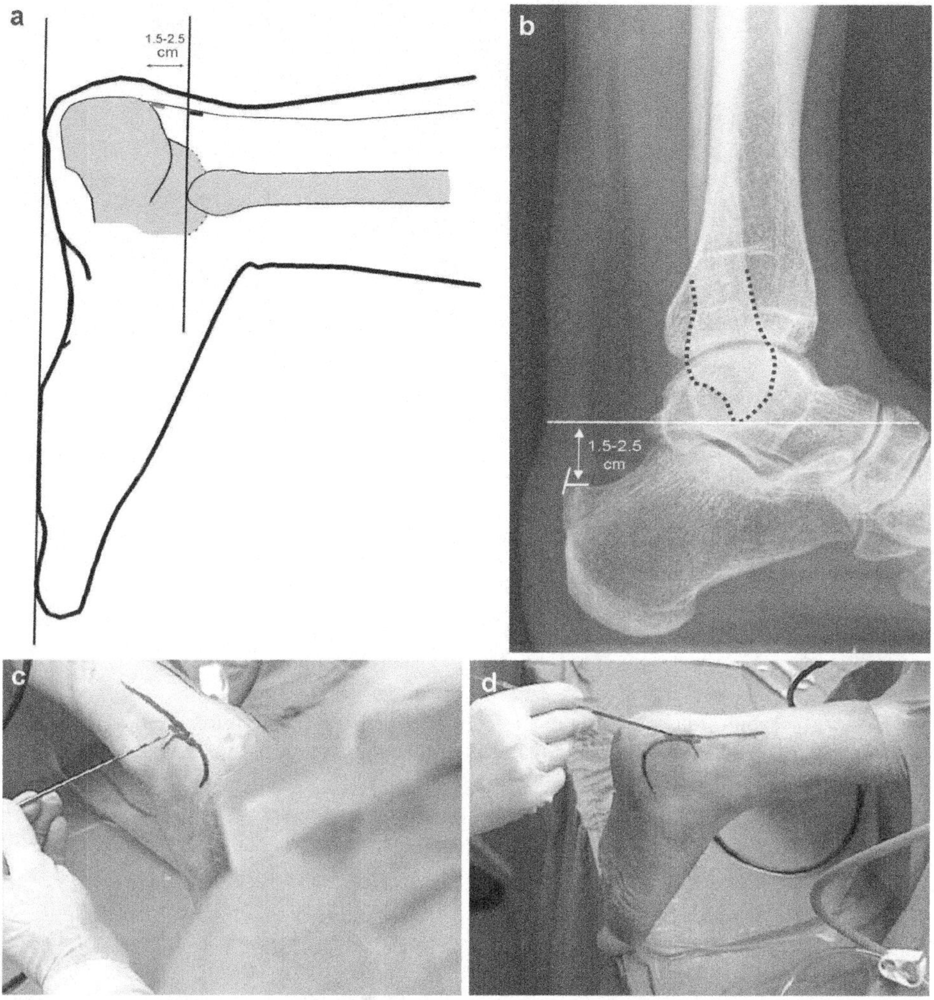

Fig. 24.4 (**a**) Schematic drawing of lateral view of the foot. The ankle is placed in plantigrade position. A line is drawn through the tip of the fibula parallel to the sole of the foot. The incision for the lateral portal in conventional posterior arthroscopy is placed directly above this line; the center of the incision in patients undergoing endoscopic calcaneoplasty is placed 1.5–2.5 cm below this line (red). (**b**) Preoperatively this can be verified by drawing these same lines on a lateral standing radiograph of the foot. (**c**) Location of lateral and medial (**d**) portal as indicated by the probe (red line)

of motion exercises for at least three times a day for 10 min each. The patient is allowed to return to wearing regular shoes as soon as tolerated. The sutures are removed after 2 weeks. A conventional lateral radiograph is made to ensure that sufficient bone has been excised (Fig. 24.10). With satisfaction of the surgeon and patient, no further outpatient department contact is necessary. Patients with limited range of motion are directed to a physiotherapist.

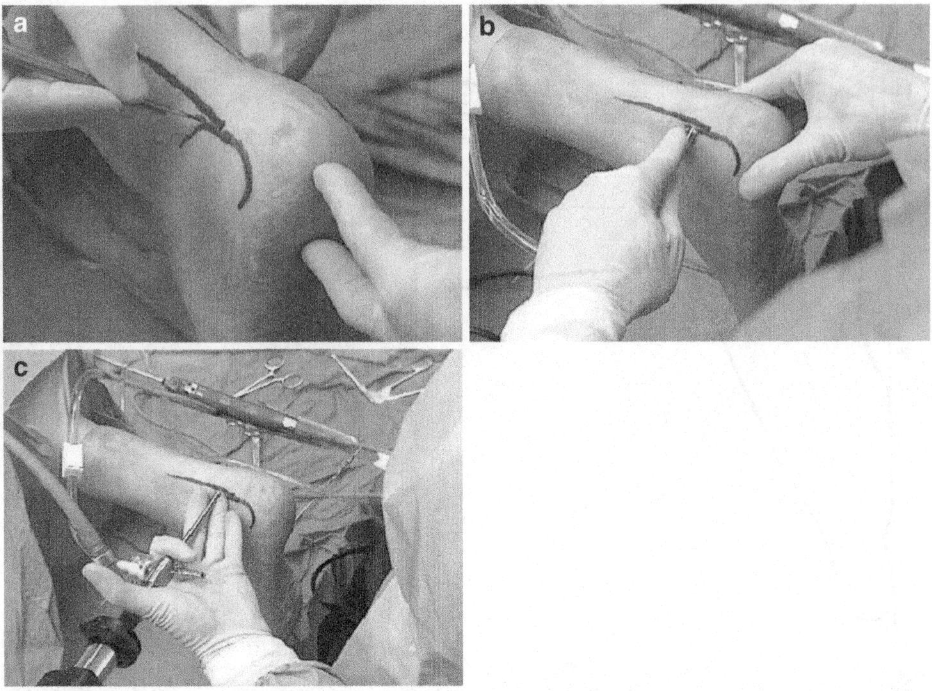

Fig. 24.5 (**a**) Incision for lateral portal in a left ankle. (**b**) Penetration of retrocalcaneal space with blunt trocar followed by blunt dissection. (**c**) Introduction of arthroscope with 30° inclination angle

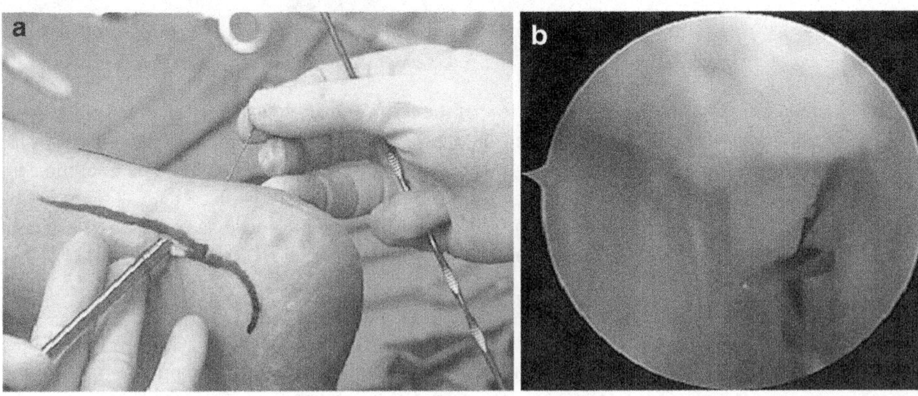

Fig. 24.6 (**a**) Introduction of spinal needle (left ankle) under direct vision (**b**) for placement of medialpor tal

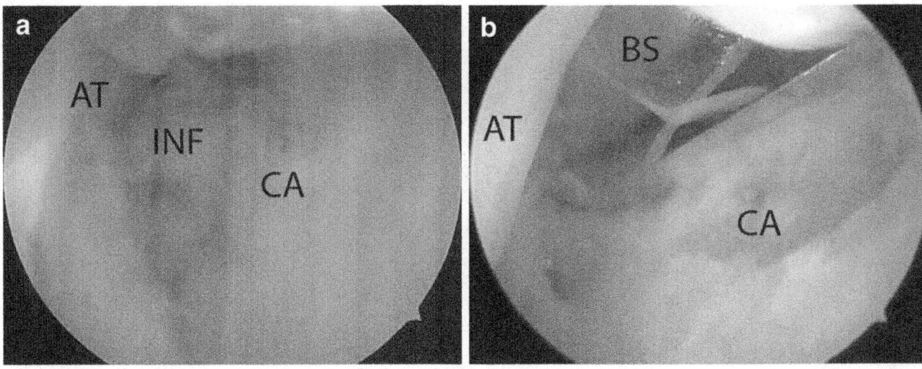

Fig. 24.7 Endoscopic calcaneoplasty of the right hindfoot of a 38-year-old female patient with retrocalcaneal bursitis. (**a**) The retrocalcaneal recess. *AT* Achilles tendon, *INF* inflamed retrocalcaneal bursa, *CA* calcaneus. (**b**) Retrocalcaneal bursa is removed with bonecutter shaver. *BS* bonecutters haver

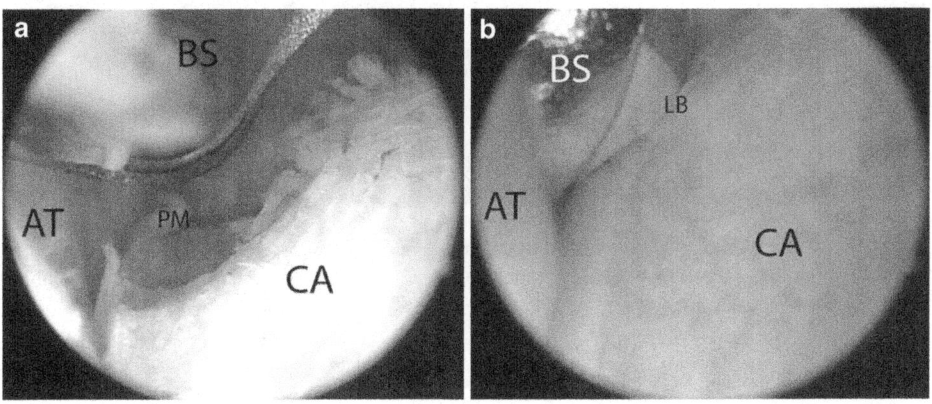

Fig. 24.8 (**a**) Removal of bone at the posteromedial border of the calcaneus with arthroscope in the lateral portal. (**b**) Removal of bone at the lateral border of the calcaneus after change of portals. *AT* Achilles tendon, *BS* bonecutter shaver, *PM* posteromedial border of calcaneus, *LB* posterolateral border of calcaneus, *CA*c alcaneus

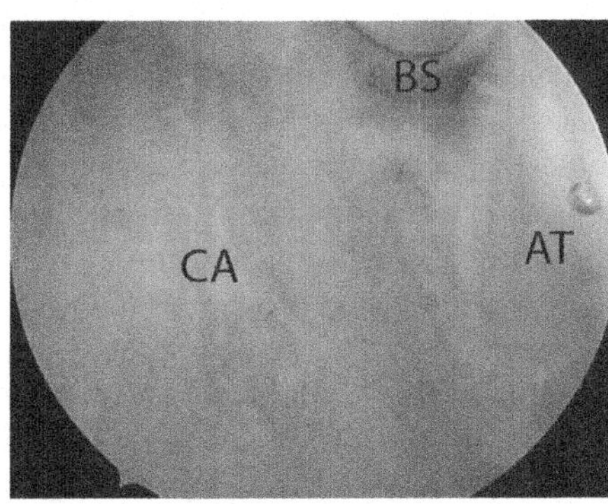

Fig.24. 9 Result at the end of procedure. *CA* calcaneus, *BS* bonecutter shaver, *AT*A chilles tendon

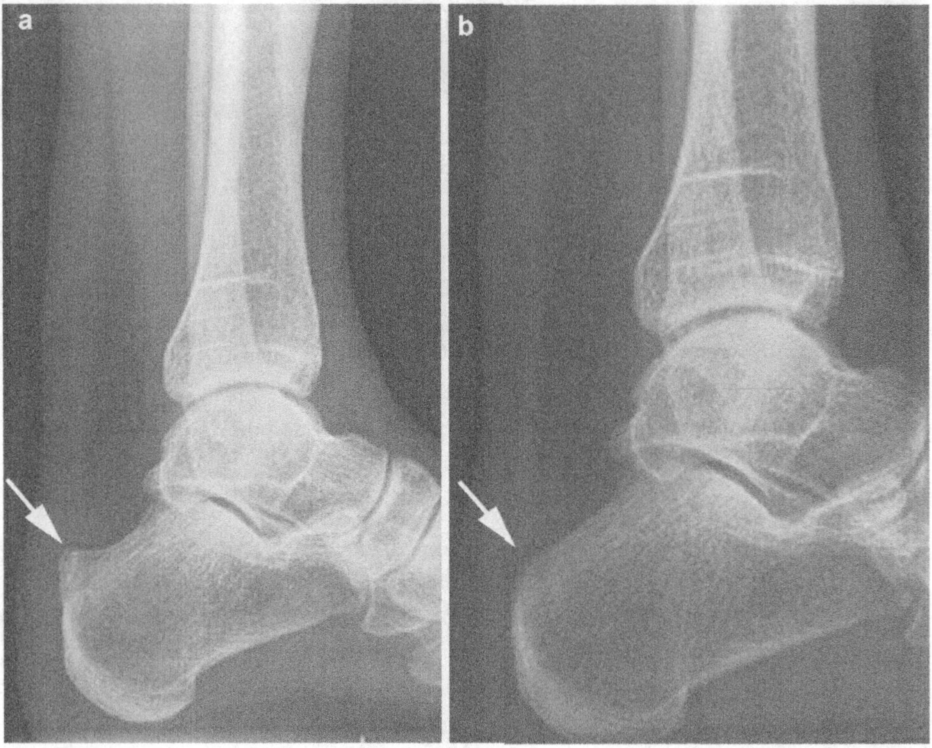

Fig. 24.10 (**a**) Preoperative X-ray, with retrocalcaneal bursitis and prominence of the posterosuperior part of the calcaneus (arrow). (**b**) postoperative X-ray. The posterosuperior part of the calcaneus is sufficientlye xcised(arrow)

24.4.4 PatientO utcome

Between 1995 and 2000 in the Academic Medical Center in Amsterdam we performed 39 procedures in 36 patients.[18] The average age was 35 years (range 16–50). Patients had a painful swelling of the soft tissue of the posterior heel, medial and lateral of the Achilles tendon on physical examination, without pain on palpation of the tendon itself. Conservative management for at least 6 months did not relieve symptoms. The conventional lateral radiograph showed a superior calcaneal angle (subtended by lines drawn from the bursal projection to the posterior calcaneal tuberosity and from the medial calcaneal tuberosity to the anterior calcaneal tuberosity) of more than 75°. An angle larger than 75° has been deemed pathologic.[3,4] The mean follow up after endoscopic calcaneoplasty was 4.5 years (range 2–7.5). There were no surgical complications except from one patient who experienced an area of hypoesthesia over the heel pad. Postoperatively there were no infections, tender or esthetically non-appealing scars and all patients were content with their small incisions. Except for two patients, all patients improved. The Ogilvie-Harris score[19] was rated fair by four patients, six rated good and 24 had excellent results. Work and sport resumption took place at an average of 5 weeks (range 10 days–6 months) and 11 weeks (range 6 weeks–6 months) respectively.[17,18]

24.5 Discussion

Conservative management for retrocalcaneal bursitis includes a single cortisone injection in the retrocalcaneal bursa.[15,20,21] Repeated injections are not advised since these can weaken the tendon with the potential danger of rupture.

The aim of surgery for retrocalcaneal bursitis, after failure of the conservative treatment, is preventing impingement between the Achilles tendon and the calcaneus. This can be accomplished by means of removing the inflamed retrocalcaneal bursa followed by either resection of the posterosuperior calcaneal rim or by a closing wedge osteotomy. Posterosuperior calcaneal resection can be performed through a posterolateral or posteromedial incision or via a combination of both.[9,13,22]

A widely used technique, especially in North America, is the midline-posterior skin incision combined with a central tendon splitting approach for debridement, retrocalcaneal bursectomy, and removal of the calcaneal bursal projection as necessary.[23] Another approach is the Cincinnati-type incision, a transverse skin incision at the level of the insertion of the Achilles tendon. With this technique, a wide exposure of the insertion of the Achilles tendon is possible, to debride the peritendinous and tendon tissue and if necessary bursectomy. The transverse skin incision at the level of the Achilles insertion also allows osteotomy of the posterosuperior corner of the calcaneus,[24] and, being in the direction of the skin creases, it has a lesser potential for healing problems than the longitudinal approaches.

Endoscopic calcaneoplasty offers a good, minimally invasive alternative to open surgery. Surgeons familiar with the endoscopic approach tend to favor this procedure, because of its better visualization as compared to the open procedure. Due to inappropriate visualization of the Achilles tendon during the open procedure, weakening or even rupture of this tendon has been reported.[12,14] Full recovery time after the open resection can take as long as 2 years. Our patient series shows a high percentage of good to excellent results based on the Ogilvie-Harris score.

Our results are comparable with other recently published reports on endoscopic treatment.

Jerosh and co-workers published a prospective study in which they described the results of endoscopic calcaneoplasty in 81 patients with an average follow-up of 35.3 months (range 12–72). Using the Ogilvie-Harris score, 41 patients presented excellent results, 34 presented good results, three had fair, and three patients showed poor results. These three patients showed an ossified area of the Achilles tendon insertion, and were revised in an open procedure. Only one patient experienced a superficial inflammation of the skin was found.[25,26] Ortmann and co-workers operated on 30 patients (32 heels) with retrocalcaneal bursitis with the endoscopic technique. The means follow-up was 35 months, and the AOFAS score averaged 62 preoperatively and 97 postoperatively. There were 26 excellent results, three good results and one poor result. One patient ruptured an Achilles tendon, one had residual pain and swelling that required reoperation through an open procedure. There were no other complications. Patients returned to work after on average of 8 weeks, and all athletes resumed their sporting activities in an average of 12 weeks.[27]

Morag and co-workers treated four patients with endoscopic calcaneoplasty, and after an average follow-up of 2 years (range 1–3.5 years), no complications, pain, disability, or range of motion deficits were reported.[28]

The advantages of the endoscopic over the open procedure are the small incisions, avoiding complications such a wound dehiscence, painful and/or ugly scars and nerve entrapment within the scar, as described for the open procedure.[10] He found a considerable amount of residual complaints in 32 clinically and radiographically examined patients treated by surgical resection of the posterosuperior calcaneal prominence for Haglund's syndrome at a mean follow-up of 18.6 years (range 2–41). 14 of these 32 patients had soft tissue problems including excessive scar formation and persistent swelling. In eight patients not enough bone was excised and two had new bone formation, both resulting in persistent painful swelling. The function of the Achilles tendon was disturbed in eight patients.[10]

There is no consensus regarding the ideal open surgical approach: medial, lateral, or both.[9,13,29] Jones and James performed ten partial calcaneal osteotomies for retrocalcaneal bursitis, followed by a short leg walking cast for 8 weeks, progressively increasing weight-bearing. Rehabilitation consisted of wearing an elevated heel of 2.5 cm. until the foot came easily to the neutral position. All patients were back to their desired level of activity within 6 months.[29] Angermann operated on 40 heels for the same indication using the posterolateral approach in 32 patients. Postoperatively 29 patients were allowed immediate weight-bearing. Complications consisted of one superficial heel infection, one hematoma and two patients with delayed skin healing. At an average follow-up of 6 years (range 1–12) 50% of the patients were cured, 20% improved, 20% remained unchanged and in 10% the pre-operative symptoms worsened.[9] The rate of poor results in this study corresponds to the results of Taylor, who reported 36% poor results after the same type of surgery.[30] Pauker and co-workers operated on 28 heels in 22 patients with Haglund's syndrome. Eighteen heels were approached laterally, and ten medially, depending on the direction of the prominent bone. All patients received a short leg walking cast for 4 weeks followed by mobilization exercises for aftertreatment. At a mean follow up of 13 years in 19 patients (range 3–20), 15 had good results, 2 fair and 2 poor. No difference in outcome between the two approaches was reported. The authors advocate using one incision, as many patients have complaints of tenderness over the operative scar up to 1 year postoperatively which might be exaggerated by a more extensive approach.[13]

Schepsis and co-workers used the medial approach in 24 patients with retrocalcaneal bursitis: 6 (25%) had a fair result requiring re-operation. In 49 heels (36 patients) operated through a lateral approach with a mean follow-up of 4.7 years (range 1–11 years), early complications were reported in 4 cases (3 hematomas and a superficial infection), and late complications in 3 cases resulting in revision surgery. Seven patients noted some improvement, one patient described no change and seven patients reported worsening of their symptoms after surgery.[31] Brunner and co-workers performed calcaneal osteotomies on 39 heels (36 patients), and reported at an average follow-up of 51 months, an average improvement of the AOFAS score of 32 points as compared to the mean pre-operative score.

Recovery time ranged from 6 months up to 2 years. Six of the 36 patients reported persisting posterior heel pain after surgery.[32]

There are two comparative studies in which both endoscopic and open procedures were performed. Leitze and co-workers compared the endoscopic approach (n = 30, 22 months follow-up) with the open surgical technique (n = 17, 42 months follow-up). The endoscopic approach revealed 19 excellent, 5 good, 3 fair and 3 poor results, which was numerically but not significantly better than the open surgical procedure. Recovery time was identical, but operation time, the amount of complications and scar tissue formation favored the endoscopic approach.[33] In a recent study by Lohrer and co-workers, a comparison was made between the endoscopic and open resection for Haglund's syndrome. In this anatomic study, nine cadaver feet were operated by means of open surgery and six were operated through endoscopic calcaneoplasty. After the procedure the ankles were dissected to determine the amount of damage following the surgery. Comparable amounts of damage were found for the sural nerve, the plantaris tendon and the medial column of the Achilles tendon.[34] Since this was an anatomic study, no data could be gathered regarding recovery time and scar healing, which seem to be the advantageous points of the endoscopic procedure. Also, cadaveric ankles could have been stiffer as compared to patients, which made the endoscopic approach more difficult to perform.

Overall, looking at the available results of open surgery, studies reported 61–83% good results and 17–36% complications or poor results requiring re-operation.[13,29,30,32,33,35] Endoscopic surgery leads up to an estimated rate of 83–93% good results, and 0.6–5% complications or poor results requiring re-operation.[10,18,26,27]

24.6 Conclusion

In summary, whether the operation is performed by endoscopic or open surgery, enough bone has to be removed to prevent impingement between the calcaneus and Achilles tendon. The endoscopic calcaneoplasty has demonstrated to show several advantages including low morbidity, functional aftertreatment, outpatient treatment, excellent scar healing, a short recovery time and quick sport resumption as compared to the results for the open technique.

References

1. Haglund P. Beitrag zur Klinik der Achillessehne. *Zeitschr Orthop Chir.* 1928; 49:49–58.
2. Dickinson PH, Coutts MB, Woodward EP, Handler D. Tendo Achillis bursitis. Report of twenty-one cases. *J Bone Joint Surg Am.* 1966; 48:77–81.
3. Fowler A. Abnormalities of the calcaneus as a cause of painful heel: its diagnosis and operative treatment. *Br J Surg.* 1945; 32:494–498.
4. Stephens MM. Haglund's deformity and retrocalcaneal bursitis. *Orthop Clin North Am.* 1994;25:41–46.

5. Alm A, Lamke LO, Liljedahl SO. Surgical treatment of dislocation of the peroneal tendons. *Injury*.1975;7:14 –19.
6. Sella EJ, Caminear DS, McLarney EA. Haglund's syndrome. *J Foot Ankle Surg*. 1997;37:110–114.
7. Vega MR, Cavolo DJ, Green RM, Cohen RS. Haglund's deformity. *J Am Podiatry Assoc*. 1984;74:129–135.
8. Fuglsang F, Torup D. Bursitis retrocalcanearis. *Acta Orthop Scand*.1961; 30:315–323.
9. Angermann P. Chronic retrocalcaneal bursitis treated by resection of the calcaneus. *Foot Ankle*.1990;10:285–287.
10. Huber HM, Waldis M. [The Haglund exostosis–a surgical indication and a minor intervention?]. *Z Orthop Ihre Grenzgeb*.1989; 127:286–290.
11. Leach RE, DiIorio E, Harney RA. Pathologic hindfoot conditions in the athlete. *Clin Orthop Relat Res*.1983;1 16–121.
12. Miller AE, Vogel TA. Haglund's deformity and the Keck and Kelly osteotomy: a retrospective analysis. *J Foot Surg*.1989; 28:23–29.
13. Pauker M, Katz K, Yosipovitch Z. Calcaneal ostectomy for Haglund disease. *J Foot Surg*. 1992;31:588–589.
14. Le TA, Joseph PM. Common exostectomies of the rearfoot. *Clin Podiatr Med Surg*. 1991;8:601–623.
15. Nesse E, Finsen V. Poor results after resection for Haglund's heel. Analysis of 35 heels in 23 patients after 3 years. *Acta Orthop Scand*.1994; 65:107–109.
16. Segesser B, Goesele A, Renggli P. [The Achilles tendon in sports]. *Orthopade*. 1995;24:252–267.
17. van Dijk CN, van Dyk GE, Scholten PE, Kort NP. Endoscopic calcaneoplasty. *Am J Sports Med*.2001;29:185–189.
18. Scholten PE, van Dijk CN. Endoscopic calcaneoplasty. *Foot Ankle Clin*. 2006;11:439–446, viii.
19. Ogilvie-Harris DJ, Mahomed N, Demaziere A. Anterior impingement of the ankle treated by arthroscopic removal of bony spurs. *J Bone Joint Surg Br*.1993; 75:437–440.
20. Myerson MS, McGarvey W. Disorders of the Achilles tendon insertion and Achilles tendinitis. *Instr Course Lect*.1999; 48:211–218.
21. Subotnick SI, Block AJ. Retrocalcaneal problems. *Clin Podiatr Med Surg*.1990; 7:323–332.
22. Kolodziej P, Glisson RR, Nunley JA. Risk of avulsion of the Achilles tendon after partial excision for treatment of insertional tendonitis and Haglund's deformity: a biomechanical study. *Foot Ankle Int*.1999; 20:433–437.
23. McGarvey WC, Palumbo RC, Baxter DE, Leibman BD. Insertional Achilles tendinosis: surgical treatment through a central tendon splitting approach. *Foot Ankle Int*.2002; 23:19–25.
24. Carmont MR, Maffulli N. Management of insertional Achilles tendinopathy through a Cincinnati incision. *BMC Musculoskelet Disord*.2007; 8:82.
25. Jerosch J, Nasef NM. Endoscopic calcaneoplasty–rationale, surgical technique, and early results: a preliminary report. *Knee Surg Sports Traumatol Arthrosc*.2003; 11:190–195.
26. Jerosch J, Schunck J, Sokkar SH. Endoscopic calcaneoplasty (ECP) as a surgical treatment of Haglund's syndrome. *Knee Surg Sports Traumatol Arthrosc*.2007; 15:927–934.
27. Ortmann FW, McBryde AM. Endoscopic bony and soft-tissue decompression of the retrocalcaneal space for the treatment of Haglund deformity and retrocalcaneal bursitis. *Foot Ankle Int*.2007;28:149 –153.
28. Morag G, Maman E, Arbel R. Endoscopic treatment of hindfoot pathology. *Arthroscopy*. 2003;19:E13.
29. Jones DC, James SL. Partial calcaneal ostectomy for retrocalcaneal bursitis. *Am J Sports Med*. 1984;12:72–73.
30. Taylor GJ. Prominence of the calcaneus: is operation justified? *J Bone Joint Surg Br*. 1986;68:467–470.

31. Schneider W, Niehus W, Knahr K. Haglund's syndrome: disappointing results following surgery – a clinical and radiographic analysis. *Foot Ankle Int.*2000; 21:26–30.
32. Brunner J, Anderson J, O'Malley M, Bohne W, Deland J, Kennedy J. Physician and patient based outcomes following surgical resection of Haglund's deformity. *Acta Orthop Belg.* 2005;71:718–723.
33. Leitze Z, Sella EJ, Aversa JM. Endoscopic decompression of the retrocalcaneal space. *J Bone Joint Surg Am.*200 3;85-A:1488–1496.
34. Lohrer H, Nauck T, Dorn NV, Konerding MA. Comparison of endoscopic and open resection for Haglund tuberosity in a cadaver study. *Foot Ankle Int.*2006; 27:445–450.
35. Schepsis AA, Wagner C, Leach RE. Surgical management of Achilles tendon overuse injuries. A long-term follow-up study. *Am J Sports Med.*1994; 22:611–619.

Part V

Ankle

Postero-medial Approach in the Supine Position for Posterior Ankle Endoscopy

25

Francesco Allegra, Filippo Spiezia, and Nicola Maffulli

25.1 Introduction

The posterior compartment of the ankle can present pathologies which can be addressed through arthroscopy. Loose bodies, osteochondral defects of talar dome or tibial plafond, bony cystic lesions, soft tissue impingement, posterior scar tissue and bony spurs are frequently found in the posterior compartment of the ankle. Symptomatic os trigonum, posterior inter-malleolar ligament impingement, talo-calcaneal joint affections, tendinopathy or impingement of the tendon of flexor hallucis longus (FHL) and pathology of the Achilles tendon and its insertion, including Haglund's syndrome, are located in the extra-articular space.

The use of thin endoscopic tools makes it possible to assess systematically the posterior compartment of the ankle from anterior portals, though reaching this area can be at times difficult because of the shape of the talus.[1,2] Pathology in the posterior compartment of the ankle, both in the intraarticular space and in the hindfoot, is frequent,[3–5] and it is usually addressed by open surgery.[6] The posterior joint compartment is reachable via anterior portals only passing along the medial and lateral aspects of the ankle[3,7]: the view of the posterior-lateral and posterior-medial gutters is not complete, and often impossible.

Some authors described safe and reproducible posterior endoscopic approaches to the ankle and the hindfoot, allowing to treat by endoscopy pathologies in this area.[1,2,8] When ankle pathology occurs in both the anterior and posterior compartments, it is not possible to operate on both compartments without using anterior and posterior portals. The surgeon therefore either limits the procedure to the anterior compartment, postponing posterior surgery to another session, or the patient is to be positioned prone, prolonging the procedure, changing the surgical set-up, risking to contaminate the surgical instruments, wasting time in surgery.

This arthroscopic procedure which allows to manage pathologies of both the anterior and posterior aspects of the ankle maintaining the patient supine.

N. Maffulli (✉)
Centre for Sports and Exercise Medicine, Queen Mary University of London, Barts and The London School of Medicine and Dentistry, Mile End Hospital, London, England, UK
e-mail: n.maffulli@keele.ac.uk

N. Maffulli and M. Easley (eds.), *Minimally Invasive Surgery of the Foot and Ankle*,
DOI: 10.1007/978-1-84996-417-3_25,

25.2 Surgical Technique

The soft spot between the posterior aspect of the medial malleolus and the anterior margin of the Achilles tendon hosts some important structures. Proceeding from superficial to deep, the tendons of *tibialis posterior* (PT), of *flexor digitorun longus* (FDL) and of *flexor hallucis longus* (FHL) are close to each other and to the posterior neurovascular bundle, with the pulsation of the tibial artery palpable behind the medial malleolus. The superficial medial calcanear nerve originates from the posterior tibial nerve 2–3 cm proximal to the tip of the medial malleolus. It runs antero-inferiorly for 2–2.5 cm, away from the Achilles tendon, curving posteriorly and medially, dividing in several cutaneous branches at the calcanear tuberosity. All these structures are at risk of lesions by surgery at the subcutaneous layer.

A right-angled triangular area nearly 25 cm^2 in the postero-medial aspect of ankle, located between the Achilles tendon, the upper calcanear tuberosity and the FHL tendon, is easily palpable. This area does not contain any neurovascular structures at risk of injury at surgery: by penetrating this area, it is possible to access is a safe fashion the postero-lateral compartment of the ankle, and to reach the posterior peroneal and tibial aspect of the ankle. A surgical instrument inserted from this area can reach the lateral malleolus without coming into contact with the medial neurovascular bundle.

Therefore, two portals placed on the anterior margin of Achilles tendon at a distance of 45–50 mm from each other allow safe insertion of endoscopic instruments, which can proceed from the inferior portal to the posterior aspect of the lateral malleolus (Fig. 25.1). As the distance from any nerve or vessel at risk is 11–14 mm, the tibial neurovascular bundle is never at risk if the instruments do not go medial to the tendon of FHL, which should always be kept under direct vision. On the other hand, the superficial medial calcanear nerve is not visualized and is potentially at risk, lying in a more superficial layer under the skin. As it maintains an antero-inferior direction until it reaches the space between the

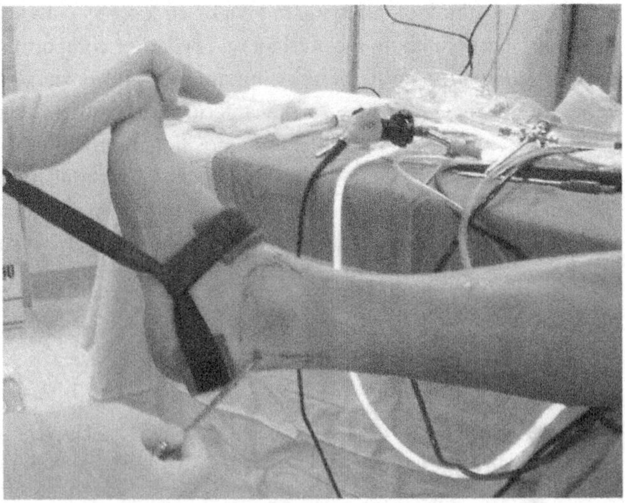

Fig.25.1 Theporta ls placement on the anterior margin of the Achilles' tendon: the picture shows the direction followed by the blunt rods to reach the posterior peroneal malleolus area and their distance from thec alcanearbr anch

calcanear tuberosity, lateral malleolus and tibia, it is sufficiently away from the Achilles tendon to prevent any contact with the instrument through the superior portal.

During the procedure, the patient is maintained supine, the hip is external rotated 15–20°, degrees and flexed to 30–35°. The upper calf is placed in a leg holder and the tourniquet, foam pads or towels are placed under the skin to prevent any pressure injury. The surgical bed is rolled slightly towards the contralateral side to keep the foot perpendicular to the floor. The leg is prepped and draped. A sterile support is clamped to the rail of the bed over the drapes and is used to hang the ring of a non-invasive string distractor device or any distraction device, if needed. The foot lies at the end of the surgical table and it can be moved up and down on the bed surface, or flexed dorsally or plantarly. At arthroscopy, the surgeon can explore the anterior joint, can visualize all the joint compartments, and can treat any anterior lesions. If necessary, a postero-lateral portal can be produced.

After the anterior arthroscopy, the bed is slightly externally rotated to enhance the external rotation of the lower limb, more than the 20° position assessed at the beginning of the procedure. By rotating the entire lower limb, the medial and postero-medial aspects of the ankle and foot are widely exposed (Fig. 25.2) with enough room to place, insert, move and withdraw the instruments. Because the medial malleolus lies more anteriorly than the lateral, the visualization of the transmalleolar axis helps to further expose the postero-medial compartment thanks to its physiological rotation of about 10–15°. This allows to increase the exposure of the triangular area, and to make it safer to insert instruments in this space.

The portals are placed medial and anterior to the Achilles tendon (Figs. 25.1 and 25.2). The first is placed at the level of the tip of the tibial malleolus. The second portal is placed 45–50 mm proximal to the first one, on the anterior margin of the Achilles tendon. Both are in a safe area 12–15 mm from the postero-medial bundle and 15–20 mm from the calcaneous sensitive branch of tibial nerve (Fig. 25.1).

After producing first the inferior portal, which is the one furthest away from the neurovascular bundle, mosquito forceps are used to split the subcutaneous layer to take gently away any nervous sensitive branches. A blunt rod is advanced anteriorly and laterally through the inferior portal, pointing to the space between the fourth and fifth toe, until

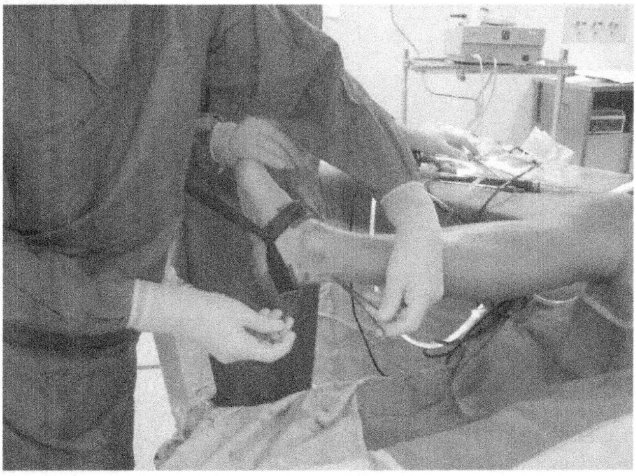

Fig.25.2 Theporta ls opening: while the blunt trochar is inserted inferiorly, a mosquito gently widens the skin of the upper portal, keeping the direction of the tip of the trochar towards the peronealma lleolus

touching bone. A prominent posterior talar process is felt as a prominence between the tibia and talus at the posterior edge of tibia and fibula. The arthroscope is then inserted. The superior portal is produced on same vertical plane of former one. Its location is in a low risk area. Also, if the ankle is dorsiflexed, the distance between the portal and the bundle increased, further preventing the risk of a lesion. A the same nick and spread technique with a mosquito clamp is used, a blunt rod is advanced inferiorly touching the shaft of the arthroscope. The rod is removed, and substituted with a shaver, advanced antero-inferiorly until it touches the sheath of the arthroscope. Triangulation of the instruments is performed on a vertical plane instead of a horizontal one.[2]

A working area is produced gently removing with the shaver the Kager's fat in the area, proceeding in a postero-anterior and medial-lateral direction, from above to below, keeping the FHL tendon under direct vision. The tip of the shaver blade is always kept lateral to the arthroscope under direct vision, visualizing the posterior talo-tibial, tibio-fibular, subtalar joints.

Loose bodies (Fig. 25.3), FHL impingement (Fig. 25.4), symptomatic os trigonum, posterior tibial bony spurs, posterior subtalar joint (Fig. 25.5), posterior calcifications are reached from a superior portal. Bony prominences of the calcaneus or the Achilles tendon

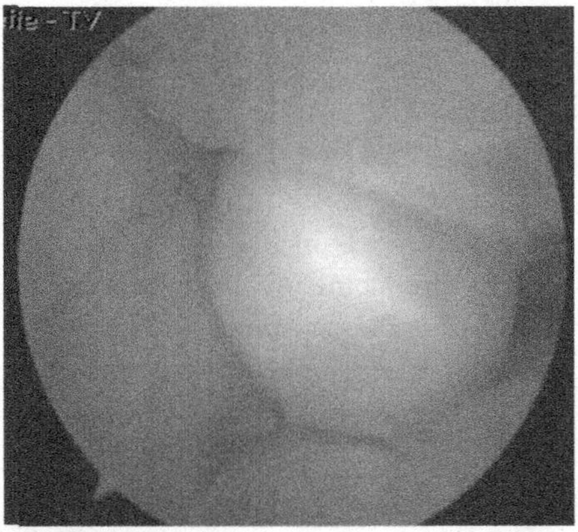

Fig.25.3 A loose body between the posterior tibialm argina ndt het alus

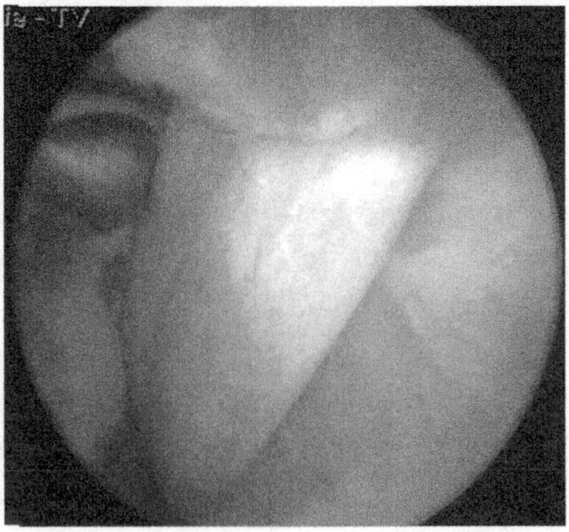

Fig.25.4 The FHL tendon appears to be the medialbor dert ot hei nstrumentss hifting

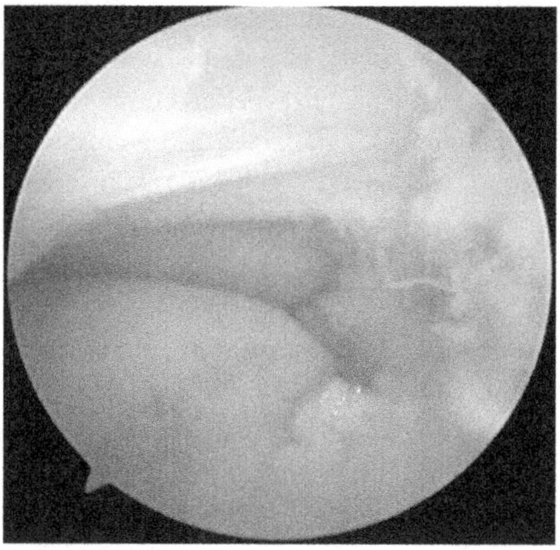

Fig.25.5 The posterior aspect of the subtalar joint: the calcaneus lies below under the talar articulars urface

are removed with the shaver in the inferior portal, moving its tip from anterior to posterior, after changing the position of the arthroscope from the superior to the inferior portal.

25.3 Discussion

Arthroscopic and endoscopic ankle portals have been widely described both anteriorly and posteriorly. Some authors[4,9,10] recommend that only the antero-lateral, antero-medial and postero-lateral portals should be used, given the proximity of the neurovascular bundle and of the tendon of tibialis posterior in the postero-medial aspect of the ankle. Other authors,[2,6,10] on the other hand, have described the endoscopic anatomy of this region, reporting on the relationship between the posterior tibial neurovascular bundle in relation to the other components of the musculo-skeletal system. A reproducible approach to the posterior area of the ankle through posterior medial and lateral portals with the patient prone allows to avoid any risk of a lesion to the neurovascular bundle.[2] These two posterior portals offer a safe complete view of the whole posterior compartment, and allow to address a pathologies in that region: again, the patient is prone. Other postero-medial portals have also been used, but several of them do not allow to deal with both intra- and extra-articular problems,[2,9,11,12] and all require the patient to be prone.

If both anterior and posterior pathologies are present, the surgeon can perform a posterior ankle arthroscopy in the prone position first, then, with the patient still prone, the surgeon can flex the knee, and operate on the anterior compartment. Obviously, in this instance the view in the anterior portal is upside-down.

The double postero-medial hindfoot approach which is propose in this chapter is located in the safe region just anterior to the anterior margin of the Achilles tendon. By maintaining the ankle in neutral or slight dorsi-flexion, the neurovascular tibial bundle lies more anteriorly, and is kept safe. This approach allows wide arthroscopic exposure of the posterior talo-tibial, talo-fibular and subtalar joints, of the upper calcanear tuberosity, of the tendons and tendon sheaths in that area, and the arthroscopic management of pathology in that region. Only in patients with limited external rotation of the hip as in hip arthritis, access to the postero-medial compartment of the ankle can be difficult if the patient is kept supine: in this instance, if the bed rotation is not sufficient to expose the triangular area, the patient will have to be positioned prone.

The double postero-medial arthroscopic approach we describe is safe, and allows full visualization and access to both intra- and extra-articular structures in the posterior aspect of the ankle.

The management of both anterior and posterior ankle disorders with the patient supine at the same sitting, and without changing position of the patient is appealing. The double postero-medial hindfoot approach allows excellent visualization of the posterior compartment of the ankle and of the structures in the hindfoot, without any neurovascular or tendinousc omplication.

References

1. Lijoi F, Lughi M, Baccarani G. Posterior arthroscopic approach to the ankle: an anatomic study. *Arthroscopy.* 2003;19:62–67. DOI:10.1053/jars.2003.50003 S0749806303500159 [pii].
2. van Dijk CN, Scholten PE, Krips R. A 2-portal endoscopic approach for diagnosis and treatment of posterior ankle pathology. *Arthroscopy.* 2000;16:871–876. DOI: S0749-8063(00)86731-6 [pii] 10.1053/jars.2000.19430.
3. Ferkel RD, Heath DD, Guhl JF. Neurological complications of ankle arthroscopy. *Arthroscopy.* 1996;12:200–208.
4. Guhl JF. New concepts (distraction) in ankle arthroscopy. *Arthroscopy.*1988; 4:160–167.
5. Parisien JS, Vangsness T. Operative arthroscopy of the ankle. Three years' experience. *Clin Orthop Relat Res.*1985; 199:46–53.
6. Maquirriain J. Posterior ankle impingement syndrome. *J Am Acad Orthop Surg.* 2005;13: 365–371.
7. Ferkel RD, Whipple TL. *Arthroscopic Surgery. The Foot and the Ankle.* Philadelphia, PA: Lippincott-Raven;1996.
8. Ljoi F, Lughi M, Baccarani G. Patologia del comparto posteriore della caviglia: trattamento artroscopico per via posteriore. *Artroscopia.*2002; 3:30–35.
9. Acevedo JI, Busch MT, Ganey TM, Hutton WC, Ogden JA. Coaxial portals for posterior ankle arthroscopy: an anatomic study with clinical correlation on 29 patients. *Arthroscopy.* 2000;16:836–845.
10. Ljoi F, Lughi M, Baccarani G. Posterior arthroscopic approach to the ankle: and anatomic study. *Arthroscopy.*2003; 19:62–67.
11. Sim JA, Lee BK, Kwak JH. 1. New posteromedial portal for ankle arthroscopy an anatomic study. *Arthroscopy.*2006; 22:799–802.
12. Sitler DF, Amendola A, Bailey CS, Than LM, Spouge A. Posterior ankle arthroscopy: an anatomic study. *J Bone Joint Surg.*2002; 84:763–769.

Ankle Equinus and Endoscopic GastrocnemiusR ecession

26

Amol Saxenaa nd Christopher DiG iovanni

26.1 Indroduction

Ankle equinus, with contracture of the Achilles tendon, may have a negative effect on foot and ankle function and morphology in the long term if left unevaluated and untreated. The gastrocnemius-soleus complex easily overpowers the other musculotendinous units and ligamentous constraints in the foot when pathologically tight. This can cause ulceration, midfoot breakdown, ankle pathology, and potential gait derangement[1–20] (Fig. 26.1). With repetitive contact between the ground and the foot any structure responsible for abnormal loading across the foot during the gait cycle, most often the Achilles tendon, hastens foot breakdown.

In the short term, a powerful, even tight (short), Achilles tendon can give an athlete the extra performance burst needed for certain sports requiring strong push-off or jumping ability. However, in the long term, this advantage might also have the undesirable impact of producing wear and tear of surrounding structures, with detrimental abnormal impacts and eccentric loading. This is possibly one of the reasons why some elite and high performance athletes may not be able to "do what they do" at a high level forever.

Although the association of Achilles tendon tightness and Achilles tendinopathy has been reported in several association studies, the actual management of the contracture with lengthening and transfer procedures has not been adequately studied in athletic patients.[4,11,21–25] Also, none of the studies adequately explain why some patients with symmetrically decreased ankle dorsiflexion are asymptomatic or present with only unilateral pathology. Furthermore, in general, activity levels of patients with Achilles tendon pathology have not been well documented. This chapter reviews present concepts of ankle equinus, what procedures are available to manage it, and a new endoscopic technique to address this pathology.

Traditionally, normal ankle range of motion is defined as 10° of ankle dorsiflexion with the foot in neutral (which is also subject to variable definitions) and the knee extended. The foot is in neutral when it is neither pronated nor supinated, based on the position of the talar head reduced on the navicular. With the knee flexed at 90° (the Silverskiold maneuver), ankle dorsiflexion should increase due to decrease of the tension of the

C. Di Giovanni (✉)
ProfessorofO rthopedicSur gery, BrownU niversityM edicalS chool, Providence, RIU SA
e-mail:he ysax@aol.com

N. Maffulli and M. Easley (eds.), *Minimally Invasive Surgery of the Foot and Ankle*,
DOI: 10.1007/978-1-84996-417-3_26, © Springer-Verlag London Limited 2011

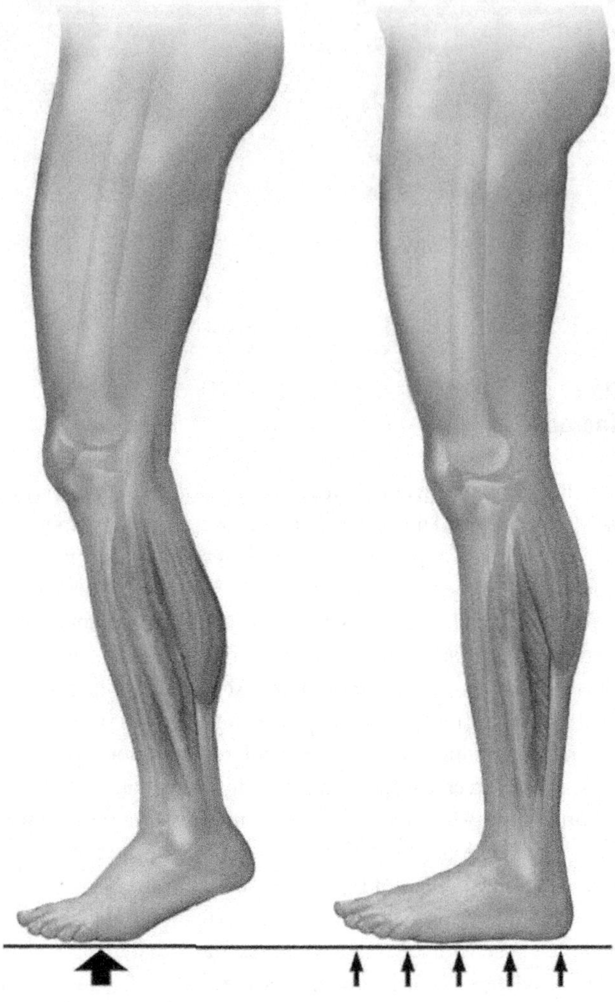

Fig. 26.1 Artist'sde pictionof the effect of a tight gastrocnemiusont hef oot

gastrocnemius. Recently, studies have shown ranges of ankle dorsiflexion with the knee extended of 0–10°, and more than 5° with the knee flexed in "normal" subjects.[3–5,11,19,21,26,27] Many of the studies have used no standardized reference points, foot position, and measuring devices. When assessing ankle equinus, one must also exclude confounding variables such as hamstring tightness, anterior ankle exostoses (visualized radiographically), posterior capsular contracture of the ankle and subtalar joints, and neuro-muscular conditions. These associated conditions can also be causative factors in patients showing limited ankle dorsiflexion with both the knee flexed and extended.

Ankle dorsiflexion has recently been more carefully researched. Tabrizi et al. studied children who sustained a unilateral lower limb injury, measuring the contralateral limb's ankle dorsiflexion without placing force on the forefoot, keeping the heel in varus. They used their patients who sustained upper extremity injuries as a control. They found 5.7° of dorsiflexion compared to 12.8° to the uninjured group. With the knee in flexion, the values were 11.2° and 21.4°, respectively.[19] DiGiovanni et al.[3] studied asymptomatic individuals and patients who were symptomatic due to forefoot/midfoot pathology. Their study showed that those subjects with less than 5° of dorsiflexion with the knee extended and less than 10° of dorsiflexion with the knee flexed were statistically more likely to be diagnosed with pathological equinus. DiGiovanni et al. labeled those with limitations with only the knee extended has having gastrocnemius tightness (Fig. 26.2a,b), and those with limited dorsiflexion with both the knee flexed and extended as having Achilles tendon tightness.[3] Saxena and Kim, in 40 adolescent athletes (average age 15 years) with no history of ankle pathology, found that the average ankle dorsiflexion was 0° with the knee extended, and 5° with the knee flexed.[28] These results may indicate that some degree of tightness of equinus may be beneficial in sport, particularly when athletes are encouraged to run on their forefoot. It is also possible that the patients in Tabrizi et al.'s study sustaining lower extremity injuries were in sports in which less ankle dorsiflexion was beneficial. Those with upper extremity injury may not participate in these types of sports. Table 26.1 summarizes these three studies.

Using DiGiovanni et al.'s definition, all the subjects in Saxena and Kim's cohort would be defined as having Achilles tendon and Gastrocnemius equinus/tightness. Tabrizi et al.'s cohort would also have borderline Gastrocnemius equinus. This may pose one to question whether these individuals, based on meeting arbitrary criteria defining them as having abnormally tight gastro-soleus complexes, should undergo a lengthening procedure.

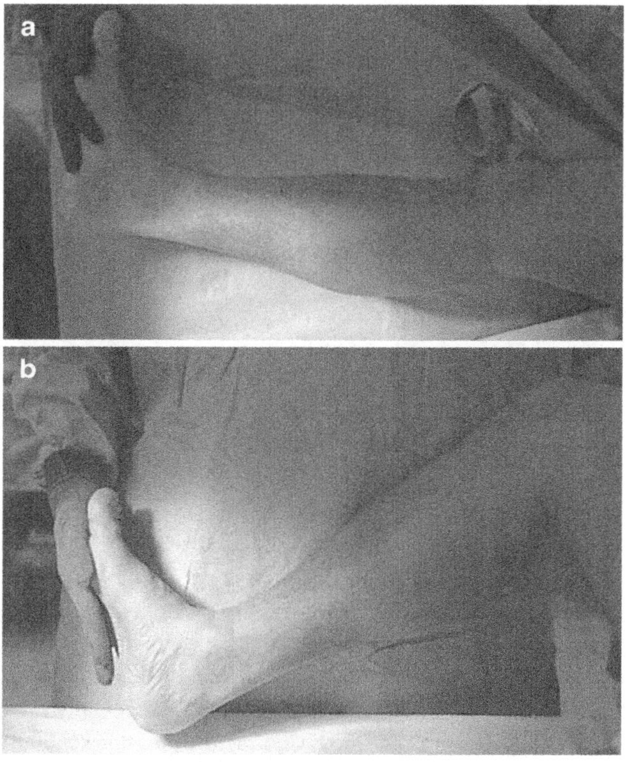

Fig. 26.2 (**a**) Silverskiold's test. With the knee extended, ankle dorsiflexion does not allow the foot to get to a 90° relationship to the leg. (**b**) With the knee bent, the foot is able to achieve 10° of dorsiflexion with respect to the leg

Table26.1 Selected studies on ankle dorsiflexion

Ankledor siflexion studies	Kneee xtended	Kneefl exed	Studygr oup
Tabrizi et al.[19]	12.8°	21.4°	Asymptomaticc ontrols
DiGiovanni et al.[3]	13.1°	22.3°	Asymptomaticc ontrols
DiGiovanni et al.[3]	<5°	<10°	Symptomaticpa tients
Saxena and Kim[28]	0°	5°	Adolescenta thletes

However, it is difficult to find a study on neurologically normal adolescents and children undergoing isolated procedures for ankle equinus.

Kaufman et al. studied 449 Navy Seals recruits with an average age of 22.5 years. They found limitations in ankle dorsiflexion with the knee extended in those recruits with Achilles tendinopathy (measured as <11.5°) together with increased hindfoot inversion.[11] Unfortunately, no longitudinal studies have been conducted in athletic individuals to ascertain whether they are likely to develop long term Achilles tendinopathy based on their limited ankle dorsiflexion. This relationship, however, has been strongly suggested in the diabetic population, as these patients are more commonly studied and almost always have Achilles tendon tightness as part of their disease process. In diabetic patients, however, pathology resulting from a tight Achilles tendon becomes more easily manifest because the patients are often neuropathic. As opposed to elite athletes with normal neurologic function, diabetic patients cannot identify nor protect themselves from this chronic, repetitive wear and tear process on surrounding structures (skin, ligaments, tendons, bone, joints). As a result, ulcers, Charcot breakdown, deformity, and instability are far more common in diabetic patients.[1–4,6,9,12,13]

Asymmetrical ankle dorsiflexion does require evaluation.[19] For athletes to be able to return to full function, ankle dorsiflexion should be within 5° of each other, or nearly symmetric.[24,29–32] Perhaps the best reason to consider treatment for ankle equinus is post-traumatic contracture.

26.2 Treatement

Initial treatment of ankle equinus has traditionally been stretching (Fig. 26.3a,b). Although it remains unclear whether a chronic stretching regimen can effectively lengthen the gastrocnemius-soleus complex, Grady and Saxena found an approximately 2° increase in ankle dorsiflexion over 6 months when subjects engaged in a stretching program. Their cohort consisted of non-athletic subjects, with an average age of 25 years, with initial dorsiflexion of 3° and 9° with the knee extended and flexed, respectively.[21] Stretching of the Achilles tendon in athletes is considered beneficial by many authors, but few outcome studies have been performed. Contractures do not generally occur through tendons them-

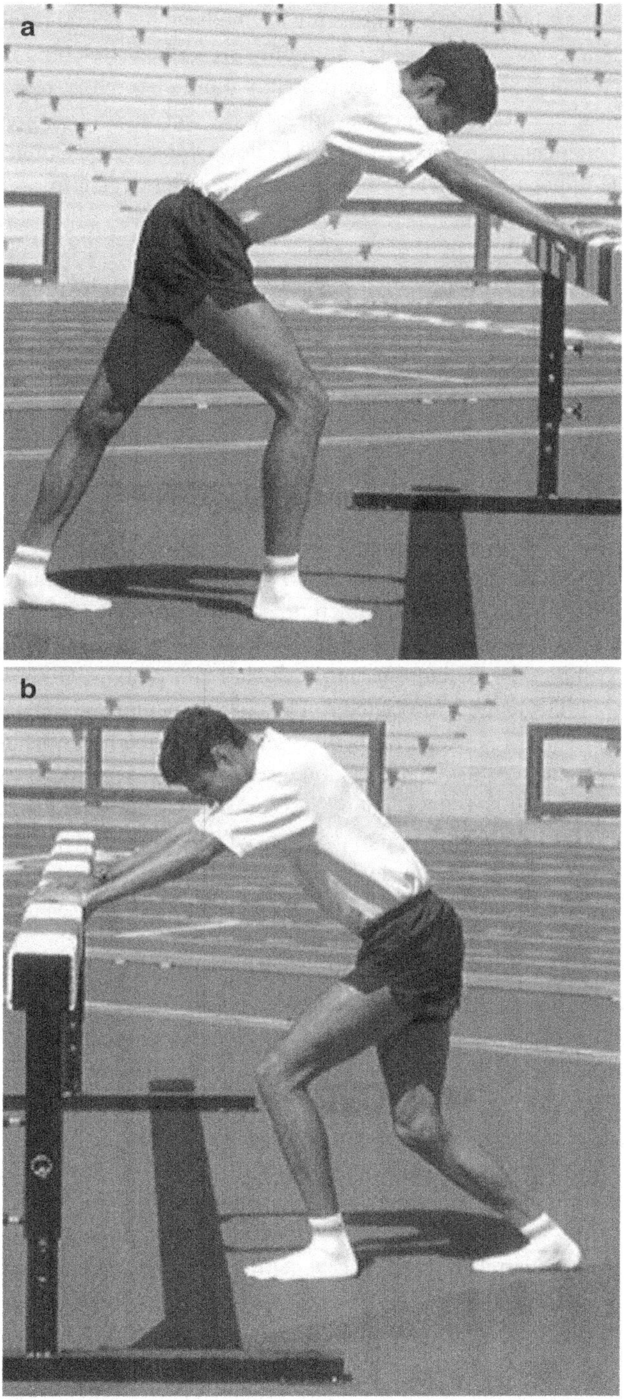

Fig.26.3 (**a**) Stretching with the knee straight creates tension on the gastrocnemius. (**b**) Stretching with the knee bent creates tension on the soleus and deep posterior musclec ompartment

selves, but rather within the muscle belly.[3] This is true for the Achilles tendon and gastro-soleus complex as well. Commonly prescribed stretching regimens designed long term to 'eliminate contracture' are probably more effective at preventing further contracture than at decreasing the tightness already present. Eccentric strengthening for up to 1 year is beneficial in reducing pain and allows for increased function in patients with Achilles tendinopathy.[33] Strengthening of the anterior leg muscles may also improve ankle dorsiflexion.

Elongation of the Achilles tendon produces disruption at 3% and complete loss of integrity at 8%.[22] Stretch likely occurs mostly in the muscle, and only a small amount in the tendon.[22,23] Other modalities of non-surgical lengthening have been casting and immobilization, though this has been predominantly studied in diabetic populations.[12]

Injections with botulinum toxin A have been used for cerebral palsy patients. A large multi-center clinical trial showed improvement in gait after botulinum injections, but the gains in ankle dorsiflexion were not reported. To date, none of the studies using botulinum injections have included athletic individuals, or neurologically normal patients.[34]

Surgical lengthening of the Achilles tendon complex was first reported by Delpech in 1816.[35] William Little, a physician with infantile paralysis and equinovarus deformity, had an Achilles tenotomy performed by Stromeyer, and became a proponent of this procedure for Achilles tendon contracture.[5,36] Throughout the twentieth century, other lengthening procedures were described. Variations of Achilles tenotomies were described by Hatt and Lampier, Hoke and Sgarlato.[4,18,37] Hatt and Lampier described a triple hemisection of the Achilles tendon, attributed to Hoke. Two medial and one lateral evenly interspaced hemi-tenotomies were performed.[4] Sgarlato described an open Z-plasty, severing the anterior two thirds of the lateral tendon distally and proximally severing the posterior two thirds of the medial Achilles tendon.[18] Posterior ankle and subtalar releases, as performed in deformities such as clubfoot, may also need to be considered as adjunctive procedures in patients with severe equinus deformity, as well as anterior ankle arthroplasty for patients with osseous equinus.

Hansen advocates open gastrocnemius recession for gastrocnemius tightness, percutaneous Achilles tendon lengthening for Achilles tendon tightness, and open Achilles tendon lengthening when precise lengthening is desired or when previous surgery has been performed on the Achilles tendon and a complete rupture of the Achilles tendon using percutaneous lengthening is a potentially greater risk.[7] Hansen and others, over a time period of almost 100 years, have recommended that Achilles tendon or gastrocnemius lengthening be performed for reconstructive foot procedures.[4,5,7,10,16–18,20,37] Unfortunately, none of these studies document patients' activity level such as participation in sports or even the ability to propulse on their toes, which would be an issue for athletes.

Post-operative regimens for Achilles tendon lengthening vary according to the procedure undertaken. However, generally the foot and ankle are protected with some form of immobilization for 4–6 weeks. Some authors allow diabetic patients to walk without any splint, and others state that protection with a below-knee cast depends on whether other concomitant procedures are performed.[1,2,4,5,9,13,16] Though tenotomy is commonly performed on the Achilles tendon, some have noted that excessive weakening or "calcaneal" deformity can occur. Delp and Zajac advised against Achilles tendon lengthening for patients with isolated gastrocnemius contracture due to excessive weakening of propulsion. One centimeter of lengthening reduces propulsive forces by almost 30%,[38] a significant amount for athletic individuals.

Other procedures to reduce Achilles tendon contracture have been described. Strayer described an open gastrocnemius recession or tenotomy as a variation of Vulpius and Stoffel's distal gastrocnemius recession that avoided the main body of the Achilles tendon, as well as "tongue-and-groove" slide techniques.[4,5,39–41] In Strayer's procedure, the distal portion of the gastrocnemius aponeurosis is transected. A posterior midline incision is made, the sural nerve is identified and protected (Fig. 26.4a). The medial and lateral margins of the gastrocnemius aponeurosis are identified and then transected. Improvement in ankle dorsiflexion is then noted (Fig. 26.4b). This procedure is occasionally performed in patients with chronic Achilles tendon ruptures to span a tissue loss of up to 5 cm. Studies on athletic individuals undergoing an open gastrocnemius recession with concomitant Achilles tendon repair are lacking.

Some of the largest studies on Achilles tendon rupture repair and surgical management for chronic tendinopathy do not show any authors' advocating a lengthening procedure at the time of surgery.[24,29–32,42] Only one recent paper by Costa et al. describes lengthening of the Achilles for tendinopathy.[43]

However, if a tight Achilles tendon is considered a potential contributing factor to the chronic tendinopathy or tear of the Achilles tendon, consideration may be given to a

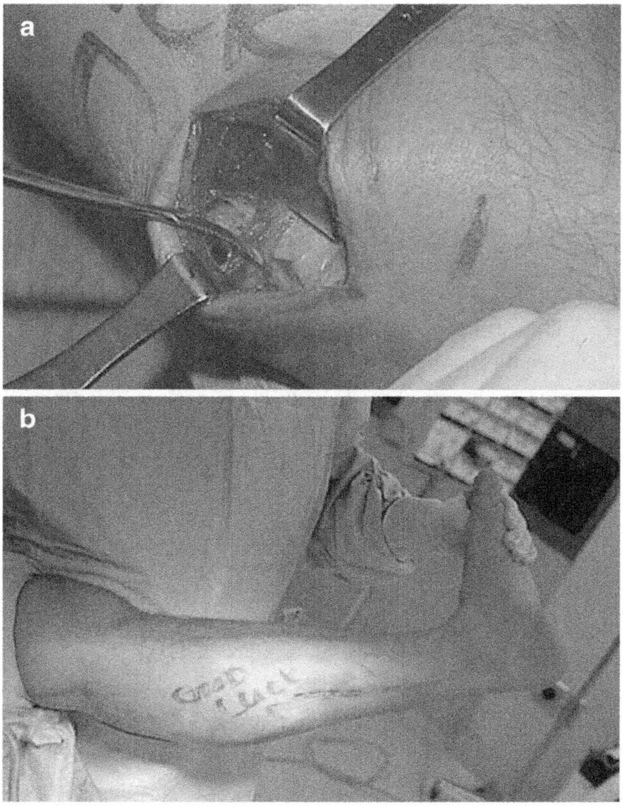

Fig.26.4 (**a**)Intra -operative view of sural nerve during an open gastrocnemius recession. (**b**)Pos t-operative view of a patient; note incisionle ngth

more proximal gastrocemius recession.[44] This technique can facilitate easier re-approximation or repair of the Achilles tendon at the site of rupture, and results in little loss of Achilles tendon strength clinically. Approximately one centimeter of length can be gained with a proximal gastrocnemius recession in such patients, which can be helpful to avoid repair under tension in the event of tissue loss after debridement or a chronic defect. This situation, however, is generally not seen in patients with an acute tear of the Achilles tendon.

For acute tendon repair, one is advised to maintain the foot in a gravity equinus position, and gradually dorsiflex it to neutral in the following post-operative weeks.[45,46] In fact, an over-lengthened position can cause deficits in athletic patients, and one paper describes surgical shortening for this situation. Cannon and Hackney recently described good results with surgical shortening on five athletic and active patients with dysfunctional Achilles tendons with prior treatment for rupture. The average age of their patients was 46 years, the tendon was shortened approximately 1 cm, and patients were protected from dorsiflexion post-operatively. There are only a few papers dealing with this subject.[47,48]

Also, a deep posterior compartment release can be added to this procedure to decrease tension of the overlying paratenon or skin repair when necessary, and can also theoretically improve vascular inflow to the repair from the well-vascularized FHL muscle belly immediately adjacent when tenodesed to the Achilles tendon.

To our knowledge, Achilles tendon lengthening or gastrocnemius recession have not been described in the context of surgery for chronic Achilles tendinopathy. Recently, Vulpiani et al. reported on 76 patients with 13 year follow-up for chronic Achilles tendinopathy, and do not mention any type of lengthening.[42] Another larger study of 91 surgeries with average 4 year follow-up also does not describe the need for lengthening in active and athletic individuals. Furthermore, post-operatively, patients are kept in an equinus position for variable periods, and some even maintain a heel raise in the shoe for several months.[29] Similar to the undocumented prevalence of contracture of the Achilles tendon in athletes, Achilles tendon lengthening for athletic individuals has also not been studied. As a result, this procedure is understandably uncommon in athletes.

Gastrocnemius recession essentially creates a surgically induced gastrocnemius tear.[49,50] This injury often is incurred without long-term sequelae, as treatment is supportive with rest, elevation and rehabilitation. In this regard, gastrocnemius recession would appear to be better tolerated than an Achilles tendon lengthening by athletic patients. Indeed, we suggest that Achilles tendon lengthening be used with much greater caution than the gastrocnemius recession in these patients. Its direct effect on the muscle tendon unit is probably much greater, and therefore its impact on direct activity of the loaded Achilles tendon can be expected to be similarly high.

Studies report the results of gastrocnemius recession and the amount of ankle dorsiflexion achieved. The 15 patients undergoing an open gastrocnemius recession had an increase of 18° 2 months after the procedure.[15] The patients are positioned prone, a 6–10 cm midline incision is made, and the medial and lateral aspects of the gastrocnemius fascia and aponeurosis distal to the muscle belly are transected. The relevant anatomy for the open technique of Strayer from a medial approach was recently studied by Pinney et al., who used a 7 cm medial incision.[40] The sural nerve was located in the superficial fascia in 42.5% of the legs operated, and deep to the fascia in the remaining 57.5%. The release site was on average 18 mm distal to the distal muscle belly of the gastrocnemius, and the gapping of the release site averaged 3 cm. Although they did not report actual data on appearance, they state "Cosmesis of the incision can also be compromised by tethering of the skin to the underlying tissue," and report that this is a "relatively frequent complication." They also relate that sural nerve injury can occur by direct trauma or excessive stretch, but do not report the actual rate of this complication. Webb et al. noted the sural nerve courses over the proximal aspect of the Achilles tendon from lateral to medial, and surgical incisions should take this into account.[51] In general, gastrocnemius recession, as compared to Achilles tendon lengthening, may result in fewer complications such as calcaneal deformity, but the larger incision and nerve injury may be a drawback.

26.3 Endoscopic technique

Endoscopic techniques include gastrocnemius recession, avoid larger incisions, and visualize the sural nerve.[16,51–53] Saxena and Widtfeldt reported on 18 patients undergoing endoscopic gastrocnemius recession. Their patients increase in ankle dorsiflexion with the knee extended statistically improved from −8.7° to 2.6° after a year ($P < 0.00001$). This is generally performed supine with the heel on a bulky towel to allow passage of instruments (Fig. 26.5). Although activity levels were not reported, patients were able to perform a single-legged heel-raise on average at 13 weeks. They generally used a two-portal technique with the patients supine and the heel on a sterile roll, a 4.0 mm endoscope, and a cannulated endoscopic blade to transect the gastrocnemius in a medial to lateral direction.[16]

Using endoscopic gastrocnemius recession, the medial incision is produced first, inferior to the medial gastrocnemius muscle belly and posterior to the great saphenous vein and saphenous nerve. A hemostat and then a fascial elevator are used to create a channel deep to the subcutaneous tissue directly posterior to the gastrocnemius aponeurosis (Fig. 26.6). A cannula is introduced with an obturator, which then replaced with a 30° 4.0 mm endoscope. The aponeurosis is visualized above (Fig. 26.7a–c). The slotted cannula should

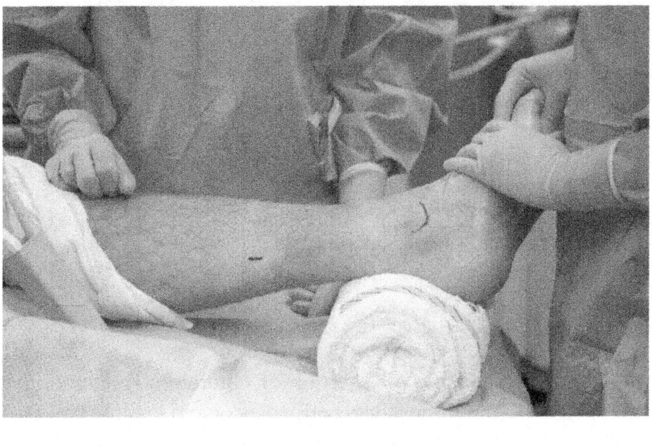

Fig.26.5 Actualpa tient before endoscopic gastrocnemiusre cession

Fig. 26.6 Creatinga fa scial pathway with elevator for thec annula

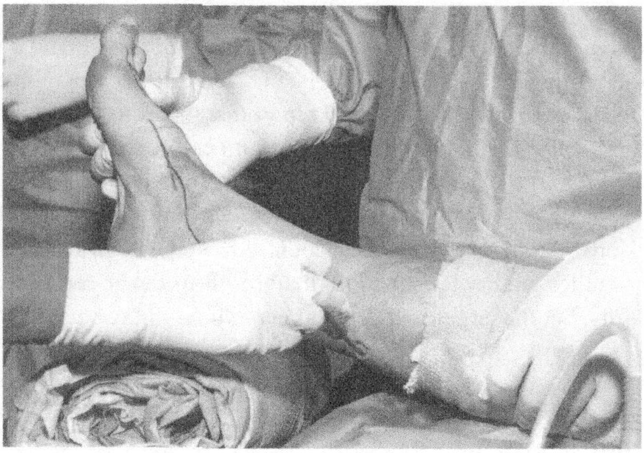

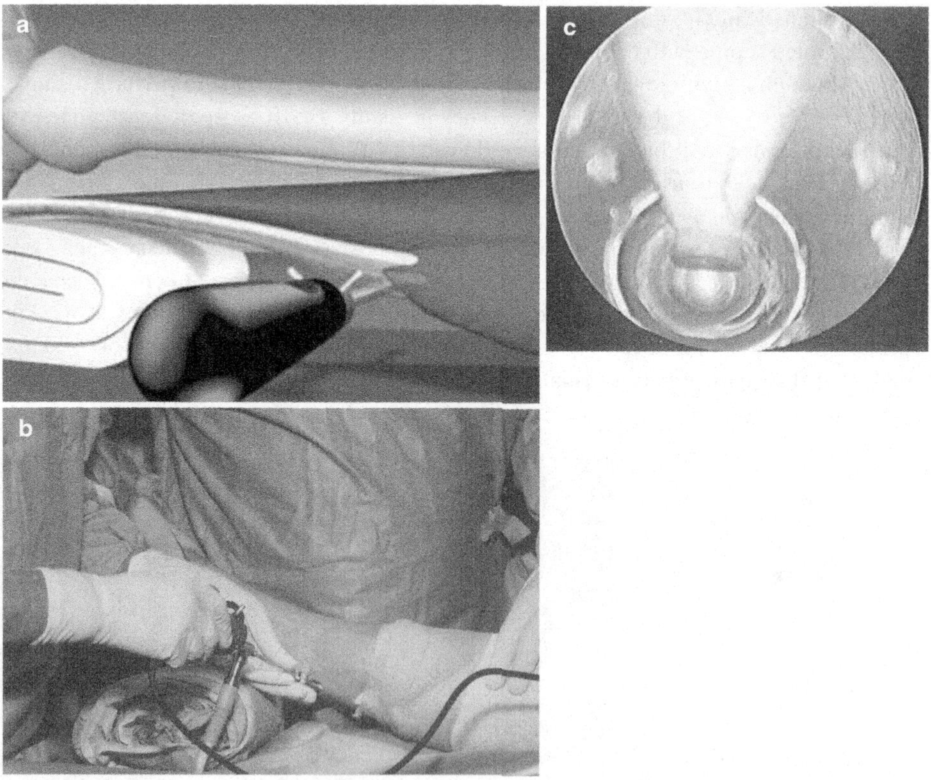

Fig. 26.7 (**a**) Schematic of insertion of obturator/cannula assembly. (**b**) Obturator removed, and replaced by 4 mm Endoscope. (**c**)E ndoscopicvi ewof ga strocnemiusa poneurosis/fascia

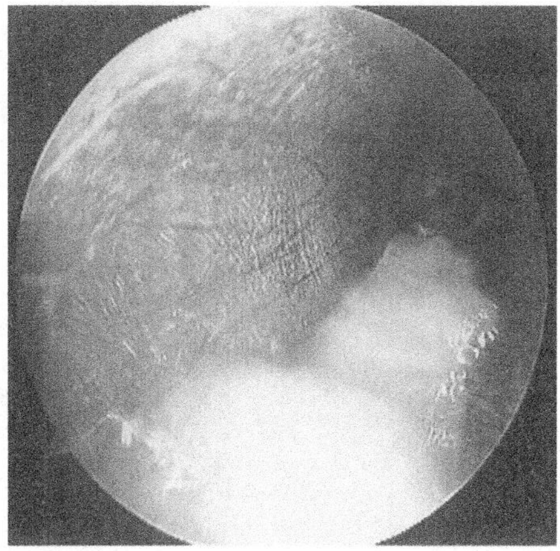

Fig.26.8 Endoscopic view of the sural nerve anda djacentve in

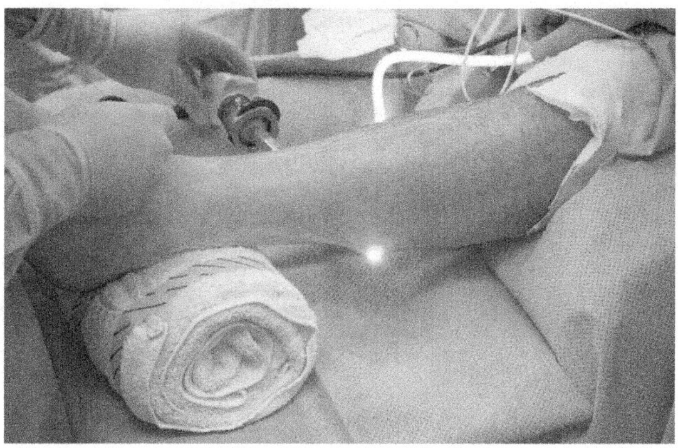

Fig.26.9 Transillumination toc reatea la teralporta l

be then rotated posteriorly to identify the sural nerve, which is generally located approximately 1 cm from the lateral border of the gastrocnemius (Fig. 26.8). After the nerve has been protected posteriorly by the cannula, a lateral portal can be created by transillumination and tenting of the skin over the cannula. A small suction-tip device can be placed within the cannula to improve visualization, which is helpful during transection (Fig. 26.9). The endoscope is then temporarily removed to visualize from lateral. The forward or reverse cutting knife (Mondeal GmBH, Germany) is carefully inserted into the cannula medially, temporarily rotating the opening to align with the skin incision (Figs. 26.10a and b). Within the knife re-positioned perpendicular to the gastrocnemius, the aponeurosis is transected from medial to lateral while dorsiflexing the foot. Hemorrhage may occur when transecting the intra-muscular septae; suction can be attached directly to the knife. Endoscopic confirmation of transection and visualization of exposed muscle is needed (Figs. 26.11a–d). Dorsiflexion should improve by at least 10°. The tendon of plantaris may also have to be transected (Figs. 26.12a and b). Routine skin sutures are used for the skin incisions. To avoid tenting of the skin due to the exposed muscle tissue, the foot can be gradually mobilized out of the equinus position post-operatively over 4 weeks. Patients are

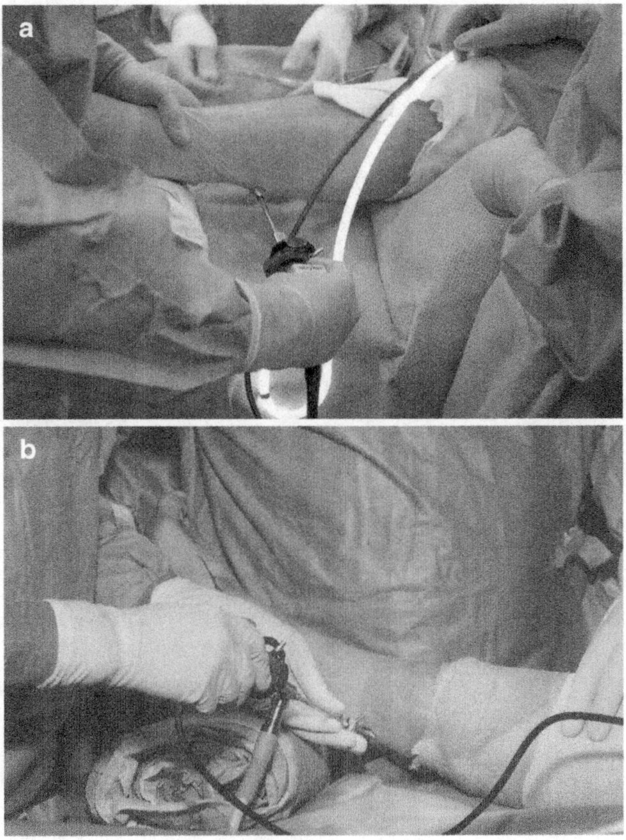

Fig.26.10 (**a**) Endoscope now being placed through lateral portal. (**b**) Insertion of endoscopic knife into the cannula in medial portal, requires a temporary rotation of 90° (in-line with the incision). Additional protection with a small retractor can be beneficial whilei nserting

maintained in a below-knee cast boot for at least 4 weeks post-operatively at 90°; longer immobilization for up to 12 weeks can be necessary if other procedures are associated. Muscle relaxants are sometimes needed post-operatively. Physical therapy to decrease fibrosis at the surgical sites and improve strength and gait is used. If endoscopic gastrocnemius recession is performed in isolation, physical therapy is started at 2 weeks. Otherwise, physical therapy is delayed according to additional procedures. In any case, patients are advised to massage the surgical sites as soon as they can access them.

Endoscopic gastrocnemius recession may produce better cosmesis and allows visualization and protection of the sural nerve. Researching endoscopic techniques on cadavers, Tashjian et al. found that the sural nerve courses within 1 cm medial to the lateral border, or about 20% of the total width of the gastrocnemius aponeurosis.[54] When a medial percutaneous gastrocnemius approach is employed, this nerve is subject to injury. A larger medial incision allows visualization of the nerve.[40] Observation and protection of this nerve during open approaches or endoscopy should reduce neural injury that could be more likely with percutaneous gastrocnemius recession techniques.[52] Sural neuritis and lateral foot dysthesia is more common when the procedure is combined with calcaneal osteotomy.[55]

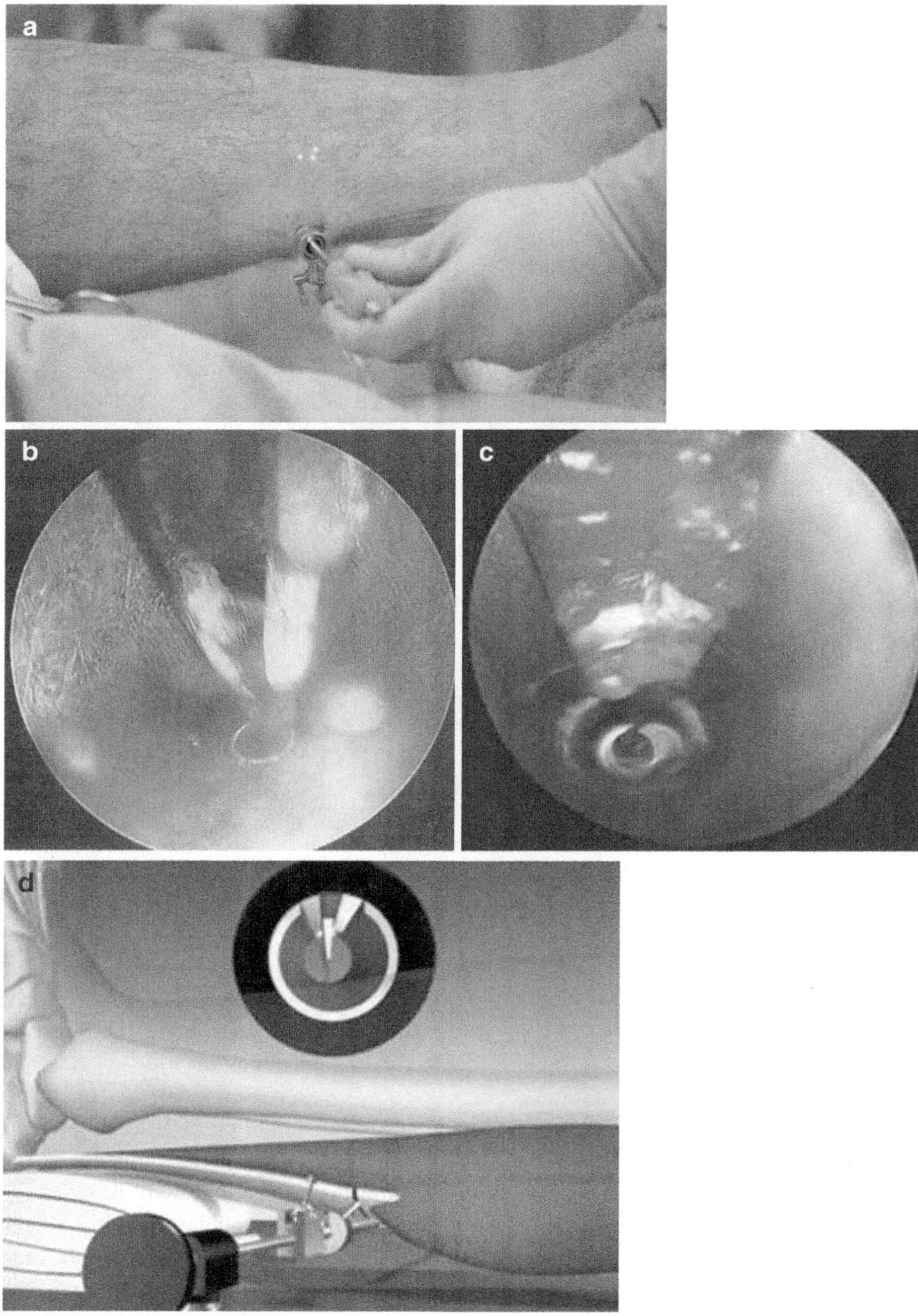

Fig. 26.11 (**a**) Schematic of endoscopic knife rotated back to perpendicular to the gastrocnemius to initiate transection. (**b**) Endoscopic view of initial transection. The foot is being dorsiflexed during this maneuver to create tension on the gastrocnemius. (**c**) Additional transection. Note further muscle exposure. (**d**) Schematic of preservation of neurovascular structures: the cannula is anterior andthe reforeprote ctsthe m

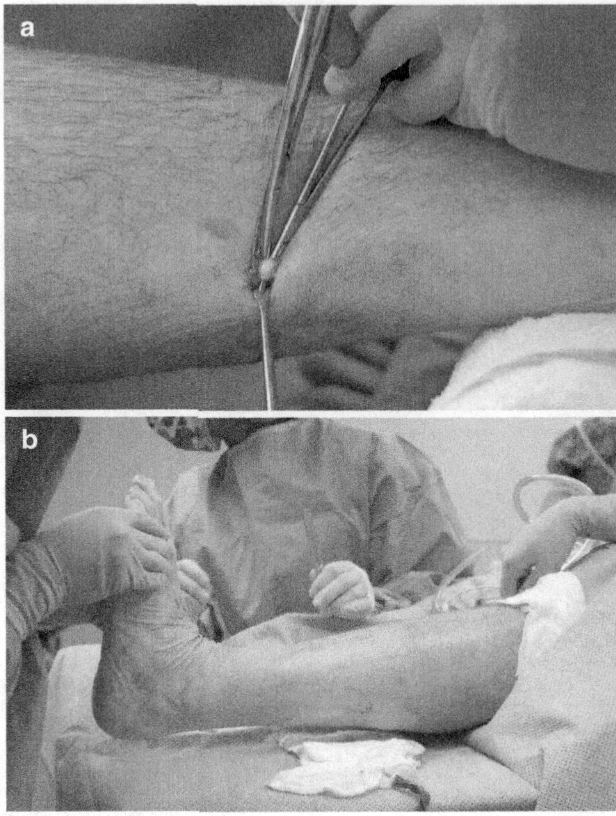

Fig. 26.12 (**a**)O pen transection of the plantaris tendon improves dorsiflexion. (**b**) Dorsiflexion should improve bya tl east10°

26.4 Discussion

Generally, Achilles tendon or gastrocnemius lengthening should be reserved to patients requiring significant foot reconstruction related to a tight gastro-soleus complex, and in those needing to avoid forefoot ulceration such as diabetics. Diabetic patients benefit from Achilles tendon lengthening, probably due to their different metabolic state and altered configuration of collagen cross-linking, but can be susceptible to over-lengthening. Perhaps, if these patients are athletic or are motivated to exercise to help control their diabetes, they could be studied for their altered biomechanics, and subsequent long-term benefits of the procedure.

Based on a current lack of data unequivocally linking a tight Achilles tendon to long term pathology of the foot and ankle, it remains difficult to justify any lengthening of this structure in asymptomatic athletes or neurologically normal individuals without foot pathology. Future studies of such patient populations will likely shed light on this subject, and longitudinal evaluation of these groups may change these recommendations, particularly if any long term pathological effects of a tight Achilles tendon left unchecked are not outweighed by any "advantages" of that tightness in the preceding years.

Repair of an Achilles tendon rupture and avulsion is typically performed with the foot in a neutral or equinus position. Scientific in vivo studies have not been performed with the Achilles tendon dorsiflexed. Therefore, until this is done, with long-term results sufficiently known, athletically active patients should proceed with caution when contemplating having an Achilles tendon positioned in a dorsiflexed position. Gastrocnemius recession is occasionally performed in conjunction with Achilles tendon rupture repair or post-ankle trauma contracture. Again, the ankle is generally maintained in an equinus position in this situation during surgery and post-operatively.

26.5 Conclusion

In summary, significantly asymmetric post-traumatic contracture is a consideration for athletic patients to undergo posterior lengthening, although only anecdotal reports are available. In some cases, the athletic foot may actually benefit from having an equinus position, and hopefully this will be better assessed in the future. Other reconstructive procedures which require posterior lengthening often include Gastrocnemius recession. The new technique of endoscopic Gastrocnemius recession is a useful technique when indicated for treating ankle equinus, particularly Gastrocnemius contracture.

References

1. Armstrong D, Stacpoole-Shea S, Nguyen H, Harkless L. Lengthening of the achilles tendon in diabetic patients who are at high risk for ulceration of the foot. *J Bone Joint Surg.* 1999;81A:535–538.
2. Barry D, Sabacinski K, Habershaw G, Giurini J, Chrzan J. Tendo achilles procedures for chronic ulcerations in diabetic patients with transmetatarsal amputations. *J Am Podiatr Assoc.* 1993;83:96–100.
3. DiGiovanni C, Kuo R, Tejwani N, Price R, Hansen T, Cziernecki J, Sangeorzan B. Isolated gastrocnemius tightness. *J Bone Joint Surg.*2002; 84A :962–970.
4. Downey M. Ankle equinus. In: McGlamry E, ed. *Comprehensive Textbook of Foot Surgery.* 2nd ed. Baltimore, MD: Williams & Wilkins; 2002:716–720.
5. Downey M. Ankle equinus. In: McGlamry E, ed. *Comprehensive Textbook of Foot Surgery.* 1st ed. Baltimore, MD: Williams & Wilkins; 1987:368–401.
6. Grant W, Sullivan R, Sonenshine D, Adam M, Slusser J, Carson K, Vinik A. Electron microscopic investigation of the effects of diabetes mellitus on the Achilles tendon. *J Foot Ankle Surg.*1997;36:272–278.
7. Hansen ST. Tendon transfers and muscle balancing techniques. Achilles tendon lengthening. In: Hansen S, ed. *Functional Reconstruction of the Foot and Ankle.* Baltimore, MD: Lippincott Williams & Wilkins; 2000:415–421.

8. Hansen ST. Midfoot arthrodesis. In: Wulker N, Stephens M, Cracchiolo A, eds. *Atlas of Foot and Ankle Surgery*. St. Louis, MO: Mosby; 1998:154.
9. Hastings M, Mueller M, Sinacore D, Salsich G, Engsberg J, Johnson J. Effects of a tendo-Achilles lengthening procedure on muscle function and gait characteristics in a patient with diabetes mellitus. *J Orthop Sports Phys Ther.*2000; 30:85–90.
10. HibbsR .M uscleboundf eet. *NY Med J.*1914; 17C:798–808.
11. Kaufman K, Brodine S, Shaffer R, Johnson C, Cullison T. The effect of foot structure and range of motion on musculoskeletal overuse injuries. *Am J Sports Med.*1999; 27:585–593.
12. Lin S, Lee T, Wapner K. Plantar forefoot ulceration with equinus deformity of the ankle in diabetic patients: the effect of tendo-Achilles lengthening and total contact casting. *Orthop.* 1996;19:465–75.
13. Mueller M, Sinacore D, Hastings M, Johnson J. The effect of Achilles tendon lengthening on neuropathic plantar ulcers: a randomized clinical trial. *J Bone Joint Surg.* 2003;85-A:1436–1445.
14. Orendurff M, Aiona M, Dorociak R, Pierce R. Length and force of the gastrocnemius and soleus during gait following tendo Achilles lengthenings in children with equinus. *Gait Posture.*2002;15 :130–135.
15. Pinney SJ, Hansen ST, Sangeorzan BJ. The effect on ankle dorsiflexion of Gastrocnemius Recession. *Foot Ankle Int.*2002; 23:26–29.
16. Saxena A, Widtfeldt A. Endoscopic gastrocnemius recession: a preliminary report on 18 cases. *J Foot Ankle Surg.*2004; 43:302–306.
17. Sgarlato T, Morgan J, Shane H, Frenkenberg A. Tendo Achilles lengthening and it's effect on foot disorders. *J Am Podiatr Assoc.*1975; 65:849–871.
18. Sgarlato TE. Medial Gastrocnemius Tenotomy to assist in body posture balancing. *J Foot Ankle Surg.*1998; 37:546–547.
19. Tabrizi P, McIntyre W, Quesnel M, Howard A. Limited ankle dorsiflexion predisposes to injuries of the ankle in children. *J Bone Joint Surg.*200 0;82-B:1103–1106.
20. Wulker N. Triple arthrodesis. In: Wulker N, Stephens M, Cracchiolo A, eds. *Atlas of Foot and Ankle Surgery*. St. Louis, MO: Mosby; 1998:262.
21. Grady J, Saxena A. The effects of stretching on gastrocnemius equinus. *J Foot Ankle Surg.* 1991;30:465–469.
22. Kannus P. Etiology and pathophysiology of chronic tendon disorders in sports. *Scand J Med Sci Sports.*1997;7: 78–85.
23. Kannus P, Jozsa L, Natri A, Jarvinen M. Effects of training, immobilization and remobilization on tendons. *Scand J Med Sci Sports.*1997; 7:67–71.
24. Schepsis A, Leach R. Surgical management of achilles tendonitis. *Am J Sports Med.* 1987;15:308–315.
25. Weber M, Niemann M, Lanz R, Muller T. Non-operative treatment of acute rupture of the Achilles tendon: results of a new protocol and comparison with operative treatment. *Am J Sports Med.*2003 ;31:685–691.
26. Silverskiold N. Reduction of the uncrossed two-joints muscles of the leg to one-joint muscles in spastic conditions. *Acta Chir Scand.*1924; 56:315–330.
27. Van Gheluwe B, Kirby KA, Roosen P, Phillips RD. Reliability and accuracy of biomechanical measurements of the lower extremities. *J Am Podiatr Med Assoc.*2002; 92:317–326.
28. Saxena A, Kim W. Ankle dorsiflexion in adolescent athletes. *J Am Podiatr Assoc.* 2003;93: 312–314.
29. Saxena A. Retrospective review of 91 surgeries for chronic Achilles pathology. *J Am Pod Med Assoc.*2003;93:2 83–291.
30. Saxena A. Results of achilles tendon surgery in elite and sub-elite track athletes. 2003;24:712–720.
31. Schepsis A, Wagner C, Leach RE. Surgical management of Achilles tendon overuse injuries. *Am J Sports Med.* 1994;22:611–619.

32. Nelen G, Martens M, Burssens A. Surgical treatment of chronic Achilles tendonitis. *Am J Sports Med.*1989;17: 754–759.
33. Alfredson H, Pietila T, Jonsson P, Lorentzon R. Heavy-load eccentric training for the treatment of chronic Achilles tendinosis. *Am J Sports Med.*1998; 26:360–366.
34. Koman L, Brashear A, Rosenfeld S, Chamber H, Russman B, Rang M, Root L, Ferrari E, Garcia de Yebenes rous J, Smith B, Turkel C, Wall J, Molloy P. Botulinum toxin Type A neuromuscular blockade in the treatment of equinus foot deformity in cerebral palsy: a multicenter open-label clinical trial. *Pediatrics.*2001; 108:1062–1071.
35. Delpech J. Tenotomie du tendon d'Achille. In: *Chirurg Clin de Montpellier: ou observations et reflexions tirees des travaux de chirurgie clinique cette ecole.* Paris: Gabon; 1823:147–231.
36. Stromeyer G. *Beitragge zur operativen Orthopädik oder Erfahrungen über die Subcutane Durchscheidung verkurzter Muskein und deren Sehnen.* Hanover, NH: Helwing; 1838.
37. Hoke M. An operation for correction of extremely relaxed feet. *J Bone Joint Surg.* 1931;13(A):773–783.
38. Delp S, Zajac F. Force- and moment-generating capacity of lower-extremity muscles before and after tendon lengthening. *Clin Orthop.*1992; 284:247–259.
39. Strayer LM. Gastrocnemius recession: a five-year report of cases. *J Bone Joint Surg.* 1958;40:1019–1030.
40. Pinney S, Sangeorzan B, Hansen S. Surgical anatomy of the Gastrocnemius recession (Strayer procedure). *Foot Ankle Int.*2004; 25:247–250.
41. Vulpius O, Stoffel A. In: *Orthopädische Operationslehre.* Stuttgart, Germany: Ferdinand Ecke;1913:29–31.
42. Vulpiani M, Guzzini M, Ferretti A. Operative treatment of chronic Achilles tendinopathy. *Int Orthop.*2003;27:307–310.
43. Costa M, Donnell S, Tucker K. Long-term outcome of tendon lengthening for chronic Achilles tendon pain. *Foot Ankle Int.*2006; 27:672–676.
44. DiGiovanni C. Proximal gastrocnemius recession (Personal Communication). 2005.
45. Maffulli N, Tallon C, Wong J, Lim K, Bleakney R. Early weightbearing and ankle mobilization after open repair of acute midsubstance tears of the achilles tendon. *Am J Sports Med.* 2003;31:692–700.
46. Mandelbaum BR, Myerson MS, Forster R. Achilles tendon ruptures: a new method of repair, early range of motion, and functional rehabilitation. *Am J Sports Med.*1995; 23:392–395.
47. Cannon L, Hackney R. Operative shortening of the elongated defunctioned Tendoachilles following previous rupture. *J Royal Nav Med Serv.*2003; 89:139–141.
48. Carmont M, Maffulli N. Z Shortening of healed Achilles tendon rupture: a technical note. *Foot Ankle Int.*200 9;30:704–707.
49. Cottrell W, Pearsall A, Hollis M. Simultaneous tears of the Achilles tendon and the medial head of the Gastrocnemius muscle. *Orthopedics.*2002; 25:685–687.
50. GilbertT ,B ullisB ,G riffiths H. Tennis calf or tennis leg. *Orthopedics.*1996; 19:179–182.
51. Webb J, Moonjani N, Radford M. Anatomy of the Sural Nerve and its relation to the Achilles Tendon. *Foot Ankle Int.*2000; 21:475–477.
52. Leversedge F, Casey P, Seiler J, Xerogeanes J. Endoscopically assisted fasciotomy: description of technique and in-vitro assessment of lower-leg compartment decompression. *Am J Sports Med.*2002;30: 272–278.
53. SaxenaA .Endos copicga strocnemiust enotomy. *J Foot Ankle Surg.*2002; 41:57–58.
54. Tashjian RZ, Appel AJ, Banerjee R, DiGiovanni CW. Anatomic study of the gastrocnemius-soleus junction and its relationship to the sural nerve. *Foot Ankle Int.*2003; 24:473–476.
55. Saxena A, Gollwitzer H, DiDomenico L, Widtfeldt A. Endoscopic Gastrocnemius Recession: a midterm report on 54 cases. *Z Orthop Unfall* .2007; 145(4):499–504.

AthroscopicA rthrodesiso ft heA nkle 27

Paul Hamilton Cooke

27.1 Abstract

Arthroscopic ankle arthrodesis (sometimes also known as arthroscopically assisted) is commonly performed to stabilise the arthritic ankle and provide pain relief.

It conveys advantages over open ankle fusion in terms of early mobilization, low non-union rates and low complication rates, and is especially useful in circumstances where there is extensive skin grafting or blood clotting disorders.

Arthroscopic fusion requires the skills of an experienced arthroscopist combined with those of the foot and ankle surgeon to obtain good results.

In the hands of a surgeon with experience, it can be used as an advanced technique in complex cases including with deformity.

27.2 History

Arthroscopic ankle arthrodesis was first performed in 1983 by Schneider.[16]

Early results were unreliable – often long procedures were associated with high rates of fibrous union.

Developments in cameras and power tools allowed surgeons to develop new skills at ankle arthroscopy, and by the 1990s articles were published[6,8] showing advantages in terms of wound and bony healing, in conjunction with early bony union, early weight bearing, and short hospital stays.

The method has continued to grow, and now about half the ankle fusions performed in the UK are performed arthroscopically. For many specialist foot and ankle surgeons the proportion is much higher.

P.H.C ooke
NuffieldO rthopaedicC entre, Headington, Oxford, UK
e-mail:oxfordfoot@ aol.com

N. Maffulli and M. Easley (eds.), *Minimally Invasive Surgery of the Foot and Ankle*,
DOI: 10.1007/978-1-84996-417-3_27,

27.3 Indicationsa ndC ontra-indications

Arthroscopic fusion is usually performed for painful ankle arthritis.

It can be used in most cases, but is especially useful when the skin is poor – when split skin grafts or flaps have been used to treat previous trauma (Fig. 27.1), when the skin has been burnt or damaged previously, or in dermatologic disease (e.g., the Koebner phenomenon in psoriasis[12]).

Also in bleeding disorders such as hemophilia.[17] Here blood loss and risks are minimized. The potential viral load (of HIV, Hepatitis B and C) is reduced to the surgeon, operating staff, and postoperative nursing, plaster room, and physiotherapy staff.

Although early advice warned against arthroscopic fusion in avascular necrosis, this is counterintuitive. This technique preserves the blood supply of the talus. It has been used successfully for the treatment of osteoarthritis in avascular necrosis, including acutely as a means of introducing a new blood supply to the talus to prevent collapse (when extensive articular cartilage damage of the ankle joint is already present)

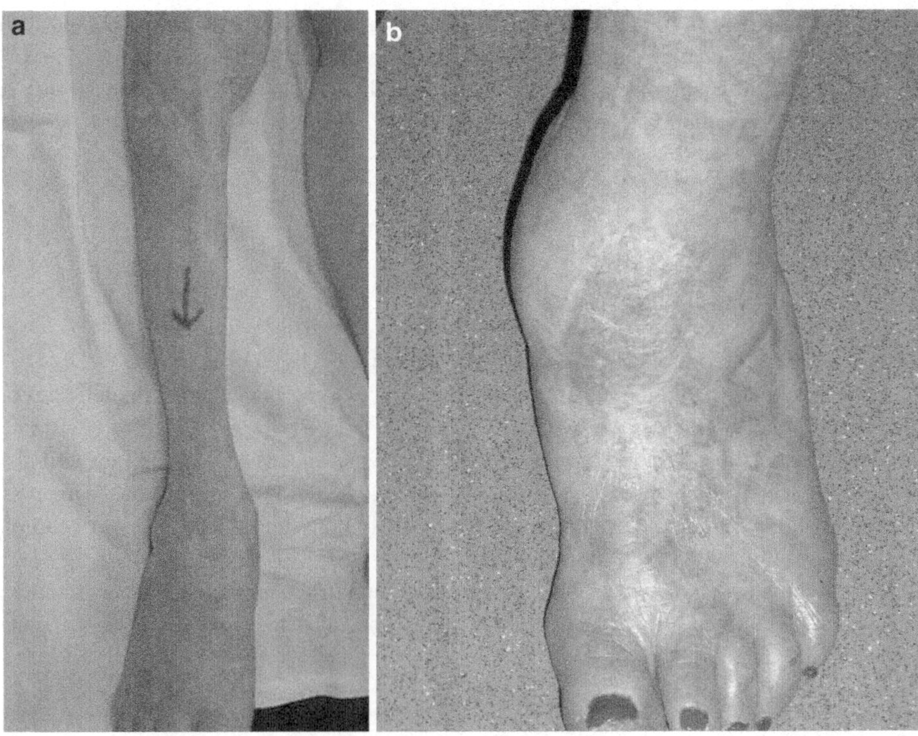

Fig. 27.1 Ankle arthrodesis may be required in the presence of split skin grafts (**a**) or skin flaps (**b**) after trauma or burns. In these situations, arthroscopic arthrodesis is much less risky (Reproduced from Cooke and Jones[3] bype rmissionof L ippincott,W illiams& W ilkins)

Although enthusiasts argue for arthroscopic fusion in all cases of ankle arthritis, there are contraindications.

All cases in the presence of infection carry high risks. Arthroscopic fusion may be performed under appropriate antibiotic suppression, but fixation-whether external or internal-may need to be removed before long-term antibiotic suppression can be stopped.

Most authors suggest that significant coronal or sagittal plane deformity (more than 5–10°) dictates against arthroscopic surgery, although Winson et al.[18] successfully corrected preoperative deformities ranging from 22° valgus and 28° varus, and others have reported similar corrections.[9]

Also large preoperative bone defects may indicate that open methods with grafting are more applicable.

Our experience has been the size of the preoperative deformity and the extent of the bone loss are as not important as the reducibility of the deformity and the experience of the surgeon(Figs. 27.2a–e).

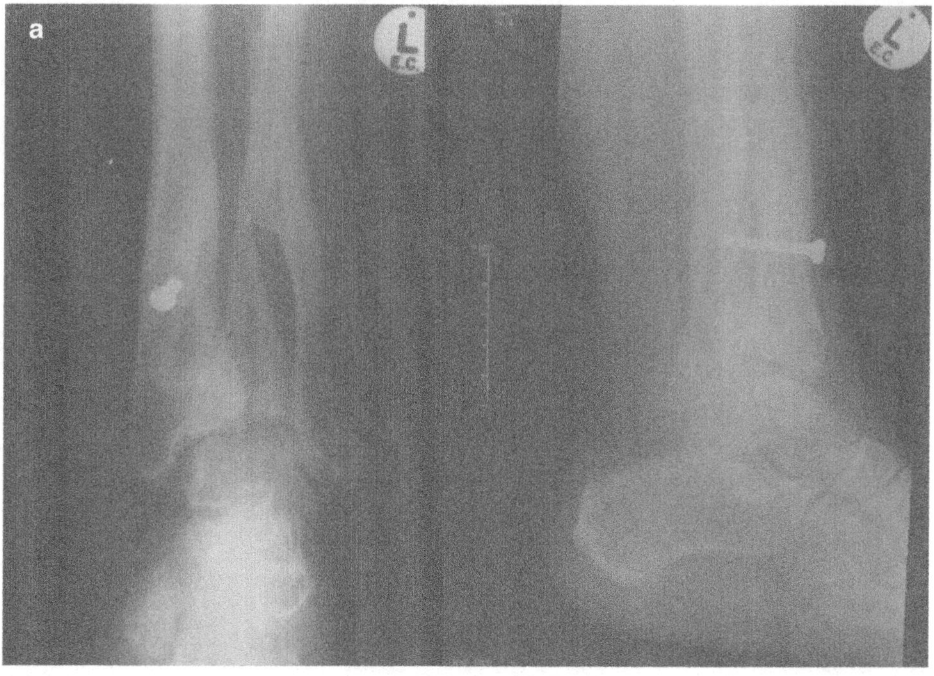

Fig. 27.2 Arthroscopic fusion can be used in cases of bone defect after trauma (**a**, **b**), and to treat bone defect and deformity as in this patient with non-union with collapse and deformity in a patient with Charcot disease (**c**, **d**, **e**). In this latter case, it is combined with arthroscopic subtalar fusion and percutaneous nailing (Reproduced from Cooke and Jones[3] by permission of Lippincott, Williams&W ilkins)

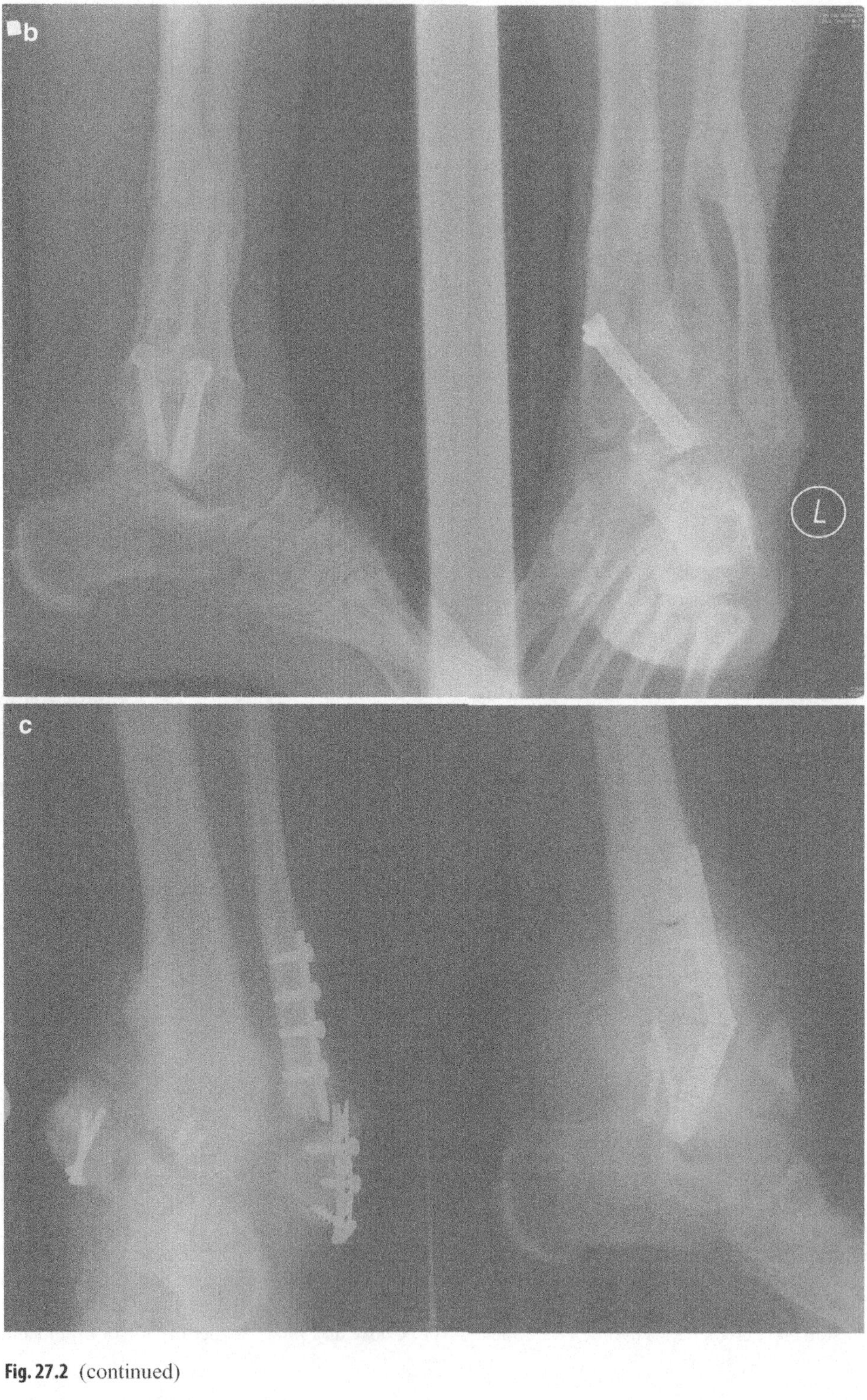

Fig. 27.2 (continued)

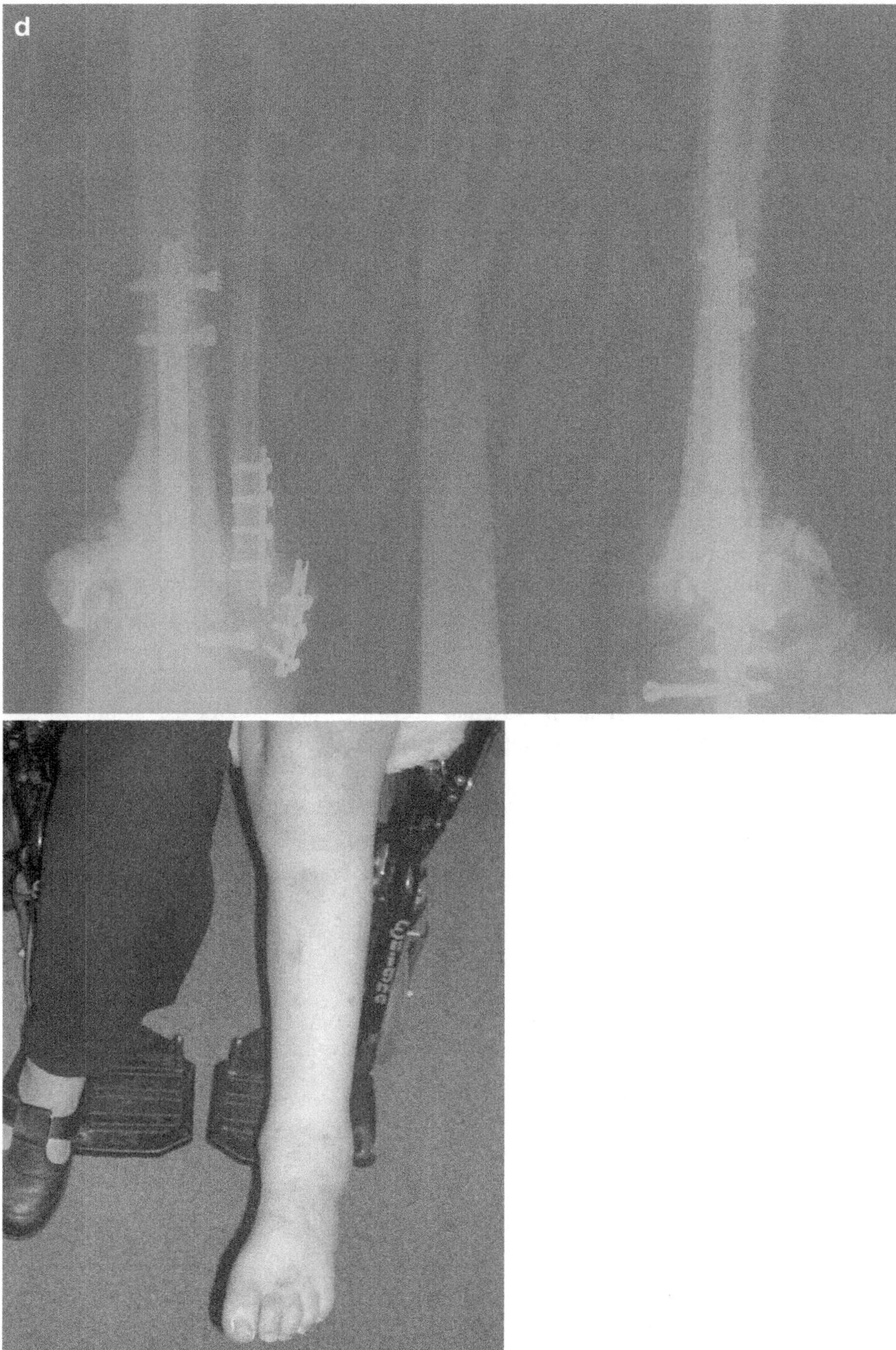

Fig. 27.2 (continued)

27.4 Examinationand A ssessment

Clinical assessment of the range of movement of the ankle is performed, ensuring that any deformities are passively correctible.

This is supplemented by careful examination of the surrounding joints.

Mobility of the surrounding compensatory joints-the lower back, hip knee, and the subtalar and other foot joints-is probably the single most important factor in the eventual outcome from technically successful fusion.

Examination of skin includes careful review of original records when a free flap has been used – to prevent inadvertent puncture of an isolated feeding vessel.

If any doubt exists as to whether the ankle is the principal focus of the pain, injection arthrogram with local anesthetic and radiopaque contrast medium is performed. Contrast medium is used because in about 10% of cases there is flow into the subtalar joint which may compromise the test.

Imaging assessment comprises anteroposterior and lateral radiographs, which may be taken weight bearing or non-weight bearing.

Weight-bearing films show possible causes of malleolar impingement, but will exaggerate deformity, and in the presence of deformity, it is difficult to confirm the radiological status of surrounding joints.

Magnetic resonance imaging or computed tomographic scans are only required in special circumstances: for example, in avascular necrosis, where doubt exists about fracture union or where large cysts or bone defects are suspected which may compromise sound fixation.

Informed consent requires communication to the patient of the common risks and problems and the normal periods to recovery. It is appropriate to remind the patient of the importance of stopping smoking since the rate of nonunion of ankle fusion is greatly increased in smokers.[2]

27.5 Equipment

Modern camera systems allow clear visualization of a distracted ankle with fluid delivered by a mechanical pump.

Surgical preparation is then performed with appropriate power and hand instruments, with fixation undertaken using cannulated compression screws under image intensifier control.

So the following equipment is needed:

1. Distraction
2. Cameras ystema ndi nstruments
3. Fixation(withi magei ntensifier)

27.5.1 Distraction

In general, soft tissue distraction is adequate, and the Smith and Nephew distractor (Acuflex, Ref 7207079) is most commonly used, but if this is not available it is possible to use distraction on a fracture table.[11]

Occasionally, especially in posttrauma cases with dense arthrofibrosis, when correcting deformity or when learning the technique, rigid distraction is easier. A simple two-fine-wire fixator gives powerful distraction, is safe and controllable, and does not impede access while allowing the foot to be plantar and dorsiflexed for access.[10]

Invasive distraction using large unilateral pins is rarely used because of the risks of damage to neurovascular or ligamentous structures associated with overdistraction, infection, pin breakage, and fracture.

27.5.2 CameraS ystem

A full-sized arthroscope (4 mm diameter) used for knee arthroscopy is appropriate and can be used in almost all patients. It has advantages over smaller instruments in terms of field of vision, clarity of vision, high fluid flow rates, and robustness. It does not matter in this situation that the joint surface may be damaged by the cannula.

The image is viewed on a screen, and images and video are easily stored.

Fluidfl ow at controlled pressure is provided by a mechanical pump.

Power tools are essential. The system should include aggressive soft tissue resectors and burrs – there are now some which combine the functions.

A small number of manual instruments are needed – mainly arthroscopic graspers to remove loose bodies and a curved ring curette to remove cartilage from the most posterior aspects of the talus.

27.5.3 Fixation

Finally, a cannulated large fragment screw set is needed with an image intensifier.

Any large fragment screw set can be used, but titanium screws have advantages (although they are more expensive). The wires can be thicker for the same screw diameter and are therefore less prone to bending. Also, computed tomographic scans can be performed around them later if non-union is suspected.

27.6 Anesthesiaand P ositioning

Arthroscopic ankle fusion requires the patient to remain still and be pain free for a period of between 1 and 2 h.

General or regional anesthesia can be used, but the best solution is to combine both-with general or spinal anesthesia supplemented by regional blocks.

Prophylactic antibiotics are administered according to local protocol. After a delay of at least 3 min from their administration, the tourniquet is applied if required. The tourniquet is not essential, and, in patients with vascular compromise, can safely be omitted.

The patient is positioned supine on the table with the knee flexed over an "arm bar," or a sand bag if soft tissue distraction is to be used, and traction applied (Fig. 27.3a–c).

After skin preparation, the leg can be draped with a collection system designed originally for use in cruciate ligament reconstruction (3M Steri-Drape). Through this the distractor is applied (Fig. 27.4). With a suction machine attached to the collection bag, all overflow irrigation fluid is removed.

27.7 Operative Technique

The ankle joint is palpated, inflated with 10–20 mL of saline and anterolateral and anteromedial (or centromedial) incisions made. The arthroscope is inserted, and the fluid pressure is set to a level of 50–70 mmHg measured in the joint.

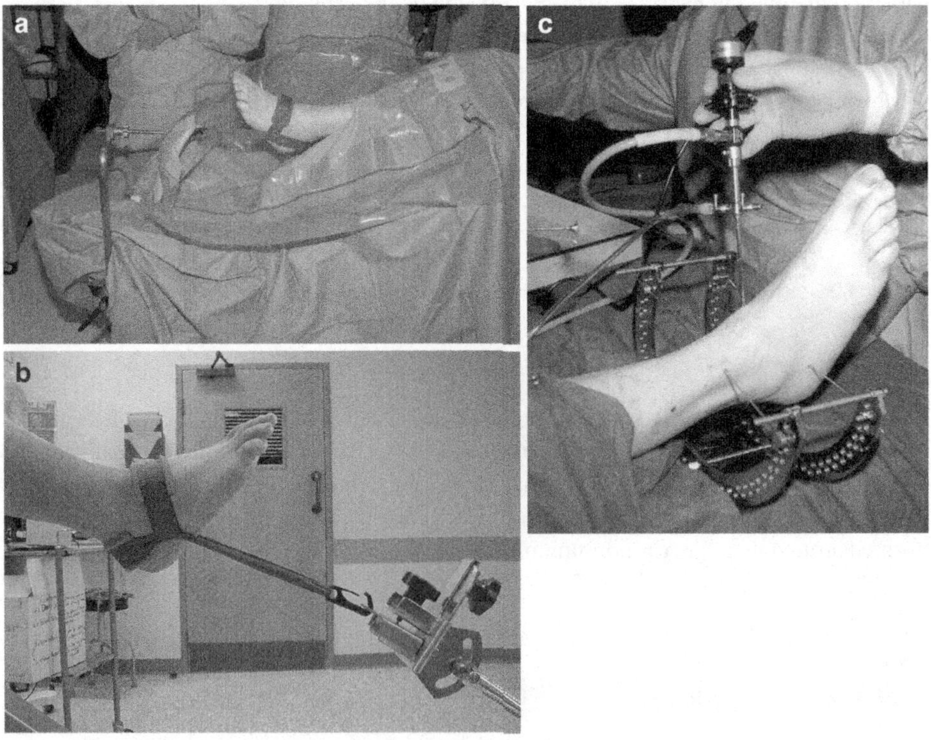

Fig. 27.3 Fixation may be achieved with a soft tissue distractor (**a**), on a fracture table (**b**) or using a two wire distractor (**c**) (Reproduced from Cooke and Jones[3] by permission of Lippincott, Williams& W ilkins)

Fig.27.4 Afl uid collection systeminus ea ts urgery.

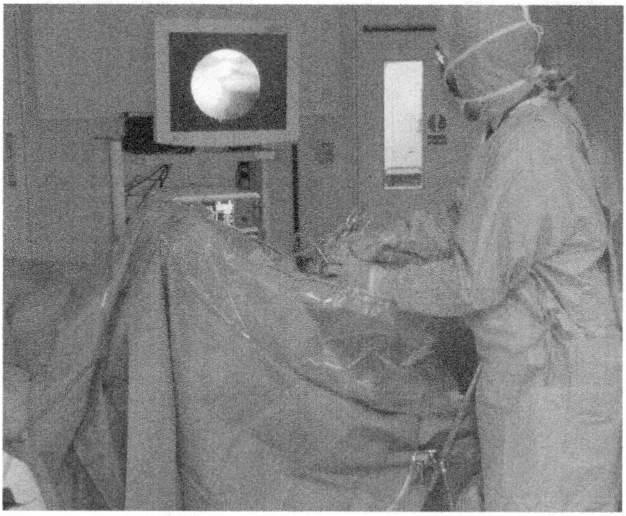

After preliminary examination of the whole joint and removal of loose bodies, anterior cheilectomy and clearance is performed to increase vision and allow reduction at the end of the procedure.

The talus is normally prepared first, although if the joint space is very tight, preliminary clearance of residual cartilage with soft tissue and bony power tools from both surfaces may allow easier access.

In turn, increasing arcs of clearance are cut from the one corner of the talus, expanding across the talus until the whole surface has been cleared.

On the first cut, residual cartilage is removed to expose the underlying bony surface.

A careful balance of burring until vision is obscured followed by gentle suction is developed to allow efficient surgery.

The burr is then used to clear down through the hard chondral bone to the softer subchondal bone, and a check is then made that bleeding subchondral bone has been exposed.

This test is known as the *suction test* (Fig. 27.5a). The inflow port on the arthroscope is closed. The suction on the burr is gradually opened, and if the correct depth of the bone has been reached, the bone surface will be seen to leak blood.

Once the correct level has been reached, arcs of clearance down to subchondral bone are again advanced until the whole of the upper surface of the accessible talus is cleared.

The suction test can be repeated up to twice in the talus, but then, the talus seems to empty of available blood, and after a maximum of three tests will always be negative.

When the accessible talus is cleared, the posterior-most portion can be cleared using the curved ring curette (Fig. 27.5b) This is not essential because, when the foot is restored to neutral at the end of the operation, the posterior-most portion of the talus will no longer be in contact with the tibia.

Throughout the operation, adequate bone preparation is more important than trying to cut flat or matching surfaces.

Once the talus is cleared, attention is turned to the tibia.

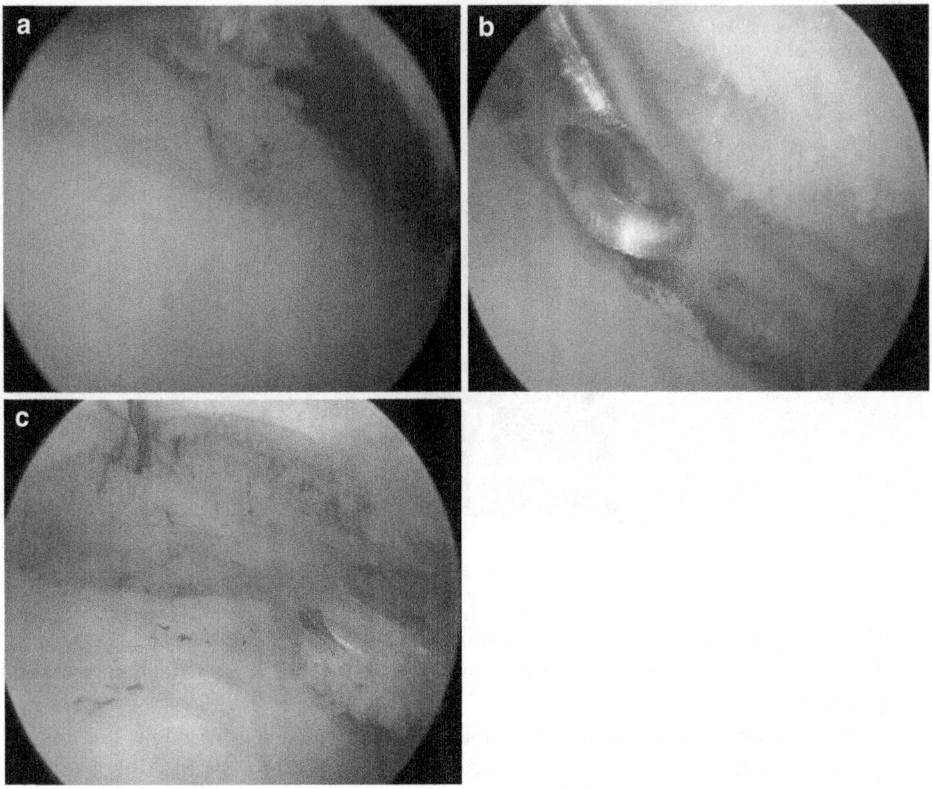

Fig. 27.5 At surgery, the tissue is burred down to bleeding subchondral bone (**a**). The posterior margin may be cleared using a curved ring curette (**b**). The level of resection may be tested using the suction test (**c**) (Reproduced from Cooke and Jones[3] by permission of Lippincott, Williams & Wilkins)

This may be performed from an anterior to posterior direction or vice versa.

When preparing the tibia, it is usually simple to tell that the right depth of cut has been made because the bone can be seen to be vascular, but if necessary, the suction test can again be applied.

After clearing the opposing horizontal surfaces of the talus and tibia, attention is turned to the medial malleolus, and again, the opposing vertical surfaces are prepared to bleeding bone using a burr smaller than that used in the main joint.

Most surgeons do not prepare the fibula or the lateral talus, preferring to preserve mobility of the fibula. The only time surgery to the fibula is necessary is if there is preexisting lateral compression or when varus deformities are corrected, and on these occasions, arthroscopic excision of the tip of the fibula prevents lateral impingement or peroneal compression after surgery.

The entry portals are then reversed to check that full clearance has been achieved (Fig. 27.5c).

No graft or biological agents need to be added because the cavity fills from the exposed and vascular cavity, allowing rapid ingrowth.

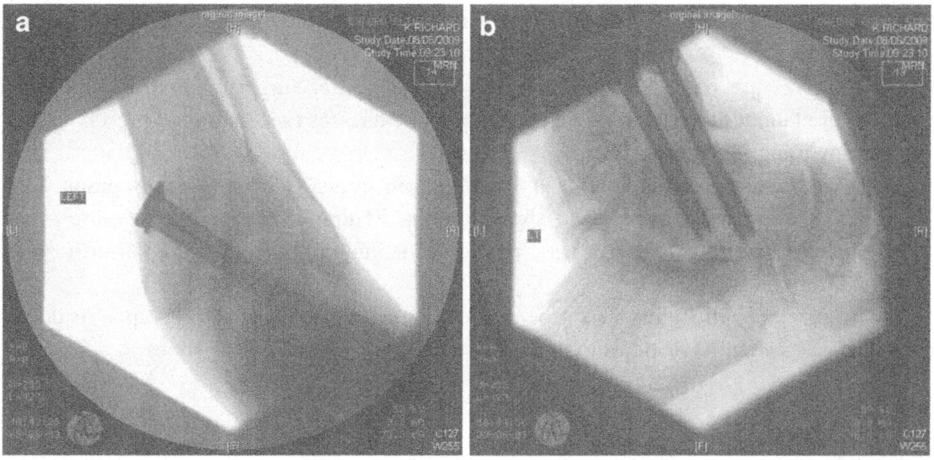

Fig.2 7.6 Cannulated screws are inserted (**a**, **b**)

Traction is removed and a bowl placed under the calf allowing access for fixation and ensuring the foot is not pushed forward relative to the tibia.

The foot is then positioned square beneath the leg and fixed using two cannulated screws. Parallel compression screws are more popular than crossed screws in the United Kingdom(Fig. 27.6).

Positioning of the foot is easier after arthroscopic fusion than open, but it is still very important to avoid deformity, especially residual equinous.

Once the foot is reduced, two wires are passed under radiograph control, and the positions are checked. Parallel screws are used inserted from medial to lateral, angulated forwards to ensure anterior compression and to minimize the risk of inadvertent perforation of the subtalar joint.

The screws are inserted using washers to prevent subsidence although prominence of these screws and washers can lead to problems.

A small gap is often seen, which although it would be unacceptable for an open fusion is acceptable immediately after arthroscopic fusion. The interval fills in rapidly. The situation is analogous to that in intramedullary nailing when gaps can be accepted on the immediate post-operative films after closed (but not open) surgery.

Some form of backslab or splint is then applied for protection, and to prevent equinus/plantaris from the hind and midfoot.

27.8 Post-operativeM anagement

Post-operative regimes vary considerably from surgeon to surgeon.

Patients mobilize using crutches initially. Some surgeons allow the patient to put as much weight as is comfortable through the operated limb. This does not appear to increase the risk of non-union as long as they are warned to avoid any painful or uncomfortable weight bearing.

The sutures are removed approximately 2 weeks after surgery, and from this time, patients are taught to perform range of movement exercises twice a day to preserve range in the remaining joints of the foot.

They are first seen in outpatients at 8 weeks from surgery for the first radiograph.

Provided they are pain-free and showing signs of union on radiograph, more active physiotherapy and full weight bearing is allowed using a light supramalleolar orthosis, if required, for confidence.

At 16 weeks from surgery, a further review is performed by physiotherapist or doctor when an assessment is made as to whether a rocker is required on the shoes.

27.9 Results, Complications and Problems

Reviewing outcomes and complication rates after ankle and hind foot surgery is difficult with problems of patient selection, methods of assessing outcome (particularly with high levels of comorbidity), and differing satisfaction based on the widely divergent desired outcomes in different patients' ages and disease groups.

In addition, the published results of arthroscopic ankle arthrodesis are almost always the results of single specialist surgeons or groups of specialist surgeons. As such, not only may they have special skills and facilities, support staff, and so on, but they may attract skewed patient populations.

Arthrodesis gives best results in young healthy patients with single joint disease and with high physical demand. These patients can expect complete relief of pain and to be able to walk without a visible limp. The further one is from this indication, the greater the likely long-term disability will be.

Gait analysis studies have shown that, for ankle fusion in general, observable gait is usually normal,[14] but the patient compensates by shortening the stride length on the affected side and presumably increasing rotation at the hips and back to compensate.

The outcome of fusion is largely dependent on the mobility of the surrounding joints, and in this respect, arthroscopic fusion has an advantage over open fusion. Decreased local tissue damage, combined with early postoperative mobilization combine to better preserve the preexisting range.

Union rates are high. Ferkel and Hewitt[7] and our own series[1] have shown union rates between 97% and 100%.

Early reports often showed lower rates of union, reflecting undeveloped equipment and technique.

Dent et al. in 1993[6] presented eight early cases with a nonunion rate of more than 50% but commented that patients with fibrous union (or fibrous nonunion) were often satisfied.

More recently, Winson et al.[18] described a higher nonunion rate and dissatisfaction rate than is generally reported, but again, this reflects the fact that they have included their first cases – when the techniques were still being developed. When the first cases are excluded, their results compare with other series, with high union rates.

Many authors have noted that not only are union rates high but that the time to union is short (Fig. 27.7). Ferkel and Hewitt[7] described mean time to union as 11.8 weeks, Glick et al.[8] as 9 weeks, Nielsen[15] as 90% union at 12 weeks with arthroscopic compared to 57% in the open group - 84 % is the figure for the open group at 12 months.

Furthermore, early weight bearing can usually be allowed. Studies have shown no difference between early and delayed weight bearing in historic review (patients with neuropathy who might not perceive pain on weight bearing were excluded from this study).[1]

No significant increase in the speed or rate of union occurs when bone-promoting factors are added to the regime.[4,5]

We have published a series without non-union,[1] but this is not typical of our results.

A more recent internal review of 100 consecutive cases[3] showed the following complication rates: nonunion, 3%; screw head prominence needing removal, 2%; and penetration of subtalar joint, 2%.

Our average surgical time in this series was 55 min compared with 65 min for open arthrodesis.

Over a period in our unit, nonunion has almost always been associated with smokers, infection, neuropathic cases, or inexperience of the operating surgeon. Delayed union occurs in approximately 10% of cases needing over 12 weeks of immobilization and 5% needing longer periods of up to 22 weeks.

Screw prominence can be troublesome early or late after surgery. The problem arises because of applying large screws and washers at an oblique angle to cross the ankle joint.

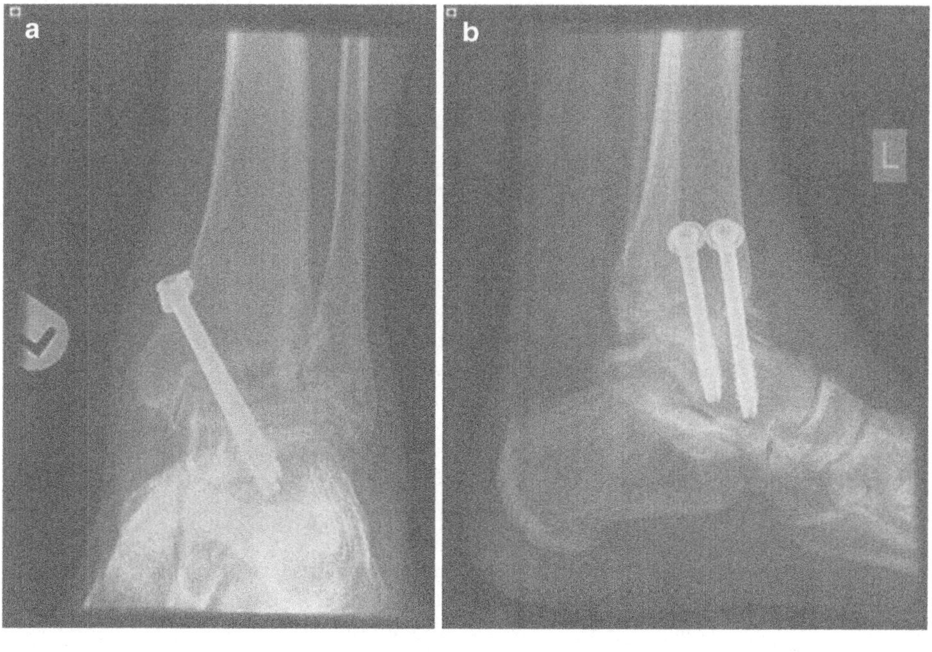

Fig. 27.7 Rapid union is shown on plain radiographs 6 weeks after surgery (the same case as Fig. 27.6)

When the bone is hard, the washers can be omitted, which avoids the problem, but in most instances, absence of the washer merely leads to sinkage of the screw head.

Most surgeons have found that intraosseous compression screws are less effective than conventional screws, so these do not offer a good alternative.

Lwin et al.[13] designed ingenious washers to allow the screw head to be countersunk, but the dimensions lead to unacceptable fracture rates.

So this remains a significant problem, and screw removal or replacement is occasionally performed when the rubbing is uncomfortable and is essential if the screw head threatens to ulcerate.

Penetration of the tip of the screw also occurs. Although this is always due to incorrect placement at the time of surgery, it is predisposed to by the length of the screw thread that approaches the total available bone depth of the talus. It can be avoided by angling the screws obliquely forward and laterally. This effectively increases the depth of the talus available, and if penetration does occur, it is into the sinus tarsi not into the posterior facet of the subtalar joint.

27.10 Conclusion

Arthroscopic ankle arthrodesis is a relatively simple technique for the modern foot and ankle surgeon with arthroscopic skills, which conveys advantages of reliable and rapid unionw ithm inimals oftt issuedi sruption.

References

1. Cannon LB, Brown J, Cooke PH. Early weight bearing is safe following arthroscopic ankle arthrodesis. *Foot Ankle Surg.*2004; 10:135–139.
2. Cobb TK, Gabrielsen TA, Campell DC, et al. Cigarette smoking and non union after ankle arthrodesis. *Foot Ankle Int.*1994; 15:64–67.
3. Cooke P, Jones I. Arthroscopic ankle arthrodesis. *Techn Foot Ankle Surg.* Dec 2007;6: 210–217.
4. Collman DR, Kass MH, Schuberth JM. Arthroscopic ankle arthrodesis: factors influencing union in 39 consecutive patients. *Foot Ankle Int.*2006; 27:1079–1085.
5. Crosby LA, Yee TC, Formanek TS, et al. Complications following ankle arthrodesis. *Foot Ankle Int.*1996;1 7:340–342.
6. Dent CM, Patil M, Fairclough JA. Arthroscopic ankle arthrodesis. *J Bone Joint Surg Br.* 1993;75:830–832.
7. Ferkel RD, Hewitt M. Long-term results of arthroscopic ankle arthrodesis. *Foot Ankle Int.* 2005;26:389–392.
8. Glick JM, Morgan CD, Myerson MS, et al. Ankle arthrodesis using an arthroscopic method: long-term follow up of 34 cases. *Arthroscopy.*1996; 12:428–434.
9. Gougoulias NE, Agathangelidis FG, Parsons SW. Arthroscopic Ankle arthrodesis. *Foot Ankle Int.*J une2007;28: 695–706.

10. Graham AJ, Hughes S, Cooke PH. Ankle arthroscopy: the use of an Ilizarov half frame to distract the ankle joint. *Foot Ankle Surg.*2000; 6:55–58.
11. Hedley D, Geary NPJ, Meda P. Ankle arthroscopy: a new technique for non-invasive ankle distraction. *Foot Ankle Surg.*2001; 7:137–139.
12. KobnerH .ZurA etiologiePps oriosis. *Vjchr Dermatol.*1 876;3:559.
13. Lwin MK, Geary NP, Zubairy AL, et al. Arthroscopic ankle fusion using two medial cannulated screws with distal washers. BOFS 2002 Proceedings. *J Bone Joint Surg Br.* 2003;85:246.
14. Mazur JM, Schwartz E, Simon SR. Ankle arthrodesis: long term follow up with gait analysis. *J Bone Joint Surg Am.*1979; 61:964–975.
15. Neilsen KK, Linde F, Jensen NC. The outcome of arthroscopic and open surgery ankle arthrodesis: a comparative retrospective study of 107 patients. *Foot Ankle Surg.*2008; 14:153–157.
16. Schneider D. Arthroscopic ankle fusion. *Arthroscopic Video J.*1983: 3.
17. Steffen RT, Bedi HS, Sharpe RJ, et al. Arthroscopic ankle arthrodesis for haemophilic arthropathy. *J Bone Joint Surg Br.*2005; 87:275–280.
18. Winson IG, Robinson DE, Allen PE. Arthroscopic ankle arthrodesis. *J Bone Joint Surg Br.* 2005;87:343–347.

Percutaneous Osteosynthesis of Distal Tibial Fractures Using Locking Plates

28

Mario Ronga, Chezhiyan Shanmugam, Umile Giuseppe Longo, Francesco Oliva, and Nicola Maffulli

28.1 Introduction

Surgical fixation of distal tibia fractures can be difficult, and requires careful preoperative planning. Fracture pattern, soft tissue injury, and bone quality critically influence the selection of fixation technique.[1] Several surgical methods have been described for the treatment of these fractures, including external fixation, intramedullary nailing, and plate fixation. Classical open reduction and internal plate fixation requires extensive soft tissue dissection and periosteal stripping, with high rates of complications, including infection, delayed and non-unions.[2,3] Moreover, the surgical dissection required to achieve anatomic reduction evacuates the osteogenic fracture ematoma. Several minimally invasive plate osteosynthesis techniques have been developed, with good results at medium term follow-up.[4–6] These techniques aim to reduce surgical trauma and to maintain a more biologically favorable environment for fracture healing.

A new advance in this field is represented by the locking plate (LP). These devices consist of plate and screw systems where the screws are locked in the plate at a fixed angle. Preliminary clinical studies report the high success rate of minimally invasive locking plate technique in the distal tibia fractures.[7–10] In this chapter, the surgical technique of the percutaneous osteosynthesis of distal tibial fractures using locking plates is presented.

28.2 Surgical Technique

The timing of surgery should be optimized to allow the soft tissues to stabilize and minimize the severe postoperative wound problems often associated with the surgical management of these complex fractures. The "wrinkle sign" is a useful test to decide the timing of

N. Maffulli (✉)
Centre for Sports and Exercise Medicine, Queen Mary University of London, Barts and The London School of Medicine and Dentistry, Mile End Hospital, London, England, UK
e-mail: n.maffulli@qmul.ac.uk

N. Maffulli and M. Easley (eds.), *Minimally Invasive Surgery of the Foot and Ankle*,
DOI: 10.1007/978-1-84996-417-3_28,

surgery. In the wrinkle sign, the ankle is dorsiflexed while the anterior aspect of the ankle is observed; the absence of a skin crease or wrinkle suggests severe swelling.[11] Temporary skeletal stabilization can be achieved by simple splintage or bridging external fixation until surgery is performed.

Good quality plain radiographs (anteroposterior, lateral, and long leg alignment views) are obtained with computed tomography (CT) scans, if necessary, to determine optimal plate location. Identification of the size and location of the articular fragments is essential before reconstruction. In the distal tibia, the plate is normally applied on the anteromedial aspect. Several precontoured plates specifically designed for these locations are commercially available. Anatomic locking plates should not be bent if possible because, bending alters the biomechanical properties of the plate leading to fatigue failure.[12]

With the patient supine on a radiolucent table, antibiotic prophylaxis is administered and standard intra-operative fluoroscopy used throughout the procedure. Great care should be taken to ensure that the fracture can be clearly visualized on both antero-posterior and lateral views. Both the injured and the noninjured limb are prepared and draped above the knee, thus allowing intraoperative alignment to be checked against the normal limb. Elevating the injured limb on radiolucent trays enables a clear lateral view and avoids interference from the other leg. The joint line of both the knee and the ankle are defined and marked on the skin. Using ankle manual traction, or through a single Steinman pin inserted into the calcaneus, the fracture is reduced (Fig. 28.1a). Depending of the quality of tibial fracture reduction reached, a fibula fracture, if present, can be plated first using a one third tubular plate to provide lateral stability and restoration of the correct length, and to prevent over-distraction at the fracture site. The main fracture fragments of the distal tibia are aligned and reduced percutaneously or through separate stab incisions using a periosteal elevator, clamps, or Kirschner wires as joysticks, and then fixed with individual lag screws. In the fractures with intra-articular extension, arthroscopy can be performed through conventional anterior portals to assess the reduction of the articular surface and to address any associated joint lesions. Several authors reported an incidence of intra-articular pathology in ankle fractures ranging between 63% and 79.2%.[13–15] Based on the minimal added time and morbidity to the surgical procedure, we use arthroscopy on a regular basis, but we limit it use to intra-articular fracture.

With the fracture adequately reduced, a small transverse or longitudinal incision is made distal to the medial malleolus, and a subcutaneous tunnel is produced using a vascular forceps (Fig. 28.1b). A LP is then passed along the tunnel, bridging the fracture site. The plate has to be long enough to bridge the metaphyseal zone and allow at least two bicortical screws insertions proximal to the fracture. Kirschner wires can be used to secure, through the ad hoc holes proximal and distal to the fracture, the plate to the bone before screw insertion. It is critical at this stage to make a thorough assessment of the limb alignment and establish that the correct rotation has been achieved by comparison with the other limb. The correct rotation is established evaluating the alignment of the proximal and distal cortices of the distal tibia and comparing at 90° of knee flexion the axis between the tibial tuberosity and the intermetatarsal spaces. As locking screws are used, the plate cannot be used to effect fracture reduction, which should therefore be achieved before the plate is applied. Additional screws are then inserted percutaneously as necessary, with a minimal of two bicortical screws at either end. Stoffel et al.[16] reported the factors that

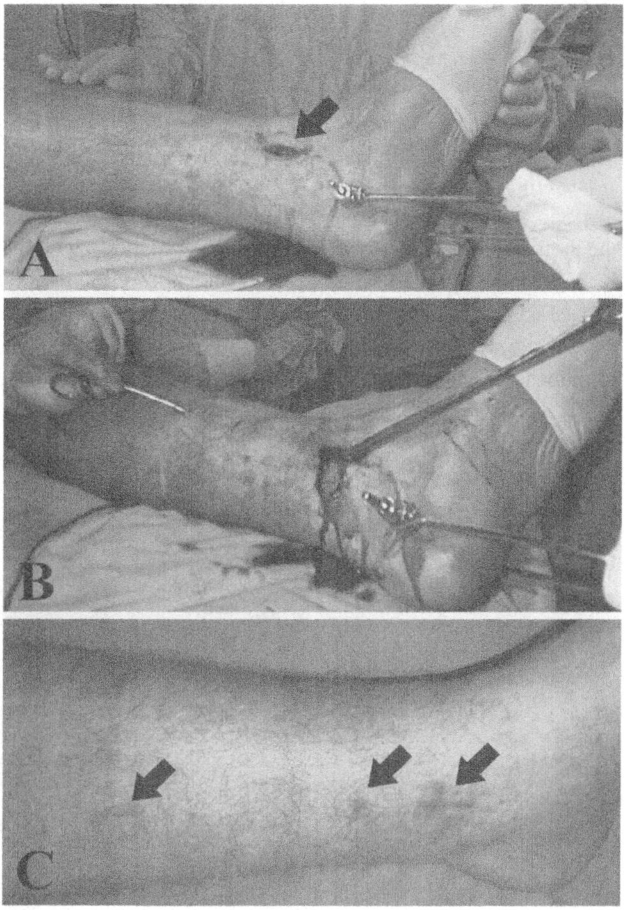

Fig.28.1 (**a**) A calcaneal Steinmann pin is applied to reduce the fracture and to maintain the length and alignment of the limb. Small longitudinal incision is distal to the medial malleolus (arrow). (**b**)The subcutaneous tunnel is fashioned using artery forceps to facilitate locking plate insertion. (**c**)Fina l scars (arrows), showing the minimal nature of the exposure

influence stability in both compression and torsion. Axial stiffness and torsional rigidity are mainly influenced by the working length, e.g., the distance of the first screw to the fracture site. By omitting one screw hole on either side of the fracture, the construct became almost twice as flexible in both compression and torsion. The number of screws also significantly affect stability. However, neither more than three screws per fragment did little to increase axial stiffness, nor did four screws increase torsional rigidity. The position of the third screw significantly affect axial stiffness, but not torsional rigidity. The other factor affecting the stability of the construct is the distance between the plate and the bone, which should be kept small, and long plates should be used to provide sufficient axial stiffness. The optimal plate distance should be 2 mm or less from the surface of the bone.[12] The stab incisions are closed in a standard fashion, the wound is dressed, and the limb is immobilized in a below knee synthetic cast (Fig. 28.1c).

28.3 RehabilitationP rotocol

Patients are allowed non-weight bearing crutch walking immediately after surgery. At 2 weeks, the below knee synthetic cast is changed to another short leg light weight cast after inspection of the wound and removal of the sutures. The weight bearing status is dependent on the individual fracture pattern, but most of the patients weight bear at least partially at 6 weeks. If the fracture is intra-articular, patients are allowed non-weight bearing for the first 2 weeks, and asked them to start toe-touch weightbearing starting from the fourth postoperative week. Outpatient physiotherapy is instituted to maximize the range of motion of the foot and ankle immediately after definitive removal of the cast. A representative case is shown in Fig. 28.2.

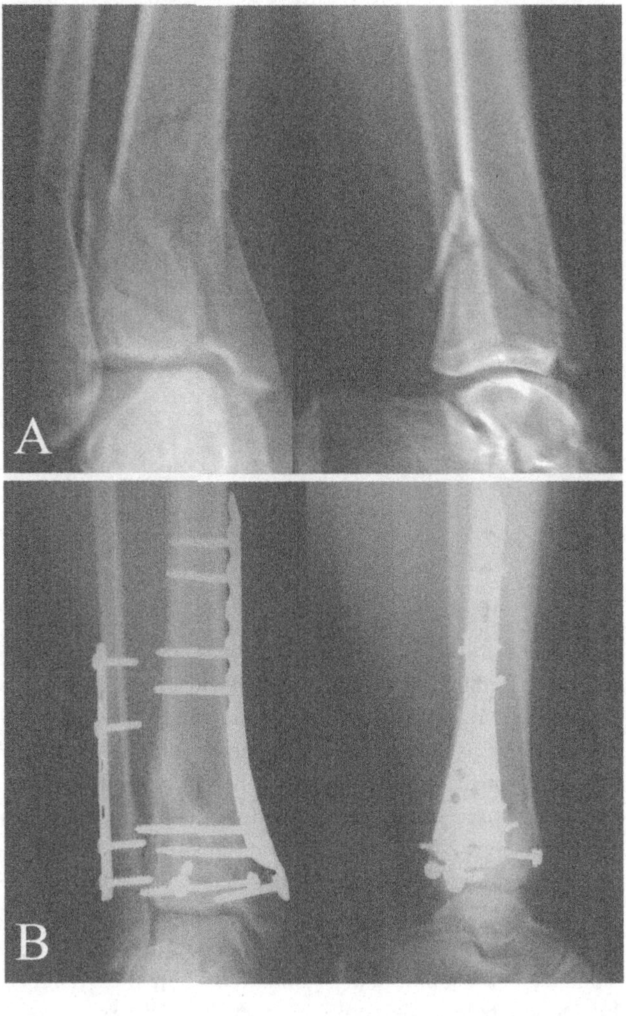

Fig.28.2 (**a**)A multifragmentary, intra-articular fracture of the distal tibia and a supra-syndesmotic fracture of fibula. (**b**) Plain radiographs after 1 year. The fracture united with no limb shortening. The patient is fully weight bearing with no aidsa ndnol imp

References

1. Bedi A, Le TT, Karunakar MA. Surgical treatment of nonarticular distal tibia fractures. *J Am Acad Orthop Surg.*2006; 14:406–416.
2. Fisher WD, Hamblen DL. Problems and pitfalls of compression fixation of long bone fractures: a review of results and complications. *Injury.*1978; 10:99–107.
3. Olerud S, Karlstrom G. Tibial fractures treated by AO compression osteosynthesis. Experiences from a five year material. *Acta Orthop Scand Suppl.*197 2;140:1–104.
4. Francois J, Vandeputte G, Verheyden F, Nelen G. Percutaneous plate fixation of fractures of the distal tibia. *Acta Orthop Belg.*2004; 70:148–154.
5. Helfet DL, Shonnard PY, Levine D, Borrelli J Jr. Minimally invasive plate osteosynthesis of distal fractures of the tibia. *Injury.* 1997;28:A42–A47, discussion A7–8.
6. Maffulli N, Toms AD, McMurtie A, Oliva F. Percutaneous plating of distal tibial fractures. *Int Orthop.*2004;28:159–162.
7. Hasenboehler E, Rikli D, Babst R. Locking compression plate with minimally invasive plate osteosynthesis in diaphyseal and distal tibial fracture: a retrospective study of 32 patients. *Injury.*2007;38:365–370.
8. Hazarika S, Chakravarthy J, Cooper J. Minimally invasive locking plate osteosynthesis for fractures of the distal tibia--results in 20 patients. *Injury.*2006; 37:877–887.
9. Lau TW, Leung F, Chan CF, Chow SP. Wound complication of minimally invasive plate osteosynthesis in distal tibia fractures. *Int Orthop.*2007; 32:697–703.
10. Ronga M, Longo UG, Maffulli N. Minimally invasive locked plating of distal tibia fractures is safe and effective. *Clin Orthop Relat Res.* 2009. DOI: 10.1007/s11999-009-0991-7.
11. Tull F, Borrelli J Jr. Soft-tissue injury associated with closed fractures: evaluation and management. *J Am Acad Orthop Surg.*2003; 11:431–438.
12. Ahmad M, Nanda R, Bajwa AS, Candal-Couto J, Green S, Hui AC. Biomechanical testing of the locking compression plate: when does the distance between bone and implant significantly reduce construct stability? *Injury.*2007; 38:358–364.
13. Hintermann B, Regazzoni P, Lampert C, Stutz G, Gachter A. Arthroscopic findings in acute fractures of the ankle. *J Bone Joint Surg Br.*2000; 82:345–351.
14. Imade S, Takao M, Nishi H, Uchio Y. Arthroscopy-assisted reduction and percutaneous fixation for triplane fracture of the distal tibia. *Arthroscopy.* 2004;20:e123–128.
15. Loren GJ, Ferkel RD. Arthroscopic assessment of occult intra-articular injury in acute ankle fractures. *Arthroscopy.*2002; 18:412–421.
16. Stoffel K, Dieter U, Stachowiak G, Gachter A, Kuster MS. Biomechanical testing of the LCP--how can stability in locked internal fixators be controlled? *Injury.*2003; 34:B11–19.

Percutaneous Supramalleolar Osteotomy Usingt hel lizarov/ TaylorS patialF rame

29

S. Robert Rozbrucha nd Austin T. Fragomen

29.1 Introduction

Malalignment of the distal tibia and ankle is a common problem that is largely left untreated even in this era of modern orthopedics. The lack of interest in treating these deformities can be attributed to the deficiency of a safe and reliable method for correction. In our hands correction of distal tibial and ankle deformities using a percutaneous osteotomy and a minimally invasive circular external fixator has yielded excellent and reproducible results with minimal complications.

Common deformities that cause malalignment include distal tibial and ankle varus, valgus, apex anterior, apex posterior, mal-rotation, and shortening. Typically, a patient will have more than one of these deformities simultaneously. A poorly aligned ankle joint experiences asymmetric forces on the articular cartilage that can lead to arthritis. Treatment of the deformity has ranged from bracing to operative reconstruction. Supramalleolar osteotomy (SMO) is a powerful method to correcting deformities of the distal tibia and ankle and re-establish normal limb alignment. The goal of surgery in patients without ankle arthritis is to re-establish a normal joint line and avoid the development of arthritis. This has been achieved primarily by using internal fixation. Problems associated with internal fixation in this location are numerous: often the skin is damaged from the original injury or from previous surgery, increasing the risk of wound breakdown and hardware contamination. Internal fixation requires an acute correction of the deformity, which may be risky for neurovascular structures, skin healing, and may require excessive soft tissue stripping. Internal fixation necessitates that an accurate correction be obtained in the operating room and therefore offers no post operative adjustability. Patients are not allowed to weight bear for several months after internal fixation.

Once the ankle joint has become arthritic, the goals change slightly. The deformity may even stem from the irregularity of the joint surface itself. The benefit of surgical realignment

S.R.R ozbruch(✉)
Limb Lengthening and Reconstruction, Hospital for Special Surgery, Weill Medical College of Cornell University, 535 East 70th Street, New York, NY 10021, USA
e-mail:R ozbruchSR@hss.edu

N. Maffulli and M. Easley (eds.), *Minimally Invasive Surgery of the Foot and Ankle*,
DOI: 10.1007/978-1-84996-417-3_29,

at that time is lessened as the cartilage has already been damaged. The goal of osteotomy is to protect and unload the intact cartilage, and then prevent further joint cartilage injury. Additional procedures are also performed concomitantly in the arthritic joint including osteophyte excision, microfracture, and, perhaps, ankle distraction arthroplasty. These adjunctive procedures are aimed at treating the arthritis once it already is present.

Circular external fixation has steadily gained popularity for foot and ankle reconstructive surgery.[23,31] Pins and wires pierce the skin and bone percutaneously, with minimal disruption of the surrounding soft tissues. This minimally invasive approach is ideal for patients with poor skin and those at risk for wound healing problems. This also makes external fixation very compatible with the percutaneous osteotomy technique. Adjustability is the hallmark of external fixation. This allows for gradual correction of large deformities to avoid neurovascular injury, limb lengthening in cases of tibial shortening, and fine-tuning of incompletely corrected deformities. The Taylor spatial frame (TSF) (Smith & Nephew, Memphis, TN) greatly simplified frame adjustments and made correcting complex deformity a routine efficient procedure. The computer program is precise and alignment can be controlled expertly. Correction of multiple deformities simultaneously is achieved with ease. External fixators are very stable and can support the bone firmly allowing early weight bearing. The external frames are modular and can be combined with additional rings for other simultaneous surgery including ankle distraction arthroplasty, high tibial osteotomy, and proximal tibial lengthening.

Percutaneous supramalleolar osteotomy (PSMO) is ideal for use in conjunction with external fixation. Both techniques require small incisions making them very compatible. A large open approach to the tibia for osteotomy could be used in conjunction with the external fixator as well, but that would defeat many of the advantages of the fixators percutaneous nature. The osteotomy itself involves only a 1 cm incision over the anterior distal tibia. We use a drill to produce multiple drill holes in one plane across the metaphyseal-diaphyseal junction of the distal tibia and an osteotome to perform the corticotomy. The fibula is osteotomised as well.

The combination of a percutaneous tibial osteotomy, a percutaneously placed fixation device, and a highly accurate computerized external fixator has made this procedure relatively simple and quite safe. It is ideal for patients with poor skin, significant deformity, a history of infection, and for those who need immediate weight bearing capabilities.[7]

This chapter will address the clinical indications, preoperative assessment, surgical technique, and postoperative care for the technique of PSMO using the Ilizarov/ TSF.

29.2 Clinical Indications

29.2.1 Malunion of Tibia Fracture

Malunion of a tibia fracture in the distal third of the leg is the most common etiology for distal tibial deformity. The resulting malalignment will cause abnormal force transmission across the ankle joint surface, and lead to post-traumatic arthrosis.[8,17,20] Varus and valgus deformities of the distal tibia both lead to increased shear stresses across the joint. While valgus deformities are more easily compensated through inversion of the subtalar joint, the deformity will lead to wear of the ankle joint. The wear pattern typically involves the lateral aspect of the joint (Fig. 29.1). Varus deformity is functionally debilitating to the patient since there is limited ability to compensate with hindfoot eversion. These deformities are more obvious, and patients often complain of walking on the lateral border of their foot. With varus the cartilage wear in the ankle is typically in the medial aspect of the joint. Recurvatum (apex posterior) deformity leads to uncovering of the talus and compensatory ankle equinus contracture (Fig. 29.2). Procurvatum (apex anterior) deformity limits dorsiflexion of the ankle and leads to anterior ankle impingement[17] (Fig. 29.3). Oblique plane deformities and rotation and translation deformities are common in malunions. External rotation deformity is particularly common after ankle fracture fixation. Patients complain of the foot pointing outward when they walk. This should not be confused with voluntary-compensatory external rotation of the foot and entire lower limb to decrease pain from and arthritic ankle during gait.

The goal of PSMO is to correct the deformity in the coronal, sagittal, and axial planes. A lateral distal tibial angle (LDTA) of 90° (Fig. 29.4a) and an anterior distal tibial angle (ADTA) of 80° are ideal[16,17] (Fig. 29.4b). The use of the Ilizarov/Taylor Spatial Frame is particularly useful for a gradual correction of a simple or large oblique plane deformity.[4,5,21] At times the osteotomy is produced at a location other than the site of the malunion. For example, a malunion of the mid-distal third of the leg that is composed of varus and translation may have a center of rotation and angulation (CORA)[16,17] or apex of deformity in the supramalleolar region. The SMO becomes a convenient way to correct this, since the supramalleolar bone is metaphyseal, previously uninjured and has better healing potential that the actual site of the malunion (Fig. 29.5a–c).

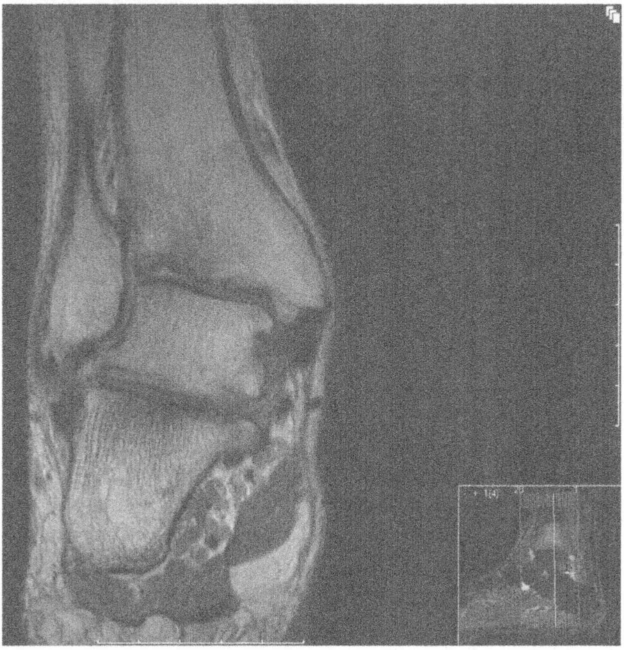

Fig.29.1 CoronalM RI: A chronic valgus deformity has caused asymmetric wear of the ankle articular cartilage with more cartilage lossla terally

Fig. 29.2 Twenty-two year old male with a malunited distal tibia with anterior translation of the foot and an apex posterior deformity. High joint contact pressure anteriorly has contributed to anterior joint space loss. The patient is not able to dorsiflex past neutral, indicating that the ankle joint has an equinus contracture (With a 10° recurvatum deformity, he should be able to dorsiflex to 10° past neutral or 20° total)

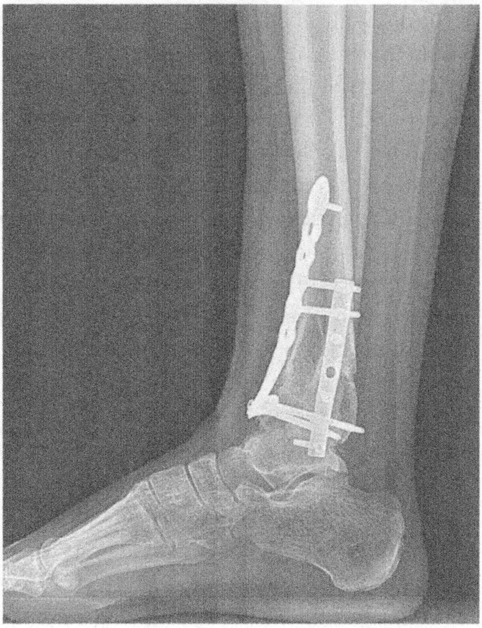

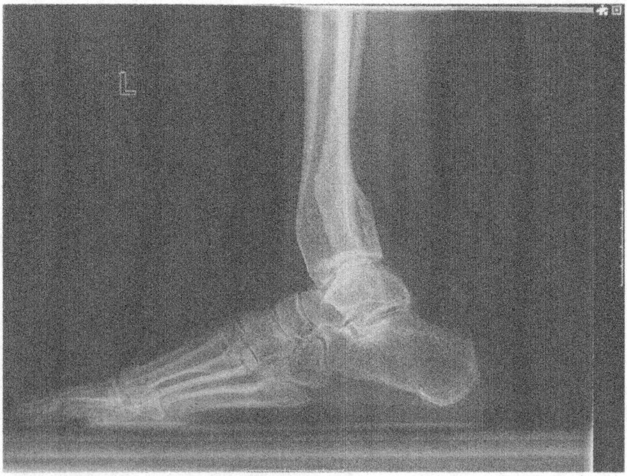

Fig. 29.3 Thisproc urvatum deformity results in symptomatic impingement of the talus on the anterior tibia with the ankle in the neutralpos ition

Associated symptomatic arthritis may be addressed as well. Ankle distraction[11,31] (Fig. 29.6) or ankle fusion (Fig. 29.7) can be performed distal to the supramalleolar osteotomy with the addition of another level of treatment. In these cases the goal of realignment is to unload the area of diseased cartilage while trying to re-build new cartilage and to assure a well aligned leg and foot in the setting of a fused ankle, respectively.

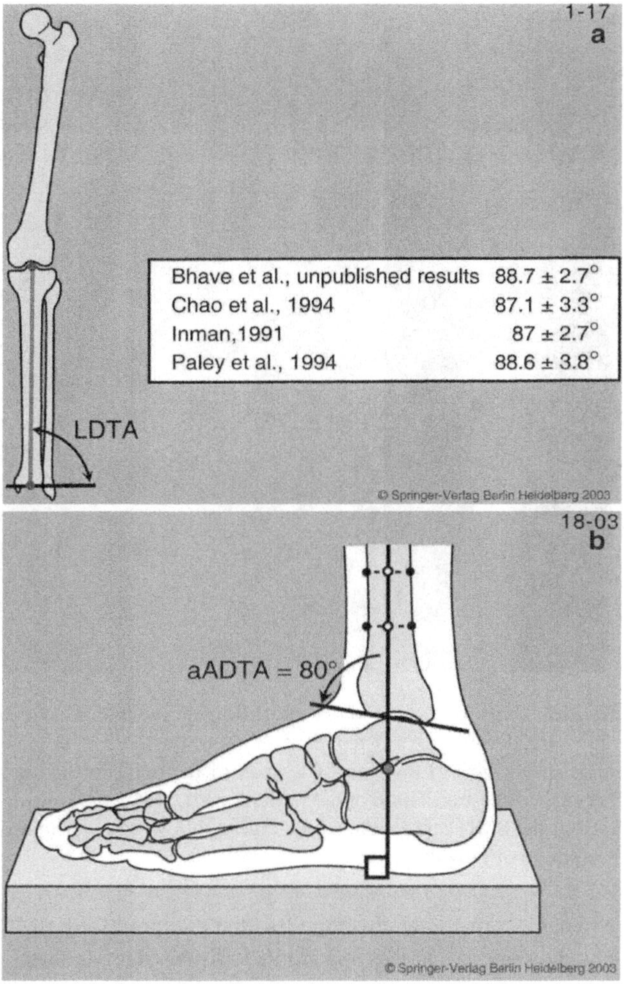

Fig.29.4 (**a**) Normal LDTA (lateral distal tibial angle) (Reprinted with permission fromD rorPa ley[33]).(**b**) Normal ADTA (anterior distal tibial angle) (Reprinted with permission from Dror Paley[33])

29.2.2 Stiff Nonunion

The same deformity types mentioned in malunions will be seen in this group. An excellent application of gradual correction is for a hypertrophic stiff nonunion with deformity.[21,23,28] This type of nonunion has fibrocartilage tissue at the nonunion site which has the biologic capacity for bony union. It lacks stability and axial alignment. Gradual distraction of this type of nonunion to achieve normal alignment results in bone formation. The nonunion acts like regenerate, and bony healing occurs. Modest lengthening of no more than 1.5 cm should be done through the nonunion. If additional lengthening is needed, a second osteotomy for lengthening is performed.[4,20,21] The principal advantages are not having to expose the nonunion site in the face of poor skin and widened callus and gaining length through an opening wedge correction. This is particularly beneficial to the region above the ankle,

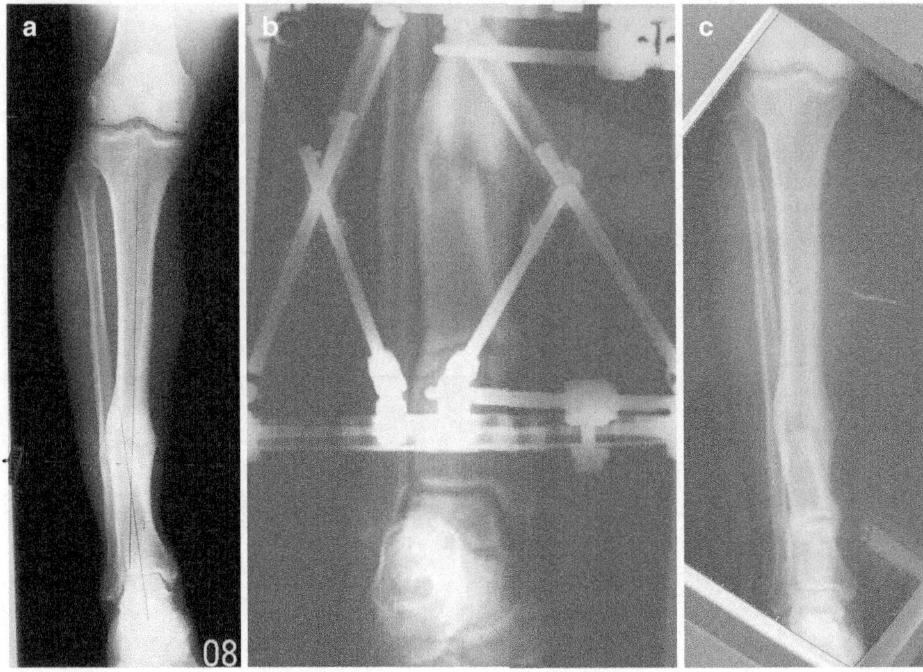

Fig. 29.5 Thirty-five year old male with 15 year old malunion of tibia who presents with ankle pain and varus deformity. (**a**) Preoperative antero-posterior radiograph showing varus deformity at the mid –distal third of the tibia. The apex of the deformity is located in the supramalleolar region because of the translation at the malunion site. (**b**) Antero-posterior radiograph at end of distraction of the SMO correction. (**c**) One year follow-up antero-posterior radiograph showing a good restorationof t het ibiala xis

where the soft-tissue envelope is often compromised. SMO is not useful for mobile atrophic nonunions and less applicable to infected nonunions.

29.2.2.1 Malunion of Ankle Fusion

An ankle fusion that is malpositioned can be very debilitating and may accelerate the degeneration of the adjacent joints.[12] Equinus malunion leads to hyperextension and pain at the knee (Fig. 29.8). A malunion positioned in calcaneous causes heel pain. Varus can lead to problems with balance, stress fracture of the fifth metatarsal, and foot pain. Valgus malunion can cause excessive stress on the subtalar joint with further valgus deformity through that joint and accelerated arthritis. Rotational malunions make gait awkward. In patients with neuropathy malunion often leads to abnormal skin pressure breakdown. Ankle fusion malunion can be corrected through a PSMO.[12,15,18,23,28] The osteotomy can be performed very distally, since wire penetration into the ankle joint is not a concern. One can correct all deformities effectively (Fig. 29.9). If some lengthening is needed, it may be done through the same osteotomy or through an osteotomy in the proximal tibia.

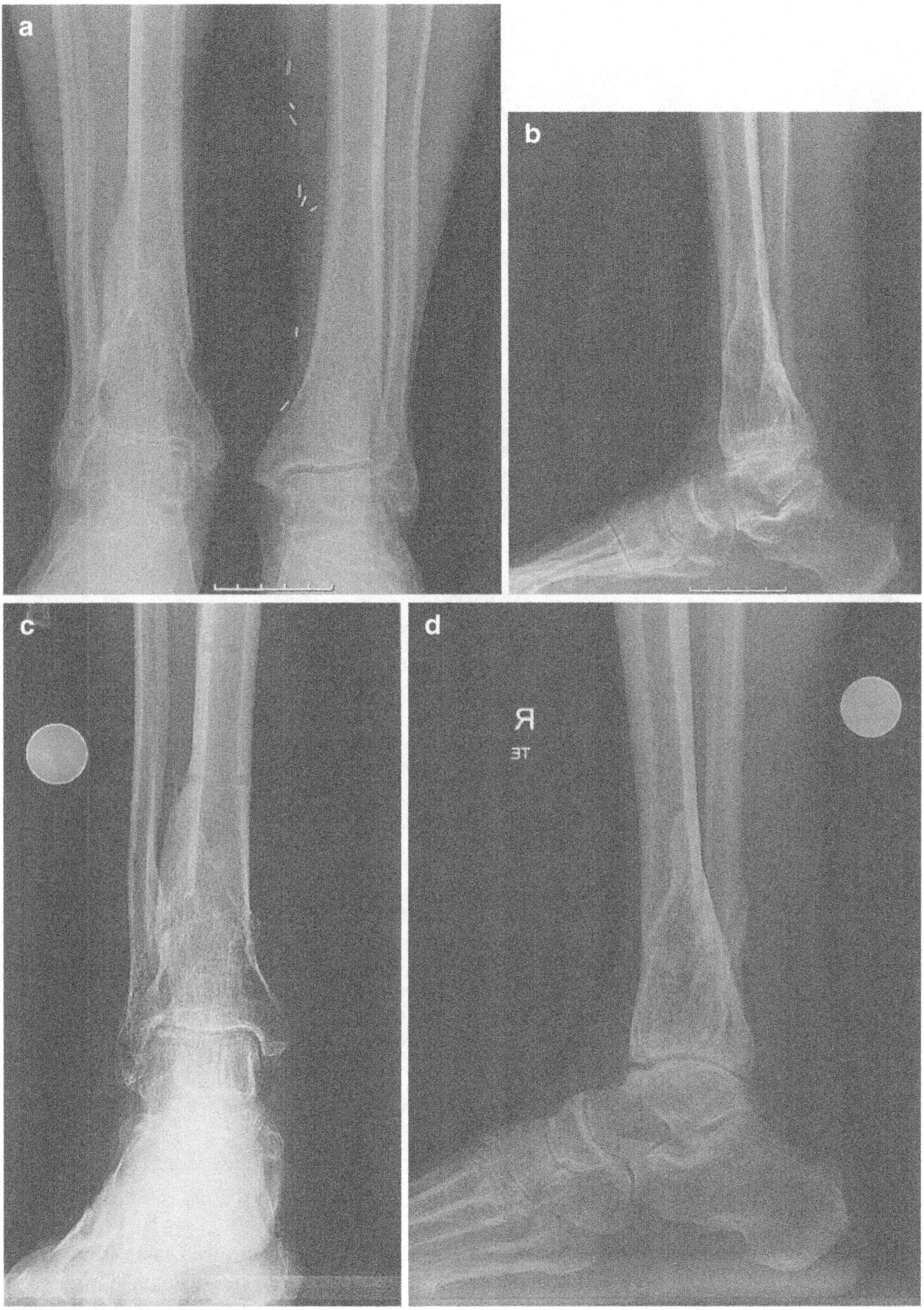

Fig. 29.6 (**a** and **b**) Pre-operative radiographs. The LDTA was 80° (valgus) and ADTA was 90° (procurvatum) pre operatively. Simultaneous PSMO and articulating ankle distraction arthroplasty was performed. (**c** and **d**) Post-operative radiographs. After PSMO the LDTA was 90° and ADTA was 80°. 29.6c showed a modest increase in joint space along the lateral aspect of the tibio-talar jointw henc omparedw ith 29.6a

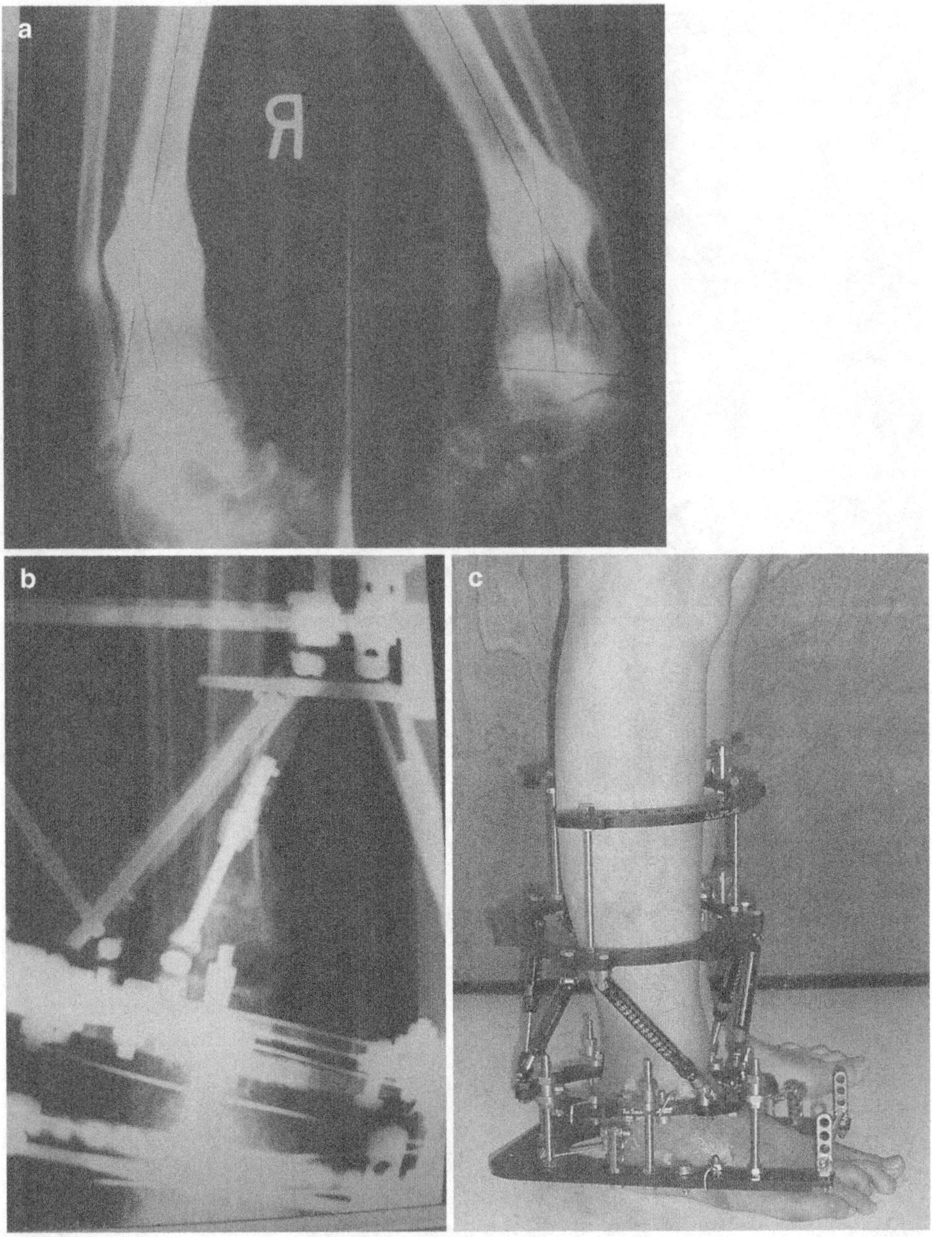

Fig. 29.7 Fifty year old woman with a malunion of the distal tibia and advanced ankle arthrosis. (**a**) Preoperative antero-posterior and lateral radiograph showing varus and recurvatum deformity with arthrosis of the ankle. (**b**), (**c**) Antero-posterior radiograph and side view showing an ankle arthrodesis and simultaneous gradual correction of the deformity with a TSF

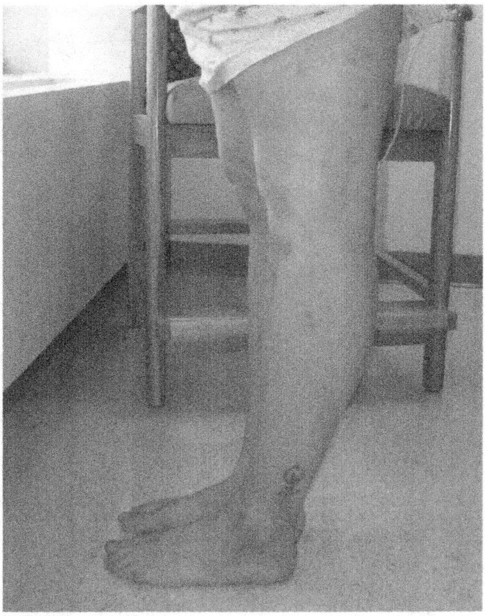

Fig.29.8 Thirty-nine year old female patient with a 10° equinus malunion of her ankle fusion and previous successful subtalar arthrodesis. She hyperextened her knee when she walked, and had debilitating knee painw ithoutothe rkne epa thology

29.2.3 Intra-articularA nkleDe formity

Ankle arthrosis may be associated with an angular deformity arising from the joint itself.[19] Tilt of the talus may develop with joint space narrowing on one side only of the ankle joint. In this situation, the SMO may be used to achieve a neutral talus relative to the axis of the tibia.[2,29,30] To achieve a talus position 90° to the tibial axis the distal tibia must often be over-corrected. This can be combined with ankle distraction to stimulate cartilage re-growth[11,23](Fig. 29.10).

29.2.4 Ankle and Foot Deformity

Combined foot and ankle deformity is common in the setting of inflammatory arthritis and neurologic disorders. These patients are often debilitated, at increased risk for infection, and need to be able to weight bear early. A combined deformity consisting of ankle valgus with foot planovalgus and forefoot abduction is often seen in rheumatoid arthritis, for example. To minimize the amount of surgery needed to correct all these deformities, a compromise may be made to correct as much as possible through the SMO. A SMO can be used to correct the ankle valgus. The ankle valgus can be overcorrected to accommodate subtalar valgus, or under corrected to accommodate forefoot supination. In addition, internal rotation at

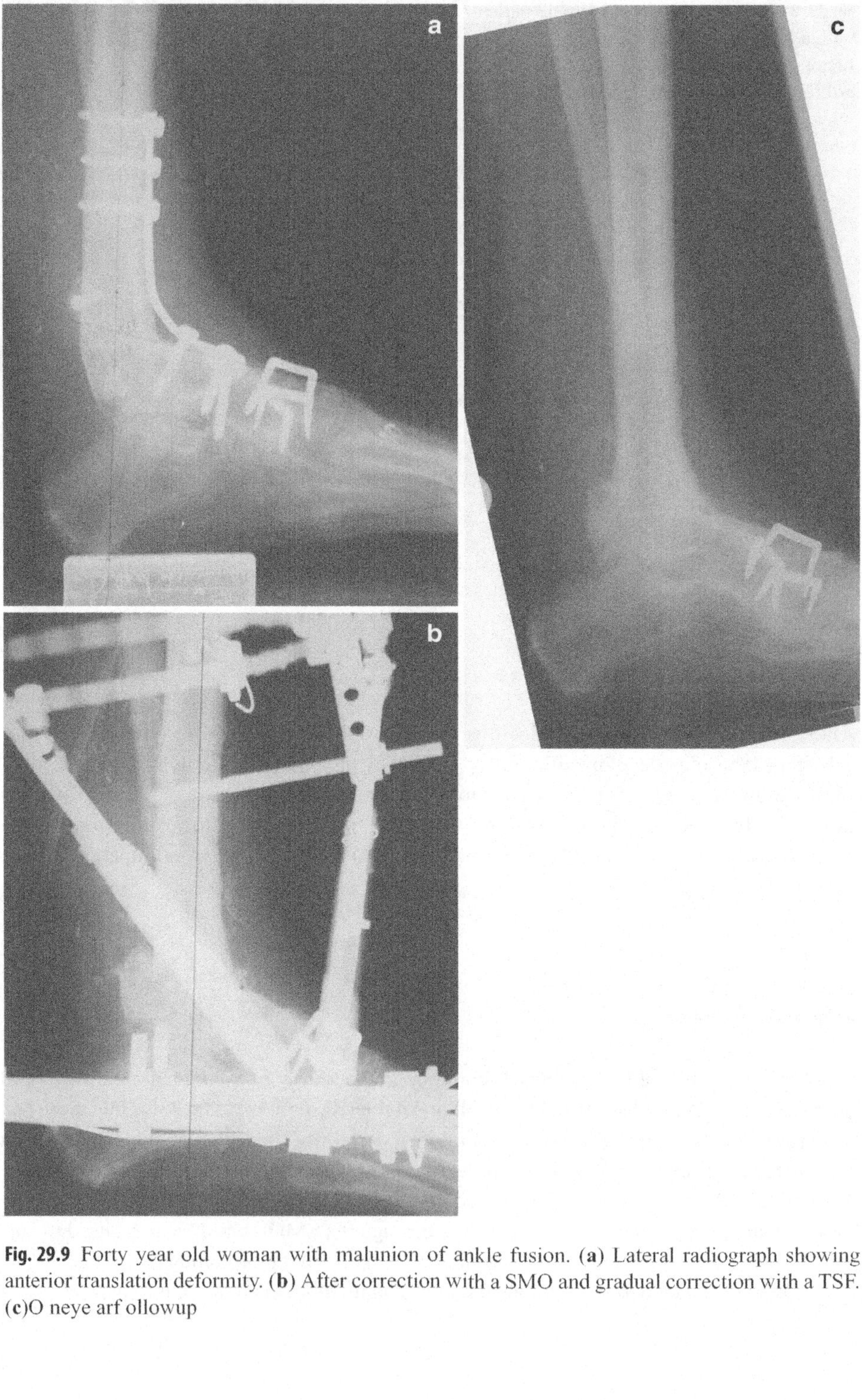

Fig. 29.9 Forty year old woman with malunion of ankle fusion. (**a**) Lateral radiograph showing anterior translation deformity. (**b**) After correction with a SMO and gradual correction with a TSF. (**c**)O neye arf ollowup

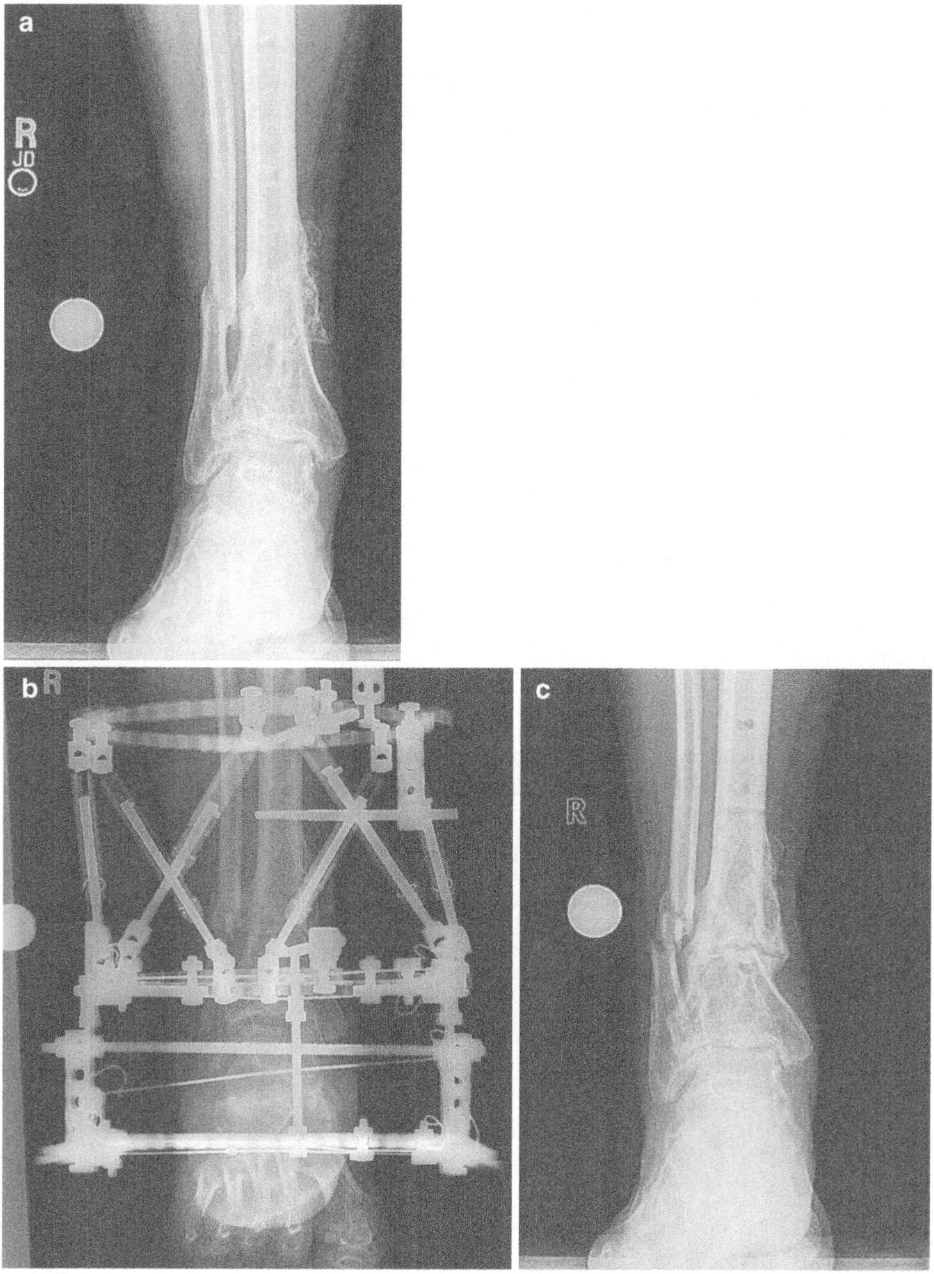

Fig. 29.10 Forty-one year old male with collapse of the lateral plafond and valgus deformity of the ankle joint (**a**). PSMO with over-correction was performed in order to realign the talus and unload the lateral cartilage (**b** and **c**)

the SMO can be used to compensate for some of the forefoot abduction.[2,27] Correction of a foot deformity above the ankle is very powerful, as a plantigrade foot can be obtained while avoiding more intricate and risky surgery to the feet in these complex cases. One is limited by the desire to avoid an oblique ankle joint line. In cases of ankle fusion or correction of ankle fusion, obliquity of the ankle fusion mass is not a significant problem.

29.2.5 GrowthA rrestD eformity

Asymmetric damage to the distal tibial growth plate can occur from trauma or infection. This will lead to deformity and shortening of the leg. The distal tibial growth plate contributes 40% of the tibial growth. PSMO can be used effectively to correct the deformity and re-establisht hel ength(Figs. 29.11a nd 29.12).

29.2.6 Congenital and Developmental Deformity

29.2.6.1 Neuromuscular

Asymmetric muscle pull can lead to deformity at the ankle.[6] This is seen in Charcot-Marie-Tooth (CMT) disease with first equinovarus of the foot and later talar tilt which further increases the varus deformity. This pattern can also be seen after nerve injury. Valgus deformities have been observed in myelomeningocele.[1,26] External rotation deformities have been observed in patients with cerebral palsy[10] and sacral agenesis.

29.2.6.2 Fibrous Dysplasia and Ollier's Disease

These tumor-like conditions are associated with deformity. This seems to occur when the lesions affect the growth plate. Deformities of the ankle related to growth disturbance at the distal tibial physis can be corrected with a SMO. When an osteotomy is performed through Ollier's bone, new normal bone will grow.[32]

29.2.6.3 Achondroplasia

In addition to varus deformities of the proximal tibiae, achondroplastic patients often have varus deformities of the distal tibiae as well. Double level tibial osteotomies including a SMO may be undertaken to correct all deformities and to divide a large lengthening betweent wos ites.

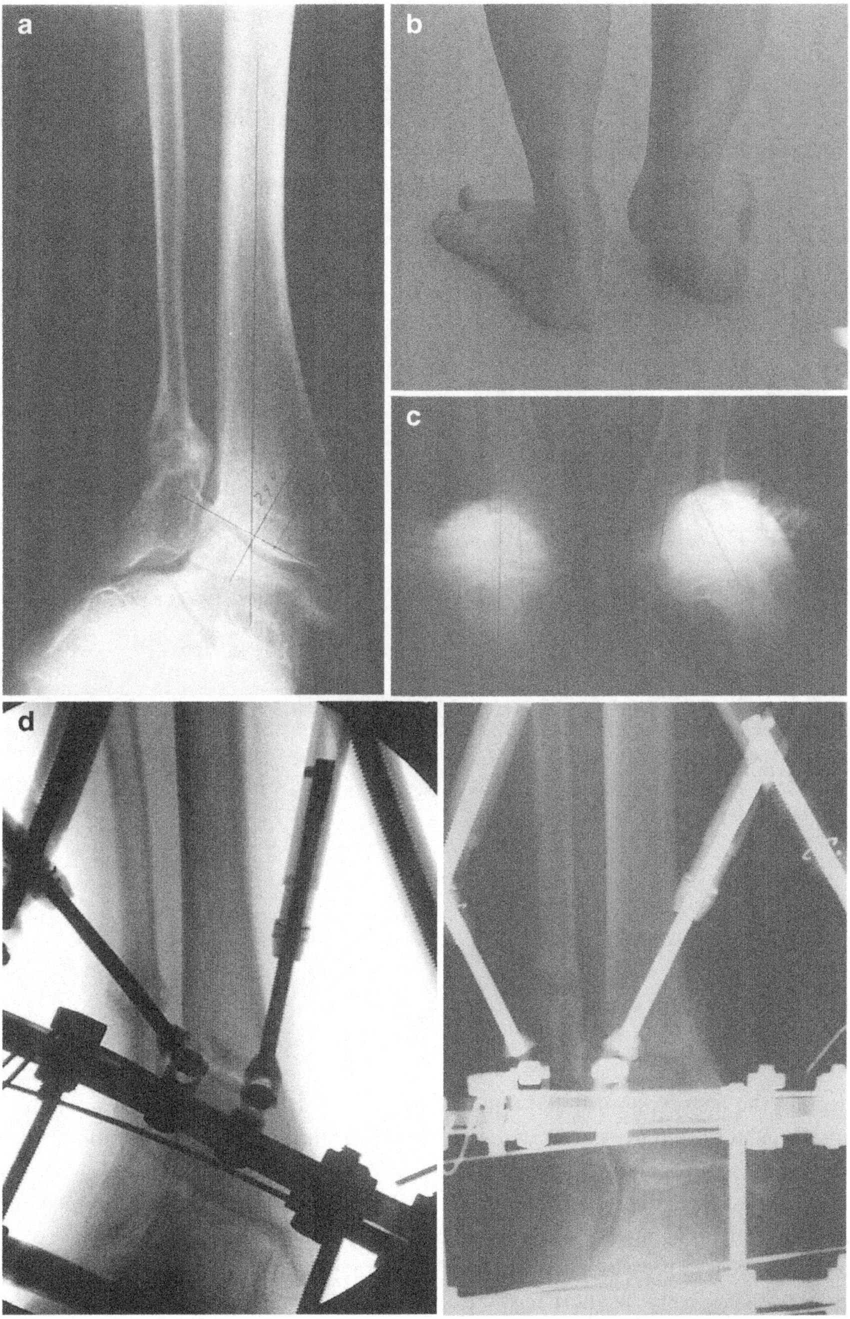

Fig. 29.11 Seventy-seven year old woman with rheumatoid arthritis with an ankle/foot deformity. (**a**) Preoperative antero-posterior radiograph showing valgus ankle deformity. (**b**) View from the back showing ankle/ hindfoot valgus and forefoot abduction. (**c**) Saltzman view illustrating the deformity. Note that the apex of deformity is in the supramalleolar region. (**d**) After SMO and application of frame to match the deformity. (**e**, **f**) After the distraction phase showing correction of the deformity. (**g**)O neye arl aters howinga he aledos teotomy

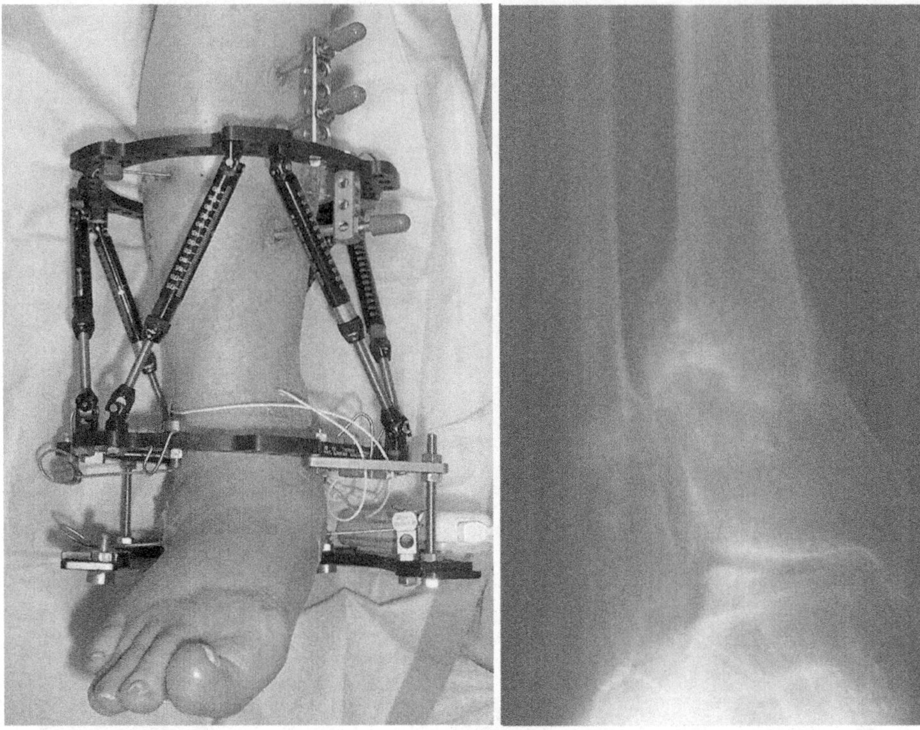

Fig. 29.11 (continued)

29.3 Preoperative Assessment

29.3.1 Clinical Evaluation

Collecting the history, one should obtain information about type of bony and soft-tissue injury, surgical procedures performed, history of infection, and the use of antibiotics. High energy injuries and open fractures are at a higher risk for infection. Information about back pain, perceived leg length discrepancy (LLD), use of a shoe lift, and deformity should be elicited from the patient. The presence of deformity will often lead patients to report of a feeling of increased pressure on the medial or lateral part of the foot with a valgus or varus deformity respectively. A short leg will often lead to complaints of low back pain and contralateral hip pain. If antibiotics are being used to manage an infected nonunion, an attempt should be made to discontinue these for 6 weeks prior to surgery in order to obtain reliable intra-operative culture samples. Discontinuation of antibiotics must be done with caution and careful observation, particularly in compromised patients like those with diabetes or on immunosuppressive medications. The current amount of pain, the use of narcotics, and the ability to walk with or without support should be noted.

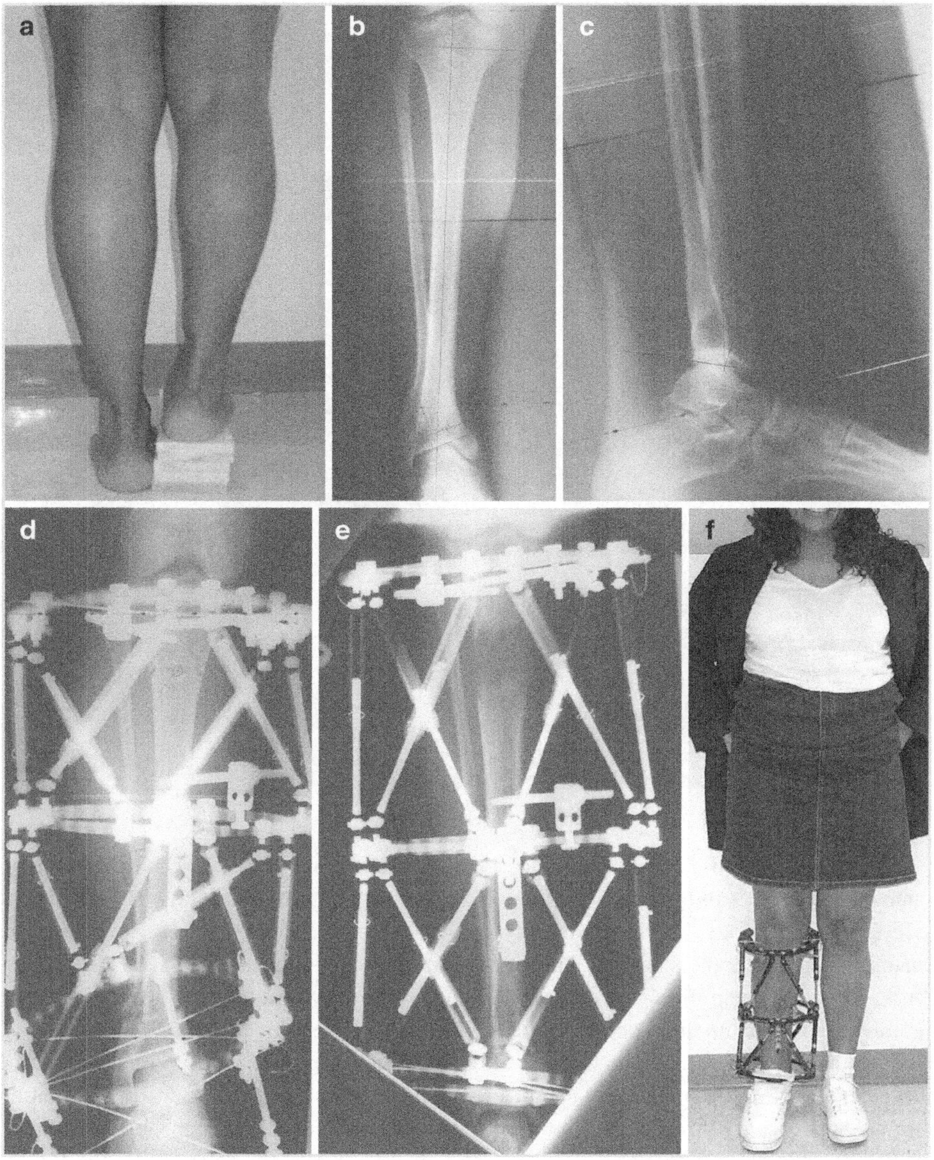

Fig. 29.12 Twenty-five year old woman with post-traumatic growth arrest of the distal tibia. (**a**) View from the back showing a LLD of 6 cm. The ankle varus is compensated by mobile hindfoot eversion. (**b**) Preoperative antero-posterior radiograph showing varus deformity. (**c**) lateral radiograph showing procurvatum deformity. The apex of deformity is periarticular. (**d**) Post-operative radiograph showing non-displaced SMO and proximal tibial osteotomy. (**e**) After distraction, showing proximal tibial lengthening and distal tibia correction. (**f**) Standing front-view at end of distraction. (**g**, **h**) Antero-posterior and lateral radiographs 1 year later showing healed osteotomies. Note the intentional medial and posterior translation of the distal fragment since the osteotomy site was away from the apex of deformity. (**i**) Standing front view showing equal leg lengths and correctionof de formity

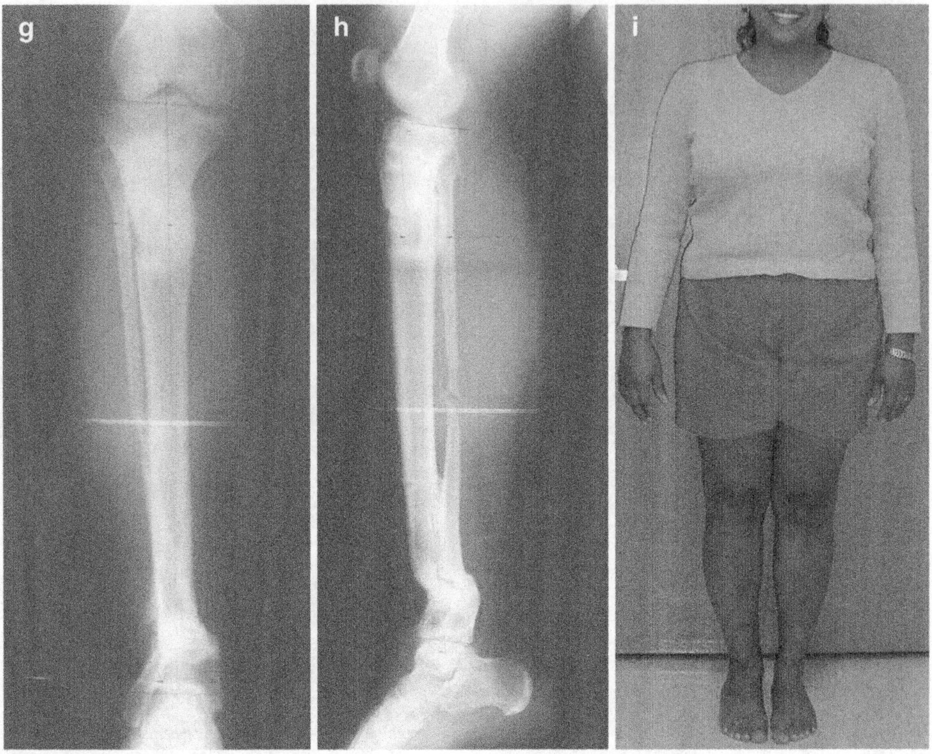

Fig. 29.12 (continued)

on physical examination, one should look for deformity and LLD with the patient standing still and walking. The inability to bear weight suggests an unstable nonunion. The view from the back is helpful to identify g coronal plane deformity. LLD is evaluated by using blocks under the short leg and by examining the level of the iliac crests. The view from the side is helpful to observe sagittal plane deformity, and equinus contracture. The combination of recurvatum deformity above the ankle and equinus contracture of the ankle will lead to a foot translated forward position, with an extension moment on the knee. The range of motion of the ankle, subtalar, forefoot, and toes should be recorded. Compensation for ankle deformity through the subtalar joint is an important factor. For varus deformity, the subtalar joint will slide into valgus. For valgus deformity, the subtalar joint will slide into varus. These compensatory deformities of the subtalar joint may become rigid and irreducible. This typically occurs with long standing ankle deformity. If this is present, it must be taken into account when correcting the ankle. The condition of the soft-tissue envelope, especially previous surgical wounds and flaps, and neurovascular findings should be recorded. This includes the posterior tibial and dorsalis pedis pulses, foot sensation, and dorsiflexion and plantarflexion motor function of the ankle and toes. Patients with poor pulses are sent for further vascular testing. Many patients with Charcot joint destruction have apparently normal sensation to light touch.

Rotational deformity is best assessed on clinical exam with the patient in the prone position. The *Thigh-foot axis* is used to assess rotational deformity of the tibia. The rotational profile of the femur is used to assess rotational deformity in the femur. CT scan can also be used for this purpose. CT scan cuts at the proximal femur, distal femur, proximal tibia, and distal tibia allow analysis of rotational deformity.[17,23]

29.3.2
RadiographicA ssessment

Radiographs should include anteroposterior (AP), lateral, and mortise views of the ankle, Saltzman's view of both feet (Figs. 29.11c and 29.13), and a 51″ bipedal erect leg x-ray including the hips to ankles with blocks under the short leg to level the pelvis. LLD and limb alignment can be measured from a standing bipedal 51″ radiograph. The short leg is placed on blocks to level the pelvis, and the height of the blocks is recorded.[16,17] This can be performed with the patient using crutches if necessary. These radiographs yield crucial information about LLD, deformity, presence of hardware, arthritis, and bony union. A supine scanogram can also be used to measure length discrepancy but this is not useful for alignment analysis. CT scan and magnetic resonance imaging (MRI) can be used for further evaluation as needed. CT scan can be helpful to obtain more information about bony union. MRI can be helpful to obtain information about the condition of cartilage in the ankle and subtalar joints, and the presence of infection. Nuclear medicine studies can also be used, but we have not found them to be very helpful in this evaluation.

Laboratory studies including white blood cell count, erythrocyte sedimentation rate, and C-reactive protein can be helpful to diagnose the presence of infection. Selective lidocaine injections into the ankle and subtalar joints may be helpful to diagnose the main source of pain.

29.3.3
SurgicalP lanning

The deformity is measured on antero-posterior radiographs (Fig. 29.4a). The proximal tibial axis is represented with a mid-diaphyseal tibial line. The distal tibial axis is

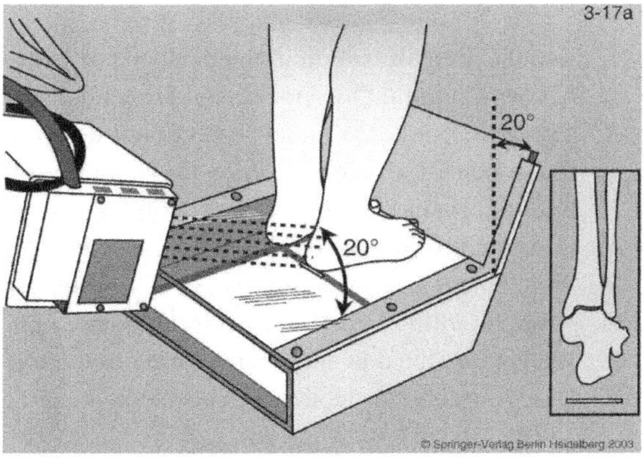

Fig.29. 13 Saltzmanvie ws chematic diagram (Reprinted with permission from Dror Paley[33])

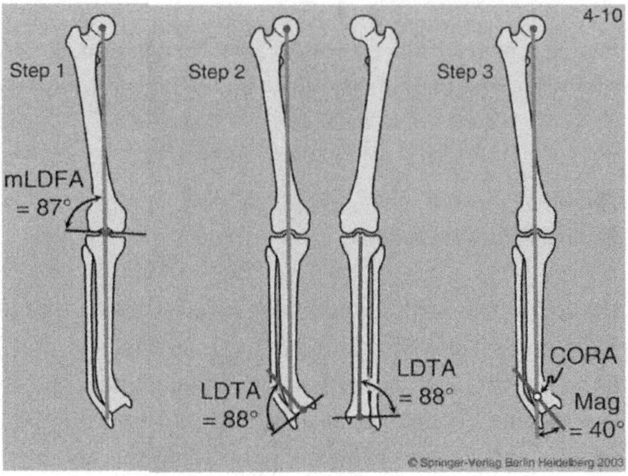

Fig.29. 14 Mechanicala xispl anning for SMO (Reprinted with permission from Dror Paley[33])

represented with a perpendicular line to the ankle joint drawn retrograde (normal LDTA is 90°). The intersection of these lines is the apex of deformity (Fig. 29.14). In the sagittal plane, the distal tibial axis is drawn 80° to the lateral joint line (a normal ADTA is 80°) (Fig. 29.4b). The intersection of these lines is the apex of deformity. The rotational deformity is assessed from the TFA measured on physical examination. If the osteotomy is at the level of the CORA, no translation is needed. If the osteotomy is done at a level that is different from the CORA, then translation at the osteotomy site will be needed to fully correct the deformity[16,17](Figs. 29.15aa ndb) .

29.4 TreatmentP rinciples

29.4.1 Features of the Ilizarov Method

The Ilizarov method is particularly useful for addressing the full spectrum of post-traumatic ankle pathology. Listed below are versatile features of the Ilizarov method.[5,11,15,22,23,28]

1. Avoidsi nternalfi xation in the presence or with a history of infection
2. Allows a minimal incision technique with a poor soft-tissue envelope
3. Usesa cutea nd/or gr adualc orrectionof de formity
4. Uses opening wedge correction avoiding need for bone resection
5. Usefulf orl argede formityc orrection
6. Post-operativea djustabilityf orc ompressionor c orrection
7. Simultaneousl engtheningi sp ossiblef oropt imizationof L LD
8. Allowsm ultiplel evelt reatment(am odulara pproach)
9. Weight bearing and ankle range of motion are encouraged
10. Usesdi stractionos teogenesist oa voidbone gr aftingt heope nw edges egment

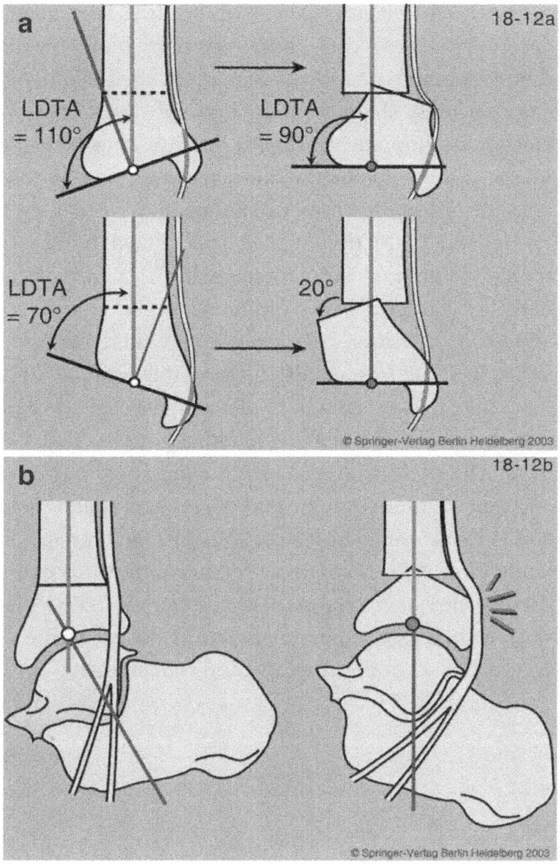

Fig.29.15 (**a**) Correction of varus can cause injury to the posterior tibial nerve with stretch and needed medial translation (Reprinted with permission from Dror Paley[33]).(**b**) Correction of procurvatum can cause injury to the posterior tibial nerve with stretch and needed posterior translation (Reprinted with permission from Dror Paley[33])

29.4.2
Acute VersusG radualC orrection

One can employ either acute or gradual correction of a nonunion or malunion.[20,21] Acute corrections can be performed in conjunction with all methods of fixation including plates,[3,26] IM nails, and external fixation frames. Gradual correction requires the use of specialized frames. The personality of the problems helps guide the surgeon toward the best method. For example, a distal tibial malunion with 15° valgus deformity and 2 cm shortening is best handled with an osteotomy to gradually correct the angular deformity and lengthen the bone with a specialized frame. The Ilizarov method allows to correct gradually all the components of deformity with distraction osteogenesis. One may choose to perform the deformity correction and lengthening at one level if bone regeneration potential is good. Alternatively, one may choose to perform a double level osteotomy – one level at the CORA[16] for deformity correction, and one level for lengthening in the proximal tibia metaphysic (Fig. 29.12). Gradual correction achieves lengthening and carries less risk of posterior tibial nerve stretch neuropraxia than if attempted with an acute correction (Figs. 29.15a–b).

The use of plates and IM nails requires an acute correction of angular and translational deformity. Acute corrections are particularly useful for modest deformity correction, mobile atrophic nonunions that are opened and bone grafted, and small bone defects that can be acutely shortened. The principle advantage of acute correction is earlier bone contact for healing and a simpler fixation construct. Acute corrections are generally better tolerated in the femur and humerus, and less well tolerated in the tibia and ankle given the possible issues of neurovascular insult.

Gradual correction with a specialized frame is useful for large deformity correction,[13,22,28] poor skin, associated limb lengthening, bone transport to treat segmental defects,[24] and stiff hypertrophic nonunion repair.[21] Gradual correction employs the principle of *distraction osteogenesis* commonly referred to as the *Ilizarov method*.[9,15] Bone and soft-tissue is gradually distracted at a rate of approximately 1 mm per day in divided increments. Bone growth in the distraction gap is called *regenerate*. The interval between osteotomy and the start of lengthening is called the *latency phase* and is usually 7–10 days. The correction and lengthening is called the *distraction phase*. The *consolidation phase* is the time from the end of distraction until bony union.[9] This phase is most variable and is most affected by patient factors such as age and health. If the *structure at risk* is a nerve such as the tibial nerve for an equinovarus deformity of the ankle, gradual correction may be the safer option. The correction can be planned so that the structure at risk is stretched slowly. If nerve symptoms do occur, the correction can be slowed or stopped. Neurolysis can be employed in select situations based on the response to gradual correction.[17]

29.5 Surgical Technique

29.5.1 Wire and Pin Configuration

Tensioned thin Kirschner wires and half pins lend approximately the same stability to the frame. The proximal ring or ring block is secured with three to four points of fixation. We will typically use one 1.2 mm Kirschner wire (1.8 mm wire for adults) as a reference wire from anterolateral to posteromedial for purposes of mounting the ring. Additional fixation is secured with half pins. Six millimeter hydroxyapatite (HA)-coated pins are our first choice for adult patients. These are inserted after drilling a 4.8 mm tract.[5]

The distal tibial ring is usually secured with two or three 1.8 mm Kirschner wires (tensioned to 130 kg) and a half-pin. The reference wire is placed in the tibia alone parallel to the ankle. Next, a fibula-tibia wire is inserted posterolateral to anteromedial to stabilize the syndesmosis and prevent fibula migration. A posteromedial to anterolateral wire can also be added. Finally, an anteromedial (medial to the tibialis anterior tendon) to posterolateral 6 mm half-pin is used to add stability in the sagittal plane (Fig. 29.16). Fixation may be extended across the ankle to the foot if additional stability of the distal segment is needed.

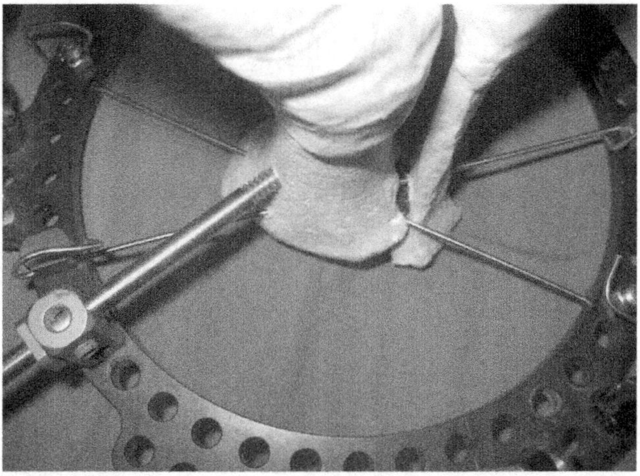

Fig. 29.16 This sawbones model shows the typical fixation arrangement for the distal tibia with two tensioned wires and one half pin

29.5.2 TaylorS patialF rame

29.5.2.1 Terminology

Rings are placed on either side of the deformity site and the anticipated lengthening site(s) (Fig. 29.17). The rings can be placed independently to optimally fit the leg. This is called the *rings first method*. One ring is chosen as the *reference ring* for each level of movement, and it is important that this ring be placed orthogonal (perpendicular) to the axis of the tibia. *Mounting parameters* are defined by the center of the reference ring and this will define the point in space where the deformity correction will occur. It is important to maintain enough distance between rings so that the struts can fit properly. In this frame, one is limited by the shortest length of strut. The advantages of this frame over the classic Ilizarov frame are numerous. The application is easier and the fit on the leg is better when using the *rings first method*. Also, residual deformity at the lengthening and docking sites can be addressed by using the same frame to correct angulation and translation simultaneously in the coronal, sagittal, and axial planes without major frame modification. This minimizes angular deformity at the lengthening sites.[4,5]

One ring is chosen to be the *reference ring*. The "virtual hinge" around which the correction occurs is defined by the origin and corresponding point. The *origin* is a point chosen on the edge of one bone segment at the defect site. A *corresponding point* (CP) on the other bone segment is chosen with the goal of reducing the CP to the origin. *Mounting parameters* define the location of the origin relative to the reference ring. Mounting parameters are defined by the spatial relationship between the center of the reference ring and the origin in the coronal, sagittal, and axial planes. This defines a virtual hinge around which the deformity correction will occur. TSF struts are used to connect the rings across the deformity.

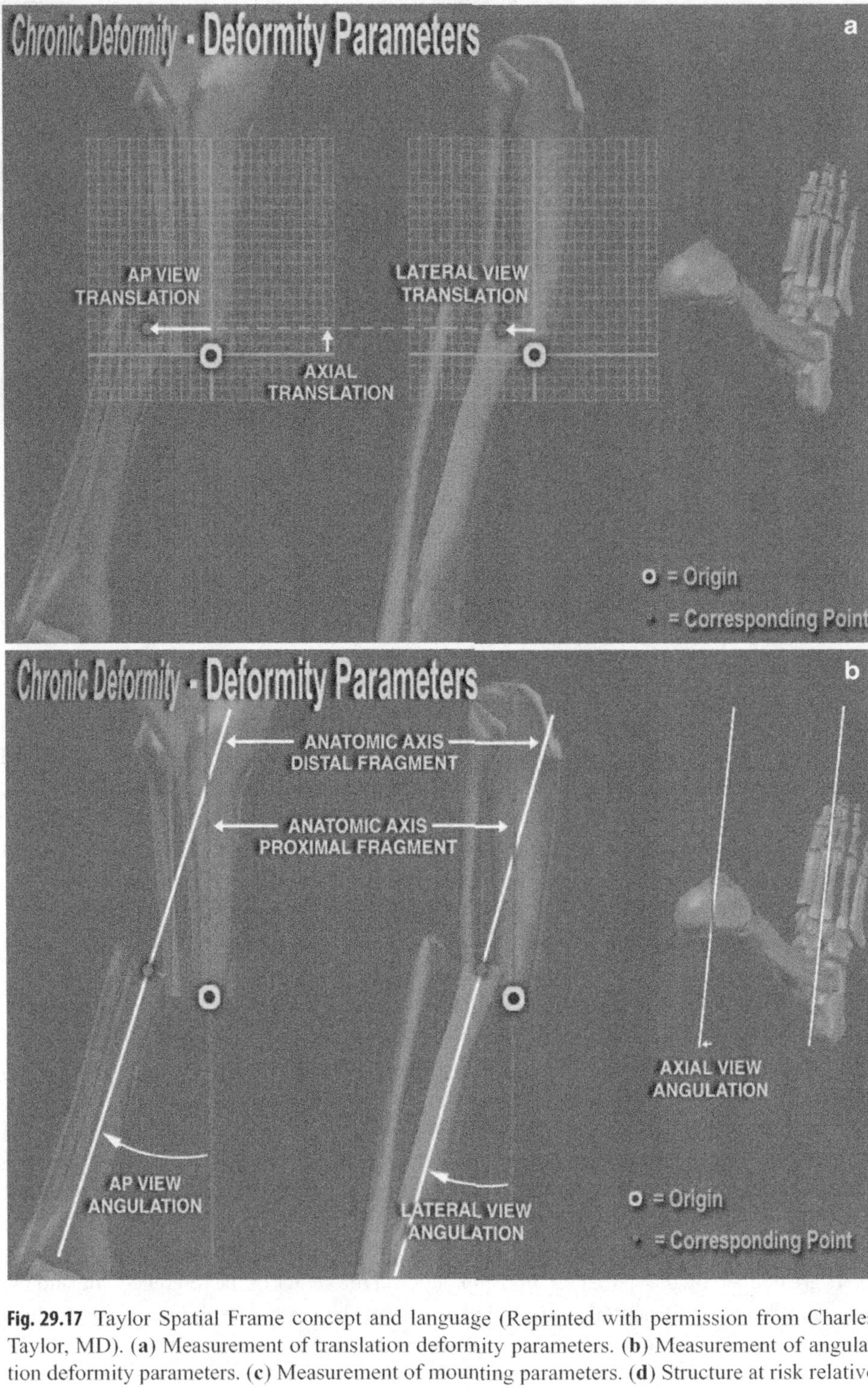

Fig. 29.17 Taylor Spatial Frame concept and language (Reprinted with permission from Charles Taylor, MD). (**a**) Measurement of translation deformity parameters. (**b**) Measurement of angulation deformity parameters. (**c**) Measurement of mounting parameters. (**d**) Structure at risk relative to origin. (**e**) Before correction. (**f**)A fterc orrection

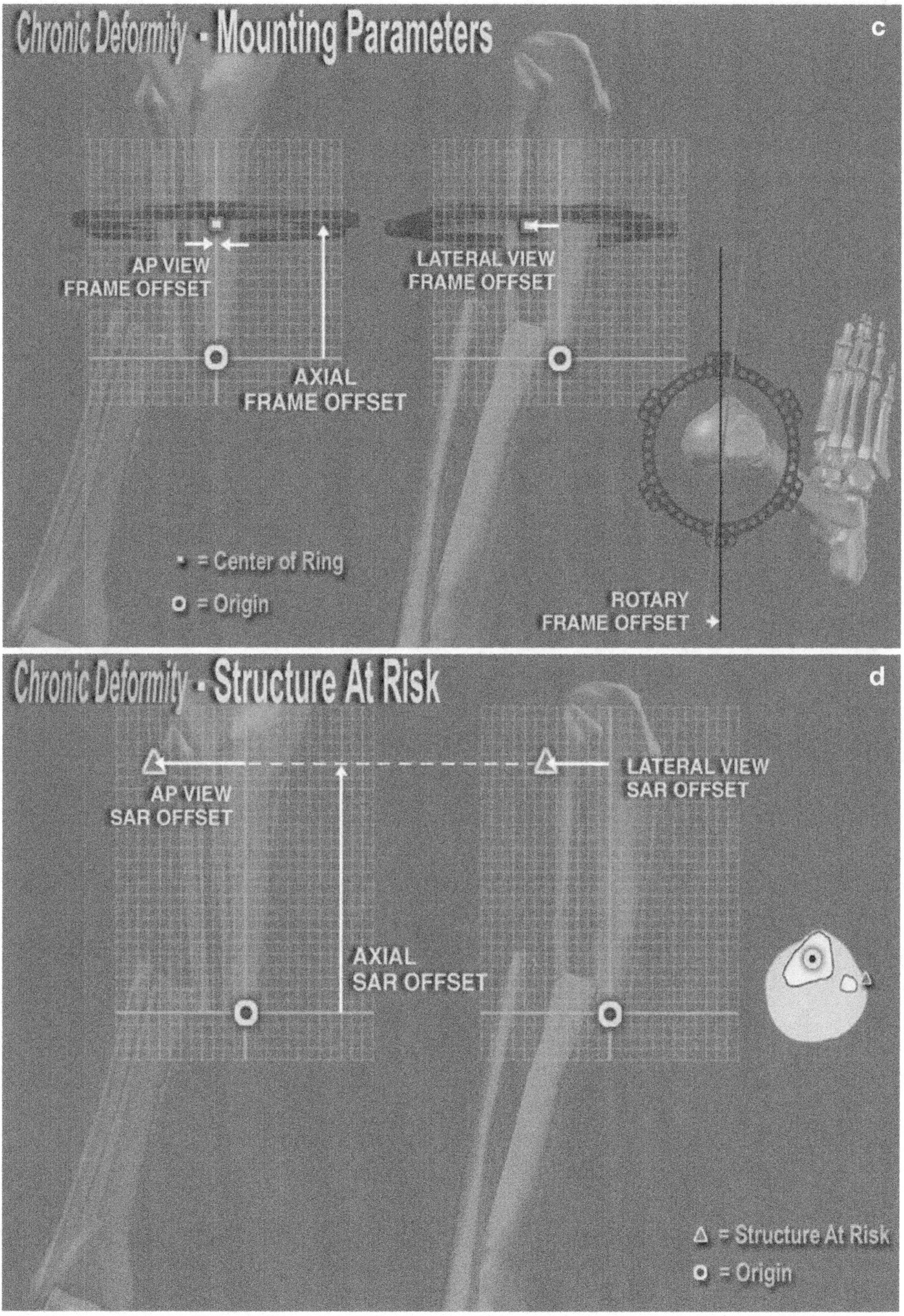

Fig. 29.17 (continued)

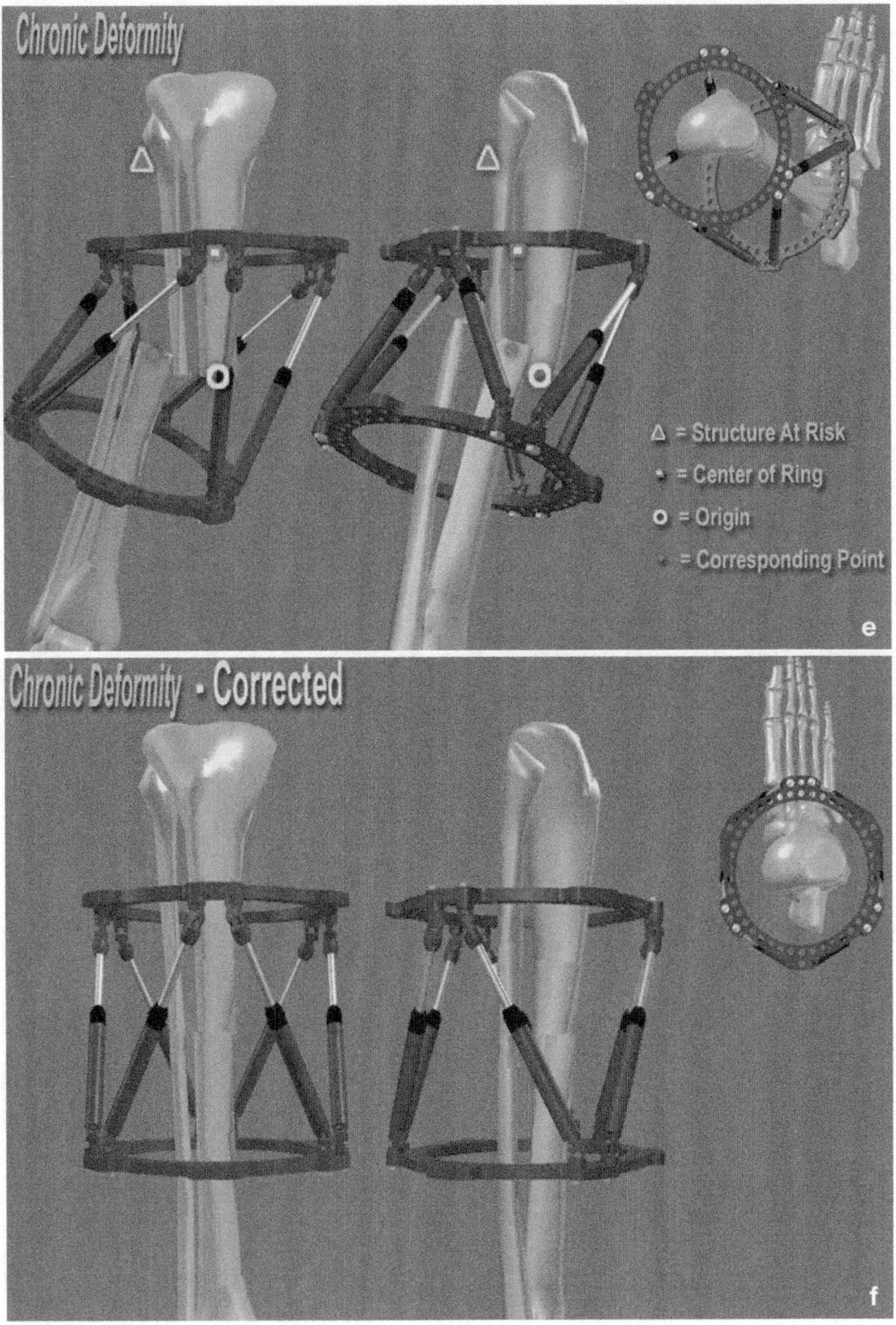

Fig. 29.17 (continued)

29.5.2.2
Deformity Parameters

There are six deformity parameters that will describe the relationship between the proximal segment and the distal segment (the reference segment has the origin and the moving segment has the corresponding point) (Figs. 29.17a, b). Deformity parameters consist of an angulation and a translation in the coronal, sagittal, and axial planes. In the coronal plane, the angulation is varus or valgus and the translation is medial or lateral. In the sagittal plane, the angulation is apex anterior or apex posterior and the translation is anterior or posterior. In the axial plane, the angulation is internal or external rotation, and the translation is short or long.

29.5.2.3
Mounting Parameters

Since the TSF enables correction around a virtual hinge, one must communicate its location (origin) to the computer program (Fig. 29.17c). A grid projected from the reference ring allows one to specify the location of the origin. The location of the origin relative to the center of the reference ring in the coronal, sagittal, and axial planes is recorded.[25] For example, the center of the reference ring may be 10 mm lateral, 25 mm posterior, and 35 mm distal to the origin.

29.5.2.4
Structure at Risk (SAR)

The speed of the correction is determined by the surgeon by choosing a structure that he or she wants to move at a determined rate (Fig. 29.17d). Typically a structure in the concavity of the deformity is the SAR. For example, if we are correcting a varus deformity, the SAR may be the medial cortex of the tibia or the posterior tibial nerve. If we are correcting a valgus, recurvatum deformity, the SAR will be the anterolateral surface of the tibia. We usually move the SAR at 1 mm per day,[25] although, this can be varied.

29.5.3
FibulaO steotomy

Osteotomy of the fibula is usually performed with the use of a tourniquet at the beginning of the procedure prior to frame application. A small lateral exposure is a simple and safe way to approach the fibula. It is best to locate the osteotomy at or near the apex of deformity, although an osteotomy should not be performed at exactly the same level of the tibia to avoid formation of a synostosis. The bone is cut with either an oscillating saw or an osteotome. Alternatively the fibula can be fractured through the tibial osteotomy site. Once the tibial osteotomy is performed, the osteotome remains in the wound and is re-directed posteriorly and laterally, toward the fibula, and advanced. This option works well when it is too risky to make a lateral incision.

The shape of osteotomy may be transverse or oblique. When correcting valgus deformity gradually, a transverse osteotomy is performed. This will be gradually distracted and the gap will fill in with regenerate. When correcting varus deformity, the fibula will need to be shortened.[8,14,22] This is accomplished with either fibula resection or an oblique osteotomy where the fragments can overlap.

29.5.4 Supramalleolar TibialO steotomy

After the frame has been mounted on the intact bone, the tibial osteotomy is performed. The strut connection between the rings are recorded and then removed. Through a 1 cm skin incision, medial to the tibialis anterior tendon and about 1 cm proximal to the distal tibial pins, the SMO is performed. The C-arm fluoroscopy is positioned in the lateral position. A multiple drill hole osteotomy technique is used. A 4.8 mm drill bit is passed three times along the plane of the planned osteotomy line (Fig. 29.18a). The SMO is then completed by passing the osteotome across the medial cortex, lateral cortex, and through the bone center to crack the posterior cortex (Fig. 29.18b). Rotation of the osteotome and ultimately rotation of the rings completes the osteotomy. Alternatively, a Gigli saw technique can be used to perform the SMO.

29.5.5 ExtensionA crossA nkle

If there is an ankle contracture, then a foot ring is placed, and gradual correction of the ankle deformity can .be performed simultaneously. Hinges are placed along the axis of the ankle joint as is done in ankle distraction arthroplasty. A pulling rod can be placed anterior or a pushing rod posterior to motor the correction (Fig 29.19).

29.5.6 Proximal TibialO steotomy

If there is shortening of the tibia, this can be addressed at the same time as the deformity correction at the apex of the deformity. An osteotomy at the proximal tibia for lengthening can be done if the bone healing potential at the apex of deformity is not optimal (Fig. 29.7).

29.6 PostoperativeC are

29.6.1 General

Patients are admitted to the hospital for 2–3 days. Non-steroidal anti-inflammatory medications are avoided in all osteotomy patients for fear of adverse affects on bone forma-

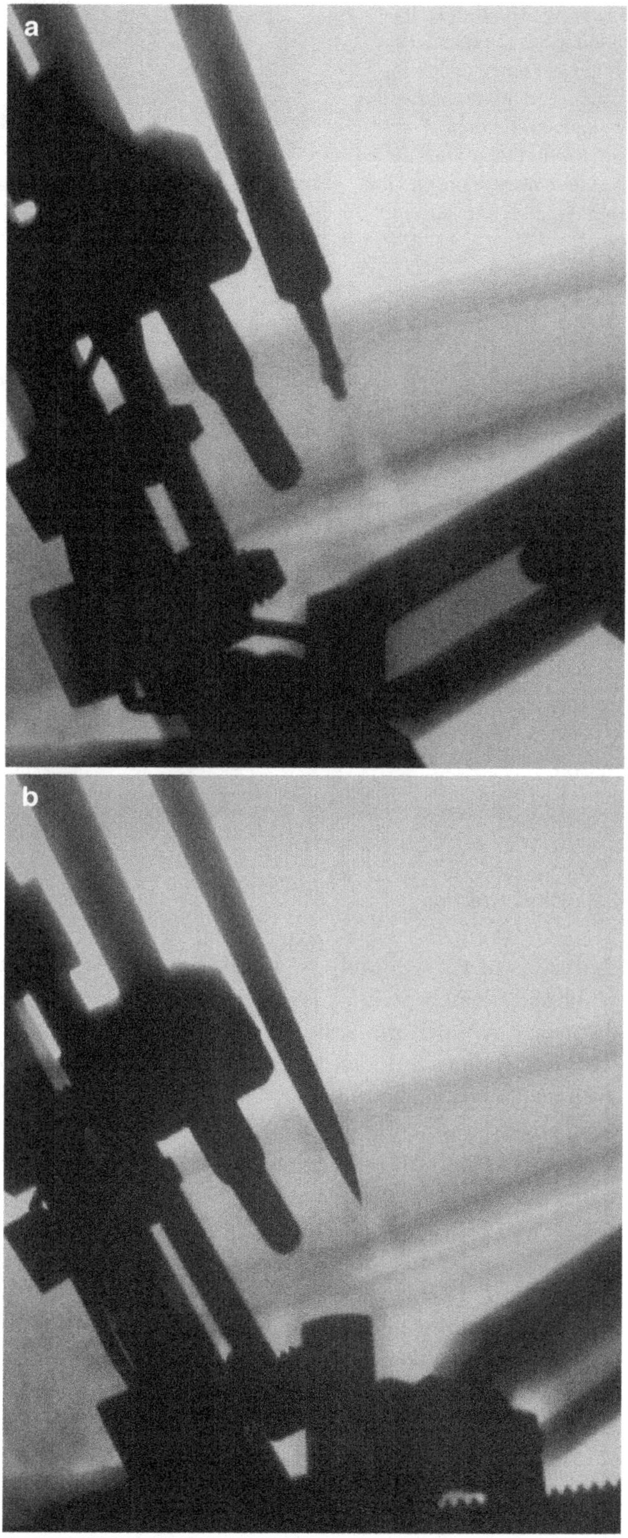

Fig.29. 18 (**a**)This intraoperative fluoroscopy film shows the 4.8 mm drill being passed in the plane of the planned osteotomy. (**b**) A 7 mm osteotome is now being inserted along the samepa tha sthe drillh oles

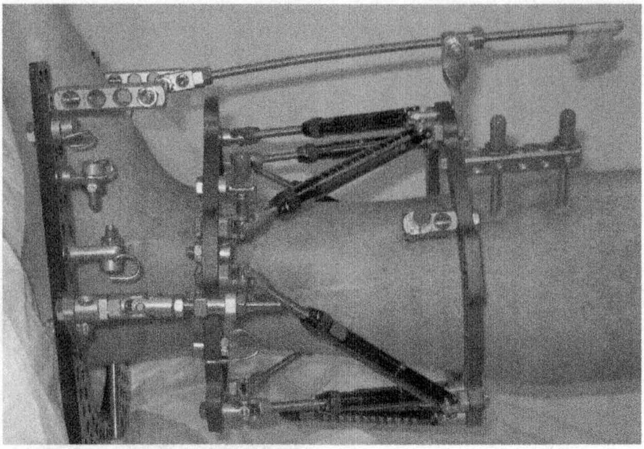

Fig.29.19 The foot ring is attached to the distal tibial ring with hinges allowing articulated ankle distraction. Note the rod "motor" anteriorly that allows the foot to move into plantarflexion and dorsiflexion

tion. The patients receive intravenous antibiotics for 24 h and are then switched to oral antibiotics. The patients are discharged on oral antibiotics for 10 days and oral pain medication. Patients return to the office 10 days post-operatively, when sutures are removed and they are educated on how to perform strut adjustments. Patients are seen every 2 weeks during this adjustment period, and then once monthly during the consolidation period.

29.6.2 DeformityC orrection

Correction of the deformity begins after a latency period of 7–10 days. The web-based Smith and Nephew program is used to generate a daily schedule for strut adjustments that the patient will perform at home. The computer requires the input of basic information including the side, the deformity parameters, the size of the rings and length of struts used, the mounting parameters measured during frame application, and rate of daily adjustment. Additionally, a structure at risk is selected and entered into the program to ensure the correct speed of gradual correction. For valgus producing osteotomy the structures a risk are the medial soft tissues, as they are in the concavity of the correction and will be stretched the greatest distance. Using this information, a clear and simplified prescription is produced for the patient to follow every day. We prescribe that struts 1 and 2 be turned in the morning, struts 3 and 4 in the afternoon, and struts 5 and 6 in the evening for a total movement of one millimeter per day.[25] The duration of the adjustment phase depends on the amount of correction needed and is typically between 14 and 28 days. The length of time in the frame is approximately 3 months.

29.6.3 PainM anagement

Transdermal wires and pins can be irritating, and we encourage patients to use appropriate oral pain medications. This is especially true during the adjustment period. Once the correction is complete, the frame is no longer moving, and the pain level decreases. Severe or atypical pain merits an evaluated for infection or deep vein thrombosis.

29.6.4 PinC are

The dressings are removed on the second post-operative day. Nurses teach proper daily pin care consisting of a mixture of half normal saline and half hydrogen peroxide applied to the pin sites with sterile cotton swabs. Pins and wires are covered with dry gauze dressings at the skin. Patients are allowed to begin showering on the fourth post operative day. They are instructed to wash the frame and pin sites with shower water daily. Antibacterial soap may be used as an adjuvant form of pin care. Problematic smooth wires can be removed in the office without anesthetic. This is commonly done after the distraction phase, or if a wire is painful and infected.

29.6.5 Rehabilitation

Ilizarov stressed the importance of early physical conditioning in conjunction with the application of circular fixators. Early motion increases blood flow to the lower extremity, prevents joint stiffness, and shortens recovery time.[11] Physical therapy assists with weight bearing as tolerated ambulation and range of motion exercises for the knee and ankle joints. Crutches are typically needed for the first 4–6 weeks after surgery. Occupational therapy provides a custom neutral foot splint to prevent the fall into equinus during sleep. Patients are encouraged to attend outpatient physical therapy where they continue with their rehabilitation programs.

29.6.6 FrameR emoval

Fixators are removed when patients are walking without pain or the use of an assistive device and when callus is seen on three cortices around the osteotomy site. This is typically 3–4 months after the index surgery. We prefer to remove the frames in the operating room. The removal of HA coated pin can be painful and is best done under sedation. We choose to curette all half pins sites in an effort to keep pin tracts clean. Transfixation wire sites are not debrided unless there is concern over a specific site. At the time of frame removal bony union and maturation of the regenerate may be evaluated with routine plain radiographs or a stress test under C-arm fluoroscopy. If there is a real concern about bony union, then the struts are removed and the rings manually compressed and distracted looking for motion at the osteotomy site. A lack of consolidation will require replacement of the struts and prolonging the time in the frame. Once the fixator is removed patients are placed into a short leg cast for 2 weeks. They are allowed 50% partial weight bearing for 2 weeks then progress to full weight bearing thereafter, first in a cam walker boot and then in a regular shoe.

29.7 Complications

29.7.1 Pin Infection

Pin site infection is common when using external fixation. Pin infections manifest with erythema, increasing pain, and drainage around the pin or wire. The vast majority of these respond well to more aggressive local pin care and oral antibiotics. If the infection does not resolve quickly, then broader spectrum antibiotics are added, or the pin or wire is removed. More advanced infections are treated with removal of the pin or wire and local bone debridement in the operating room, and intravenous antibiotics as needed. Loose pins and wires are removed, and the pin sites debrided even in the absence of infection. The use of HA coated half pins has decreased problems with pin loosening and infection.

29.7.2 Premature Consolidation

Incomplete corticotomy can complicate SMO. A circumferential division of the tibial cortex may be ensured by rotating the proximal and distal rings in opposite directions and witnessing free motion at the corticotomy site. Other methods have been described including acute distraction and angulation at the osteotomy site, but these techniques are more disruptive to the periosteum and not recommended.

True premature consolidation of the osteotomy is rare in adult patients. Once the osteotomy is performed, there is a latency period of 7–10 days before correction is started. If the latency period is prolonged, the osteotomy site will consolidate prematurely. Similarly if the correction is carried out too slowly the osteotomy site may heal preventing further correction.

29.7.3 Patient Related

The success of any gradual correction system is based on the patient's ability to participate in their own care. Patients are responsible for performing their own strut adjustment three times a day at the outset of treatment. The TSF has simplified this process through color coordination and a precise numbering system. Even so, patients do make strut adjustment errors. These mistakes are usually quickly acknowledged and remedied. Patients need to be seen frequently (every 10–14 days) during the adjustment period to avoid errors.

29.7.4 Nonunion

Bony nonunion can complicate any osteotomy procedure. Causes may include inadequate fixation, lack of weight bearing, smoking and other causes of poor blood flow to the extremity, patient comorbidities, too rapid a correction, poor osteotomy technique, and an osteotomy through diaphyseal bone. Nonunions are treated aggressively with a variety of methods, including compression across the osteotomy site, percutaneous periosteal and endosteal stimulation, and additional points of fixation. Nonunions are rare when using the TSF technique. In fact, when there is impaired healing, this specialized frame is ideal for effective treatment.

29.7.5 Nervel njury

Direct injury to a nerve can occur during surgery from pin or wire insertion during the osteotomy. A more common mechanism is stretch injury during distraction. This is discussed above in "acute versus gradual correction." Gradual correction is much safer than acute correction and avoids stretching the nerves too rapidly.

29.7.6 Deep Vein Thrombosis(DVT)

DVT is always a concern with surgery of the lower extremity. Treatment is aimed at prevention. Patients are enrolled into early rehabilitation programs emphasizing immediate mobility to avoid venous stasis. There is no restriction to movement at the ankle, knee, or hip, and frame stability allows comfortable weight bearing early in the post operative period. While in hospital, patients receive subcutaneous low molecular weight heparin. After discharge, patients continue a 3 week course of subcutaneous low molecular weight heparin. The patient can then be switched to aspirin if they are still not walking well. With this regimen, we have not had any cases of DVT or pulmonary embolism.

29.7.7 SepticA rthritis

This is a rare complication that needs to be recognized and treated quickly. The best way to avoid this is prevention. One must be careful not to insert the wires too close to the ankle joint capsule. In general, if the wires and pins are inserted proximal to the epiphyseal scar, there is little risk of an intra-articular wire. If ankle distraction is being performed simultaneously, then the talus wire is intra-articular and should be monitored. One should aspirate the joint immediately in the office, and send cultures before giving any antibiotics. Septic arthritis is treated with removal of the infected intra-articular wire and open or arthroscopic joint lavage. The lavages are repeated until negative cultures are obtained. Appropriate systemic antibiotics are given once a culture has been taken.

29.7.8 Other

Complications we have *not* experienced secondary to PSMO include necrotizing fasciitis, compartments yndrome,a ndos teomyelitis.

References

1. Abraham E, Lubicky JP, Songer MN, Millar EA. Supramalleolar osteotomy for ankle valgus in myelomeningocele. *J Pediatr Orthop.*1996; 16:774–781.
2. Benthien RA, Myerson MS. Supramalleolar osteotomy for ankle deformity and arthritis. *Foot Ankle Clin.*2004 ;9:475–487,vi ii.
3. Best A, Daniels TR. Supramalleolar tibial osteotomy secured with the Puddu plate. *Orthopedics.*2006; 29:537–540.
4. Feldman DS, Shin SS, Madan S, Koval KJ. Correction of tibial malunion and nonunion with six-axis analysis deformity correction using the Taylor Spatial Frame. *J Orthop Trauma.* 2003;17:549–554.
5. Fragomen A, Ilizarov S, Blyakher A, Rozbruch SR. Proximal tibial osteotomy for medial compartment osteoarthritis of the knee using the Taylor spatial frame. *Techn Knee Surg.* September2005;4: 175–185.
6. Fraser RK, Menelaus MB. The management of tibial torsion in patients with spina bifida. *J Bone Joint Surg Br.*1993; 75:495–497.
7. Gessmann J, Seybold D, Baecker H, et al. Correction of supramalleolar deformities with the Taylor spatial frame. *Z Orthop Unfall.*2009; 147:314–320.
8. Graehl PM, Hersh MR, Heckman JD. Supramalleolar osteotomy for the treatment of symptomatic tibial malunion. *J Orthop Trauma.*1987; 1:281–292.
9. Ilizarov GA. Clinical application of the tension-stress effect for limb lengthening. *Clin Orthop Relat Res.*1990;250: 8–26.
10. Inan M, Ferri-de Baros F, Chan G, Dabney K, Miller F. Correction of rotational deformity of the tibia in cerebral palsy by percutaneous supramalleolar osteotomy. *J Bone Joint Surg Br.* 2005;87:1411–1415.
11. Inda JI, Blyakher A, O'Malley MJ, Rozbruch SR. Distraction arthroplasty for the ankle using the Ilizarov frame. *Tech Foot Ankle Surg.*2003; 2:249–253.
12. Katsenis D, Bhave A, Paley D, Herzenberg JE. Treatment of malunion and nonunion at the site of an ankle fusion with the ilizarov apparatus. *J Bone Joint Surg Am.*2005; 87:302.
13. Mangone PG. Distal tibial osteotomies for the treatment of foot and ankle disorders. *Foot Ankle Clin.*2001; 6:583–597.

14. Mendicino RW, Catanzariti AR, Reeves CL. Percutaneous supramalleolar osteotomy for distal tibial (near articular) ankle deformities. *J Am Podiatr Med Assoc.*2005; 95:72–84.
15. Paley D. The correction of complex foot deformities using Ilizarov's distraction osteotomies. *Clin Orthop Relat Res.*1993; 293:97–111.
16. Paley D, Herzenberg JE, Tetsworth K, McKie J, Bhave A. Deformity planning for frontal and sagittal plane corrective osteotomies. *Orthop Clin North Am.*1994; 25:425–465.
17. PaleyD . *Principles of Deformity Correction.* 1st ed. Berlin, Germany: Springer; 2005.
18. Paley D, Lamm BM, Katsenis D, et al. Treatment of malunion and nonunion at the site of an ankle fusion with the Ilizarov apparatus. Surgical technique. *J Bone Joint Surg Am.* 2006;88:119–134.
19. Pearce MS, Smith MA, Savidge GF. Supramalleolar tibial osteotomy for haemophilic arthropathy of the ankle. *J Bone Joint Surg Br.*1994; 76:947–950.
20. Pugh K, Rozbruch SR. Nonunions and malunions. In: Baumgaertner MR, Tornetta P, eds. *Orthopaedic Knowledge Update Trauma 3.* Rosemont, IL: American Academy of Orthopaedic Surgeons;2005:1 15–130.
21. Rozbruch SR, Helfet DL, Blyakher A. Distraction of hypertrophic nonunion of tibia with deformity using Ilizarov/Taylor Spatial Frame. Report of two cases. *Arch Orthop Trauma Surg.*2002;122:295–298.
22. Rozbruch SR, Blyakher A, Haas SB, Hotchkiss R. Correction of large bilateral tibia vara with the Ilizarov method. *J Knee Surg.*2003; 16:34–37.
23. Rozbruch SR. Post-traumatic Reconstruction of the Ankle using the Ilizarov Method. *J Hosp Special Surg.*2005 ;1:68–88.
24. Rozbruch SR, Weitzman AM, Watson JT, Freudigman P, Katz HV, Ilizarov S. Simultaneous treatment of tibial bone and soft-tissue defects with the Ilizarov method. *J Orthop Trauma.* 2006;20:197–205.
25. Rozbruch SR, Fragomen A, Ilizarov S. Correction of tibial deformity with use of the Ilizarov/Taylor Spatial Frame. *JBJS-Am.*2006; 88-A:156–174.
26. Selber P, Filho ER, Dallalana R, Pirpiris M, Nattrass GR, Graham HK. Supramalleolar derotation osteotomy of the tibia, with T plate fixation. Technique and results in patients with neuromuscular disease. *J Bone Joint Surg Br.*2004; 86:1170–1175.
27. Sen C, Kocaoglu M, Eralp L, Cinar M. Correction of ankle and hindfoot deformities by supramalleolar osteotomy. *Foot Ankle Int.*2003; 24:22–28.
28. Shtarker H, Volpin G, Stolero J, Kaushansky A, Samchukov M. Correction of combined angular and rotational deformities by the Ilizarov method. *Clin Orthop Relat Res.* 2002;402: 184–195.
29. Stamatis ED, Myerson MS. Supramalleolar osteotomy: indications and technique. *Foot Ankle Clin.*2003;8:317–3 33.
30. Stamatis ED, Cooper PS, Myerson MS. Supramalleolar osteotomy for the treatment of distal tibial angular deformities and arthritis of the ankle joint. *Foot Ankle Int.*2003; 24:754–764.
31. Tellisi N, Fragomen AT, Kleinman D, et al. Joint preservation of the osteoarthritic ankle using distration arthroplasty. *Foot Ankle Int.*2009; 30:318–325.
32. Tellisi N, Ilizarov S, Fragomen A, et al. Humeral lengthening and deformity correction in Ollier's disease: distraction osteogenesis with a multiaxial correction frame. *J Pediatr Orthop B.*M ay2008;17:152–157.
33. PaleyD . *Principles of Deformity Correction.*B erlin,G ermany:S pringer;2003.

Minimally Invasive Management ofS yndesmoticl njuries

30

Stefan Buchmann, Umile Giuseppe Longo,a nd Andreas B. Imhoff

30.1 Introduction

Ankle sprains are one of the most common foot injuries, and the severity and degree of these injuries vary greatly.[18] Their complexity remains a diagnostic and therapeutic challenge.[11] Syndesmotic injuries occur less often in the general and sport populations when compared with lateral ankle sprains, with a reported incidence from 1% to 11% of all ankle injuries.[21] They usually require a longer recovery period than lateral ankle sprains.[21] Though the injury of the syndesmosis is the most important predictive factor for chronic ankle dysfunction 6 months after ankle sprains,[14,19] diagnostic protocols, which include physical examination, radiographs, stress examinations and MRI, do not completely quantify the extent of ligament damage.[13]

Stabilizing structures of the distal tibiofibular syndesmosis include the anterior inferior tibiofibular ligament, the posterior inferior tibiofibular ligament, the inferior transverse ligament, the interosseous ligament and the distal interosseous membrane. The anterior and posterior tibiofibular ligament serve as main stabilizing structures, whereas the interosseus portion provides the anatomic elasticity of the syndesmotic complex.[15] The intact distal tibiofibular joint allows up to 5° external rotation of the fibula. In maximal external rotation, a posterior and medial translation of the fibula (up to 3.1 and 2.5 mm) can be measured.[2] In anatomic studies, insufficiency of the syndesmotic complex manifests as increased external rotation of the talus under dynamic stress, and a loss of congruence of the talo-crural joint.[4,39]

The classical described injury mechanism is the ankle being subjected to an external rotation moment with the foot in a dorsiflexed, pronated position.[39] The talus rotates externally in the tibia, possibly injuring the medial deltoid ligament. Given the mechanism of injury, an associated high grade lesion of the lateral ligaments (Grade II-IV) seldom occurs, but isolated concomitant lesions of the anterior talofibular ligament are described in up to 83% of patients.[6,33] The severity and the time of the applied force determine how proximal

S.B uchmann(✉)
Department of Orthopaedic Sports Medicine, Klinikum Rechts der Isar, UniversityofM unich, 32,C onnollySt reet, Munich 80809, Germany
e-mail:s _buchmann17@hotmail.com

N. Maffulli and M. Easley (eds.), *Minimally Invasive Surgery of the Foot and Ankle*,
DOI: 10.1007/978-1-84996-417-3_30, © Springer-Verlag London Limited 2011

the syndesmotic and interosseous injury extends. The proximal extent of the injury can result in distal fractures of the tibia.[33]

Involvement of the syndesmosis in ankle injuries is described in up to 15% of cases, whereas Grade III lesions with diastasis of the tibio-fibular joint occur only in 0.25% of all ankle sprains.[14]

30.2 Clinical and Imaging Examination

There is controversy as to the most effective evaluation of syndesmosis sprains.[21] In a patient with a syndesmosic injury without any mortise widening, physical examination is fundamental for diagnosis. External rotation is one of the most common mechanisms of injury. Therefore, the external rotation test can be useful to confirm suspicions of syndesmosis injury (Fig. 30.1a). The stability of the ankle joint may be examined by asking the patient to toe raise, walking, and jumping.[21] Amendola described the "stabilization test," which is performed by tightly taping the leg of the patient just above the ankle joint in an attempt to stabilize the syndesmosis.[36] If toe raises, walking, and/or jumping are less painful upon taping, this would indicate a positive test result (Fig. 30.1b).[36] The Cotton test, performed by translating the talus medial to lateral within the mortise, may also indicate deltoid ligament injury associated with the syndesmosis sprain if increased translation or pain is noted.[7]

Standard radiographic examination following ankle trauma should include a weight bearing lateral, antero-posterior and mortise view of the ankle. Diastasis is identified by an

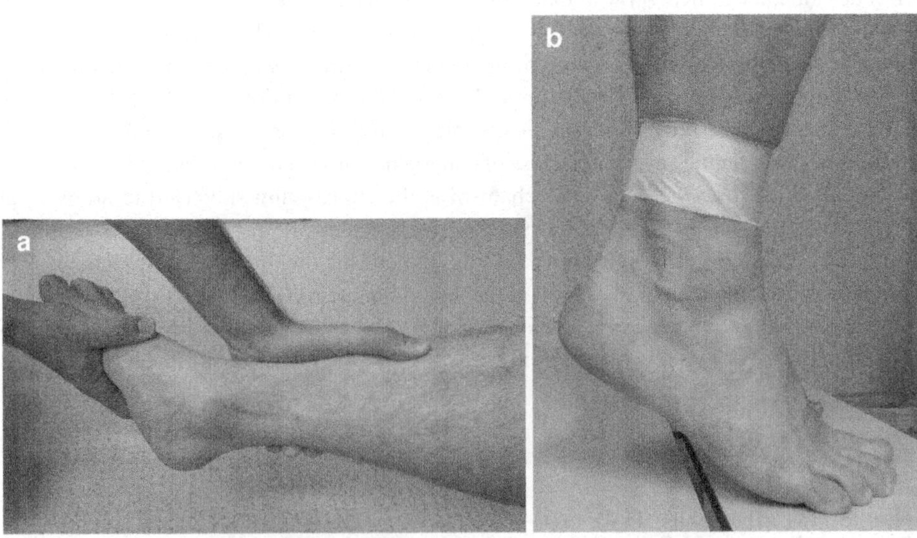

Fig. 30.1 (**a**) Frick-Test (**b**) Stabilization Test with applied tape

increased tibiofibular clear space on an antero-posterior and radiographs to a value of 6 mm or greater.[17] Avulsion fractures from the anterior or posterior tibia can occur in up to 50% of syndesmosis injuries and aid in identifying disrupted structures[12](Fig. 30.2).

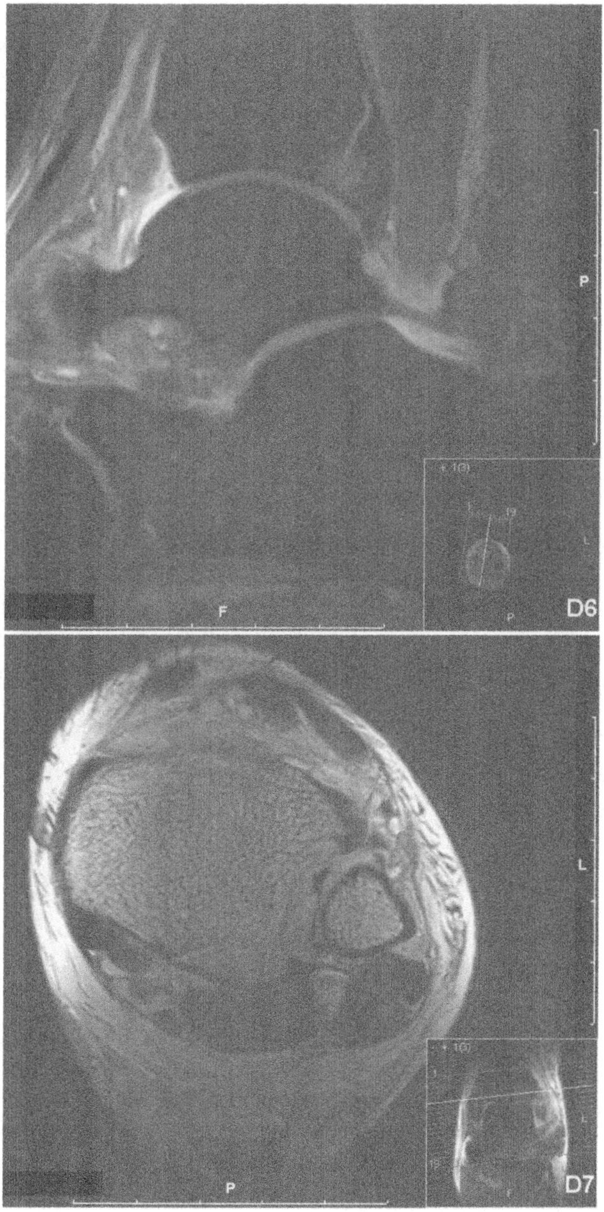

Fig.30. 2 Sagittala nda xial MRI (T2) of syndesmotic injury with non dislocated fractureofthe pos teriort ibia

Some authors recommend stress radiographs under external rotation. However, a cadaveric study of Beumer et al. showed only minimal differences in medial-lateral and anterior-posterior translation so that this technique does not provide further diagnostic information.[3] According to the West Point Ankle Grading System, a grade I injury indicates a lesion without laxity at clinical and radiographic examination, but tenderness over the syndesmosis and pain during weight bearing. Grade II is described as clinical evidence of laxity without defined diastasis under radiographic control. Grade III injuries are defined by widening of the ankle mortise on radiographs, with or without external rotation stress.[14]

Dynamic ultrasound examination (0°, IR, ER) of the torn anterior inferior tibiofibular ligament is a sensitive and specific method for imaging and diagnosing a syndesmotic sprain.[23] To exclude concomitant injuries and evaluation of the injured structures MRI examination gives more detailed information (Fig. 30.2).[6] When correlated to arthroscopy, MRI showed a high sensitivity and specificity for lesions of the anterior and posterior tibiofibular ligaments of 93–100%.[28] In conclusion, diagnosing syndesmotic injuries and grading their severity is a challenge for every practitioner, and needs careful consideration with a combined clinical and radiological approach.

30.3 Managementl ndications

In syndesmotic injuries without diastasis, aggressive/conservative management produces satisfying clinical results and a quick return to sports.[10] However, Ogilvie-Harris et al. described patients with chronic lateral ankle pain from scar tissue and syndesmotic ligament stumps flipped in the lateral compartment of the ankle, requiring secondary arthroscopic management.[22] For Grade III injuries, primary surgical management to stabilize the distal tibio-fibular joint is recommended.[24,29] Additionally, we recommend surgical management when there is evidence of osteo-chondral intraarticular lesions.

30.4 OperativeM anagement

30.4.1 Tightrope™ System (Arthrex, Naples)

The Tightrope™ Systems is a minimally invasive system that combines a less rigid fixation of the distal tibio-fibular joint without material removal.[30,31]

It consists of a four-holed round button (lateral button) and a two-holed oblong button (medial button). They are connected with a Fiberwire No. 5 so that four strands of suture span between the two buttons. Comparable to a pulley system, traction on the two trailing ends of the lateral sutures pulls the buttons closer together. Two pull-through sutures are looped through the eccentric aperture holes of the oblong button, and they are attached to

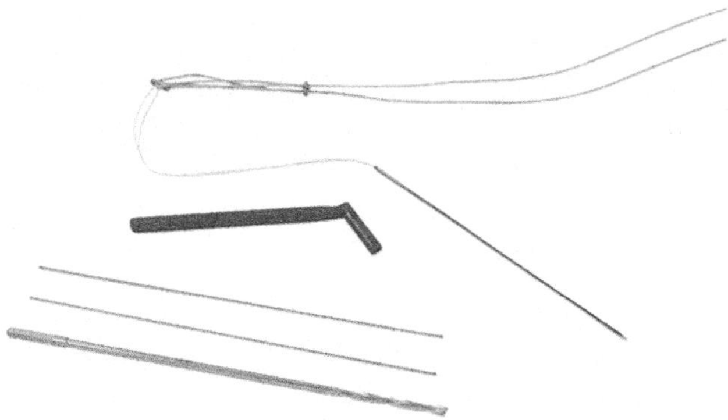

Fig.30.3 TightR opeSys temw ithc annulateddr ill(Arthrex,N aples,U SA)

a long straight needle (Fig. 30.3). These sutures are only used for pulling through the system and to flip the medial button easily over the tibial cortex. After inserting the implant, the needle and the pulling sutures have to be removed.

The Tightrope™ Kit includes two Kirschner wires and a cannulated 4 mm drill bit with drill sleeve, as well as the Tightrope™ system itself.[1]

Thornes at al. showed that a Suture-Endobutton construct in a cadaver syndesmosis injury model showed comparable results to a single four-cortex 4.5 mm A.O. screw fixation, with more persistent reduction in the Endobutton group.[31] A more recent cadaver study showed significant differences in translation and rotation of the fibula between Tightrope™ and 3.5 mm screw fixation, whereas the screw had a significant higher failure torque.[26]

The system is also used for minimally invasive reconstruction of the coraco-clavicular ligaments, and biomechanical studies show a sufficient stabilization in comparison to native coraco-clavicular ligaments.[25,35]

30.4.2
Acute Syndesmotic Lesions (<2 Weeks Posttraumatic)

The patient is placed supine on a radiolucent operating table, and the contralateral leg is lowered for intraoperative fluoroscopy in the sagittal and coronary plane. A pillow is placed under the ipsilateral gluteal area to internally rotate the limb. After marking the bony and soft tissue landmarks (fibula, tibia, joint line, and superficial veins), the tourniquet is insufflated.

The ankle can be examined pre- and intra-operatively under fluoroscopy to perform a dynamic test of laxity. According to preoperative MRI, a diagnostic or therapeutic arthroscopy of the ankle joint can be performed.[27]

Under fluoroscopy, the insertion area in the central portion of the lateral aspect of the fibula is placed about 2 cm proximal to the joint line. The skin is incised vertically over about 2 cm, and the bony surface of the fibula is prepared and exposed. The leg is now placed in 30° of internal rotation to prevent posterior placement of the tibial button with concomitant danger of nerve and vessel injuries. The fibular insertion point of the Tightrope™ device is marked with the electro-cautery, and the Tightrope™ system is prepared.

Thefi bula should be formally reduced before drilling. Therefore, a reverse mechanism of injury (internal rotation) is performed. The ankle should be placed in moderate plantar flexion, which facilitates accurate fibular reduction into the incisural notch of the tibia.[30] Under fluoroscopy, the reduction in all planes is controlled carefully, and, if an anatomic repositioning cannot be performed, open reduction is indicated.[8]

The Kirschner wire is now inserted about 2 cm proximal of the tibio-talar joint.[20] A parallel insertion to the joint line and the tibial and fibular entrance position is controlled under fluoroscopy in antero-posterior and lateral views.[34] The Kirschner wire is over drilled using the 4 mm cannulated drill, the Tightrope™ device is inserted, and the long needle brought trough the skin on the medial side without skin incision. Under palpation, the medial button is pulled out of the tibia. With help of the two shuttle sutures, the button can be flipped easily under the skin, and the lateral button is pulled down to the bone. After removal of the medial needle, including the sutures, the pulley is tightened to complete the reduction of the tibio-fibular joint with slight plantar-flexion and internal rotation of the foot.[30] It is not possible to over tighten the syndesmosis.[32] The repositioning of the fibula and direct contact of the buttons to the bone of the tibia and the fibula is checked under fluoroscopy (Fig. 30.4). The Tightrope™ is fixed with five alternating knots, the sutures are cut, and the lateral incision is sutured in a routine fashion.

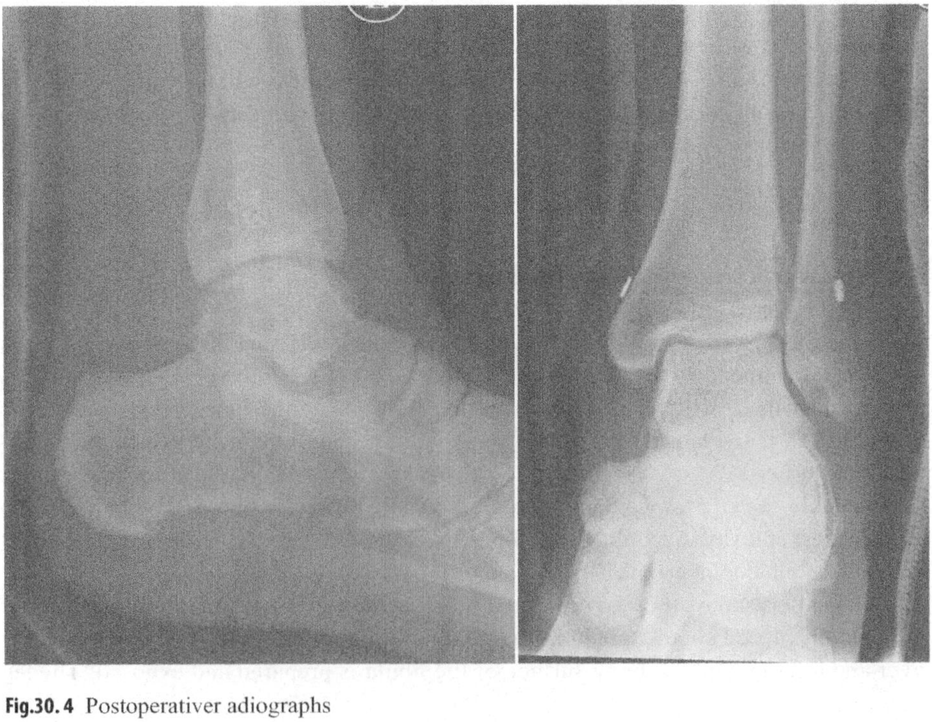

Fig.30.4 Postoperativer adiographs

The system can also be used in combination with osteosynthesis of fibular fractures through a distal hole of the fibular plate. In Maisonneuve fractures, the use of two Tightrope™ Systems 2 and 4 cm proximal of the tibia plafond is recommended.[30]

30.4.3 Chronic Syndesmotic Lesions

In case of chronic syndesmosis insufficiency, the above described surgical technique is modified with a 3 cm anterior vertical incision slightly medial to the syndesmosis. The anterior tibia is exposed and a periosteal flap of about 2 on 3 cm for a modified Brostrom Procedure is prepared.[5] Before performing the Tightrope™ procedure the syndesmotic space is debrided to prevent malreduction because of the hypertrophic scar tissue and to produce bleeding surfaces to induce healing. The repositioning of the fibula is evaluated under fluoroscopy, and the reduction using the Tightrope™ device is performed as described above. Finally, the periosteal flap is sutured to the fibula, and transosseous sutures can be used.

The debridement of the syndesmotic space can also be performed arthroscopically with a combined evaluation and management of intraarticular pathologies.[38] Several surgical techniques are available for the management of chronic syndesmotic lesions, but most of them are performed using a more invasive approach (tendon transfer, bone block transfer).[2,16] The technique described allows also a biological augmentation of the Tightrope™ stabilisation via this minimally invasive approach.

30.5 Postoperative Management

After reconstruction of the syndesmosis, the foot and ankle are placed in a short-leg splint in neutral position, and no weight bearing is allowed for 2 weeks. After suture removal at 2 weeks, the splint is removed, and a pneumatic cam boot is applied. For 6 weeks, the ROM is restricted to plantarflexion/dorsalextension 20°/0°/0° and no pronation, supination and rotation exercises are allowed. After 6 weeks, weight bearing anteroposterior and lateral views are obtained, and the boot is removed with a following full mobilisation of the ankle. Cutting activities are usually allowed after 3 months.

30.6 Clinical Results

The first clinical results of the Tightrope™ system included 12 patients with nine Weber C and three Maisonneuve fractures.[30] After a minimum follow up of 6 months, the mean AOFAS score was 87. There were no complications and no patient required secondary surgery for any reason, including hardware removal.

Willmott et al. showed good clinical results in a very heterogeneous study with fractures and isolated syndesmotic injuries, with complete weight bearing after 6 weeks and sufficient radiographic stability of the distal tibio-fibular joint. In this group, mechanical irritation over the buttons was documented in two of six patients, and the implants were removed after 6 months without radiographic evidence of loss of stability.[37]

In a recent study of 25 patients with disruption of the distal tibiofibular joint that underwent management with the Tightrope™ device,[9] a single Tightrope™ was placed in 21 cases, and in four cases two Tightrope™ devices were used. Associated ankle fractures were treated using standard internal fixation techniques. After a follow up of 10.8 months, radiographs demonstrated no evidence of re-displacement of the syndesmotic complex and good clinical results. In our own experience we followed 15 patients after Tightrope™ procedure . The heterogenic group (isolated syndesmosis lesions and combined fractures) showed a mean AOFAS Hindfoot score of 87.5 points and pain score (VAS) of 1.0 after a minimum follow up of 1 year. There was one patient with irritations over the buttons while wearing a skiing boot, so that the implants were removed without loss of stability after 8 months.

In conclusion, the Tightrope™ technique is an option in patients with diastasis of the syndesmotic complex. The placement of the device is quick, can be performed in a minimally invasive fashion, and obviates the need for hardware removal. Current literature shows excellent reduction of the syndesmosis, with encouraging clinical results and a low rate of complications.[9,30,37]

References

1. Arthrex. Tight rope syndesmosis fixation - surgical technique. Available at: http://www.ankle-tightrope.com.2009
2. Beumer A, Heijboer R, Fontijne WP, Swierstra BA. Late reconstruction of the anterior distal tibiofibular syndesmosis: good outcome in 9 patients. *Acta Orthop Scand.*2000; 71:519–521.
3. Beumer A, Valstar ER, Garling EH. External rotation stress imaging in syndesmotic injuries of the ankle: comparison of lateral radiography and radiostereometry in a cadaveric model. *Acta Orthop Scand.*2003; 74:201–205.
4. Bridgman SA, Clement D, Downing A, Walley G, Phair I, Maffulli N. Population based epidemiology of ankle sprains attending accident and emergency units in the West Midlands of England, and a survey of UK practice for severe ankle sprains. *Emerg Med J.* 2003;20:508–510.
5. Brostrom L. Sprained ankles. V. Treatment and prognosis in recent ligament ruptures. *Acta Orthop Scand.*1966; 132:537–550.
6. Brown KW, Morrison WB, Schweitzer ME, Parellada JA, Nothnagel H. MRI findings associated with distal tibiofibular syndesmosis injury. *Am J Roentgenol.*2004; 182:131–136.
7. Capasso G, Maffulli N, Testa V. Ankle taping: support given by different materials. *Br J Sports Med.*1989; 23:239–240.
8. Coetzee JC, Ebeling P. Treatment of syndesmosis disruptions with tightrope fixation. *Techn Foot Ankle Surg.*2008; 7:196–202.

9. Cottom JM, Hyer CF, Philbin TM, Berlet GC. Treatment of syndesmotic disruptions with the Arthrex Tightrope: a report of 25 cases. *Foot Ankle Int.*2 008;29:773–780.
10. Nussbaum ED, Hosea TM, Sieler SD, Incremona BR, Kessler DE. Prospective evaluation of syndesmotic ankle sprains without diastasis. *Am. J. Sports Med.*2001; 29:31–35.
11. Ferran NA, Maffulli N. Epidemiology of sprains of the lateral ankle ligament complex. *Foot Ankle Clin.*2006;1 1:659–662.
12. Frey C.A nkle sprains. *Instr Course Lect.*2001; 50:515–520.
13. Gardner MJ, Demetrakopoulos D, Briggs SM, Helfet DL, Lorich DG. Malreduction of the tibiofibular syndesmosis in ankle fractures. *Foot Ankle Int.*2006; 27:788–792.
14. Gerber JP, Williams GN, Scoville CR, Arciero RA, Taylor DC. (1998) Persistent disability associated with ankle sprains: a prospective examination of an athletic population. *Foot Ankle Int.*2006;19:653–6 60.
15. Grass R, Herzmann K, Biewener A, Zwipp H. [Injuries of the inferior tibiofibular syndesmosis]. *Unfallchirurg.*2000; 103:520–532.
16. Grass R, Rammelt S, Biewener A, Zwipp H. Peroneus longus ligamentoplasty for chronic instability of the distal tibiofibular syndesmosis. *Foot Ankle Int.*2003; 24:392–397.
17. Harper M. An anatomic and radiologic investigation of the tibiofibular clear space. *Foot Ankle Int.*1993;14:455–4 58.
18. Malliaropoulos N, Ntessalen M, Papacostas E, Longo UG, Maffulli N. Reinjury after acute lateral ankle sprains in elite track and field athletes. *Am J Sports Med.*2009; 37:1755–1761.
19. Malliaropoulos N, Papacostas E, Papalada A, Maffulli N. Acute lateral ankle sprains in track and field athletes: an expanded classification. *Foot Ankle Clin.*2006; 11:497–507.
20. McBryde A, Chiasson B, Wilhelm A, Donovan F, Ray T, Bacilla P. Syndesmotic screw placement: a biomechanical analysis. *Foot Ankle Int.*1997; 18:262–266.
21. Molinari A, Stolley M, Amendola A. High ankle sprains (syndesmotic) in athletes: diagnostic challenges and review of the literature. *Iowa Orthop J.*2 009;29:130–138.
22. Ogilvie-Harris DJ, Gilbart MK, Chorney K. Chronic pain following ankle sprains in athletes: the role of arthroscopic surgery. *Arthroscopy.*1997; 13:564–574.
23. Mei-Dan O, Kots E, Barchilon V, Massarwe S, Nyska M, Mann G. A dynamic ultrasound examination for the diagnosis of ankle syndesmotic injury in professional athletes. *Am J Sports Med.* 2009;37:1009–1016.
24. Press CM, Gupta A, Hutchinson MR. Management of ankle syndesmosis injuries in the athlete. *Curr Sports Med Rep.*2009; 8:228–233.
25. Salzmann GM, Walz L, Schoettle PB, Imhoff AB. Arthroscopic anatomical reconstruction of the acromioclavicular joint. *Acta Orthop Belg.*2008; 74:397–400.
26. Soin SP, Knight TA, Dinah AF, Mears SC, Swierstra BA, Belkoff SM. Suture-button versus screw fixation in a syndesmosis rupture model: a biomechanical comparison. *Foot Ankle Int.* 2009;30:346–352.
27. Takao M, Ochi M, Naito K. Arthroscopic diagnosis of the tibiofibular syndesmosis disruption. *Arthroscopy.*2001; 17:836–843.
28. Takao M, Ochi M, Oae K, Naito K, Uchio Y. Diagnosis of a tear of the tibiofibular syndesmosis: the role of arthroscopy of the ankle. *J Bone Joint Surg Br.*2003; 85:324–329.
29. Taylor DC, Tenuta JJ, Uhorchak JM, Arciero RA. Aggressive surgical treatment and early return to sports in athletes with grade III syndesmosis sprains. *Am J Sports Med.* 2007;35:1833–1838.
30. Thornes B, McCartan D. Ankle syndesmosis injuries treated with the tightRope Suture-Button kit. *Tech Foot Ankle Surg.*2006; 5:45–53.
31. Thornes B, Walsh A, Hislop M, Murray P, O'Brien M. Suture-Endobutton fixation of ankle tibio-fibular diastasis: a Cadaver study. *Foot Ankle Int.*2 003;24:142–146.
32. Tornetta P 3rd, Spoo JE, Reynolds FA, Lee C. Overtightening of the ankle syndesmosis: is it really possible? *J Bone Joint Surg Am.*2001; 83:489–492.

33. Uys HD, Rijke AM. Clinical association of acute lateral ankle sprain with syndesmotic involvement: a stress radiography and magnetic resonance imaging study. *Am J Sports Med.* 2002;30:816–822.
34. van den Bekerom MP, Hogervorst M, Bolhuis HW, van Dijk CN. Operative aspects of the syndesmotic screw: review of current concepts. *Injury.*2008; 39:491–498.
35. Walz L, Salzmann GM, Fabbro T, Eichhorn S, Imhoff AB. The anatomic reconstruction of acromioclavicular joint dislocations using 2 TightRope devices: a biomechanical study. *Am J Sports Med.*2008 ;36:2398–2406.
36. Williams GN, Jones MH, Amendola A. Syndesmotic ankle sprains in athletes. *Am J Sports Med.*2007;35:1 197–1207.
37. Willmott HJ, Singh B, David LA. Outcome and complications of treatment of ankle diastasis with tightrope fixation. *Injury.*2009; 40:1204–1206
38. Wolf BR, Amendola A. Syndesmosis injuries in the athlete: when and how to operate. *Curr Opin Orthop.*20 02;13:151–154.
39. Xenos JS, Hopkinson WJ, Mulligan ME, Olson EJ, Popovic NA. The tibiofibular syndesmosis: evaluation of the ligamentous structures, methods of fixation, and radiographic assessment. *J Bone Joint Surg Am.*1995; 77:847–856.

Part VI

The Achilles Tendon

Endoscopic Assisted Percutaneous Achilles TendonR epair

31

Mahmut Nedim Doral, Murat Bozkurt, Egemen Turhan,a nd Ozgür Ahmet Atay

The Achilles tendon is the strongest tendon in the human body.[1] Hippocrates said "this tendon, if bruised or cut, causes the most acute fevers, induces choking, deranges the mind and at length brings death."[2] Achilles tendon rupture has been the focus of many studies since Ambroise Paré initially described it in 1575.[3] Achilles tendon ruptures are the third most frequent major tendon ruptures, following rotator cuff and quadriceps ruptures.[4,5] Nevertheless, there is no consensus on the optimal management, and management is still determined by the preferences of the surgeon and the patient. Cast immobilization may lead to suboptimal healing, with elongation of the tendon, reduced strength of the calf muscles, and an unacceptably high rate of re-rupture.[6–10]

Open surgical repair of the Achilles tendon carries specific risks including adhesions between the tendon and the skin, infection, and particularly wound breakdown.[11–14] Although Ma and Griffith introduced the percutaneous repair technique to avoid these complications, percutaneous repair may not achieve satisfactory contact of the tendon stumps and adequate initial fixation.[15] In addition, sural nerve entrapment is a reported complication of this technique.[16,17] Only recently have safe and sound techniques been developed, and some are described Prof Maffulli in other chapters of this book by.

Percutaneous repair has become popular. The advantages of the operative and conservative methods are combined in minimally invasive percutaneous repair techniques, but these techniques do not allow direct visualization of the tendon ends. This may be overcome by performing the percutaneous repair under endoscopic control.[18,19]

31.1 The Technique of Endoscopy Assisted Percutaneous Repair

The operation is performed with the patients in prone position with infiltration of local anaesthesia in the area to be operated on. No tourniquet is used, and we do not use antibiotic or antithrombotic prophylaxis. Before starting the procedure, the rupture site is marked

M.N.D oral(✉)
Department of Orthopedics and Traumatology, Hacettepe University, Faculty of Medicine, Sihhiye, Ankara, 06100 Turkey
e-mail:mn-dora l@bim.net.tr

N. Maffulli and M. Easley (eds.), *Minimally Invasive Surgery of the Foot and Ankle*,
DOI: 10.1007/978-1-84996-417-3_31, © Springer-Verlag London Limited 2011

(Figs. 31.1 and 31.2). Then, to minimize local bleeding, proximal (about 5 cm) and distal (about 4 cm) to the palpated gap, the skin, subcutaneous tissues, and peritendon are infiltrated with 20–50 mL 0.9% saline solution with local anesthetic (1% Citanest® 5 mL + 0.5% Marcain® 5 mL) around the eight planned stab wounds, four medial and four lateral tto the tendon, distributed evenly proximally and distal to the rupture (Fig. 31.3), These stab wounds are later enlarged with the nick and spread technique, and used for needle

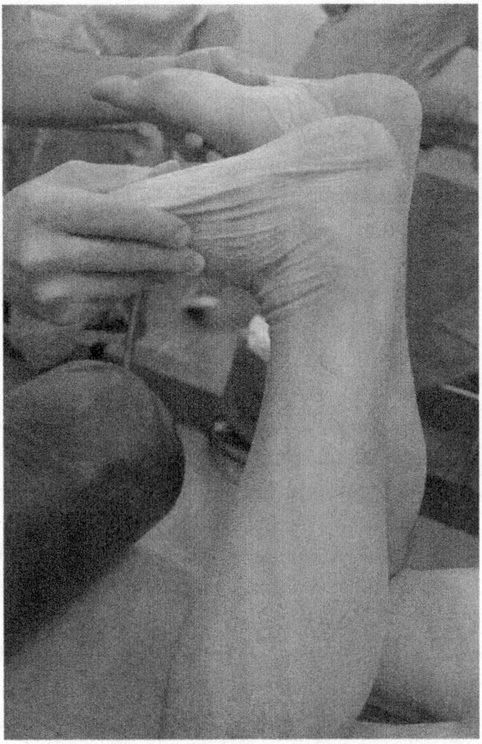

Fig.31.1 Greaterdors iflexion on the ruptureds idet hanont hehe althys ide

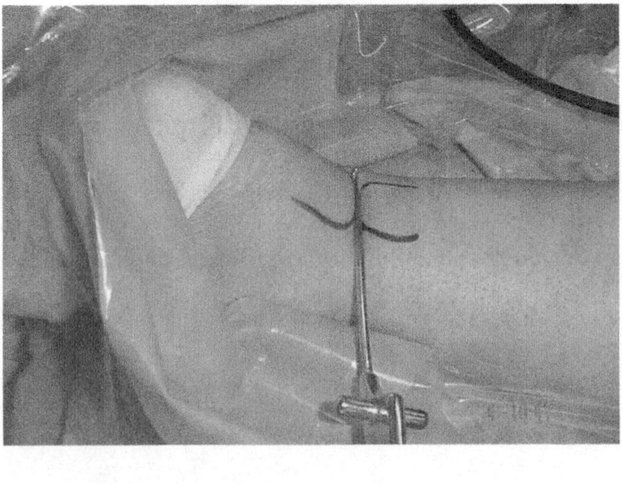

Fig.31.2 Palpation of the gap between the ruptured tendon ends using an arthroscopic probe

entry. Special attention is paid to the area lateral to the Achilles tendon, especially proximally, where the sural nerve lies close to and crosses the Achilles tendon. The patient is prompted to report any paraesthesiae or pain in the area of distribution of the sural nerve at any time during the injection of local anaesthetic or during the procedure. If this is experienced, the injection site is moved 0.5–1 cm toward the midline. The injured foot is positioned in approximately 15° of plantar flexion. The tendon and paratenon are examined with a 30° arthroscope (Smith-Nephew, London) via the distal medial incision (Fig. 31.4). After the level of the rupture has been determined, the continuity of the surrounding tissues together with their consistency and vascularization are evaluated. The torn ends of the

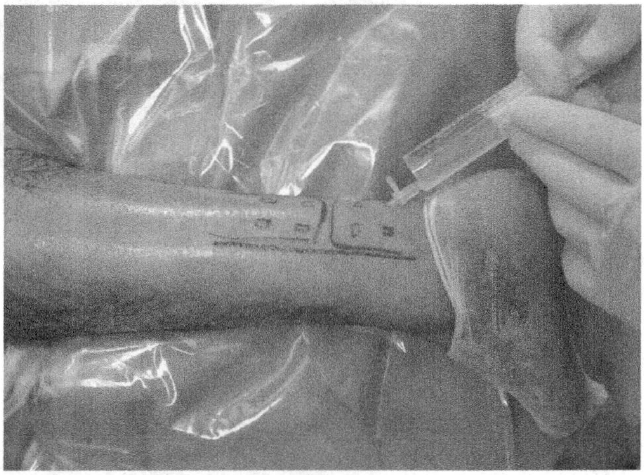

Fig.31.3 Locala naesthetic injection to the subcutaneous tissues from the stab incisions

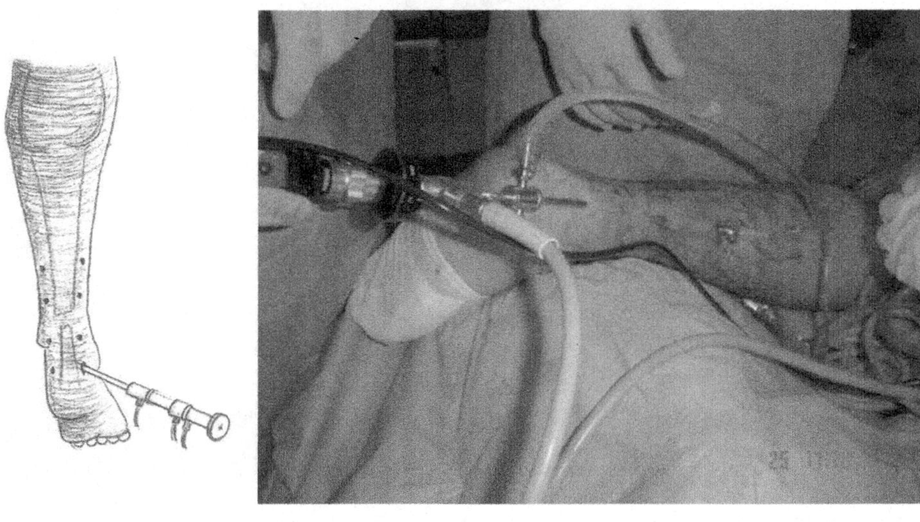

Fig.31.4 Thepla cementof t hea rthroscopef romdi stalm ediali ncision

Achilles tendons are inspected, and, if necessary, are manipulated within the paratenon. The passing of the suture through the Achilles tendon is also controlled with the scope. We use an Ethibond No.5 or PDS No. 5 (Ethicon Inc, Johnson & Johnson, Somerville, NJ) suture with a modified Bunnell configuration.

The needle with the PDS or Ethibond suture is first introduced through the upper medial portal (shown as "1" in Fig. 31.5a). The Achilles tendon is gently palpated between the

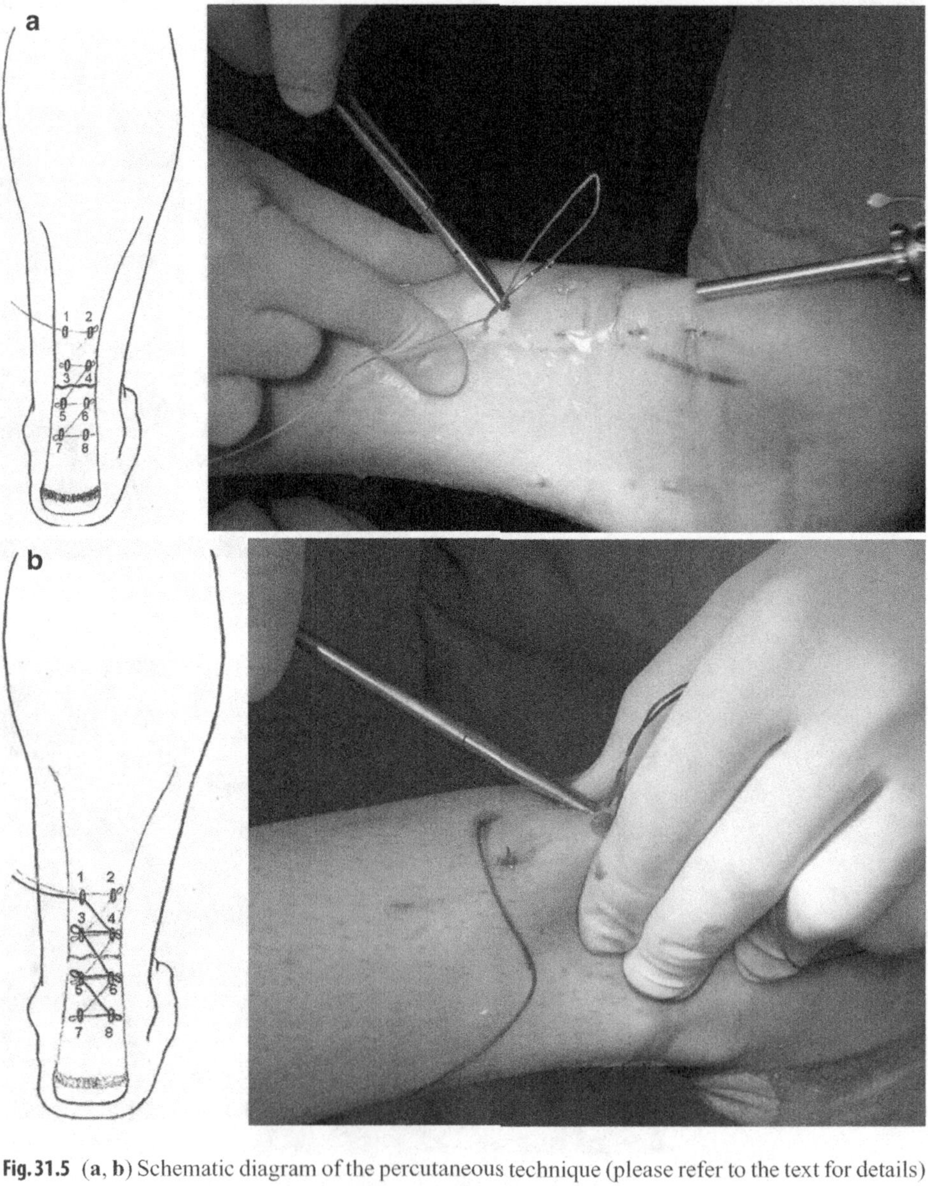

Fig. 31.5 (**a**, **b**) Schematic diagram of the percutaneous technique (please refer to the text for details) (**c**) The sutures are tied with the ankle in the neutral position

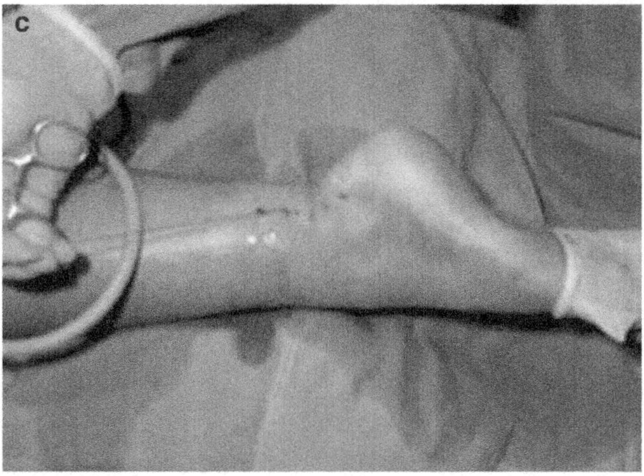

Fig. 31.5 (continued)

thumb and the index finger of the opposite hand to make sure that it is caught fully by the needle. This first bite is a transverse one, and the needle emerges from the upper lateral portal (shown as "2" in Fig. 31.5a). The needle is then retrieved, introduced again through it and passed through the upper lateral portal towards portal 3. The procedure is repeated in a proximal to distal direction going from portal 3 to portal 4, from portal 4 to portal 5, from portal 5 to portal 6, from portal 6 to portal 7, and from portal 7 to portal 8, the distal most lateral portal. At this point, the needle is retrieved from portal 8, introduced through it and passed through the distal most lateral portal towards portal 5, and the procedure described above repeated backward in a distal to proximal direction until the needle is finally returned to the upper medial portal (shown as "1" in Fig. 31.5b).

First, we pass the suture from the proximal medial incision and out from the medial incision just above the ruptured tendon, making sure that the body of the proximal stump of the tendon is squeezed between the thumb and index (Fig. 31.5a). Second, we pass the suture from the same incision and out from the lateral stab incision just above the tendon (Fig. 31.5a). Finally, as in the first step, the suture is passed through this stab incision and out from the distal medial side (Fig. 31.5a).

During suture passage, the arthroscope is placed alternatively in the various entry portals, and the Achilles tendon is inspected from the medial and lateral aspects, and the proximal and distal stumps are inspected from proximal and distal to make sure that the tendon stumps are juxtaposed. Also, through the endoscope we make sure that the sutures are introduced in the tendon at different levels on the coronal plane, so that the chance of them cutting through during the process of tensioning is minimised.

Finally, the sutures are tensioned, and tied in the proximal medial entry portal with the ankle in neutral position whilst checking the tendon approximation through the arthroscope. Before tying the sutures with the ankle in neutral position, the patient is instructed to actively dorsi- and plantar-flex the ankle with the knee at 90° of flexion (Fig. 31.5c) to make sure that appropriate tension is imparted to the suture. A final check is performed, and the suture is knotted fully.

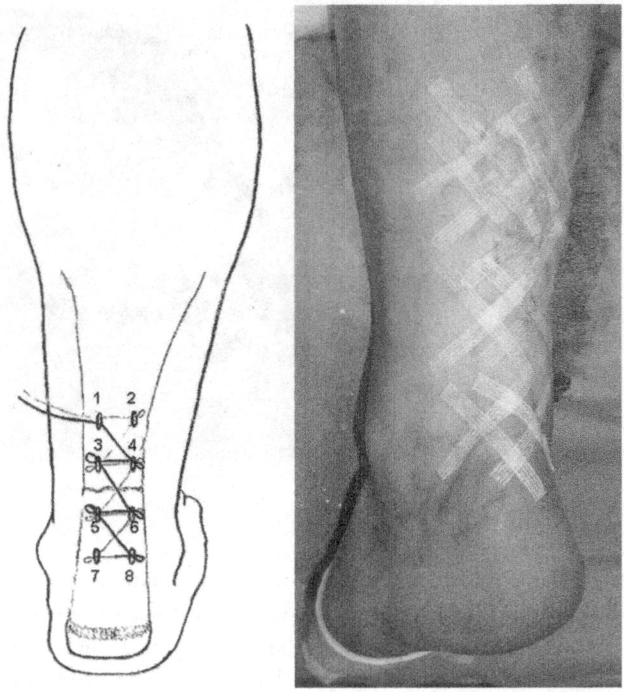

Fig. 31.6 Finals tabw ound closurew iths terisrtips

The skin stab incisions are closed with subcutaneous suture and steristrips are used for initial dressing, and a walking brace with the ankle in neutral is applied for at least 3 weeks (Fig. 31.6).

Immediate weight-bearing as tolerated with a walking brace is initiated (for 3 weeks only), alternating with passive range of motion exercises. Physiotherapy includes electrical stimulation of the gastrosoleus complex; cryotherapy and therapeutic ultrasound are applied around the Achilles tendon for reduction of edema. Transverse friction massage is used to promote scar and tendon re-formation.

Patients are instructed to move the ankle four times a day between 20° of plantar flexion and 10° of dorsiflexion. The patients complete gentle isometric, eccentric and concentric exercises of the ankle several times a day, with flexion and extension of the toes in a supine position, and full plantar flexion and dorsiflexion of the ankle to neutral in a supine position; extension of the knee in a sitting position; flexion of the knee in a prone position; and extension of the hip in a prone position within first 3 weeks. The walking brace is discontinued after 3 weeks. From the sixth week to tenth week, rehabilitation progresses to using elastic resistance bands; rotation of the ankles; standing on the toes and heels; ankle stretching exercises to flexion with the help of a rubber band; stretching of the calf muscle by standing with the leg to be stretched straight behind and the other leg bent in front and leaning the body forward, with support from a wall or physiotherapist; stretching exercises for the toes and ankle against manual resistance in a sitting position; balance and proprioception exercises on different surface progress from bilateral to unilateral; controlled squats, lunges, bilateral calf raise (progressing to unilateral), toe raises, controlled slow eccentrics versus body-weight. After 10 weeks, patients start training jogging/running, jumping and eccentric loading exercises, non-competitive sporting activities, sports-specific exercises, and return to physically demanding sports and/or work.

RehabilitationProc ess	
0–3 weeks:	Range of motion: 20° of plantar flexion and 10° of dorsiflexion
0–6 weeks:	Gentle isometric, eccentric and concentric exercises with flexion and extension of the toes, full plantar flexion and dorsiflexion of the ankle to neutral in a supine position; extension of the knee in a sitting position; flexion of the knee in a prone position; and extension of the hip in a prone position.
6–10 weeks:	Resistance exercises, rotation of the ankles; standing on the toes and heels; ankle stretching exercises for calf muscles, the toes and ankle, balance and proprioception exercises on different surface progress from bilateral to unilateral; controlled squats, lunges, bilateral calf raise (progressing to unilateral), toe raises, controlled slow eccentrics vs. body-weight.
10- ↑ weeks:	Start training jogging/running, jumping and eccentric loading exercises, non-competitive sporting activities, sports-specific exercises, and return to physically demanding sports and/or work.

Endoscopy-assisted percutaneous repair allows direct observation of the process of suturing the Achilles tendon. This eliminates some of the disadvantages of the percutaneous repair techniques, especially the evaluation of the juxtaposition of the torn ends.[20–23] Endoscopy-assisted percutaneous repair allows early active ankle mobilization and weight bearing after a short period of cast immobilization and thereby, prevents complications due to the prolonged immobilization such as arthrofibrosis, joint stiffness, calf atrophy, damage to the articular cartilage, and deep vein thrombosis. Buchgraber and Pässler[24] compared the results of immobilization and functional postoperative treatment after percutaneous repair of Achilles tendon rupture and found that functional postoperative rehabilitation with early weight-bearing was associated with significantly less severe calf muscle work by the injured leg than postoperative immobilization. Considering these advantages, endoscopy-assisted percutaneous repair of AT may prevent some of the negative issues associated with open, conservative, or percutaneous techniques. Also, this technique could help to prevent the risk of damage to the sural nerve by allowing its direct visualisation. However, we stress that knowledge of the local anatomy is necessary to place the stab wounds in the areas less likely to damage this nerve.[25–27]

In endoscopic repair, the paratenon is protected, providing a biological advantage to the mechanical strength of the repair furnished by the suture material. Also, preservation of the paratenon decreases the gliding resistance of the extrasynovial tendons after repetitive motion *in vitro*.[25] Achilles tendoscopy allows direct observation of the haematoma and the stab wounds, and controlled juxtaposition of the tendon ends without damaging the paratenon.[26]

Any technique may result in lengthening of the Achilles tendon, possibly from not having closely approximated the tendon ends. Carmont and Maffulli recommend a mini open technique, with a 1.2–1.5 cm transverse incision at the level of the rupture, to directly

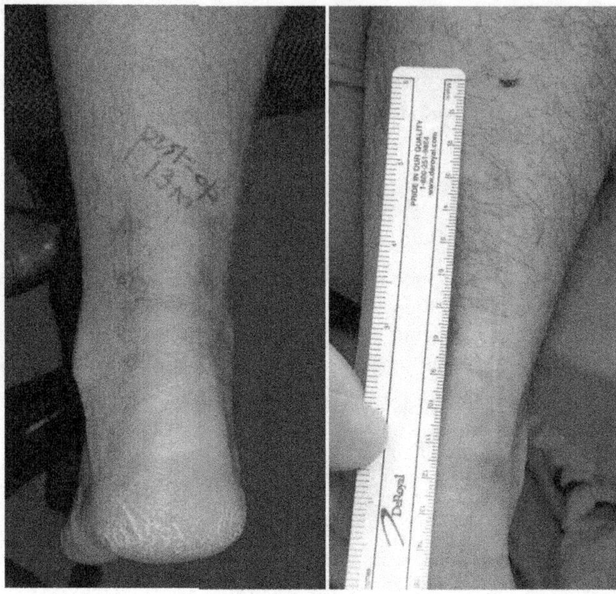

Fig.31. 7 Bilaterallyo perated patient of AT rupture. Left side is operated with percutaneous method and right side was operated with open surgery previously. The appearance of the wound is cosmetic with percutaneous method

observe that appropriate juxtaposition of the ruptured tendon ends had been achieved.[28] Direct visualization of the tendon ends by endoscope through the stab incisions allows this without any additional incision.

Obviously, the procedure requires experience in soft tissue endoscopy. Percutaneous repair of the Achilles tendon under endoscopic control results excellent wound appearance (Fig. 31.7), This technique resulted in a cosmetic wound appearance, endurable to early-active mobilization and satisfactory clinical recovery without any severe complication,. Furthermore, this procedure protects the paratenon, and should enhance biologic recovery. Direct visualization and manipulation of the tendon ends also provide stable repair that allows early weight-bearing and ambulation, and we have used in athletic individuals. Percutaneous repair is likely more cost effective than open techniques, and, in some settings, endoscopic control carries no additional costs.[29]

Acknowledgements We would like to thank to Professor Nicola Maffulli for his support and Dr. M. Ayvaz and Dr. G. Dönmez for archiving and pictures.

References

1. MaffulliN .R upture oft heA chillest endon. *J Bone Joint Surg (Am).*1999; 81:1019–1036.
2. Carden DG, Noble J, Chalmers J et al. Rupture of the calcaneal tendon. The early and late management. *J Bone Joint Surg (Br).*1987; 69:416–420.
3. Cetti R, Christensen SE, Ejsted R et al. Operative versus nonoperative treatment of Achilles tendon rupture. A prospective randomized study and review of the literature. *Am J Sports Med.* 1993;21:791–799.

4. Hattrup SJ, Johnson KA. A review of ruptures of the Achilles tendon. *Foot Ankle.* 1985;6: 34–38.
5. Weiner AD, Lipscomb PR Rupture of muscles and tendons. *Minn Med.*1956; 39:731–736.
6. Edna TH. Non-operative treatment of Achilles tendon ruptures. *Acta Orthop Scand.* 1980;51: 991–993.
7. Fierro N, Sallis R Achilles tendon rupture: is casting enough? *Postgrad Med.* 1995;98: 145–151.
8. Inglis AE, Scott WN, Sculco TP et al. Ruptures of the tendo Achillis. *J Bone Joint Surg (Am).* 1976;58:990–993.
9. Jacobs D, Martens M, Van Audekercke R et al. Comparison of conservative and operative treatment of Achilles tendon ruptures. *Am J Sports Med.*1978; 6:107–111.
10. Leppilahti J, Puranen J, Orava S. Incidence of Achilles tendon rupture. *Acta Orthop Scand.* 1996;67:277–279.
11. Aoki M, Ogiwara N, Ohta T, Nabeta Y Early active motion and weightbearing after cross-stitch achilles tendon repair. *Am J Sports Med.*N ov–Dec1998; 26:794–800.
12. Bhandari M, Guyatt GH, Siddique F et al. Treatment of acute Achilles tendon ruptures a systematic overview and meta-analysis. *Clin Orthop.*2002; 400:190–200.
13. Kangas J, Pajala A, Siira P et al. Early functional treatment versus early immobilization in tension of the musculotendinous unit after Achilles rupture repair: a prospective, randomized, clinical study. *J Trauma.*2003; 54:1171–1180.
14. Mortensen NHM, Skov O, Jensen PE. Early motion of the ankle after operative treatment of a rupture of the Achilles tendon: a prospective randomized clinical and radiographic study. *J Bone Joint Surg (Am).*1999; 81:983–990.
15. Ma GWC, Griffith TG. Percutaneous repair of acute closed ruptured Achilles tendon. A new technique. *Clin Orthop.*1977; 128:247–255.
16. Klein W, Lang DM, Saleh M. The use of the Ma-Griffith technique for percutaneous repair of fresh ruptured tendo Achillis. *Chir Organi Mov.* July–Sept 1991;76:223–228 (English, Italian).
17. Rowley DI, Scotland TR. Rupture of the Achilles tendon treated by a simple operative procedure. *Injury.*1982;14: 252–254.
18. Tang KL, Thermann H, Dai G, Chen GX, Guo L, Yang L. Arthroscopically assisted percutaneous repair of fresh closed Achilles tendon rupture by Kesslers suture. *Am J Sports Med.* 2007;35:589–596.
19. Thermann H, Tibesku CO, Mastrokalos DS, Pässler HH. Endoscopically assisted percutaneous achilles tendon suture. *Foot Ankle Int.*2001; 22:158–160.
20. Halasi T, Tállay A, Berkes I. Percutaneous Achilles tendon repair with and without endoscopic control. *Knee Surg Sports Traumatol Arthrosc.*20 03;11:409–414.
21. Rebeccato A, Santini S, Salmaso G, Nogarin L. Repair of the achilles tendon rupture: a functional comparison of three surgical techniques. *J Foot Ankle Surg.*2001; 40:188–194.
22. Tang KL, Thermann H, Dai G, Chen GX, Guo L, Yang L. Arthroscopically assisted percutaneous repair of fresh closed achilles tendon rupture by Kesslers suture. *Am J Sports Med.* 2007;35:589–596.
23. Webb JM, Bannister GC. Percutaneous repair of the ruptured tendo Achillis. *J Bone Joint Surg (Br).*1999;81:877– 880.
24. Buchgrabber A, Pässler HH. Percutaneous repair of Achilles tendon rupture. Immobilization versus functional postoperative treatment. *Clin Orthop.*1997; 341:113–122.
25. McClelland D, Maffulli N. Percutaneous repair of ruptured Achilles tendon. *J R Coll Surg Edinb.*2002;47:613–618.
26. Momose T, Amadio PC, Zobitz ME, Zhao C, An KN. Effect of paratenon and repetitive motion on the gliding resistance of tendon of extrasynovial origin. *Clin Anat.* 2002;15:199–205.
27. Doral MN, Tetik O, Atay OA, Leblebicioğlu G, Oznur A. Achilles tendon diseases and its management. *Acta Orthop Traumatol Turc.* 2002;36:42–46.

28. Carmont MR, Maffulli N. Modified percutaneous repair of ruptured Achilles tendon. *Knee Surg Sports Traumatol Arthrosc.*2008; 16:199–203.
29. Ebinesan AD, Sarai BS, Walley GD, Maffulli N. Conservative, open or percutaneosus repair for acute rupture of the Achilles tendon. *Disabil Rehabil.*2008; 30:1721–1725.

Percutaneous Repair of Acute Achilles Tendon Ruptures

32

Nicola Maffulli, Francesco Oliva, and Mario Ronga

32.1 Introduction

The Achilles tendon (AT) is the strongest tendon in the human body, but despite its strength, is the most frequently ruptured tendon in the body. Ruptures usually occur between 2 and 6 cm of its insertion into the superior surface of the calcaneus, a relatively hypovascular area.[8,17] The major blood supply to tendons is from the mesotendon, and the largest supply is from the anterior mesentery.[2] The tendon is at the greatest risk of rupture when the it is obliquely loaded, the muscle is contracting maximally, and tendon length is short.[5] This usually occurs as a result of pushing off with the foot against resistance, and occurs most frequently in males in their fourth decade.

The diagnosis of acute AT rupture is generally made clinically. There is usually a palpable defect in the AT. Patients will often report that they felt as though they had been struck at the back of the heel and may have heard a snapping sound. They are usually unable to weight bear on the affected limb because of pain and/or weakness. If some time has elapsed since the rupture, the diagnosis can be more difficult, as the gap fills in with oedema and palpation is unreliable. Various tests can be employed to aid diagnosis,[12–14] such as calf squeeze test,[13] the Matles test can also be used,[12] and the needle test. The neurovascular status of the limb should be assessed, in particular the sensation over the distribution of the sural nerve, and documented.

Open surgical management of patients with ruptured ATs allows accurate apposition of the ruptured tendon ends, earlier motion, has a low risk of re-rupture, but is associated with a significant rate of wound healing problems.

Advocates of minimally invasive AT surgery cite faster recovery times, shorter hospital stays, and improved functional outcomes as the principal reasons for adopting these new approaches when compared to traditional open techniques.

In this chapter we describe a minimally invasive technique to repair acute AT rupture.

N. Maffulli (✉)
Centre for Sports and Exercise Medicine, Queen Mary University of London, Barts and The London School of Medicine and Dentistry, Mile End Hospital, London, England, UK
e-mail: n.maffulli@qmul.ac.uk

N. Maffulli and M. Easley (eds.), *Minimally Invasive Surgery of the Foot and Ankle*,
DOI: 10.1007/978-1-84996-417-3_32,

32.2 Surgical Technique

The patient is positioned prone.[3] Areas 4–6 cm proximal and distal to the palpable tendon defect and the skin over the defect are infiltrated with 20 mL of 1% Lignocaine. Ten milliliters of Chirocaine 0.5% are infiltrated deep to the tendon defect. A calf tourniquet, skin preparation and steridrapes are applied.

A 1 cm transverse incision is made over the defect using a size 11 blade. Four longitudinal stab incisions are made lateral and medial to the tendon 6 cm proximal to the palpable defect. Two further longitudinal incisions on either side of the tendon are made 4–6 cm distal to the palpable defect. Forceps are then used to mobilise the tendon from beneath the subcutaneous tissues. A 9 cm Mayo needle (BL059N, #B00 round point spring eye, B Braun, Aesculap, Tuttlingen, Germany) is threaded with two double loops of Number 1 Maxon (Tyco Healthcare, Norwalk, CT, USA), and this is passed transversely between the proximal stab incisions through the bulk of the tendon (Fig. 32.1). The bulk of the tendon is surprisingly superficial. The loose ends of the suture are held with a clip. In turn, each of the ends is then passed distally from just proximal to the transverse Maxon passage through the bulk of the tendon to pass out of the diagonally opposing stab incision. A subsequent diagonal pass is then made to the transverse incision over the ruptured tendon. To prevent entanglement, both ends of the Maxon are held in separate clips. This suture is then tested for security by pulling with both ends of the Maxon distally. Another double loop of Maxon is then passed between the distal stabs incisions through the tendon (Fig. 32.2), and in turn through the tendon and out of the transverse incision starting distal to the transverse passage in a half Kessler configuration (Fig. 32.3). The ankle is held in full plantar flexion, and in turn opposing ends of the Maxon thread are tied together with a double throw knot, and then three further throws before being buried using the forceps. A clip is used to hold the first throw of the lateral side to maintain the tension of the suture.

A subcuticular Biosyn suture 3.0 (Tyco Healthcare) is used to close the transverse incision, and Steri-strips (3M Health Care, St Paul, MN, USA) are applied to the stab

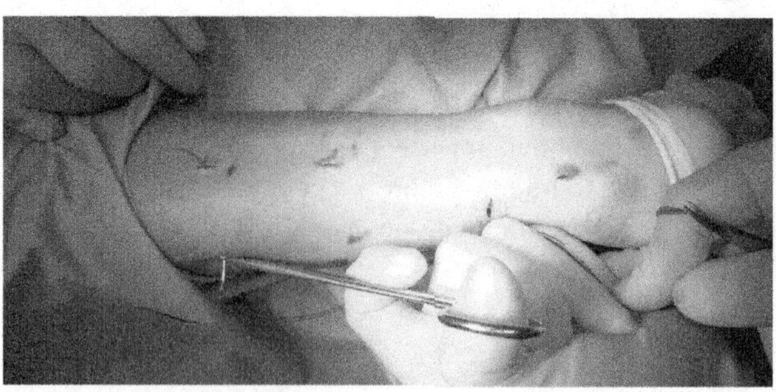

Fig. 32.1 A 9 cm Mayo needle (BL059N, #B00 round point spring eye, B Braun, Aesculap, Tuttlingen, Germany) is threaded with two double loops of Number 1 Maxon (Tyco Healthcare, Norwalk, CT, USA), and this is passed transversely between the proximal stab incisions through thebul kof t het endon

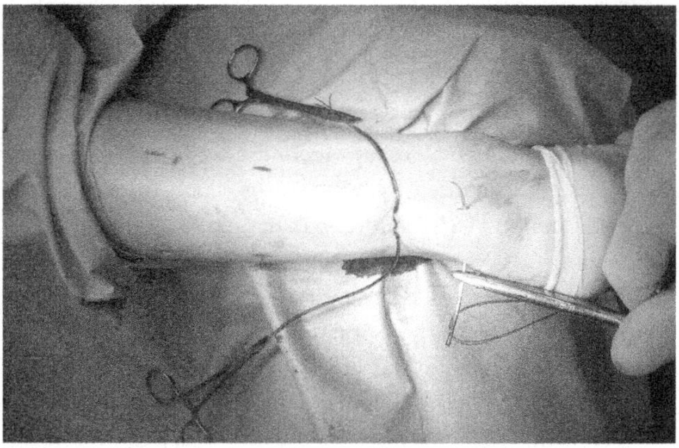

Fig.32.2 Anotherdoubl e loop of Maxon is then passed between the distal stabs incisions through the tendon

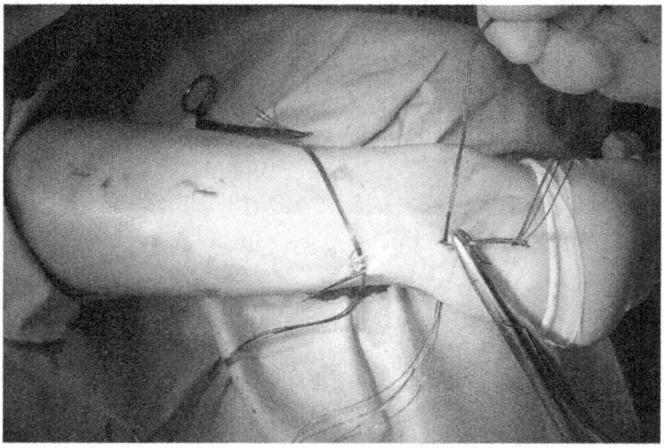

Fig.32.3 The double loop of Maxon is passed in turn through the tendon and out of the transverse incision starting distal to the transversepa ssage

incisions. Finally, a Mepore dressing (Molnlycke Health Care, Gothenburg, Sweden) is applied, and a bivalved removable scotch cast in full plantar flexion is applied being held in place with Velcro straps.

32.3 PostoperativeR egimen

The patient is allowed home on the day of surgery, and fully weight bears as able in the cast in full plantar flexion. At 2 weeks, the wounds are inspected, and the back shell is removed allowing proprioception, plantar flexion, inversion and eversion exercises. The front shell remains in place for 6 weeks to prevent forced inadvertent dorsiflexion of the ankle.

32.4 Discussion

Several percutaneous repair techniques have been described.[4,6,10,15,16] Ma and Griffith described a technique of percutaneous repair of the AT in 18 patients using stab incisions over the tendon.[10] The suture was passed through stab incisions and crisscrossed through the tendon.

Gorschewsky et al. described a technique using barbed suture wires passed from proximal to distal to pull the retracted proximal stump distally and approximate the ruptured tendon ends. Fibrin glue was then applied to the repair. The wires were removed at 3 weeks. At 1 year follow-up in 20 patients there was one re-rupture and no other complications.[6]

Webb and Bannister described a new percutaneous technique that reduced the potential risk to the sural nerve by placing the most proximal of the incisions to the medial side, away from the nerve.[13] We described a percutaneous technique of repair of the ruptured ATs similar to that described by Webb and Bannister,[16] but using a more secure suture configuration. Recently, several authors reported on the Achillon mini-incision technique, comparing the basic mechanical properties of the tendon suture performed using the Achillon method with those of the Kessler method, and assesses whether the strength of the repair was related to tendon diameter. The Achillon repair had comparable tensile strength to the Kessler repair. When compared to the Achillon repair the present technique[3] is cheaper, and allows a stronger repair, as it allows to use a greater number of suture strands (eight) for the repair of the AT.

Complications of this surgery can be early, intermediate or late, and are outlined in Table 32.1.[3]

Early possible post-operative complications of this surgery are sural nerve damage and hematoma formation.

Hockenbury and John noted sural nerve entrapment in three of five cases treated using a percutaneous technique in cadaveric specimens with divided ATs.[2] The positioning of the incisions and the configuration of the stitch reduces the risk of damage to the sural nerve.

The risk of hematoma formation is reduced as the procedure is carried out without tourniquet so that the surgeon will be able to deal with any bleeding at the time of operation.

Intermediate superficial and deep wound infections can occur. Open repair is associated with a significant risk of wound breakdown. Percutaneous repair reduces this risk (Table 32.2).

The most important late complication is re-rupture.

Table32.1 Complications which can occur following a ruptured AT

Early(peri-operative)	Sural nerve damage
	Hematoma
Intermediate (<6 weeks)	Infection
	Wound healing complications
Late (6 weeks to 6 months)	Re-rupture of tendon

Table32.2 Key points of rupture and repair

Patients election
Pronepos ition
Locala nesthesia
Incisions made to avoid sural nerve
Four and if necessary eight strand repair
Splintage to protect repair for total of 6 weeks

Bradley and Tibone[1] reported a higher risk of re-rupture in percutaneous repairs compared with open repair. Lim et al. more recently, however, in a prospective multicentre randomized controlled study comparing open and percutaneous repair techniques reported a higher rate of re-rupture in patients treated by an open technique (6% versus 3%, using a percutaneous technique). The difference, however, was not statistically significant. Bradley and Tibone[1] compared 15 patients treated with a gastrocsoleus fascial graft and 12 patients treated using a percutaneous technique. Strength, power and endurance measurements of both groups showed no statistical difference. Two of 12 (13%) percutaneous repairs re-ruptured up to a follow-up of 1.8 years, compared with none in the open repair group (follow-up 4.6 years). They recommended percutaneous repair in the recreational athlete and open repair in the competitive athlete. Martinelli[11] reported 30 cases of percutaneous repair of ATs in which all athletes returned to preinjury levels of sport by 150 days post-injury. Wound healing problems associated with open repair can be reduced by using percutaneous techniques, and the incidence of adhesion of the skin to the underlying tendon, as can occur in open repair, is also lower with percutaneous techniques.[9,16]

Kauranen and Leppilahti[7] reviewed the motor performance of 90 patients following operative repair (mean of 3.1 years post surgery) of a ruptured AT. They observed the performance of the unloaded lower extremity, and compared the operated limbs with the unoperated side, and to age and gender-matched control subjects. They found no statistical difference between any of the groups, and concluded that the motor performance of the unloaded lower limb had fully recovered in the tested parameters.

References

1. Bradley JP, Tibone JE. Percutaneous and open surgical repairs of Achilles tendon ruptures. A comparative study. *Am J Sports Med.* 1990; 18:188–195.
2. Maffulli N, Longo UG, Hüfner T, Denaro V. Surgical treatment for pain syndromes of the Achilles tendon. *Unfallchirurg*. Sep 2010;113(9):721–725.
3. Carmont MR, Maffulli N. Modified percutaneous repair of ruptured Achilles tendon. *Knee Surg Sports Traumatol Arthrosc.* 2008; 16:199–203.
4. Cretnik A, Zlajpah L, Smrkolj V, et al. The strength of percutaneous methods of repair of the Achilles tendon: a biomechanical study. *Med Sci Sports Exerc.* 2000; 32:16–20.

5. McMaster PE. Tendon and muscle ruptures: clinical and experimental studies on the causes and location of subcutaneous ruptures. *J Bone Joint Surg.* 1933; 15:705–722.
6. Gorschewsky O, Vogel U, Schweizer A, et al. Percutaneous tenodesis of the Achilles tendon. A new surgical method for the treatment of acute Achilles tendon rupture through percutaneous tenodesis. *Injury.* 1999; 30:315–321.
7. Kauranen KJ, Leppilahti JI. Motor performance of the foot after Achilles rupture repair. *Int J Sports Med.* 2001 ;22:154–158.
8. Langergren C, Lindholni A. Vascular distribution in the Achilles tendon. *Acta Chir Scand.* 1958;116:491–495.
9. Lim J, Dalal R, Waseem M. Percutaneous vs. open repair of the ruptured Achilles tendon - a prospective randomized controlled study. *Foot Ankle Int.* 2001; 22:559–568.
10. Ma GW, Griffith TG. Percutaneous repair of acute closed ruptured achilles tendon: a new technique. *Clin Orthop Relat Res.* 1977; 128:247–255.
11. Martinelli B. Percutaneous repair of the Achilles tendon in athletes. *Bull Hosp Jt Dis.* 2000;59: 149–152.
12. Matles AL. Rupture of the tendo Achilles. Another diagnostic sign. *Bull Hosp Joint Dis.* 1975;36:48–51.
13. Simmonds FA. The diagnosis of the ruptured Achilles tendon. *Practitioner.* 1957; 179:56–58.
14. O'Brien T. The needle test for complete rupture of the Achilles tendon. *J Bone Joint Surg (A).* 1984;66:1099–1101.
15. Webb J, Moorjani N, Radford M. Anatomy of the sural nerve and its relation to the Achilles tendon. *Foot Ankle Int.* 2000; 21:475–477.
16. Webb JM, Bannister GC. Percutaneous repair of the ruptured tendo Achillis. *J Bone Joint Surg Br.* 1999;81:877– 880.
17. Williams PL, Warwick R, Dyson M, Bannister LH. *Grays Anatomy.* 37th ed. Edinburgh, UK/ NewY ork,N Y:C hurchillLi vingstone;1989.

Minimally Invasive Semitendinosus Tendon Graft Augmentation for Reconstruction of Chronic Tears of the Achilles Tendon

33

Nicola Maffulli, Umile Giuseppe Longo, Filippo Spiezia, and Vincenzo Denaro

33.1 Introduction

The management of chronic ruptures of tendo Achillis often requires augmentation techniques. These can be performed using a turn down flap, a tendon transfer, tendon graft, or synthetic materials. Open procedures on the Achilles tendon can lead to difficulty with wound healing because of the tenuous blood supply and increased chance of wound breakdown and infection. In this chapter we describe a method of minimally invasive semitendinosus reconstruction for the Achilles tendon. This technique uses one proximal para-midline incision and one distal midline incision preserving skin integrity over the site most prone to wound breakdown. The first incision is a 5 cm longitudinal incision, made 2 cm proximal and just medial to the palpable end of the residual tendon. The second incision is 3 cm long and is also longitudinal but is 2 cm distal and in the midline to the distal end of the tendon rupture. The distal and proximal Achilles tendon stumps are mobilised. After trying to reduce the gap of the ruptured Achilles tendon, if the gap produced is greater than 6 cm despite maximal plantar flexion of the ankle and traction on the Achilles tendon stumps, the ipsilateral semitendinosus tendon is harvested. The semitendinosus tendon is passed through small incisions in the substance of the proximal stump of the Achilles tendon, and it is sutured to the Achilles tendon. It is then passed beneath the intact skin bridge into the distal incision, and passed from medial to lateral through a transverse tenotomy in the distal stump. With the ankle in maximal plantar flexion, the semitendinosus tendon is sutured to the Achilles tendon at each entry and exit point. This minimally invasive technique allows reconstruction of the Achilles tendon using the tendon of semitendinosus preserving skin integrity over the site most prone to wound breakdown, and can be especially used to reconstruct the Achilles tendon in the presence of large gap (greater than 6 cm).

N. Maffulli (✉)
Centre for Sports and Exercise Medicine, Queen Mary University of London, Barts and The London School of Medicine and Dentistry, Mile End Hospital, London, England, UK
e-mail: n.maffulli@qmul.ac.uk

N. Maffulli and M. Easley (eds.), *Minimally Invasive Surgery of the Foot and Ankle*,
DOI: 10.1007/978-1-84996-417-3_33, © Springer-Verlag London Limited 2011

33.2 Surgical Technique

The patient is positioned prone with a calf tourniquet. Skin preparation is performed in the usual fashion, and sterile drapes are applied. Pre-operative anatomical markings include the palpable tendon defect and both malleoli. Two skin incisions are made (Fig. 33.1), and accurate haemostasis by ligation of the larger veins and diathermy of the smaller ones is performed. The first incision is a 5 cm longitudinal incision, made 2 cm proximal and just medial to the palpable end of the residual tendon. The second incision is 3 cm long and is also longitudinal but is 2 cm distal and in the midline over the distal end of the tendon rupture. Care is taken to prevent damage to the sural nerve. At the level of the Achilles tendon insertion, the sural nerve is 18.8 mm lateral to the tendon but, as it progresses proximally, the nerve gradually traverses medially crossing the lateral border of the tendon 9.8 cm proximal to the calcaneum.[6] Thus, the second incision avoids the sural nerve by being placed medial and posterior to the nerve.

The proximal and distal Achilles tendon stump are mobilised, freeing them of all the peritendinous adhesions. It should be possible to palpate the medial tubercle of the calcaneum. The ruptured tendon end is then resected back to healthy tendon, and a Number 1 Vicryl (Ethicon, Edinburgh) locking suture is run along the free tendon edge to prevent separation of the bundles (Fig. 33.2).

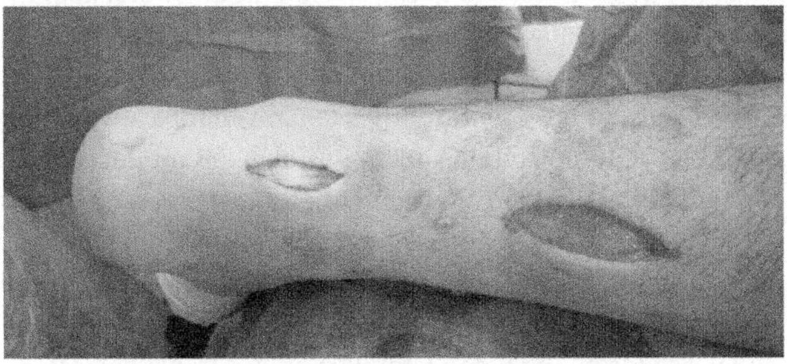

Fig. 33.1 Two skin incisions are made. The first incision is a 5 cm longitudinal incision, made 2 cm proximal and just medial to the palpable end of the residual tendon. The second incision is 3 cm long and is also longitudinal but is 2 cm distal and in the midline over the distal end of the tendon rupture

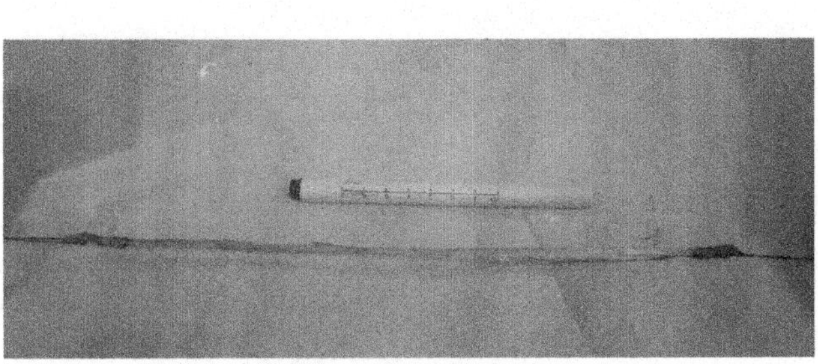

Fig. 33.2 A locking suture is run along the free tendon edge to prevent separation of thebundl es

The proximal tendon is then mobilised from the proximal wound, any adhesions are divided, and further soft tissue release anterior to the soleus and gastrocnemius allows maximal excursion, minimising the gap between the two tendon stumps. A Vicryl locking suture is run along the free tendon edge to allow adequate exposure and to prevent separation of the bundles.

After trying to reduce the gap of the ruptured Achilles tendon, if the gap produced is greater than 6 cm despite maximal plantar flexion of the ankle and traction on the Achilles tendon stumps, the ipsilateral semitendinosus tendon is harvested through a vertical 2.5–3 cm long incision over the pes anserinus (Fig. 33.3). The semitendinosus tendon is passed through a small incision in the substance of the proximal stump of the Achilles tendon (Fig. 33.4), and it is sutured to the Achilles tendon at the entry and exit point using 3–0 Vicryl (Polyglactin 910 braided absorbable suture; Johnson & Johnson, Brussels, Belgium). The semitendinosus tendon is then passed beneath the intact skin bridge into the distal incision and passed from medial to lateral through a transverse tenotomy in the distal stump (Fig. 33.5). With the ankle in maximal plantar flexion, the semitendinosus tendon is sutured to the Achilles tendon at each entry and exit point using 3–0 Vicryl (Polyglactin 910 braided absorbable suture; Johnson & Johnson, Brussels, Belgium). The repair is tensioned to maximal equinus.

One extremity of the semitendinosus tendon is then passed again beneath the intact skin bridge into the proximal incision, and passed from medial to lateral through a transverse tenotomy in the proximal stump (Fig. 33.6). The other extremity of the semitendinosus tendon is then passed again from medial to lateral through a transverse tenotomy in the distal stump. The reconstruction may be further augmented using a Maxon (Tyco Health Care, Norwalk, CT) suture. The wounds are closed with 2.0 Vicryl, 3,0 Biosyn (Tyco Health Care, Norwalk, CT) and Steri-strips (3 M Health Care, St Paul, MN) (Fig. 33.7). A previously prepared removable scotch cast support with Velcro straps is applied.

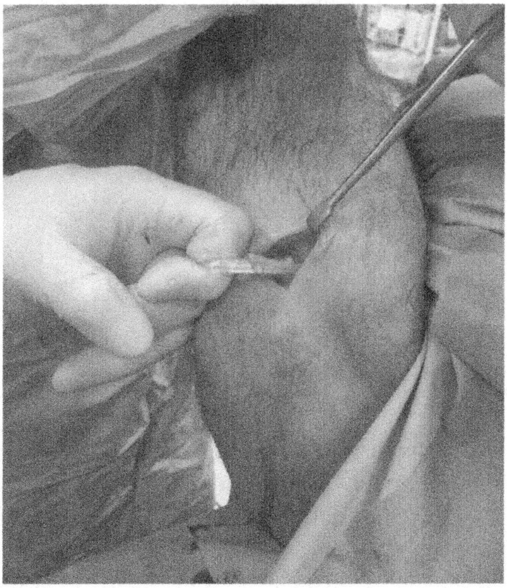

Fig. 33.3 The tendon of the semitendinosus is harvested through a vertical, 2.5–3 cm longitudinalinc isionove rt hepe sa nserinus

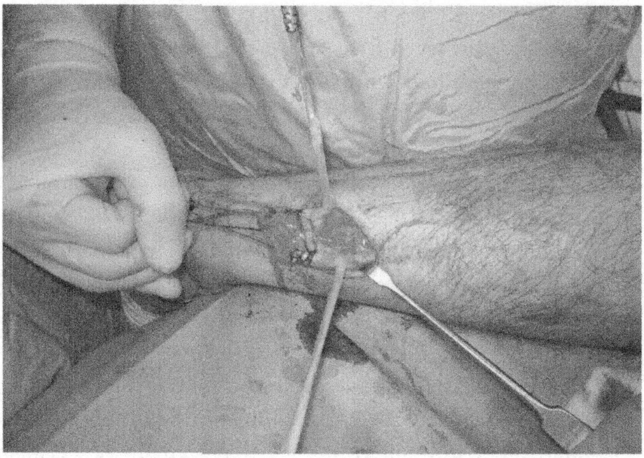

Fig.33. 4 Thes emitendinosus tendon is passed through a small incision in the substance of the proximal stumpof t heA chillest endon

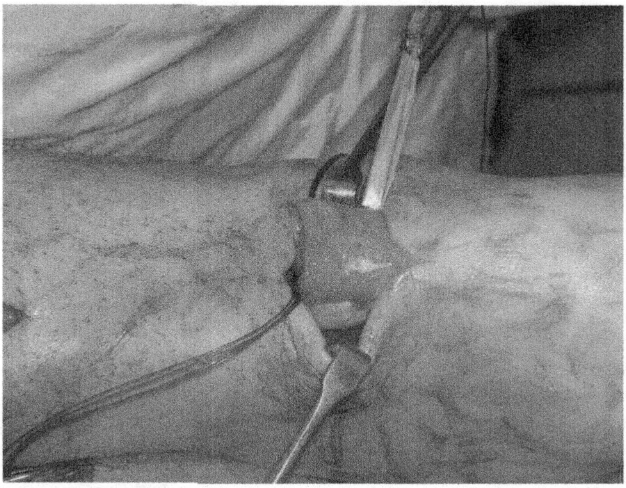

Fig.33. 5 Thes emitendinosus tendon is passed from medial to lateral through a transverse tenotomy in the distals tump

33.3 PostoperativeM anagement

Post operatively, patients are allowed to weight bear as comfort allows with the use of elbow crutches.[2,3] It would be unusual for a patient to weight bear fully at this stage. After 2 weeks, the back shell is removed, and physiotherapy is commenced with the front shell in situ preventing dorsiflexion of the ankle, focusing on proprioception, plantar-flexion of the ankle, inversion and eversion.[2,3] During this period of rehabilitation, the patient is

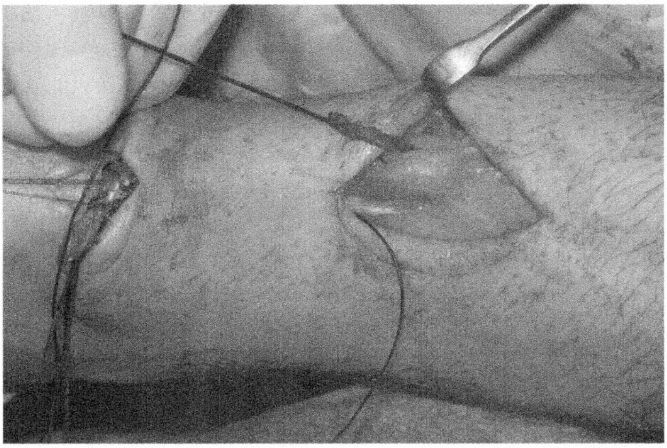

Fig.33.6 Onee xtremityof the semitendinosus tendon is passed from medial to lateral through a transverse tenotomy in the proximal stump

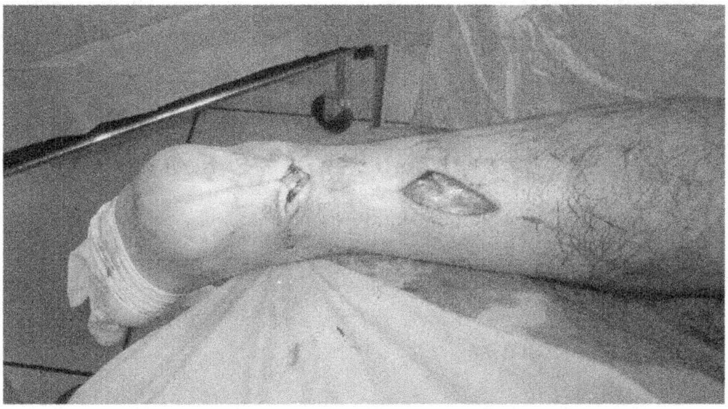

Fig.33.7 Thefi nalre sult

permitted to weight bear as comfort allows with the front shell in situ although full weight bearing rarely occurs on account of balance difficulties and patients usually still require the assistance of a single elbow crutch as this stage. The front shell may be finally removed after 6 weeks. We do not use a heel raise after removal of the cast, and patients normally regain a plantigrade ankle over 2 or 3 weeks.[2,3]

33.4 Discussion

The main complication the surgeon may encounter is sural nerve injury. Care is taken to prevent damage to the sural nerve. At the level of the Achilles tendon insertion, the sural nerve is 18.8 mm lateral to the tendon but, as it progresses proximally, the nerve gradually traverses medially crossing the lateral border of the tendon 9.8 cm proximal to the calcaneum.[6] Thus, the second incision avoids the sural nerve by being placed medial to the nerve.

Wound breakdown is a challenging complications in Achilles tendon reconstruction surgery, with open techniques having a 9% superficial infection rate.[5] The great advantage of this technique is that it allows to perform a semitendinosus tendon augmentation in a minimally invasive fashion, preserving skin integrity. In patients with chronic ruptures, the skin over the gap retracts over several weeks, and remains so until the operation. In open surgery, this skin is incised, and is then stretched out in a relatively acute fashion to accommodate the reconstructed tendon. Therefore, following the reconstruction, the skin over the gap may well be stretched so much that vascular supply is impaired.[4] The reconstructed gastro-soleus Achilles tendon complex will stretch with increased loading and range of movement exercises during rehabilitation.[1] Preservation of skin cover during reconstruction procedures is clearly an advantage, as the skin is not injured by the operation, and protects the reconstruction beneath. As with all surgery performed through minimally invasive incisions, this procedure is technically demanding. Careful incision placement is required together with skin retraction to allow visualisation of the tendon ends and to permit the reconstruction. This technique is designed to preserve skin cover of the reconstruction site, and, although reconstruction is always risky, it may extend the indications for surgery in patients prone to wound complications such as vasculopaths and diabetics who present with a large gap.

In conclusion, this technique allows minimally invasive reconstruction of the Achilles tendon using semitendinosus tendon preserving skin integrity, and can be especially used to reconstruct the Achilles tendon in the presence of large gap (greater than 6 cm).

33.5 Competingl nterests

The authors declare that they have no competing interests.

References

1. Carmont MR, Maffulli N. Less invasive Achilles tendon reconstruction. *BMC Musculoskelet Disord.*2007;8:10 0.
2. Maffulli N, Tallon C, Wong J, et al. Early weightbearing and ankle mobilization after open repair of acute midsubstance tears of the achilles tendon. *Am J Sports Med.*2003; 31:692–700.
3. Maffulli N, Tallon C, Wong J, et al. No adverse effect of early weight bearing following open repair of acute tears of the Achilles tendon. *J Sports Med Phys Fitness.*2003; 43:367–379.
4. McClelland D, Maffulli N. Neglected rupture of the Achilles tendon: reconstruction with peroneus brevis tendon transfer. *Surgeon.*2004; 2:209–213.
5. Pintore E, Barra V, Pintore R, et al. Peroneus brevis tendon transfer in neglected tears of the Achilles tendon. *J Trauma.*2001; 50:71–78.
6. Webb J, Moorjani N, Radford M. Anatomy of the sural nerve and its relation to the Achilles tendon. *Foot Ankle Int.*2000; 21:475–477.

Minimally Invasive Achilles Tendon Reconstruction Using the Peroneus Brevis TendonG raft

34

Nicola Maffulli, Filippo Spiezia, Umile Giuseppe Longo,a nd Vincenzo Denaro

34.1 Introduction

Minimally invasive peroneus brevis reconstruction for the Achilles tendon (AT) overcome the problems with an open procedure, namely difficulty with wound healing because of the tenuous blood supply and increased chance of wound breakdown and infection. In this chapter we presented a technique which uses two para-midline incisions preserving skin integrity over the site most prone to wound breakdown. This minimally invasive technique allows reconstruction of the Achilles tendon using the tendon of peroneus brevis preserving skin integrity over the site most prone to wound breakdown, and can be especially used to reconstruct the Achilles tendon in the presence of gap less than 6 cm.

The ideal candidate to minimally invasive semitendinosus tendon graft augmentation is a patient with a chronic tear of the Achilles tendon with a gap, during surgery less than 6 cm with the ankle kept in maximal plantar flexion and traction on the AT stumps.[7] This technique is designed to preserve skin cover of the reconstruction site, and, although reconstruction is always risky, it may extend the indications for surgery to patients prone to wound complications such as those with peripheral vasculopathy and diabetes who present with a tendon gap. Gap grater than 6 cm are better managed with semitendinosus transfer.[3]

There are no specific contraindications for minimally invasive ipsilateral tendon. Obviously this is not possible in patients previously undergone peroneus tendon harvesting for other procedure.

N.M affulli(✉)
Centre for Sports and Exercise Medicine, Queen Mary University of London, Barts and The London School of Medicine and Dentistry, Mile End Hospital, London, England, UK
e-mail:n.ma ffulli@qmul.ac.uk

N. Maffulli and M. Easley (eds.), *Minimally Invasive Surgery of the Foot and Ankle*,
DOI: 10.1007/978-1-84996-417-3_34, © Springer-Verlag London Limited 2011

34.2 Surgical Technique

The patient is positioned prone with a calf tourniquet. Skin preparation is performed in the usual fashion, and sterile drapes are applied. Pre-operative anatomical markings include the palpable tendon defect, both malleoli, and the base of the fifth metatarsal.

Three skin incisions are made, and accurate hemostasis by ligation of the larger veins and diathermy of the smaller ones is performed. The first incision is a 5 cm longitudinal incision, made 2 cm proximal and just medial to the palpable end of the proximal stump. The second incision is 3 cm long and is also longitudinal, but is 2 cm distal and lateral to the distal stump. Care is taken to prevent damage to the sural nerve by making this incision as close as possible to the anterior aspect of the lateral border of the Achilles tendon to avoid the nerve. At the level of the Achilles tendon insertion, the sural nerve is 18.8 mm lateral to the tendon but, as it progresses proximally, the nerve gradually traverses medially crossing the lateral border of the tendon 9.8 cm proximal to the calcaneum. Thus, the second incision avoids the sural nerve by being placed on the lateral side of the Achilles tendon but posterior to the nerve. The third incision is a 2 cm longitudinal incision at the base of the fifth metatarsal.

The distal Achilles tendon stump is mobilized, freeing it of all the peritendinous adhesions, particularly on its lateral aspect (Fig. 34.1). This allows access to the base of the lateral aspect of the distal tendon close to it insertion. It should be possible to palpate the medial tubercle of the calcaneum. The ruptured tendon end is then resected back to healthy tendon, and a Number 1 Vicryl (Ethicon, Edinburgh) locking suture is run along the free tendon edge to prevent separation of the bundles.

The proximal tendon is then mobilized from the proximal wound, any adhesions are divided, and further soft tissue release anterior to the soleus and gastrocnemius allows maximal excursion, minimizing the gap between the two tendon stumps (Fig. 34.2). A Vicryl locking suture is run along the free tendon edge to allow adequate exposure and to prevent separation of the bundles (Fig. 34.3).

The tendon of peroneus brevis is harvested (Fig. 34.4). The tendon is identified through the incision on the lateral border of the foot at its insertion at the base of the fifth metatarsal.

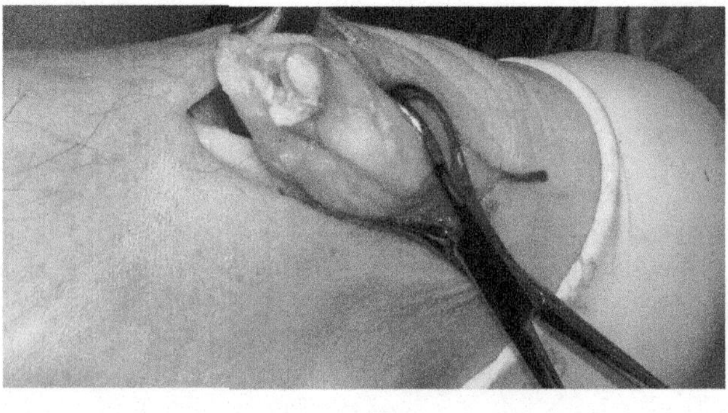

Fig.34. 1 Thedis talA chilles tendon stump is mobilized, freeing it of all the peritendinousa dhesions

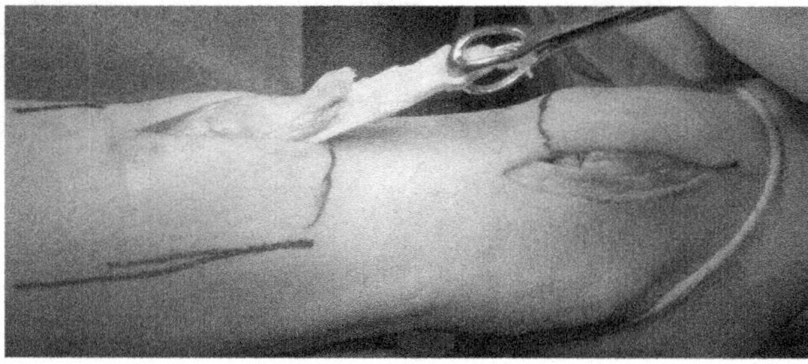

Fig. 34.2 The proximal tendon is then mobilized from the proximal wound, any adhesions are divided, and further soft tissue release anterior to the soleus and gastrocnemius allows maximal excursion, minimizing the gap between the two tendon stumps

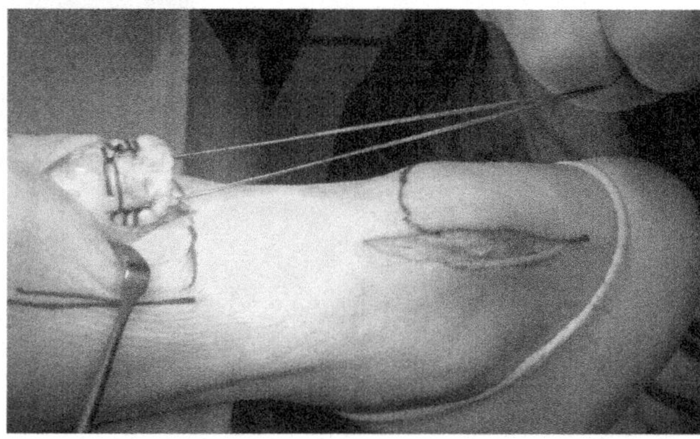

Fig.3 4.3 AV icryll ocking suture is run along the free tendon edge to allow adequate exposure and to prevent separation of the bundles

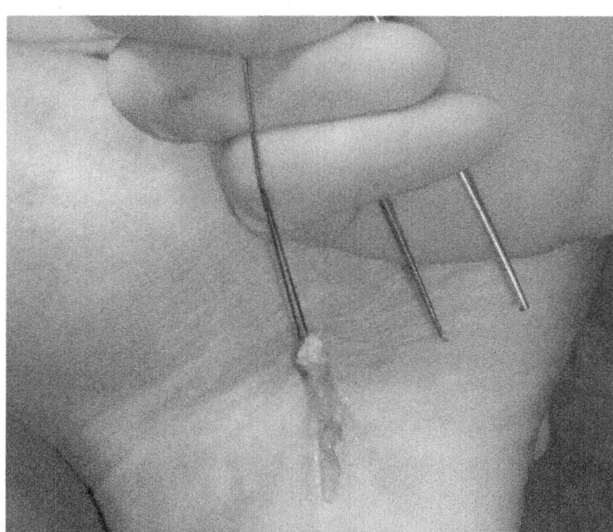

Fig.34. 4 Thete ndonof peroneusbre visis ha rvested

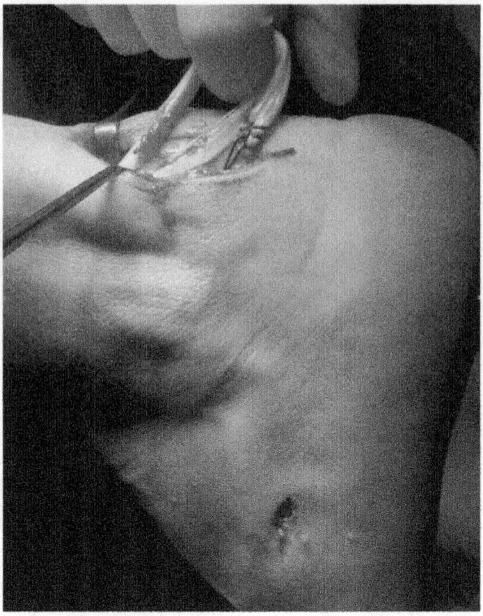

Fig.34. 5 The tendon of peroneus brevis is thenw ithdrawnt hrought hedi stalw ound

The tendon is exposed, and a No.1 Vicryl locking suture is applied to the tendon end before release from the metatarsal base. The tendon of peroneus brevis is identified at the base of the distal incision of the Achilles tendon following incision of the deep fascia overlying the peroneal muscles compartment. The tendon of peroneus brevis is then withdrawn through the distal wound (Fig. 34.5). This may take significant force, as there may be tendinous strands between the two peroneal tendons distally. The muscular portion of peroneus brevis is then mobilized proximally to allow increased excursion of the tendon of peroneus brevis.

A longitudinal tenotomy parallel to the tendon fibres is made through both stumps of the tendon. A clip is used to develop the plane, from lateral to medial, in the distal stump of the Achilles tendon, and the peroneus brevis graft is passed through the tenotomy (Fig. 34.6). With the ankle in maximal plantar flexion, a No.1 Vicryl suture is used to suture the peroneus brevis to both sides of the distal stump. The tendon of peroneus brevis is then passed beneath the intact skin bridge into the proximal incision, and passed from medial to lateral through a transverse tenotomy in the proximal stump, and further secured with No 1 Vicryl. Finally, the tendon of peroneus brevis is sutured back onto itself on the lateral side of the proximal incision. The reconstruction may be further augmented using a Maxon (Tyco Health Care, Norwalk, CT) suture.

The wounds are closed with 2.0 Vicryl, 3.0 Biosyn (Tyco Health Care, Norwalk, CT) and Steri-strips (3 M Health Care, St Paul, MN), taking care to avoid the risk of post operative hematoma and minimize wound breakdown. A previously prepared removable scotch cast support with Velcro straps is applied.

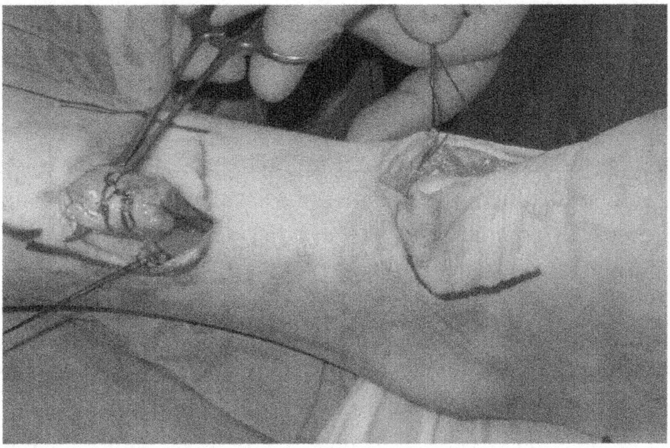

Fig. 34.6 A clip is used to develop the plane, from lateral to medial, in the distal stump of the Achilles tendon, and the peroneus brevis graft is passed through the tenotomy

34.3 PostoperativeM anagement

Post operatively, patients are allowed to weight bear as comfort allows with the use of elbow crutches.[9,10] It would be unusual for a patient to weight bear fully at this stage. After 2 weeks, the back shell is removed, and physiotherapy is commenced with the front shell in situ preventing dorsiflexion of the ankle, focusing on proprioception, plantar-flexion of the ankle, inversion and eversion.[9,10] During this period of rehabilitation, the patient is permitted to weight bear as comfort allows with the front shell in situ, although full weight bearing rarely occurs on account of balance difficulties and patients usually still require the assistance of a single elbow crutch as this stage. The front shell may be finally removed after 6 weeks. We do not use a heel raise after removal of the cast, and patients normally regain a plantigrade ankle over 2 or 3 weeks.[9,10]

34.4 Discussion

The main complication the surgeon may encounter is sural nerve injury. Care is taken to prevent damage to the sural nerve. At the level of the AT insertion, the sural nerve is 18.8 mm lateral to the tendon but, as it progresses proximally, the nerve gradually traverses medially crossing the lateral border of the tendon 9.8 cm proximal to the calcaneum.[13] Thus, the second incision avoids the sural nerve by being placed medial to the nerve.

Wound breakdown is a challenging complications in AT reconstruction surgery, with open techniques having a 9% superficial infection rate.[12] The great advantage of this technique is that it allows to perform a peroneus brevis tendon augmentation in a minimally invasive fashion, preserving skin integrity. In patients with chronic ruptures, the skin over the gap retracts over several weeks, and remains so until the operation. In open surgery, this skin is incised, and is then stretched out in a relatively acute fashion to accommodate the reconstructed tendon.[1] Therefore, following the reconstruction, the skin over the gap may well be stretched so much that its vascular supply is impaired.[11] The reconstructed gastro-soleus AT complex will stretch with increased loading and range of movement exercises during rehabilitation.[2] Preservation of skin cover during reconstruction procedures is clearly an advantage, as the skin is not injured by the operation, and protects the reconstruction beneath.[4-6,8] As with all surgery performed through minimally invasive incisions, this procedure is technically demanding. Careful incision placement is required together with skin retraction to allow visualization of the tendon ends and to permit the reconstruction. This technique is designed to preserve skin cover of the reconstruction site, and, although reconstruction is always risky, it may extend the indications for surgery in patients prone to wound complications such as vasculopaths and diabetics who present with a tendinous gap.

In conclusion, this technique allows minimally invasive reconstruction of the AT using peroneus brevis tendon preserving skin integrity, and can be especially used to reconstruct the AT in the presence of gap less than 6 cm.

34.5 Competingl nterests

The authors declare that they have no competing interests.

References

1. Ames PR, Longo UG, Denaro V, et al. Achilles tendon problems: not just an orthopaedic issue. *Disabil Rehabil.*2008; 30:1646–1650.
2. Carmont MR, Maffulli N. Less invasive Achilles tendon reconstruction. *BMC Musculoskelet Disord.*2007;8:100.
3. Crisp T, Khan F, Padhiar N, et al. High volume ultrasound guided injections at the interface between the patellar tendon and Hoffa's body are effective in chronic patellar tendinopathy: a pilot study. *Disabil Rehabil.*2008; 30:1625–1634.
4. Longo UG, Ramamurthy C, Denaro V, et al. Minimally invasive stripping for chronic Achilles tendinopathy. *Disabil Rehabil.*2008; 30:1709–1713.
5. Longo UG, Ronga M, Maffulli N. Achilles tendinopathy. *Sports Med Arthrosc.* 2009;17: 112–126.
6. Longo UG, Ronga M, Maffulli N. Acute ruptures of the achilles tendon. *Sports Med Arthrosc.* 2009;17:127–138.
7. Maffulli N, Ajis A, Longo UG, et al. Chronic rupture of tendo Achillis. *Foot Ankle Clin.* 2007; 12:583–596,vi.

8. Maffulli N, Longo UG, Ronga M, et al. Favorable outcome of percutaneous repair of achilles tendon ruptures in the elderly. *Clin Orthop Relat Res.*2010; 468:1039–1046.
9. Maffulli N, Tallon C, Wong J, et al. Early weightbearing and ankle mobilization after open repair of acute midsubstance tears of the achilles tendon. *Am J Sports Med.* 2003;31:692–700.
10. Maffulli N, Tallon C, Wong J, et al. No adverse effect of early weight bearing following open repair of acute tears of the Achilles tendon. *J Sports Med Phys Fitness.*2003; 43:367–379.
11. McClelland D, Maffulli N. Neglected rupture of the Achilles tendon: reconstruction with peroneus brevis tendon transfer. *Surgeon.*2004; 2:209–213.
12. Pintore E, Barra V, Pintore R, et al. Peroneus brevis tendon transfer in neglected tears of the Achilles tendon. *J Trauma.*2001; 50:71–78.
13. Webb J, Moorjani N, Radford M. Anatomy of the sural nerve and its relation to the Achilles tendon. *Foot Ankle Int.*2000; 21:475–477.

Free Hamstrings Tendon Transfer and Interference Screw Fixation for Less Invasive Reconstruction of Chronic Avulsionsoft heA chilles Tendon

35

Nicola Maffulli, Umile Giuseppe Longo, Filippo Spiezia,a nd Vincenzo Denaro

35.1 Introduction

Chronic avulsions of the Achilles tendon from the calcaneus are infrequent.[1,13,19,26] Achilles "sleeve" avulsions are a surgical challenge, as the Achilles tendon sleeves from its insertion into the calcaneus leaving virtually no tendinous tissue on the posterior calcaneus to facilitate a repair to the free end of the Achilles tendon.[22] Therefore, reconstruction of chronic avulsions of the Achilles tendon can be technically difficult. Hence, can be necessary a tendon graft because may be not possible to directly reattach the Achilles tendon. The free hamstrings tendon transfer and interference screw fixation for less invasive reconstruction of chronic avulsions of the Achilles tendon is a less invasive technique using a free semitendinosus tendon graft with interference screw fixation in the calcaneus through a Cincinnati incision. This approach permits a wide exposure of the insertion of the Achilles tendon, preserving the integrity of the skin overlying the site most decreasing the risk of wound breakdown.

Open reduction and fixation is possible only when a large bony fragment is avulsed.

Bibbo et al.[2] described a transcalcaneal suture technique for repair of the Achilles tendon sleeve avulsion, through a longitudinal extensile incision. This technique, to be used in patients without a large tendon defect, allows reinsertion of the tendon to the calcaneus. However, when a large tendon defect is present, the surgeon must consider a tendon graft to bridge the gap and produce a strong construct.[8,12,14,25,28] Moreover, open procedures on the Achilles tendon can lead to difficulty with wound healing because of the tenuous blood supply and increased chance of wound breakdown and infection.[20,21,24] The broad exposure

N.M affulli(✉)
Centre for Sports and Exercise Medicine, Queen Mary University of London, Barts and The London School of Medicine and Dentistry, Mile End Hospital, London, England, UK
e-mail:n.ma ffulli@qmul.ac.uk

N. Maffulli and M. Easley (eds.), *Minimally Invasive Surgery of the Foot and Ankle*,
DOI: 10.1007/978-1-84996-417-3_35, © Springer-Verlag London Limited 2011

given by open procedures may cause extensive iatrogenic disruption of the subcutaneous tissues and paratenon, increasing the potential for peritendinous adhesions.[10,11] For this reason, less invasive surgical approaches have been developed.[4,6,9,15,18,27] Advocates of less invasive AT surgery cite faster recovery times, shorter hospital stays, and improved functional outcomes as the principal reasons for adopting these new approaches when compared to traditional open techniques.[4,6,7,9,18]

This technique uses one proximal para-midline incision and one distal Cincinnati incision to respectively expose the proximal Achilles tendon stump and the Achilles tendon insertion. Using this approach, a wide exposure of the insertion of the Achilles tendon is possible.

35.2 Surgical Technique

The patient is positioned prone with a calf tourniquet. Skin preparation is performed in the usual fashion, and sterile drapes are applied. Pre-operative anatomical markings include the palpable tendon defect and the tuberosity of the calcaneus. Two skin incisions are made, and accurate hemostasis by ligation of the larger veins and diathermy of the smaller ones is performed. The first incision is a 5 cm longitudinal incision, made 2 cm proximal and just medial to the palpable end of the residual tendon. The second incision is 5–7 cm semicircular Cincinnati skin incision,[5] made over the area of Achilles tendon insertion.

The proximal and distal Achilles tendon stumps are mobilized, freeing them of all the peritendinous adhesions. After trying to reduce the gap of the ruptured Achilles tendon, if the gap does not allow the tendon to reach the bone despite maximal plantar flexion of the ankle and traction on the AT stump, the ipsilateral semitendinosus is harvested through a vertical 2.5–3 cm long incision over the pes anserinus. The tendon is prepared in the usual fashion.[15]

A cannulated headed reamer corresponding to the grafts diameter is used to perforate the calcaneus to allow the passage of the double-looped semitendinosus tendon graft (Fig. 35.1). A wire is then passed through the tunnel (Fig. 35.2).

The proximal tendon is then mobilized from the proximal wound, any adhesions are divided, and further soft tissue release anterior to the soleus and gastrocnemius allows maximal excursion, minimizing the gap between the two tendon stumps. The semitendinosus tendon is passed through a small incision in the substance of the proximal stump of the AT (Fig. 35.3), and it is sutured to the AT at the entry and exit point using 3–0 Vicryl (Polyglactin 910 braided absorbable suture; Johnson & Johnson, Brussels, Belgium). The semitendinosus tendon is then passed beneath the intact skin bridge into the distal incision, and then through the calcaneus tunnel (Fig. 35.4). With the ankle in maximal plantar flexion, the semitendinosus tendon is fixed to the calcaneus using a bioabsorbable interference screw (Fig. 35.5) inserted over a guide wire into the calcaneus.

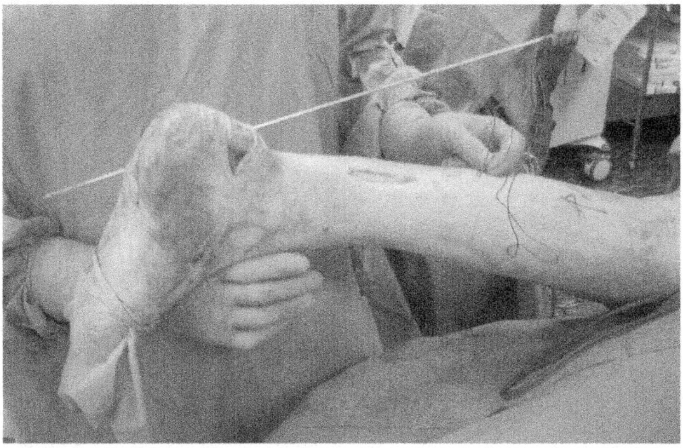

Fig.35. 1 Ac annulated headed reamer corresponding to the grafts diameter is used to perforate the calcaneus to allow the passage of the double-looped semitendinosus tendongra ft

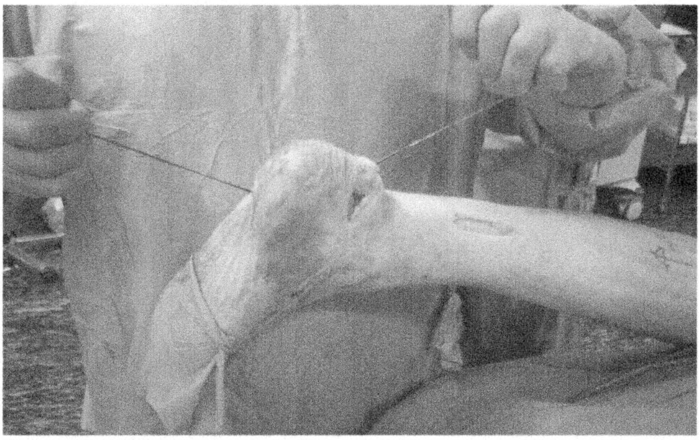

Fig.35. 2 A wire is passed throughthe tunne l

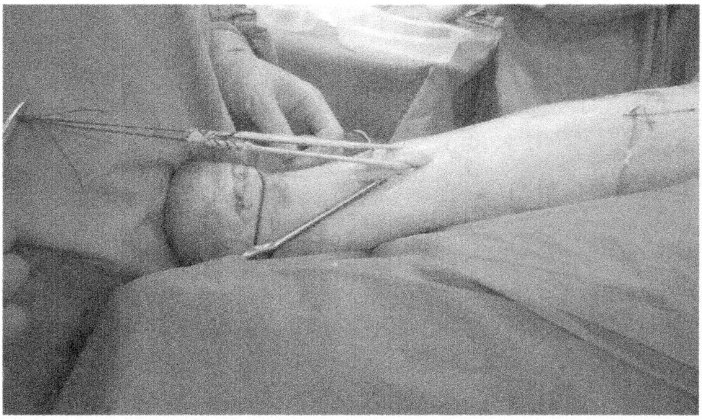

Fig.35. 3 Thes emitendinosus tendon is passed through a small incision in the substance of the proximal stumpofthe A T

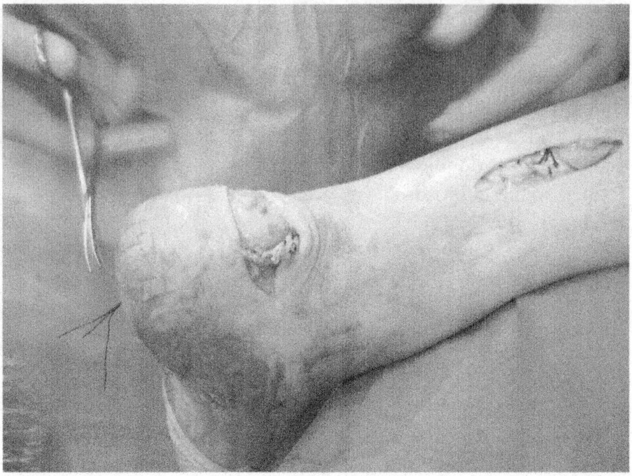

Fig.35.4 Thes emitendinosus tendon is passed into the calcaneust unnel

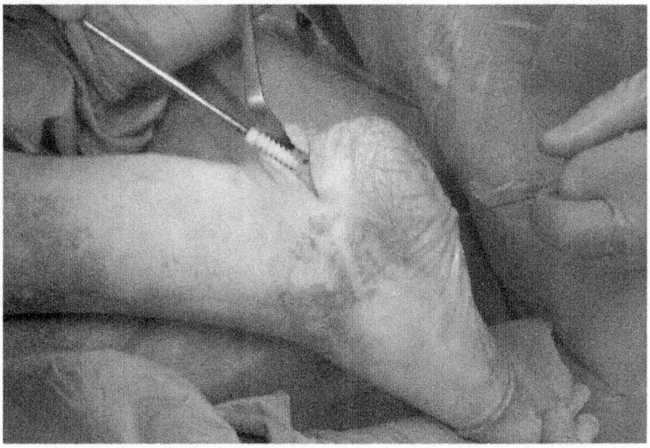

Fig.35.5 Thebioa bsorbable interference screw is insertedove ra gui dew ire

35.3 PostoperativeR egimen

The patient immobilized in a below knee weight bearing synthetic cast boot. Postoperatively, patients are allowed to weight bear as comfort allows with the use of elbow crutches.[16,17] It would be unusual for a patient to weight bear fully at this stage. After 2 weeks, the cast is removed and an Aircast boot with five heel wedges (XP Walker, DJO Ltd, Guilford, England) is applied, and physiotherapy is commenced preventing dorsiflexion of the ankle, focusing on proprioception, plantar-flexion of the ankle, inversion and eversion.[16,17] During this period of rehabilitation, the patient is permitted to weight bear as comfort allows with the boot in situ, although full weight bearing rarely occurs and patients usually still require the assistance of a single elbow crutch as this stage. One heel wedge is removed every other week, and the boot may be finally removed after 6 weeks. We do not use a heel raise after removal of the boot, and patients normally regain a plantigrade ankle over 2 or 3 weeks.[16,17]

35.4 Discussion

Wound breakdown is a challenging complications in AT reconstruction surgery, with open techniques having a 9% superficial infection rate.[23] To minimize the rate of infection after AT reconstruction, two less invasive techniques of reconstruction of AT have been already described using peroneus brevis[4] and semitendinous autologus tendon graft.[14]

These techniques allow reconstruction of the AT using tendon autografts preserving skin integrity, and can be especially used to reconstruct the AT in the presence of previous surgery.[4] When a chronic avulsion occurs at the tendon insertion, a reconstruction of the enthesis is required. When the tendon avulses from the posterior calcaneus, it may do so without bony element. The tendon of semitendinosus is long and strong, and provides a robust reconstruction to the AT. It has showed good integration rate when used in anterior cruciate ligament surgery with interference screws.[29] A free semitendinosus graft does not deprive the knee of motor strength and power, is safe, and, given its length, can be used to bridge large gaps.[3] The great advantage of this technique is that it allows to perform a semitendinosus tendon transfer preserving skin integrity.

Preservation of skin cover during reconstruction procedures is clearly an advantage, as the skin is not injured by the operation, and protects the reconstruction beneath. As with all surgery performed through small incisions, the procedure is technically demanding. Careful incision placement is required together with skin retraction to allow visualization of the tendon ends and to permit the reconstruction. This technique preserve skin cover of the reconstruction site, and, although reconstruction is always risky, it may extend the indications for surgery in patients prone to wound complications such as vasculopathy and diabetic patients who present with a large gap.

References

1. Ames PR, Longo UG, Denaro V, Maffulli N. Achilles tendon problems: not just an orthopaedic issue. *Disabil Rehabil.*2008; 30:1646–1650.
2. Bibbo C, Anderson RB, Davis WH, Agnone M. Repair of the Achilles tendon sleeve avulsion: quantitative and functional evaluation of a transcalcaneal suture technique. *Foot Ankle Int.* 2003;24:539–544.
3. Capuano L, Hardy P, Longo UG, Denaro V, Maffulli N. No difference in clinical results between femoral transfixation and bio-interference screw fixation in hamstring tendon ACL reconstruction. A preliminary study. *Knee.*2008; 15:174–179.
4. Carmont MR, Maffulli N. Less invasive Achilles tendon reconstruction. *BMC Musculoskelet Disord.*2007;8:100 .

5. Carmont MR, Maffulli N. Management of insertional Achilles tendinopathy through a Cincinnati incision. *BMC Musculoskelet Disord.*2007; 8:82.
6. Carmont MR, Maffulli N. Modified percutaneous repair of ruptured Achilles tendon. *Knee Surg Sports Traumatol Arthrosc.*2008; 16:199–203.
7. Elliot RR, Calder JD. Percutaneous and mini-open repair of acute Achilles tendon rupture. *Foot Ankle Clin.*2007; 12:573–582,vi .
8. Franceschi F, Longo UG, Ruzzini L, Rizzello G, Maffulli N, Denaro V. Soft tissue tenodesis of the long head of the biceps tendon associated to the Roman Bridge repair. *BMC Musculoskelet Disord.*2008;9:7 8.
9. Longo UG, Ramamurthy C, Denaro V, Maffulli N. Minimally invasive stripping for chronic Achilles tendinopathy. *Disabil Rehabil.*2008; 30:1709–1713.
10. Longo UG, Ronga M, Maffulli N. Achilles tendinopathy. *Sports Med Arthrosc.* 2009;17:112–126.
11. Longo UG, Ronga M, Maffulli N. Acute ruptures of the achilles tendon. *Sports Med Arthrosc.* 2009;17:127–138.
12. Lui TH. Endoscopic assisted flexor hallucis tendon transfer in the management of chronic rupture of Achilles tendon. *Knee Surg Sports Traumatol Arthrosc.*2007; 15:1163–1166.
13. Maffulli N, Ajis A, Longo UG, Denaro V. Chronic rupture of tendo Achillis. *Foot Ankle Clin.* 2007;12:583–596,vi .
14. Maffulli N, Longo UG, Gougoulias N, Denaro V. Ipsilateral free semitendinosus tendon graft transfer for reconstruction of chronic tears of the Achilles tendon. *BMC Musculoskelet Disord.* 2008;9:100.
15. Maffulli N, Longo UG, Ronga M, et al. Favorable outcome of percutaneous repair of achilles tendon ruptures in the elderly. *Clin Orthop Relat Res.*2 010;468:1039–1046.
16. Maffulli N, Tallon C, Wong J, Lim KP, Bleakney R. Early weightbearing and ankle mobilization after open repair of acute midsubstance tears of the achilles tendon. *Am J Sports Med.* 2003;31:692–700.
17. Maffulli N, Tallon C, Wong J, Peng Lim K, Bleakney R. No adverse effect of early weight bearing following open repair of acute tears of the Achilles tendon. *J Sports Med Phys Fitness.* 2003;43:367–379.
18. Maffulli N, Testa V, Capasso G, et al. Results of percutaneous longitudinal tenotomy for Achilles tendinopathy in middle- and long-distance runners. *Am J Sports Med.* 1997;25:835–840.
19. Maffulli N, Testa V, Capasso G, et al. Surgery for chronic Achilles tendinopathy produces worse results in women. *Disabil Rehabil.*2008; 30:1714–1720.
20. Nilsson-Helander K, Thurin A, Karlsson J, Eriksson BI. High incidence of deep venous thrombosis after Achilles tendon rupture: a prospective study. *Knee Surg Sports Traumatol Arthrosc.*2009;17: 1234–1238.
21. Paavola M, Orava S, Leppilahti J, et al. Chronic Achilles tendon overuse injury: complications after surgical treatment. An analysis of 432 consecutive patients. *Am J Sports Med.* 2000;28:77–82.
22. Pavlou G, Roach R, Salehi-Bird S. Repair of the achilles tendon sleeve avulsion: a transcalcaneal suture technique. *Foot Ankle Int.*2009; 30:65–67.
23. Pintore E, Barra V, Pintore R, Maffulli N. Peroneus brevis tendon transfer in neglected tears of the Achilles tendon. *J Trauma.*2001; 50:71–78.
24. Saxena A, Maffulli N, Nguyen A, Li A. Wound complications from surgeries pertaining to the Achilles tendon: an analysis of 219 surgeries. *J Am Podiatr Med Assoc.*2008; 98:95–101.
25. Sebastian H, Datta B, Maffulli N, Neil M, Walsh WR. Mechanical properties of reconstructed achilles tendon with transfer of peroneus brevis or flexor hallucis longus tendon. *J Foot Ankle Surg.*2007;46:42 4–428.

26. Silbernagel KG, Nilsson-Helander K, Thomee R, et al. A new measurement of heel-rise endurance with the ability to detect functional deficits in patients with Achilles tendon rupture. *Knee Surg Sports Traumatol Arthrosc.*2010; 18:258–264.
27. Testa V, Capasso G, Benazzo F, Maffulli N. Management of Achilles tendinopathy by ultrasound-guided percutaneous tenotomy. *Med Sci Sports Exerc.*2002; 34:573–580.
28. Wagner E, Gould JS, Kneidel M, Fleisig GS, Fowler R. Technique and results of Achilles tendon detachment and reconstruction for insertional Achilles tendinosis. *Foot Ankle Int.* 2006;27:677–684.
29. Weiler A, Peine R, Pashmineh-Azar A, Abel C, Sudkamp NP, Hoffmann RF. Tendon healing in a bone tunnel. Part I: biomechanical results after biodegradable interference fit fixation in a model of anterior cruciate ligament reconstruction in sheep. *Arthroscopy.*2002; 18:113–123.

Percutaneous Longitudinal Tenotomies for ChronicA chilles Tendinopathy

36

Jonathan S. Young, Murali Krishna Sayana, Vittorino Testa, Filippo Spiezia, Umile Giuseppe Longo,a nd Nicola Maffulli

36.1 Introduction

Athletic tendinopathy is an overuse condition causing pain and swelling in and around tendons,[8] not only restricted to athletes, but 25–30% of patients are nonathletes.[1]

The Achilles tendon is commonly affected by this condition, due to continuous prolonged intense functional demands imposed on it especially in sportsman.[2,14,17,23] Surgery is recommended for patients in whom non-operative management has proved ineffective for at least 6 months. Twenty-four percent to 45.5% of the patients with Achilles tendon problem fail to respond to conservative treatment and eventually require surgical intervention.[3,6,12]

Each patient should be managed on an individual basis, and appropriate work up for theatre should be instituted. All patients should have a full history and examination and the diagnosis of Achilles tendinopathy should be established.

Patients can complain of burning pain in the posterior aspect of the calf and ankle, often worse at the beginning of a training session, and after exercise. Some patients have difficulty taking the first few steps in the morning. Pain during activities of daily living, include prolonged walking and stair climbing. Clinical diagnosis is mostly based on palpation and on the use of the painful arc sign.[21] In paratendinopathy, the area of tenderness and thickening remains fixed in relation to the malleoli when the ankle is moved from full dorsiflexion into plantarflexion. If the lesion lies within the tendon, the point of tenderness and any swelling associated with it move with the tendon as the ankle is brought from full dorsiflexion into plantarflexion. In mixed lesions, both motion and fixation of the swelling and of the tenderness can be detected in relation to the malleoli.[10,19]

N.M affulli(✉)
Centre for Sports and Exercise Medicine, Queen Mary University of London, Barts and The LondonSc hoolofM edicinea ndD entistry, MileEndH ospital, London, England, UK
e-mail:n.ma ffulli@qmul.ac.uk

N. Maffulli and M. Easley (eds.), *Minimally Invasive Surgery of the Foot and Ankle*,
DOI: 10.1007/978-1-84996-417-3_36, © Springer-Verlag London Limited 2011

36.2 Surgical Technique

There are different surgical techniques for tendinopathy,[4,5,11,15,16,18,20] but the objective is to excise fibrotic adhesions, remove degenerated nodules and make multiple longitudinal incisions in the tendon to detect intratendinous lesions and to restore vascularity, and possibly stimulate the remaining viable cells to initiate cell matrix response and healing.[13]

Management of paratendinopathy includes releasing the crural fascia on both sides of the tendon. Adhesions around the tendon are then trimmed; the hypertrophied adherent portions of the paratenon are excised.[3] In tenolysis, classically longitudinal tenotomies are made along the longitudinal axis of the tendon in the abnormal tendon tissues, excising areas of mucinoid degeneration. Reconstruction procedure may be required if large lesions are excised.[7]

The paratenon and crural fascia are incised and dissected from the underlying tendon. If necessary, the tendon is freed from adhesions on the posterior, medial and lateral aspects. The paratenon should be excised obliquely as transverse excision may produce a constriction ring, which may require further surgery.[21] Areas of thickened, fibrotic and inflamed tendon are excised. The pathology is identified by the change in texture and color of the tendon. The lesions are then excised, and the defect can either be sutured in a side-to-side fashion or left open. Open procedures on the Achilles tendon can lead to difficulty with wound healing due to the tenuous blood supply and increased chance of wound breakdown and infection. Hemostasis is important, since the reduction of postoperative bleeding speeds up recovery, diminishes the chance of wound infection and diminishes any possible fibrotic inflammatory reaction.

In patients with isolated Achilles tendinopathy with no paratendinous involvement and a well-defined nodular lesion less that 2.5 cm long, multiple percutaneous longitudinal tenotomies can be used when conservative management has failed. An ultrasound scan can be used to confirm the precise location of the area of tendinopathy.

In this chapter two techniques for the percutaneous management of Achilles tendinopathy are discussed.[10,20] Although the techniques reported in this article are performed under local anesthesia, there is a small chance that general anesthesia may be necessary, and therefore baseline investigations such as blood tests, ECG and chest radiographs should be undertaken if deemed necessary. Patients should have DVT prophylaxis. Valid informed consent should be achieved prior to the operation, and the patient should be aware of risks of infection, bleeding, wound and scar problems, operation failure, and that further surgery may be required.

36.3 MultipleP ercutaneousL ongitudinal Tenotomies

Patients are operated as day cases. The patient lies prone on the operating table with the feet protruding beyond the edge, and the ankles resting on a sandbag. A bloodless field is not necessary. The tendon is accurately palpated, and the area of maximum swelling and/or tenderness marked, and checked again by US scanning. The skin and the subcutaneous tissues over the Achilles tendon are infiltrated with 10–15 mL of plain 1% lignocaine (Lignocaine Hydrochloride, Evans Medical Ltd, Leatherhead, England).

A number 11 surgical scalpel blade is inserted parallel to the long axis of the tendon fibres in the marked area(s) with the cutting edge pointing cranially. Keeping the blade still, a full passive ankle dorsi-flexion movement is produced. After reversing the position of the blade, a full passive ankle plantar-flexion movement is produced. A variable, but probably in the region of 3 cm long, area of tenolysis is thus obtained through a stab wound. The procedure is repeated 2 cm medial and proximally, medial and distally, lateral and proximally and lateral and distally to the site of the first stab wound. The five wounds are closed with steristrips, dressed with cotton swabs, and a few layers of cotton wool and a crepe bandage are applied.

36.4 UltrasoundG uidedP ercutaneous Tenotomy

Patients are operated as outpatients. The patient lies prone on the examination couch with the feet protruding beyond the edge, and the ankles resting on a sandbag. A bloodless field is not necessary. The tendon is accurately palpated, and the area of maximum swelling and/or tenderness marked, and checked by US scanning. The skin is prepped with an antiseptic solution, and a sterile longitudinal 7.5 MHz probe is used to image again the area of tendinopathy. Before infiltrating the skin and the subcutaneous tissues over the Achilles tendon with 10 mL of 1% Carbocaina (Pierrel, Milan, Italy), 7 mL of 0.5% Carbocaina are used to infiltrate the space between the tendon and the paratenon, to try and distend the paratenon and break the adherences that may be present between the tendon and the paratenon.

Under US control, a number 11 surgical scalpel blade (Swann-Morton, England) is inserted parallel to the long axis of the tendon fibres in the centre of the area of tendinopathy, as assessed by high resolution US imaging (Fig. 36.1). The cutting edge of the blade points caudally, and penetrates the whole thickness of the tendon (Fig. 36.2a, b). Keeping the blade still, a full passive ankle flexion is produced (Fig. 36.3). The scalpel blade is then retracted to the surface of the tendon, inclined 45° on the sagittal axis, and the blade is

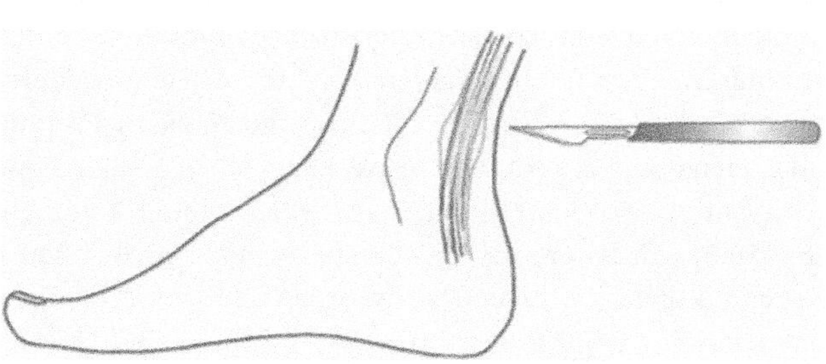

Fig.36.1 11-scalpelbla de inserted into the predetermined area with sharpe dgepointingc audally

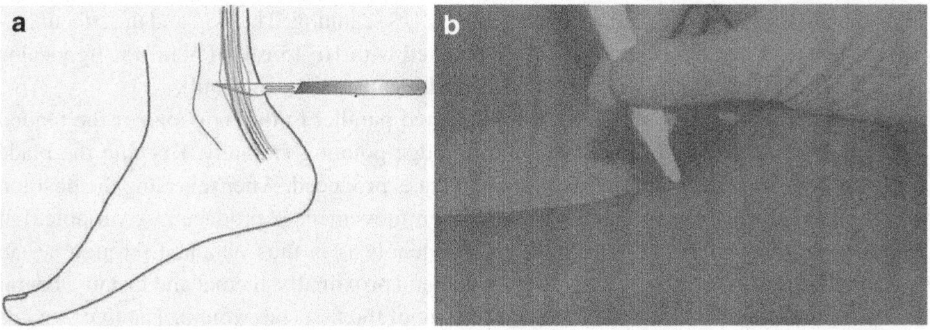

Fig.36.2 ((**a**) and (**b**)) The blade penetrating the whole thickness of the Achilles tendon

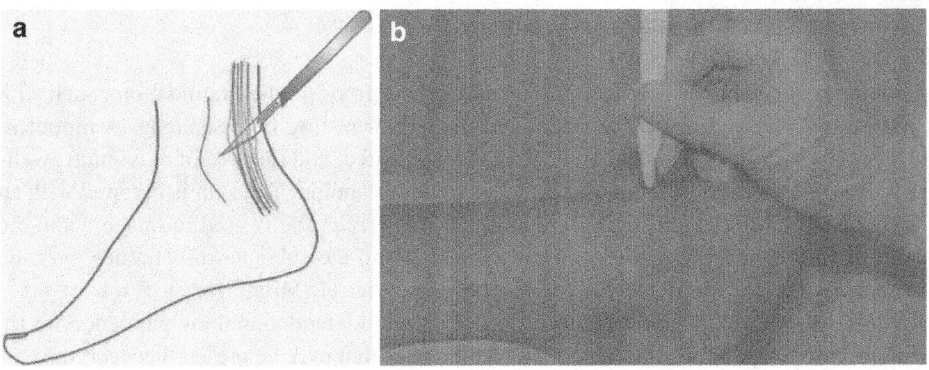

Fig.36.3 ((**a**) and (**b**)) Passive ankle flexioni spr oduced

inserted medially through the original tenotomy (Fig. 36.4). Keeping the blade still, a full passive ankle flexion is produced. The whole procedure is repeated inclining the blade 45° laterally to the original tenotomy, inserting it laterally through the original tenotomy (Fig. 36.4). Keeping the blade still, a full passive ankle flexion is produced. The blade is then partially retracted to the posterior surface of the Achilles tendon, reversed 180°, so that its cutting edge now points cranially, and the whole procedure repeated, taking care to dorsiflex the ankle passively (Figs. 36.5a, b and 36.6a, b). Preliminary cadaveric studies showed that a tenotomy 2.8 cm long on average is thus obtained through a stab wound in the main body of the tendon.[10] A steristrip (3M United Kingdom PLC, Bracknell, Berkshire, England) can be applied on the stab wound, or the stab wound can be left open.[9] The wound is dressed with cotton swabs, and a few layers of cotton wool and a crepe bandage area pplied.

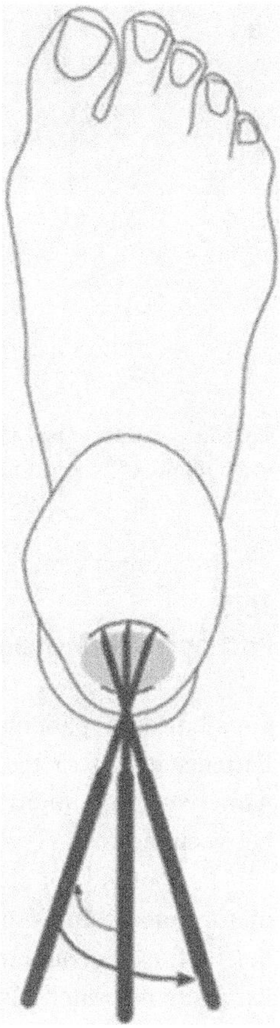

Fig. 36.4 Procedure repeated with blade inclining the 45° medial and 45° lateral to the original tenotomy

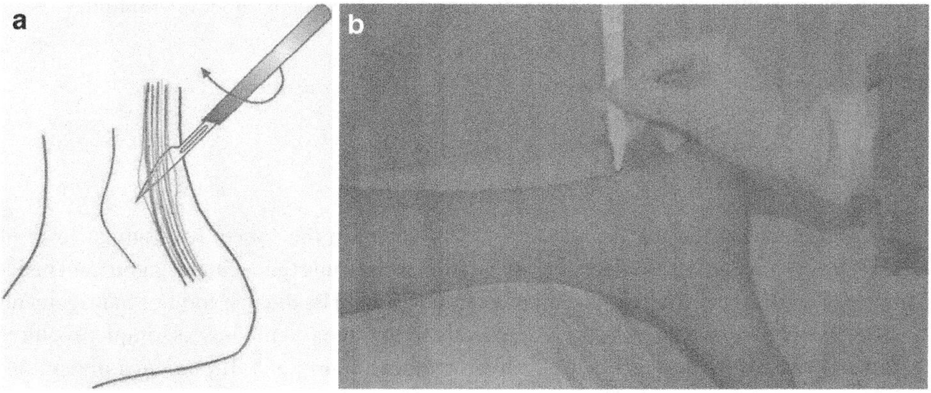

Fig. 36.5 ((**a**) and (**b**))T hebl adei sr eversed180°

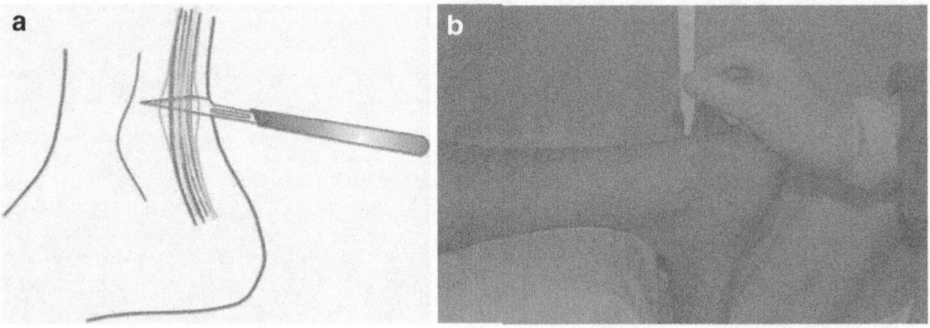

Fig. 36.6 ((**a**) and (**b**)) The sequence of tenotomies repeated with ankle dosriflexion and the 45° medial and 45° lateral inclination to the initial tenotomy

36.5 Post-operativeM anagement

On admission, patients are taught to perform isometric contractions of their triceps surae. Patients are instructed to perform the isometric strength training at three different angles, namely at maximum dorsi-flexion, maximum plantar flexion and at a point midway between the two.

The foot is kept elevated on the first postoperative day, and non-steroidal anti-inflammatory medications are given for pain control. Early active dorsi- and plantar-flexion of the foot are encouraged.[22] On the second postoperative day, patient are allowed to walk using elbow crutches weight-bearing as able. Full weight-bearing was allowed after 2 or 3 days, when the bandage is reduced to a simple adhesive plaster over the wounds. Stationary bicycling and isometric, concentric and eccentric strengthening of the calf muscles are started under physiotherapy guidance after 4 weeks. Swimming and water running are encouraged from the second week. Gentle running is started 4–6 weeks after the procedure, and mileage gradually increased.

Patients normally discontinue physiotherapy by the sixth post-operative month.

36.6 Discussion

The management of Achilles tendinopathy aims to return the patient to a similar level of activity prior to acquiring tendinopathy in the shortest possible time without significant residual pain. Physiotherapy and conservative treatment should be the first form of management.

If conservative measures fail, percutaneous longitudinal tenotomy is simple, requires only local anesthesia, and can be performed without a tourniquet. If post-operative mobilization is carried out early, preventing the formation of adhesions, this will allow the return to high levels of activity in the majority.

References

1. Astrom M. Partial rupture in chronic achilles tendinopathy. A retrospective analysis of 342 cases. *Acta Orthop Scand.* 1998; 69:404–407.
2. James SL, Bates BT, Osternig LR. Injuries to runners. *Am J Sports Med.* 1978; 6:40–50.
3. Kvist M. Achilles tendon injuries in athletes. *Sports Med.* 1994; 18:173–201.
4. Leach RE, Schepsis AA, Takai H. Long-term results of surgical management of Achilles tendinitis in runners. *Clin Orthop Relat Res.* 1992; 282:208–212.
5. Leadbetter WB, Mooar PA, Lane GJ, Lee SJ. The surgical treatment of tendinitis. Clinical rationale and biologic basis. *Clin Sports Med.* 1992; 11:679–712.
6. Leppilahti J, Orava S, Karpakka J, et al. Overuse injuries of the Achilles tendon. *Ann Chir Gynaecol.* 1991;80: 202–207.
7. Ljungqvist R. Subcutaneous partial rupture of the Achilles tendon. *Acta Orthop Scand.* 1967;113:1–86.
8. Maffulli N, Khan KM, Puddu G. Overuse tendon conditions: time to change a confusing terminology. *Arthroscopy.* 1998; 14:840–843.
9. Maffulli N, Pintore E, Petricciuolo F. Arthroscopy wounds: to suture or not to suture. *Acta Orthop Belg.* 1991 ;57:154–156.
10. Maffulli N, Testa V, Capasso G, et al. Results of percutaneous longitudinal tenotomy for Achilles tendinopathy in middle- and long-distance runners. *Am J Sports Med.* 1997;25:835–840.
11. Nelen G, Martens M, Burssens A. Surgical treatment of chronic Achilles tendinitis. *Am J Sports Med.* 1989;17: 754–759.
12. Paavola M, Kannus P, Paakkala T, et al. Long-term prognosis of patients with achilles tendinopathy. An observational 8-year follow-up study. *Am J Sports Med.* 2000; 28:634–642.
13. Rolf C, Movin T. Etiology, histopathology, and outcome of surgery in achillodynia. *Foot Ankle Int.* 1997;18 :565–569.
14. Rovere GD, Webb LX, Gristina AG, et al. Musculoskeletal injuries in theatrical dance students. *Am J Sports Med.* 1983; 11:195–198.
15. Schepsis AA, Leach RE. Surgical management of Achilles tendinitis. *Am J Sports Med.* 1987;15:308–315.
16. Subotnick SI, Sisney P. Treatment of Achilles tendinopathy in the athlete. *J Am Podiatr Med Assoc.* 1986;76:55 2–557.
17. Teitz CC, Garrett WE Jr, Miniaci A, et al. Tendon problems in athletic individuals. *Instr Course Lect.* 1997; 46:569–582.
18. Testa V, Capasso G, Maffulli N, et al. Ultrasound-guided percutaneous longitudinal tenotomy for the management of patellar tendinopathy. *Med Sci Sports Exerc.* 1999; 31:1509–1515.
19. Testa V, Capasso G, Benazzo F, et al. Management of Achilles tendinopathy by ultrasound-guided percutaneous tenotomy. *Med Sci Sports Exerc.* 2002; 34:273–280.
20. Testa V, Maffulli N, Capasso G, et al. Percutaneous longitudinal tenotomy in chronic Achilles tendonitis. *Bull Hosp Joint Dis.* 1996; 54:241–244.
21. Williams JG. Achilles tendon lesions in sport. *Sports Med.* 1986; 3:114–135.
22. Williams JG, Sperryn PN, Boardman S, et al. Post-operative management of chronic achilles tendon pain in sportsmen. *Physiotherapy.* 1976; 62:256–259.
23. Winge S, Jorgensen U, Lassen Nielsen A. Epidemiology of injuries in Danish championship tennis. *Int J Sports Med.* 1989; 10:368–371.

Minimally Invasive Stripping for Chronic Achilles Tendinopathy

37

Nicola Maffulli, Umile Giuseppe Longo, Chandrusekar Ramamurthy, and Vincenzo Denaro

37.1 Introduction

The aetiology of pain in Achilles tendinopathy is widely debated, with recent evidence that neo-vascularisation and neo-innervation may be responsible.[2,4,5,9,11,13,16] Neo-vascularisation is often present in patients with tendinopathy, and the area in which patients perceive most pain correlates with the area where most neo-vascularisation occurs on power Doppler ultrasound scan (US).[16]

During eccentric calf-muscle contraction, the flow in the neovessels disappears on ankle dorsiflexion.[2] The good clinical effects with eccentric training may result from the interference on the neovessels and accompanying nerves. Also, local anesthetic injected in the area of neo-vascularisation outside the tendon resulted in a pain-free tendon, indicating that this area is involved in pain generation.[2,17]

A pilot study injecting a commercially available sclerosing agent into and around the neo-vessels[2,15] significantly reduced pain in eight of ten patients. A similar study of patellar tendinopathy, which has a similar histological picture to Achilles tendinopathy, gave equally encouraging results.[1,3]

Recently, the same group has developed an arthroscopic approach to this issue. They proposed arthroscopic shaving of the area with neovessels and nerves on the posterior aspect of the patellar tendon in patients with patellar tendinopathy.[19]

In this chapter we describe a minimal invasive technique of stripping of neovessels from the Kager's triangle of the AT is performed. This achieves safe and secure breaking of neo-vessels and the accompanying nerve supply.

N.M affulli(✉)
Centre for Sports and Exercise Medicine, Queen Mary University of London, Barts and The LondonSc hoolofM edicinea ndD entistry, MileEndH ospital, London, England, UK
e-mail:n.ma ffulli@keele.ac.uk

N. Maffulli and M. Easley (eds.), *Minimally Invasive Surgery of the Foot and Ankle*,
DOI: 10.1007/978-1-84996-417-3_37,

37.2 Surgical Technique

The patient undergoes local or general anesthesia, according to surgeon or patient preferences. The patient is positioned prone with a calf tourniquet which is inflated to 250 mmHg after exsanguination. Skin preparation is performed in the usual fashion.

Four skin incisions are made. The first two incisions are 0.5 cm longitudinal incisions at the proximal origin of the Achilles tendon, just medial and lateral to the origin of the tendon. The other two incisions are also 0.5 cm long and longitudinal, but 1 cm distal to the distal end of the tendon insertion on the calcaneus.

A mosquito is inserted in the proximal incisions (Fig. 37.1) , and the Achilles tendon is freed of the peritendinous adhesions. A Number 1 unmounted Ethibond (Ethicon, Somerville, NJ) suture thread is inserted proximally, passing through the two proximal incision (Fig. 37.2). The Ethibond is retrieved from the distal incisions (Fig. 37.3), over the

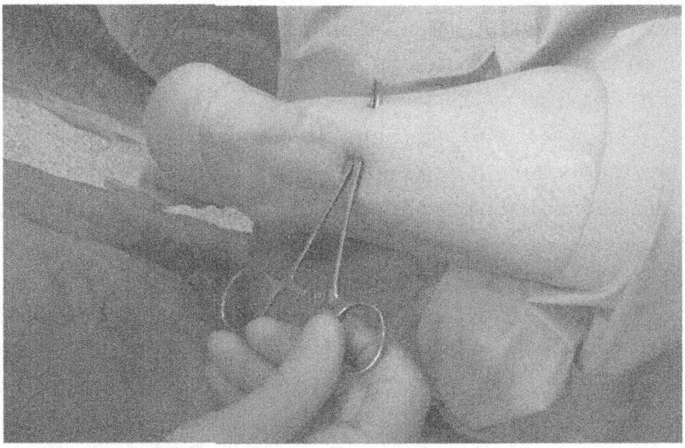

Fig.37.1 Amos quitoi s inserted in the proximal incisions

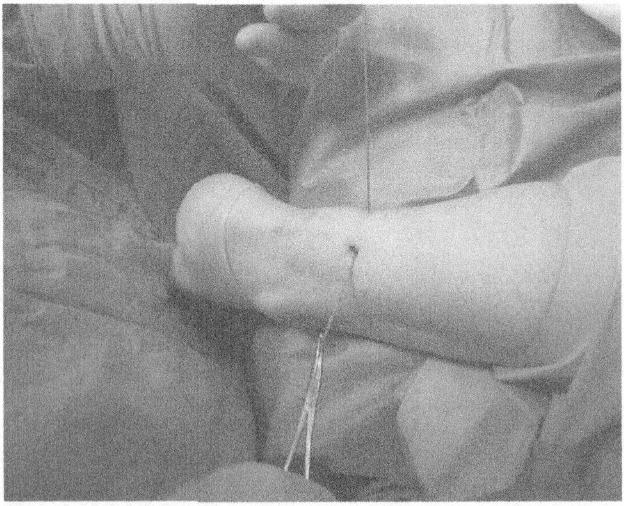

Fig.37.2 AN umber1 Ethibond (Ethicon, Somerville, NJ) is inserted proximally, passing through the two proximal incision over the anterior aspect of theA chillest endon

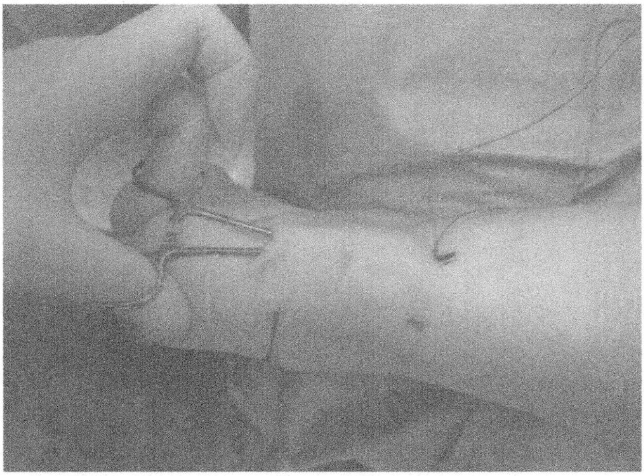

Fig. 37. 3 The Ethibond is retrieved from the distal incisions

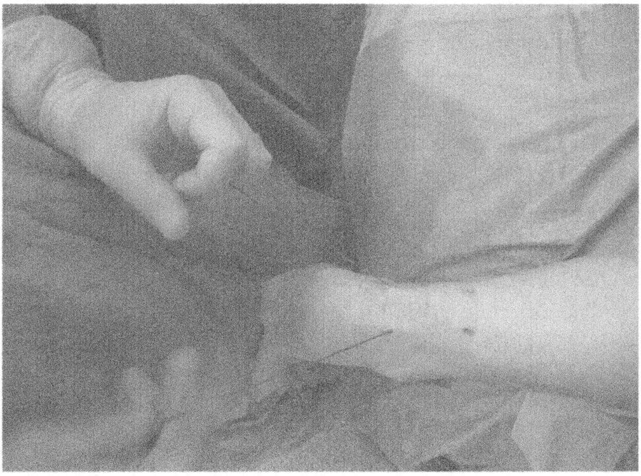

Fig. 37. 4 The Ethibond is slid over the anterior aspect of the Achilles tendon with a gentle see-saw motion. The whole process is repeated over the posterior aspect of the tendon

posterior aspect of the Achilles tendon. Using a gentle see-saw motion, similar to using a Gigli saw, the Ethibond suture thread is made to slide posterior to the tendon (Fig. 37.4), which is stripped and freed from the fat of Kager's triangle.

The procedure is repeated for the posterior aspect of the Achilles tendon.

If necessary, using an 11 blade, longitudinal percutaneous tenotomies parallel to the tendon fibres are made.[10,14,18]

The subcutaneous and subcuticular tissues are closed in a routine fashion, and Mepore (Molnlycke Health Care, Gothenburg, Sweden) dressings are applied to the skin. A removable scotch cast support with Velcro straps can be applied if deemed necessary.

37.3 PostoperativeR egimen

Post-operatively, patients are allowed to mobilize fully weight bearing. After 2 weeks, the cast, if used is removed, and physiotherapy is commenced, focusing on proprioception, plantar-flexion of the ankle, inversion and eversion.

37.4 Discussion

The source of pain and the background to the pain mechanisms associated with chronic AT have not been scientifically clarified.[9]

In ATs with chronic painful tendinopathy, but not in normal pain-free tendons, there is neo-vascularization outside and inside the ventral part of the tendinopathic area.[1,2,9,11,13]

The pathogenetic significance of the neo-vascularisation is unknown, but several theories can be proposed. The increased vascularization often seen in biopsies from patients with AT who underwent surgery is a part of a reparative response in the tendon.[7,11,12] Reparative processes associated with neovascularisation are probably inadequate.[1,2]

Surgery should be offered to patients with chronic recalcitrant tendinopathy.[8]

The percentage of patients requiring surgery is around 25%,[6] depending on poorly understood biochemical and molecular events leading to AT.[9] Surgery is successful in up to 85% of patients,[7] even though postoperative ultrasound examination often shows a widened tendon with hypo-echoic areas. This has led to hypotheses of a possible denervation of the tendon as one of the explanations to the frequently favorable effect of surgery.[7]

The rationale behind this technique is that the sliding of the Ethibond breaks the neovessels and the accompanying nerve supply, therefore decreasing the pain in patients with chronic Achilles tendinopathy.

Classically, open surgery for midsubstance tendinopathy of the AT has provided good results.[9] However, wound complications can occur with these procedures.[9] One possible advantage of this minimal invasive technique could be reduction of infection risks. It is, furthermore, technically easy to master, and inexpensive. It may provide greater potential for the management of recalcitrant AT by breaking neo-vessels and the accompanying nerve supply to the tendon. It can be associated with other minimally invasive procedures toopt imizer esults.

References

1. Alfredson H, Ohberg L. Neovascularisation in chronic painful patellar tendinosis–promising results after sclerosing neovessels outside the tendon challenge the need for surgery. *Knee Surg Sports Traumatol Arthrosc.* 2005; 13:74–80.

2. Alfredson H, Ohberg L, Forsgren S. Is vasculo-neural ingrowth the cause of pain in chronic Achilles tendinosis? An investigation using ultrasonography and colour Doppler, immunohistochemistry, and diagnostic injections. *Knee Surg Sports Traumatol Arthrosc.* 2003;11:334–338.
3. Kannus P. Structure of the tendon connective tissue. *Scand J Med Sci Sports.* 2000;10:312–320.
4. Knobloch K, Kraemer R, Lichtenberg A, et al. Achilles tendon and paratendon microcirculation in midportion and insertional tendinopathy in athletes. *Am J Sports Med.* 2006;34:92–97.
5. Kristoffersen M, Ohberg L, Johnston C, et al. Neovascularisation in chronic tendon injuries detected with colour Doppler ultrasound in horse and man: implications for research and treatment. *Knee Surg Sports Traumatol Arthrosc.*2005; 13:505–508.
6. Kvist M. Achilles tendon injuries in athletes. *Ann Chir Gynaecol.*1991; 80:188–201.
7. Longo UG, Ramamurthy C, Denaro V, Maffulli N. Minimally invasive stripping for chronic Achilles tendinopathy. *Disabil Rehabil.*2008; 30(20-22):1709–13.
8. Maffulli N, Kenward MG, Testa V, et al. Clinical diagnosis of Achilles tendinopathy with tendinosis. *Clin J Sport Med.*2003; 13:11–15.
9. Maffulli N, Sharma P, Luscombe KL. Achilles tendinopathy: aetiology and management. *J R Soc Med.*2004 ;97:472–476.
10. Maffulli N, Testa V, Capasso G, et al. Results of percutaneous longitudinal tenotomy for Achilles tendinopathy in middle- and long-distance runners. *Am J Sports Med.* 1997;25:835–840.
11. Maffulli N, Testa V, Capasso G, et al. Similar histopathological picture in males with Achilles and patellar tendinopathy. *Med Sci Sports Exerc.*2004; 36:1470–1475.
12. Maffulli N, Testa V, Capasso G, et al. Surgery for chronic Achilles tendinopathy yields worse results in nonathletic patients. *Clin J Sport Med.*2006; 16:123–128.
13. Maffulli N, Wong J, Almekinders LC. Types and epidemiology of tendinopathy. *Clin Sports Med.*2003;22:675 –692.
14. MaffulliN ,A lmekindersLC . *The Achilles Tendon.* New York, NY: Springer; 2007:83–92.
15. Ohberg L, Alfredson H. Ultrasound guided sclerosis of neovessels in painful chronic Achilles tendinosis: pilot study of a new treatment. *Br J Sports Med.* 2002;36:173–175, discussion 6–7.
16. Ohberg L, Lorentzon R, Alfredson H. Neovascularisation in Achilles tendons with painful tendinosis but not in normal tendons: an ultrasonographic investigation. *Knee Surg Sports Traumatol Arthrosc.*2001; 9:233–238.
17. Sayana MK, Maffulli N. Eccentric calf muscle training in non-athletic patients with Achilles tendinopathy. *J Sci Med Sport.*2007; 10:52–58.
18. Testa V, Capasso G, Benazzo F, et al. Management of Achilles tendinopathy by ultrasound-guided percutaneous tenotomy. *Med Sci Sports Exerc.*2002; 34:573–580.
19. Willberg L, Sunding K, Ohberg L, et al. Treatment of Jumper's knee: promising short-term results in a pilot study using a new arthroscopic approach based on imaging findings. *Knee Surg Sports Traumatol Arthrosc.*2007; 15:676–681.

Index

C

G

H

I

R

S

T

Made in the USA
Monee, IL
13 September 2026

62976967R00269